More information about this series at http://www.springer.com/series/7412

Lecture Notes in Computer Science 11768

Founding Editors

Gerhard Goos
  Karlsruhe Institute of Technology, Karlsruhe, Germany
Juris Hartmanis
  Cornell University, Ithaca, NY, USA

More information about this series at http://www.springer.com/series/7412

Dinggang Shen · Tianming Liu ·
Terry M. Peters · Lawrence H. Staib ·
Caroline Essert · Sean Zhou ·
Pew-Thian Yap · Ali Khan (Eds.)

Medical Image Computing and Computer Assisted Intervention – MICCAI 2019

22nd International Conference
Shenzhen, China, October 13–17, 2019
Proceedings, Part V

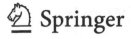 Springer

Editors
Dinggang Shen
University of North Carolina
at Chapel Hill
Chapel Hill, NC, USA

Terry M. Peters (iD)
Western University
London, ON, Canada

Caroline Essert (iD)
University of Strasbourg
Illkirch, France

Pew-Thian Yap
University of North Carolina
at Chapel Hill
Chapel Hill, NC, USA

Tianming Liu
University of Georgia
Athens, GA, USA

Lawrence H. Staib (iD)
Yale University
New Haven, CT, USA

Sean Zhou
United Imaging Intelligence
Shanghai, China

Ali Khan
Western University
London, ON, Canada

ISSN 0302-9743   ISSN 1611-3349   (electronic)
Lecture Notes in Computer Science
ISBN 978-3-030-32253-3   ISBN 978-3-030-32254-0   (eBook)
https://doi.org/10.1007/978-3-030-32254-0

LNCS Sublibrary: SL6 – Image Processing, Computer Vision, Pattern Recognition, and Graphics

This Springer imprint is published by the registered company Springer Nature Switzerland AG
The registered company address is: Gewerbestrasse 11, 6330 Cham, Switzerland

Preface

We are pleased to present the proceedings for the 22nd International Conference on Medical Image Computing and Computer-Assisted Intervention (MICCAI), which was held at the InterContinental Hotel, Shenzhen, China, October 13–17, 2019. The conference also featured 34 workshops, 13 tutorials, and 22 challenges held on October 13 or 17. MICCAI 2019 had an approximately 63% increase in submissions and accepted papers compared with MICCAI 2018. These papers, which comprise six volumes of *Lecture Notes in Computer Science* (LNCS) proceedings, were selected after a thorough double-blind peer-review process. Following the example set by the previous program chairs of MICCAI 2018 and 2017, we employed Microsoft's Conference Managing Toolkit (CMT) for paper submissions and double-blind peer-reviews, and the Toronto Paper Matching System (TPMS) to assist with automatic paper assignment to area chairs and reviewers.

From 2625 original intentions to submit, 1809 full submissions were received and sent out to peer-review. Of these, 63% were considered as pure Medical Image Computing (MIC), 5% as pure Computer-Assisted Interventions (CAI), and 32% as both MIC and CAI. The MICCAI 2019 Program Committee (PC) comprised 69 area chairs, with 25 from the Americas, 21 from Europe, and 23 from Asia/Pacific/Middle East. Each area chair was assigned ~25 manuscripts, with up to 15 suggested potential reviewers using TPMS scoring and self-declared research areas. Subsequently, over 1200 invited reviewers were asked to bid for the papers for which they had been suggested. Final reviewer allocations via CMT took account of PC suggestions, reviewer bidding, and TPMS scores, finally allocating 5–6 papers per reviewer. Based on the double-blinded reviews, 306 papers (17%) were accepted immediately, and 920 papers (51%) were rejected, with the remainder being sent for rebuttal. These decisions were confirmed by the area chairs. During the rebuttal phase, two additional area chairs were assigned to each rebuttal paper using CMT and TPMS scores, who then independently scored them to accept or reject, based on the reviews, rebuttal, and manuscript, resulting in clear paper decisions using majority voting. This process resulted in the acceptance of further 234 papers for an overall acceptance rate of 30%. Regional PC teleconferences were held in late June to confirm the final results and collect PC feedback on the peer-review process.

For the MICCAI 2019 proceedings, 538 accepted papers have been organized in six volumes as follows:

Part I, LNCS Volume 11764: Optical Imaging; Endoscopy; Microscopy
Part II, LNCS Volume 11765: Image Segmentation; Image Registration; Cardiovascular Imaging; Growth, Development, Atrophy, and Progression
Part III, LNCS Volume 11766: Neuroimage Reconstruction and Synthesis; Neuroimage Segmentation; Diffusion-Weighted Magnetic Resonance Imaging; Functional Neuroimaging (fMRI); Miscellaneous Neuroimaging

Part IV, LNCS Volume 11767: Shape; Prediction; Detection and Localization; Machine Learning; Computer-Aided Diagnosis; Image Reconstruction and Synthesis
Part V, LNCS Volume 11768: Computer-Assisted Interventions; MIC Meets CAI
Part VI, LNCS Volume 11769: Computed Tomography; X-ray Imaging

We would like to thank everyone who contributed to the success of MICCAI 2019 and the quality of its proceedings, particularly the MICCAI Society for support, insightful comments, and providing funding for Kitty Wong to be the ongoing Conference System Manager. Given the increase in workload for this year's meeting, the Program Committee simply could not have functioned effectively without her, and she will provide ongoing oversight of the review process for future MICCAI conferences. Without the dedication and support of all of the organizers of the workshops, tutorials, and challenges, under the guidance of Kenji Suzuki, together with satellite event chairs Hongen Liao, Qian Wang, Luping Zhou, Hayit Greenspan, and Bram van Ginneken, none of these peripheral events would have been feasible.

Also, the Industry Forum (led by Xiaodong Tao and Yiqiang Zhan), the Industry Session (led by Sean Zhou), as well as the Doctoral Symposium (led by Junzhou Huang and Dajiang Zhu) brought new events to MICCAI 2019. The publication chairs, Li Wang and Gang Li, undertook the onerous task of assembling the camera-ready proceedings for publication by Springer.

Behind the scenes, MICCAI secretariat personnel, Janette Wallace and Johanne Langford, kept a close eye on logistics and budgets, while Doris Lam and her team from Momentous Asia, this year's Professional Conference Organization, along with the Local Organizing Committee chair, Dong Ni (together with Jing Qin, Qianjin Feng, Dong Liang, Xiaoying Tang), handled the website and local organization. The Student Travel Award Committee chaired by Huiguang He, Jun Shi, and Xi Jiang evaluated numerous applications, including awards for undergraduate students, which is new in the history of MICCAI. We also thank our sponsors for their financial support and presence on site. We are especially grateful to all members of the Program Committee for their diligent work in the reviewer assignments and final paper selection, as well as the reviewers for their support during the entire process. Finally, and most importantly, we thank all authors, co-authors, students/postdocs, and supervisors, for submitting and presenting their high-quality work that made MICCAI 2019 a greatly enjoyable, informative, and successful event. We are indebted to those reviewers and PC members who helped us resolve issues relating to last-minute missing reviews. Overall, we thank all of the authors and attendees for making MICCAI 2019 a spectacular success. We look forward to seeing you in Lima, Peru at MICCAI 2020!

October 2019

Dinggang Shen
Tianming Liu
Terry M. Peters
Lawrence H. Staib
Caroline Essert
Sean Zhou
Pew-Thian Yap
Ali Khan

Organization

General Chairs

Dinggang Shen	The University of North Carolina at Chapel Hill, USA
Tianming Liu	The University of Georgia, USA

Program Executive

Terry Peters	Robarts Research Institute, Western University, Canada
Lawrence H. Staib	Yale University, USA
Sean Zhou	United Imaging Intelligence (UII), China
Caroline Essert	University of Strasbourg, France
Pew-Thian Yap	The University of North Carolina at Chapel Hill, USA
Ali Khan	Robarts Research Institute, Western University, Canada

Submissions Manager

Kitty Wong	Robarts Research Institute, Western University, Canada

Workshops/Challenges/Tutorial Chairs

Kenji Suzuki	Illinois Institute of Technology, USA
Hayit Greenspan	Tel Aviv University, Israel
Bram van Ginneken	Radboud University Medical Center, The Netherlands
Qian Wang	Shanghai Jiao Tong University, China
Luping Zhou	The University of Sydney, Australia
Hongen Liao	Tsinghua University, China

MICCAI Society, Board of Directors

Leo Joskowicz (President)	The Hebrew University of Jerusalem, Israel
Stephen Aylward (Treasurer)	Kitware, Inc., NY, USA
Josien Pluim (Secretary)	Eindhoven University of Technology, The Netherlands
Wiro Niessen (Past President)	Erasmus Medical Centre, The Netherlands
Marleen de Bruijne	Erasmus Medical Centre, The Netherlands and University of Copenhagen, Denmark
Hervé Delinguette	Inria, Sophia Antipolis, France
Caroline Essert	University of Strasbourg, France
Alejandro Frangi	University of Leeds, UK
Lena Maier-Hein	German Cancer Research Center, Germany

Shuo Li	Western University, London, Canada
Tianming Liu	University of Georgia, USA
Anne Martel	University of Toronto, Canada
Daniel Racoceanu	Pontifical Catholic University of Peru, Peru
Julia Schnabel	King's College, London, UK
Guoyan Zheng	Institute for Surgical Technology & Biomechanics, Switzerland
Kevin Zhou	Chinese Academy of Sciences, China

Industry Forum

Xiaodong Tao	iFLYTEK Health, China
Yiqiang Zhan	United Imaging Intelligence (UII), China

Publication Committee

Gang Li	The University of North Carolina at Chapel Hill, USA
Li Wang	The University of North Carolina at Chapel Hill, USA

Finance Committee

Dong Ni	Shenzhen University, China
Janette Wallace	Robarts Research Institute, Western University, Canada
Stephen Aylward	Kitware, Inc., USA

Local Organization Chairs

Dong Ni	Shenzhen University, China
Jing Qin	The Hong Kong Polytechnic University, SAR China
Qianjin Feng	Southern Medical University, China
Dong Liang	Shenzhen Institutes of Advanced Technology, Chinese Academy of Sciences, China
Xiaoying Tang	Southern University of Science and Technology, China

Sponsors and Publicity Liaison

Kevin Zhou	Institute of Computing Technology, Chinese Academy of Sciences, China
Hongen Liao	Tsinghua University, China
Wenjian Qin	Shenzhen Institutes of Advanced Technology, Chinese Academy of Sciences, China

Keynote Lectures Chairs

Max Viergever   University Medical Center Utrecht, The Netherlands
Kensaku Mori   Nagoya University, Japan
Gözde Ünal   Istanbul Technical University, Turkey

Student Travel Award Committee

Huiguang He   Institute of Automation, Chinese Academy of Sciences,
                               China
Jun Shi   Shanghai University, China
Xi Jiang   University of Electronic Science and Technology
                               of China, China

Student Activities Liaison

Julia Schnabel   King's College London, UK
Caroline Essert   University of Strasbourg, France
Dimitris Metaxas   Rutgers University, USA
MICCAI Student Board Members

Area Chairs

Purang Abolmaesumi   The University of British Columbia, Canada
Shadi Albarqouni   The Technical University of Munich (TUM), Germany
Elsa Angelini   Imperial College London, UK
Suyash Awate   Indian Institute of Technology (IIT) Bombay, India
Ulas Bagci   University of Central Florida (UCF), USA
Kayhan Batmanghelich   University of Pittsburgh, USA
Christian Baumgartner   Swiss Federal Institute of Technology Zurich,
                               Switzerland
Ismail Ben Ayed   Ecole de Technologie Superieure (ETS), Canada
Weidong Cai   The University of Sydney, Australia
Xiaohuan Cao   United Imaging Intelligence (UII), China
Elvis Chen   Robarts Research Institute, Western University, Canada
Xinjian Chen   Soochow University, China
Jian Cheng   Beihang University, China
Jun Cheng   Cixi Institute of Biomedical Engineering, Chinese
                               Academy of Sciences, China
Veronika Cheplygina   Eindhoven University of Technology, The Netherlands
Elena De Momi   Politecnico di Milano, Italy
Ayman El-Baz   University of Louisville, USA
Aaron Fenster   Robarts Research Institute, Western University, USA
Moti Freiman   Philips Healthcare, The Netherlands
Yue Gao   Tsinghua University, China

Daoqiang Zhang   Nanjing University of Aeronautics and Astronautics,
                                   China
Miaomiao Zhang   Washington University in St. Louis, USA
Tuo Zhang   Northwestern Polytechnical University, China
Guoyan Zheng   Shanghai Jiao Tong University, China
S. Kevin Zhou   Institute of Computing Technology, Chinese Academy
                                   of Sciences, China
Dajiang Zhu   The University of Texas at Arlington, USA

Reviewers

Abdi, Amir   Barbu, Adrian
Abduljabbar, Khalid   Bardosi, Zoltan
Adeli, Ehsan   Bateson, Mathilde
Aganj, Iman   Bathula, Deepti
Aggarwal, Priya   Batmanghelich, Kayhan
Agrawal, Praful   Baumgartner, Christian
Ahmad, Ola   Baur, Christoph
Ahmad, Sahar   Baxter, John
Ahn, Euijoon   Bayramoglu, Neslihan
Akbar, Shazia   Becker, Benjamin
Akhondi-Asl, Alireza   Behnami, Delaram
Akram, Saad   Beig, Niha
Al-Kadi, Omar   Belyaev, Mikhail
Alansary, Amir   Benkarim, Oualid
Alghamdi, Hanan   Bentaieb, Aicha
Ali, Sharib   Bernal, Jose
Allan, Maximilian   Beyeler, Michael
Amiri, Mina   Bhatia, Parmeet
Anton, Esther   Bhole, Chetan
Anwar, Syed   Bhushan, Chitresh
Armin, Mohammad   Bi, Lei
Audigier, Chloe   Bian, Cheng
Aviles-Rivero, Angelica   Bilinski, Piotr
Awan, Ruqayya   Bise, Ryoma
Awate, Suyash   Bnouni, Nesrine
Aydogan, Dogu   Bo, Wang
Azizi, Shekoofeh   Bodenstedt, Sebastian
Bai, Junjie   Bogunovic, Hrvoje
Bai, Wenjia   Bozorgtabar, Behzad
Balbastre, Yaël   Bragman, Felix
Balsiger, Fabian   Braman, Nathaniel
Banerjee, Abhirup   Bridge, Christopher
Bano, Sophia   Broaddus, Coleman

Bron, Esther
Brooks, Rupert
Bruijne, Marleen
Bühler, Katja
Bui, Duc
Burlutskiy, Nikolay
Burwinkel, Hendrik
Bustin, Aurelien
Cabeen, Ryan
Cai, Hongmin
Cai, Jinzheng
Cai, Yunliang
Camino, Acner
Cao, Jiezhang
Cao, Qing
Cao, Tian
Carapella, Valentina
Cardenes, Ruben
Cardoso, M.
Carolus, Heike
Castro, Daniel
Cattin, Philippe
Chabanas, Matthieu
Chaddad, Ahmad
Chaitanya, Krishna
Chakraborty, Jayasree
Chakraborty, Rudrasis
Chang, Ken
Chang, Violeta
Charaborty, Tapabrata
Chatelain, Pierre
Chatterjee, Sudhanya
Chen, Alvin
Chen, Antong
Chen, Cameron
Chen, Chao
Chen, Chen
Chen, Elvis
Chen, Fang
Chen, Fei
Chen, Geng
Chen, Hanbo
Chen, Hao
Chen, Jia-Wei
Chen, Jialei
Chen, Jianxu

Chen, Jie
Chen, Jingyun
Chen, Lei
Chen, Liang
Chen, Min
Chen, Pingjun
Chen, Qingchao
Chen, Xiao
Chen, Xiaoran
Chen, Xin
Chen, Xuejin
Chen, Yang
Chen, Yuanyuan
Chen, Yuncong
Chen, Zhiqiang
Chen, Zhixiang
Cheng, Jun
Cheng, Li
Cheng, Yuan
Cheng, Yupeng
Cheriet, Farida
Chong, Minqi
Choo, Jaegul
Christiaens, Daan
Christodoulidis, Argyrios
Christodoulidis, Stergios
Chung, Ai
Çiçek, Özgün
Cid, Yashin
Clarkson, Matthew
Clough, James
Collins, Toby
Commowick, Olivier
Conze, Pierre-Henri
Cootes, Timothy
Correia, Teresa
Coulon, Olivier
Coupé, Pierrick
Courtecuisse, Hadrien
Craley, Jeffrey
Crimi, Alessandro
Cury, Claire
D'souza, Niharika
Dai, Hang
Dalca, Adrian
Das, Abhijit

Das, Dhritiman
Deeba, Farah
Dekhil, Omar
Demiray, Beatrice
Deniz, Cem
Depeursinge, Adrien
Desrosiers, Christian
Dewey, Blake
Dey, Raunak
Dhamala, Jwala
Ding, Meng
Distergoft, Alexander
Dobrenkii, Anton
Dolz, Jose
Dong, Liang
Dong, Mengjin
Dong, Nanqing
Dong, Xiao
Dong, Yanni
Dou, Qi
Du, Changde
Du, Lei
Du, Shaoyi
Duan, Dingna
Duan, Lixin
Dubost, Florian
Duchateau, Nicolas
Duncan, James
Duong, Luc
Dvornek, Nicha
Dzyubachyk, Oleh
Eaton-Rosen, Zach
Ebner, Michael
Ebrahimi, Mehran
Edwards, Philip
Egger, Bernhard
Eguizabal, Alma
Einarsson, Gudmundur
Ekin, Ahmet
Elazab, Ahmed
Elhabian, Shireen
Elmogy, Mohammed
Eltanboly, Ahmed
Erdt, Marius
Ernst, Floris
Esposito, Marco

Esteban, Oscar
Fan, Jingfan
Fan, Xin
Fan, Yong
Fan, Yonghui
Fang, Xi
Farag, Aly
Farzi, Mohsen
Fauser, Johannes
Fawaz, Hassan
Fedorov, Andrey
Fehri, Hamid
Feng, Chiyu
Feng, Jun
Feng, Xinyang
Feng, Yuan
Fenster, Aaron
Ferrante, Enzo
Feydy, Jean
Fischer, Lukas
Fischer, Peter
Fishbaugh, James
Fletcher, Tom
Flores, Kevin
Forestier, Germain
Forkert, Nils
Fotouhi, Javad
Fountoukidou, Tatiana
Franz, Alfred
Frau-Pascual, Aina
Freysinger, Wolfgang
Fripp, Jurgen
Fu, Huazhu
Funka-Lea, Gareth
Funke, Isabel
Funke, Jan
Fürnstahl, Philipp
Furukawa, Ryo
Gahm, Jin
Galassi, Francesca
Galdran, Adrian
Gan, Yu
Gao, Fei
Gao, Mingchen
Gao, Siyuan
Gao, Zhifan

Gardezi, Syed
Ge, Bao
Gerber, Samuel
Gerig, Guido
Gessert, Nils
Gevaert, Olivier
Gharabaghi, Sara
Ghesu, Florin
Ghimire, Sandesh
Gholipour, Ali
Ghosal, Sayan
Giraud, Rémi
Glocker, Ben
Goceri, Evgin
Goetz, Michael
Gomez, Alberto
Gong, Kuang
Gong, Mingming
Gonzalez, German
Gopal, Sharath
Gopinath, Karthik
Gordon, Shiri
Gori, Pietro
Gou, Shuiping
Granados, Alejandro
Grau, Vicente
Green, Michael
Gritsenko, Andrey
Grupp, Robert
Gu, Lin
Gu, Yun
Gu, Zaiwang
Gueziri, Houssem-Eddine
Guo, Hengtao
Guo, Jixiang
Guo, Xiaoqing
Guo, Yanrong
Guo, Yong
Gupta, Kratika
Gupta, Vikash
Gutman, Boris
Gyawali, Prashnna
Hacihaliloglu, Ilker
Hadjidemetriou, Stathis
Haldar, Justin
Hamarneh, Ghassan

Hamze, Noura
Han, Hu
Han, Jungong
Han, Xiaoguang
Han, Xu
Han, Zhi
Hancox, Jonny
Hanson, Erik
Hao, Xiaoke
Haq, Rabia
Harders, Matthias
Harrison, Adam
Haskins, Grant
Hatamizadeh, Ali
Hatt, Charles
Hauptmann, Andreas
Havaei, Mohammad
He, Tiancheng
He, Yufan
Heimann, Tobias
Heldmann, Stefan
Heller, Nicholas
Hernandez-Matas, Carlos
Hernandez, Monica
Hett, Kilian
Higger, Matt
Hinkle, Jacob
Ho, Tsung-Ying
Hoffmann, Nico
Holden, Matthew
Hong, Song
Hong, Sungmin
Hou, Benjamin
Hsu, Li-Ming
Hu, Dan
Hu, Kai
Hu, Xiaowei
Hu, Xintao
Hu, Yan
Hu, Yipeng
Huang, Heng
Huang, Huifang
Huang, Jiashuang
Huang, Kevin
Huang, Ruobing
Huang, Shih-Gu

Huang, Weilin
Huang, Xiaolei
Huang, Yawen
Huang, Yixing
Huang, Yufang
Huang, Zhongwei
Huaulmé, Arnaud
Huisman, Henkjan
Huo, Xing
Huo, Yuankai
Husch, Andreas
Hussein, Sarfaraz
Hutter, Jana
Hwang, Seong
Icke, Ilknur
Igwe, Kay
Ingalhalikar, Madhura
Irmakci, Ismail
Ivashchenko, Oleksandra
Izadyyazdanabadi, Mohammadhassan
Jafari, Mohammad
Jäger, Paul
Jamaludin, Amir
Janatka, Mirek
Jaouen, Vincent
Jarayathne, Uditha
Javadi, Golara
Javer, Avelino
Jensen, Todd
Ji, Zexuan
Jia, Haozhe
Jiang, Jue
Jiang, Steve
Jiang, Tingting
Jiang, Weixiong
Jiang, Xi
Jiao, Jianbo
Jiao, Jieqing
Jiao, Zhicheng
Jie, Biao
Jin, Dakai
Jin, Taisong
Jin, Yueming
John, Rogers
Joshi, Anand
Joshi, Shantanu

Jud, Christoph
Jung, Kyu-Hwan
Jungo, Alain
Kadkhodamohammadi, Abdolrahim
Kakileti, Siva
Kamnitsas, Konstantinos
Kang, Eunsong
Kao, Po-Yu
Kapoor, Ankur
Karani, Neerav
Karayumak, Suheyla
Kazi, Anees
Kerrien, Erwan
Kervadec, Hoel
Khalifa, Fahmi
Khalili, Nadieh
Khallaghi, Siavash
Khalvati, Farzad
Khan, Hassan
Khanal, Bishesh
Khansari, Maziyar
Khosravan, Naji
Kia, Seyed
Kikinis, Ron
Kim, Geena
Kim, Hosung
Kim, Hyo-Eun
Kim, Jae-Hun
Kim, Jinman
Kim, Jinyoung
Kim, Minjeong
Kim, Namkug
Kim, Seong
Kim, Young-Ho
Kitasaka, Takayuki
Klein, Stefan
Klinder, Tobias
Kolli, Kranthi
Kong, Bin
Kong, Xiang-Zhen
Konukoglu, Ender
Koo, Bongjin
Koohbanani, Navid
Kopriva, Ivica
Kose, Kivanc
Koutsoumpa, Christina

Kozinski, Mateusz
Krebs, Julian
Krishnan, Anithapriya
Krishnaswamy, Pavitra
Krivov, Egor
Kruggel, Frithjof
Krupinski, Elizabeth
Kuang, Hulin
Kügler, David
Kuijper, Arjan
Kulkarni, Prachi
Kumar, Arun
Kumar, Ashnil
Kumar, Kuldeep
Kumar, Neeraj
Kumar, Nitin
Kumaradevan, Punithakumar
Kunz, Manuela
Kunze, Holger
Kuo, Weicheng
Kurc, Tahsin
Kurmann, Thomas
Kwak, Jin
Kwon, Yongchan
Laadhari, Aymen
Ladikos, Alexander
Lalonde, Rodney
Lamata, Pablo
Langs, Georg
Lartizien, Carole
Lasso, Andras
Lau, Felix
Laura, Cristina
Le, Ngan
Ledig, Christian
Lee, Hansang
Lee, Hyekyoung
Lee, Jong-Hwan
Lee, Kyong
Lee, Minho
Lee, Soochahn
Léger, Étienne
Leger, Stefan
Lei, Baiying
Lekadir, Karim
Lenga, Matthias

Leow, Wee
Lessmann, Nikolas
Li, Annan
Li, Bin
Li, Fuhai
Li, Gang
Li, Guoshi
Li, Hongwei
Li, Hongying
Li, Huiqi
Li, Jian
Li, Jianning
Li, Ke
Li, Minli
Li, Quanzheng
Li, Rongjian
Li, Shaohua
Li, Shulong
Li, Shuyu
Li, Wenqi
Li, Xiang
Li, Xianjun
Li, Xiaojie
Li, Xiaomeng
Li, Xiaoxiao
Li, Xiuli
Li, Yang
Li, Yuexiang
Li, Zhang
Li, Zhi-Cheng
Li, Zhiyuan
Li, Zhjin
Lian, Chunfeng
Liang, Jianming
Liang, Shanshan
Liang, Yudong
Liao, Ruizhi
Liao, Xiangyun
Licandro, Roxane
Lin, Hongxiang
Lin, Lanfen
Lin, Muqing
Lindner, Claudia
Lippert, Christoph
Lisowska, Aneta
Litjens, Geert

Liu, Bin
Liu, Daochang
Liu, Dong
Liu, Dongnan
Liu, Fang
Liu, Feihong
Liu, Feng
Liu, Hong
Liu, Hui
Liu, Jianfei
Liu, Jiang
Liu, Jin
Liu, Jing
Liu, Jundong
Liu, Kefei
Liu, Li
Liu, Mingxia
Liu, Na
Liu, Peng
Liu, Shenghua
Liu, Siqi
Liu, Siyuan
Liu, Tianming
Liu, Tiffany
Liu, Xianglong
Liu, Yixun
Liu, Yong
Liu, Yue
Liu, Zhe
Loddo, Andrea
Lopes, Daniel
Lorenzi, Marco
Lou, Bin
Lu, Allen
Lu, Donghuan
Lu, Jiwen
Lu, Le
Lu, Weijia
Lu, Yao
Lu, Yueh-Hsun
Luo, Gongning
Luo, Jie
Lv, Jinglei
Lyu, Ilwoo
Lyu, Junyan
Ma, Benteng

Ma, Burton
Ma, Da
Ma, Kai
Ma, Xuelin
Mahapatra, Dwarikanath
Mahdavi, Sara
Mahmoud, Ali
Maicas, Gabriel
Maier-Hein, Klaus
Maier, Andreas
Makrogiannis, Sokratis
Malandain, Grégoire
Malik, Bilal
Malpani, Anand
Mancini, Matteo
Manhart, Michael
Manjon, Jose
Mansoor, Awais
Mao, Yunxiang
Martel, Anne
Martinez-Torteya, Antonio
Mathai, Tejas
Mato, David
Mcclelland, Jamie
Mcleod, Jonathan
Medrano-Gracia, Pau
Mehta, Ronak
Meier, Raphael
Melbourne, Andrew
Meng, Qingjie
Meng, Xianjing
Meng, Yu
Menze, Bjoern
Mi, Liang
Miao, Shun
Michielse, Stijn
Midya, Abhishek
Milchenko, Mikhail
Min, Zhe
Miyamoto, Tadashi
Mo, Yuanhan
Molina, Rafael
Montillo, Albert
Moradi, Mehdi
Moreno, Rodrigo
Mortazi, Aliasghar

Rad, Reza
Rafii-Tari, Hedyeh
Rajpoot, Kashif
Ramachandram, Dhanesh
Ran, Lingyan
Raniga, Parnesh
Rashwan, Hatem
Rathore, Saima
Ratnarajah, Nagulan
Raval, Mehul
Ravikumar, Nishant
Raviprakash, Harish
Raza, Shan
Reaungamornrat, Surreerat
Rekik, Islem
Remeseiro, Beatriz
Rempfler, Markus
Ren, Jian
Ren, Xuhua
Ren, Yudan
Reyes-Aldasoro, Constantino
Reyes, Mauricio
Riedel, Brandalyn
Rieke, Nicola
Risser, Laurent
Rittner, Leticia
Rivera, Diego
Ro, Yong
Robinson, Emma
Robinson, Robert
Rodas, Nicolas
Rodrigues, Rafael
Rohr, Karl
Roohani, Yusuf
Roszkowiak, Lukasz
Roth, Holger
Rouco, José
Roy, Abhijit
Ruijters, Danny
Rusu, Mirabela
Rutter, Erica
S., Sharath
Sabuncu, Mert
Sachse, Frank
Safta, Wiem
Saha, Monjoy

Saha, Pramit
Sahu, Manish
Samani, Abbas
Samek, Wojciech
Sánchez-Margallo, Francisco
Sánchez-Margallo, Juan
Sankaran, Sethuraman
Sanroma, Gerard
Sao, Anil
Sarhan, Mhd
Sarikaya, Duygu
Sarker, Md.
Sato, Imari
Saut, Olivier
Savardi, Mattia
Savitha, Ramasamy
Scarpa, Fabio
Scheinost, Dustin
Scherf, Nico
Schirmer, Markus
Schlaefer, Alexander
Schmid, Jerome
Schnabel, Julia
Schultz, Thomas
Schwartz, Ernst
Sdika, Michael
Sedai, Suman
Sekou, Taibou
Sekuboyina, Anjany
Selvan, Raghavendra
Semedo, Carla
Senouf, Ortal
Seoud, Lama
Sermesant, Maxime
Serrano, Carmen
Sethi, Amit
Shaban, Muhammad
Shaffie, Ahmed
Shah, Meet
Shalaby, Ahmed
Shamir, Reuben
Shan, Hongming
Shao, Yeqin
Sharma, Harshita
Shehata, Mohamed
Shen, Haocheng

Shen, Li
Shen, Mali
Shen, Yiru
Sheng, Ke
Shi, Bibo
Shi, Jun
Shi, Kuangyu
Shi, Xiaoshuang
Shi, Yonggang
Shi, Yonghong
Shigwan, Saurabh
Shin, Hoo-Chang
Shin, Jitae
Shontz, Suzanne
Signoroni, Alberto
Siless, Viviana
Silva, Carlos
Silva, Wilson
Simonovsky, Martin
Simson, Walter
Sinclair, Matthew
Singh, Vivek
Soans, Rajath
Sohel, Ferdous
Sokooti, Hessam
Soliman, Ahmed
Sommen, Fons
Sommer, Stefan
Song, Ming
Song, Yang
Sotiras, Aristeidis
Sparks, Rachel
Spiclin, Ziga
St-Jean, Samuel
Steinbach, Peter
Stern, Darko
Stimpel, Bernhard
Strait, Justin
Studholme, Colin
Styner, Martin
Su, Hai
Su, Yun-Hsuan
Subramanian, Vaishnavi
Subsol, Gérard
Sudre, Carole
Suk, Heung-Il

Sun, Jian
Sun, Li
Sun, Tao
Sung, Kyunghyun
Suter, Yannick
Tajbakhsh, Nima
Tan, Chaowei
Tan, Jiaxing
Tan, Wenjun
Tang, Min
Tang, Sheng
Tang, Thomas
Tang, Xiaoying
Tang, Youbao
Tang, Yuxing
Tang, Zhenyu
Tanner, Christine
Tanno, Ryutaro
Tao, Qian
Tarroni, Giacomo
Tasdizen, Tolga
Thung, Kim
Tian, Jiang
Tian, Yun
Toews, Matthew
Tong, Yubing
Topsakal, Oguzhan
Torosdagli, Neslisah
Toussaint, Nicolas
Troccaz, Jocelyne
Trzcinski, Tomasz
Tulder, Gijs
Tustison, Nick
Tuysuzoglu, Ahmet
Ukwatta, Eranga
Unberath, Mathias
Ungi, Tamas
Upadhyay, Uddeshya
Urschler, Martin
Uslu, Fatmatulzehra
Uyanik, Ilyas
Vaillant, Régis
Vakalopoulou, Maria
Valindria, Vanya
Varela, Marta
Varsavsky, Thomas

Vedula, S.
Vedula, Sanketh
Veeraraghavan, Harini
Vega, Roberto
Veni, Gopalkrishna
Verma, Ujjwal
Vetter, Thomas
Vialard, Francois-Xavier
Villard, Pierre-Frederic
Villarini, Barbara
Virga, Salvatore
Vishnevskiy, Valery
Viswanath, Satish
Vlontzos, Athanasios
Vogl, Wolf-Dieter
Voigt, Ingmar
Vos, Bob
Vrtovec, Tomaz
Wang, Bo
Wang, Changmiao
Wang, Chengjia
Wang, Chunliang
Wang, Dadong
Wang, Guotai
Wang, Haifeng
Wang, Haoqian
Wang, Hongkai
Wang, Hongzhi
Wang, Hua
Wang, Huan
Wang, Jiazhuo
Wang, Jingwen
Wang, Jun
Wang, Junyan
Wang, Kuanquan
Wang, Kun
Wang, Lei
Wang, Li
Wang, Liansheng
Wang, Manning
Wang, Mingliang
Wang, Nizhuan
Wang, Pei
Wang, Puyang
Wang, Ruixuan
Wang, Shanshan

Wang, Sheng
Wang, Shuai
Wang, Wenzhe
Wang, Xiangxue
Wang, Xiaosong
Wang, Xuchu
Wang, Yalin
Wang, Yan
Wang, Yaping
Wang, Yuanjun
Wang, Ze
Wang, Zhe
Wang, Zhinuo
Wang, Zhiwei
Wang, Zilei
Weber, Jonathan
Wee, Chong-Yaw
Weese, Jürgen
Wei, Benzheng
Wei, Dong
Wei, Donglai
Wei, Dongming
Weigert, Martin
Wein, Wolfgang
Wels, Michael
Wemmert, Cédric
Werner, Rene
Wesierski, Daniel
Williams, Bryan
Williams, Jacqueline
Williams, Travis
Williamson, Tom
Wilms, Matthias
Wiskin, James
Wittek, Adam
Wollmann, Thomas
Wolterink, Jelmer
Wong, Ken
Woo, Jonghye
Wu, Guoqing
Wu, Ji
Wu, Jian
Wu, Jiong
Wu, Pengxiang
Wu, Xi
Wu, Ye

Wu, Yicheng
Wuerfl, Tobias
Xi, Xiaoming
Xia, Jing
Xia, Wenfeng
Xiao, Deqiang
Xiao, Yiming
Xie, Hai
Xie, Hongtao
Xie, Jianyang
Xie, Long
Xie, Weidi
Xie, Yiting
Xie, Yuanpu
Xie, Yutong
Xing, Fuyong
Xiong, Tao
Xu, Chenchu
Xu, Jiaofeng
Xu, Jun
Xu, Kele
Xu, Rui
Xu, Ting
Xu, Yan
Xu, Yongchao
Xu, Zheng
Xu, Zhenlin
Xu, Zhoubing
Xu, Ziyue
Xue, Jie
Xue, Wufeng
Xue, Yuan
Yahya, Faridah
Yan, Chenggang
Yan, Ke
Yan, Weizheng
Yan, Yu
Yan, Yuguang
Yan, Zhennan
Yang, Guang
Yang, Guanyu
Yang, Hao-Yu
Yang, Jie
Yang, Lin
Yang, Shan
Yang, Xiao

Yang, Xiaohui
Yang, Xin
Yao, Dongren
Yao, Jianhua
Yao, Jiawen
Ye, Chuyang
Ye, Jong
Ye, Menglong
Ye, Xujiong
Yi, Jingru
Yi, Xin
Ying, Shihui
Yoo, Youngjin
Yousefi, Bardia
Yousefi, Sahar
Yu, Jinhua
Yu, Kai
Yu, Lequan
Yu, Renping
Yu, Weichuan
Yushkevich, Paul
Zanjani, Farhad
Zenati, Marco
Zeng, Dong
Zeng, Guodong
Zettinig, Oliver
Zhan, Liang
Zhang, Baochang
Zhang, Chuncheng
Zhang, Dongqing
Zhang, Fan
Zhang, Haichong
Zhang, Han
Zhang, Haopeng
Zhang, Heye
Zhang, Jianpeng
Zhang, Jiong
Zhang, Jun
Zhang, Le
Zhang, Lichi
Zhang, Mingli
Zhang, Pengyue
Zhang, Pin
Zhang, Qiang
Zhang, Rongzhao
Zhang, Shengping

Zhang, Shu
Zhang, Songze
Zhang, Tianyang
Zhang, Tong
Zhang, Wei
Zhang, Wen
Zhang, Wenlu
Zhang, Xiang
Zhang, Xin
Zhang, Yi
Zhang, Yifan
Zhang, Yizhe
Zhang, Yong
Zhang, Yongqin
Zhang, You
Zhang, Yu
Zhang, Yue
Zhang, Yueyi
Zhang, Yungeng
Zhang, Yunyan
Zhang, Yuyao
Zhang, Zizhao
Zhao, Haifeng
Zhao, Jun
Zhao, Qingyu
Zhao, Rongchang
Zhao, Shijie
Zhao, Shiwan
Zhao, Tengda
Zhao, Wei
Zhao, Yitian
Zhao, Yiyuan

Zhao, Yu
Zhao, Zijian
Zheng, Shenhai
Zheng, Yalin
Zheng, Yinqiang
Zhong, Zichun
Zhou, Bo
Zhou, Jianlong
Zhou, Luping
Zhou, Niyun
Zhou, S.
Zhou, Shoujun
Zhou, Tao
Zhou, Wenjin
Zhou, Yuyin
Zhou, Zhiguo
Zhu, Hancan
Zhu, Junjie
Zhu, Qikui
Zhu, Weifang
Zhu, Wentao
Zhu, Xiaofeng
Zhu, Xinliang
Zhu, Yingying
Zhu, Yuemin
Zhu, Zhuotun
Zhuang, Xiahai
Zia, Aneeq
Zimmer, Veronika
Zolgharni, Massoud
Zou, Ju
Zuluaga, Maria

Accepted MICCAI 2019 Papers

By Region of First Author

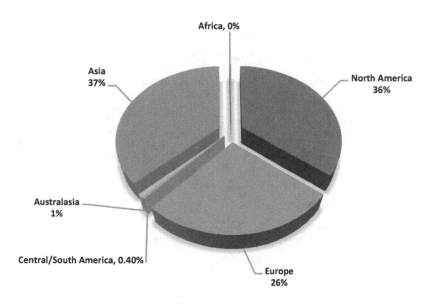

Africa, 0%

Asia 37%

North America 36%

Australasia 1%

Central/South America, 0.40%

Europe 26%

By Technical Keyword

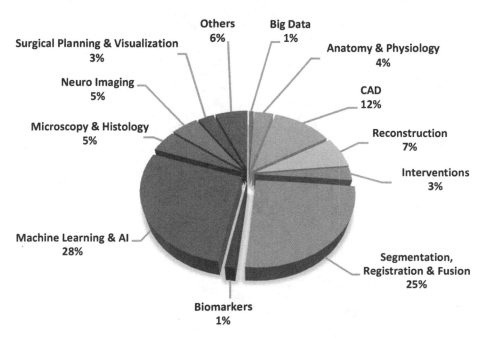

Others 6%

Big Data 1%

Surgical Planning & Visualization 3%

Anatomy & Physiology 4%

Neuro Imaging 5%

CAD 12%

Microscopy & Histology 5%

Reconstruction 7%

Interventions 3%

Machine Learning & AI 28%

Segmentation, Registration & Fusion 25%

Biomarkers 1%

Awards Presented at MICCAI 2018, Granada, Spain

MICCAI Society Enduring Impact Award: The Enduring Impact Award is the highest award of the MICCAI Society. It is a career award for continued excellence in the MICCAI research field. The 2018 Enduring Impact Award was presented to Sandy Wells, Brigham and Women's Hospital/Harvard Medical School, USA.

MICCAI Society Fellowships: MICCAI Fellowships are bestowed annually on a small number of senior members of the society in recognition of substantial scientific contributions to the MICCAI research field and service to the MICCAI community. In 2018, fellowships were awarded to:

- Pierre Jannin (Université de Rennes, France)
- Anne Martel (University of Toronto, Canada)
- Julia Schnabel (King's College London, UK)

Medical Image Analysis Journal Award Sponsored by Elsevier: Jianyu Lin, for his paper entitled "Dual-modality Endoscopic Probe for Tissue Surface Shape Reconstruction and Hyperspectral Imaging Enabled by Deep Neural Networks," authored by Jianyu Lin, Neil T. Clancy, Ji Qi, Yang Hu, Taran Tatla, Danail Stoyanov, Lena Maier-Hein, and Daniel S. Elson.

Best Paper in *International Journal of Computer-Assisted Radiology and Surgery* (IJCARS) journal: Arash Pourtaherian for his paper entitled "Robust and Semantic Needle Detection in 3D Ultrasound Using Orthogonal-Plane Convolutional Neural Networks," authored by Arash Pourtaherian, Farhad Ghazvinian Zanjani, Svitlana Zinger, Nenad Mihajlovic, Gary C. Ng, Hendrikus H. M. Korsten, and Peter H. N. de With.

Young Scientist Publication Impact Award: MICCAI papers by a young scientist from the past 5 years were eligible for this award. It is made to a researcher whose work had an impact on the MICCAI field in terms of citations, secondary citations, subsequent publications, h-index. The 2018 Young Scientist Publication Impact Award was given to Holger R Roth: "A New 2.5D Representation for Lymph Node Detection Using Random Sets of Deep Convolutional Neural Network Observations" authored by Holger R. Roth, Le Lu, Ari Seff, Kevin M. Cherry, Joanne Hoffman, Shijun Wang, Jiamin Liu, Evrim Turkbey, and Ronald M. Summers.

MICCAI Young Scientist Awards: The Young Scientist Awards are stimulation prizes awarded for the best first authors of MICCAI contributions in distinct subject areas. The nominees had to be full-time students at a recognized university at, or within, two years prior to submission. The 2018 MICCAI Young Scientist Awards were given to:

- Erik J. Bekkers for the paper entitled: "Roto-Translation Covariant Convolutional Networks for Medical Image Analysis"
- Bastian Bier for the paper entitled: "X-ray-transform Invariant Anatomical Landmark Detection for Pelvic Trauma Surgery"

- Yuanhan Mo for his paper entitled: "The Deep Poincaré Map: A Novel Approach for Left Ventricle Segmentation"
- Tanya Nair for the paper entitled: "Exploring Uncertainty Measures in Deep Networks for Multiple Sclerosis Lesion Detection and Segmentation"
- Yue Zhang for the paper entitled: "Task-Driven Generative Modeling for Unsupervised Domain Adaptation: Application to X-ray Image Segmentation"

Contents – Part V

MIC Meets CAI

Computer-Assisted Interventions

Computer-Assisted Interventions

Robust Cochlear Modiolar Axis Detection in CT

Wilhelm Wimmer[1,2,3](✉) [ID], Clair Vandersteen[1,4], Nicolas Guevara[1,4],
Marco Caversaccio[2,3,4], and Hervé Delingette[4] [ID]

[1] Université Côte d'Azur, Inria, Epione, Sophia Antipolis, France
wilhelm.wimmer@inria.fr
[2] Department of Otolaryngology, Inselspital, University of Bern,
Bern, Switzerland
[3] Hearing Research Laboratory, ARTORG Center, University of Bern,
Bern, Switzerland
[4] Université Côte d'Azur, Centre Hospitalier Universitaire de Nice,
Institut Universitaire de la Face et du Cou, Nice, France

Abstract. The cochlea, the auditory part of the inner ear, is a spiral-shaped organ with large morphological variability. An individualized assessment of its shape is essential for clinical applications related to tonotopy and cochlear implantation. To unambiguously reference morphological parameters, reliable recognition of the cochlear modiolar axis in computed tomography (CT) images is required. The conventional method introduces measurement uncertainties, as it is based on manually selected and difficult to identify landmarks. Herein, we present an algorithm for robust modiolar axis detection in clinical CT images. We define the modiolar axis as the rotation component of the kinematic spiral motion inherent in the cochlear shape. For surface fitting, we use a compact shape representation in a 7-dimensional kinematic parameter space based on extended Plücker coordinates. It is the first time such a kinematic representation is used for shape analysis in medical images. Robust surface fitting is achieved with an adapted approximate maximum likelihood method assuming a Student-t distribution, enabling axis detection even in partially available surface data. We verify the algorithm performance on a synthetic data set with cochlear surface subsets. In addition, we perform an experimental study with four experts in 23 human cochlea CT data sets to compare the automated detection with the manually found axes. Axes found from co-registered high resolution μCT scans are used for reference. Our experiments show that the algorithm reduces the alignment error providing more reliable modiolar axis detection for clinical and research applications.

Keywords: Kinematic surface recognition · Approximate maximum likelihood · Natural growth

© Springer Nature Switzerland AG 2019
D. Shen et al. (Eds.): MICCAI 2019, LNCS 11768, pp. 3–10, 2019.
https://doi.org/10.1007/978-3-030-32254-0_1

1 Introduction

The cochlea is a spiral structure in the inner ear that transduces acoustic waves into electrical nerve impulses to enable hearing. The morphology of the human cochlea is complex and highly variable. Therefore, an unambiguous description of the morphological parameters for both modeling and clinical applications is required. Of great importance is the modiolar axis, the central axis of the spiral shape, as it is used to define the z-axis of cylindrical cochlear coordinate reference systems [1]. Due to the tonotopic organization of the cochlea, the modiolar axis connects anatomical features with physiological parameters, mapping spatial positions along the spiral with the perceived characteristic frequencies. In cochlear implantation, in which an electrode array is inserted into the cochlea to restore hearing, radiological parameters referenced by the modiolar axis are used for preoperative planning (selection of suitable implant lengths), for postoperative evaluation (array insertion depth assessment) and for audio processor programming (patient-specific tonotopic stimulation maps). They are also used to investigate the effects of tonotopic mismatch between different stimulation channels on speech rehabilitation in bilateral cochlear implant users.

A common definition of the modiolar axis is based on anatomical landmarks that can only be identified imprecisely in computed-tomography (CT) images: the helicotrema and the center of the modiolus in the basal turn of the cochlea [2]. This leads to misalignment and inter-observer variability, even when using multiplanar reconstructions. As a consequence, outcome measures that are referenced by modiolus-based coordinate systems are distorted. Furthermore, misclassification of cochlear morphology can be caused by inaccurate modiolar axis estimation [3]. Previous detection algorithms use center-line based methods, however either requiring fully segmented image data of the cochlea [3] or knowledge of additional extrinsic parameters [4].

Herein, we present a novel approach for modiolar axis detection suitable for clinical resolution CT images. The spiral shape of the cochlea is modelled as a kinematic surface to mimic its natural growth. Kinematic surfaces are defined as the location of surface points that are tangent to a parameterized stationary velocity field. Then, the modiolar axis is determined as the rotation component of the intrinsic spiral motion. Our contribution lies in the first application of a compact seven-dimensional kinematic surface representation for medical image analysis. Furthermore, we extend the method by a robust maximum likelihood scheme based on a Student-t distribution. The algorithm output is verified using a synthetic data set. Finally, we perform an experimental validation study to compare the modiolar axis detection results between the conventional landmark-based method and our algorithm under consideration of μCT reference data.

2 Methods

2.1 Kinematic Modiolar Axis Detection

To find the modiolar axis, we aim to determine the rotation component of the intrinsic kinematic spiral motion forming the cochlea. We base our work on a line element geometry approach for kinematic surface recognition [5]. A kinematic surface is a surface consisting of oriented points (with position $\mathbf{p}_i$ and unit surface normals $\mathbf{n}_i$) that is tangent to a parametric velocity field $\mathbf{v}(\mathbf{p})$, i.e. $\mathbf{v}(\mathbf{p}) \cdot \mathbf{n} = 0$. Kinematic surfaces somewhat extend the notion of implicit surfaces $S(\mathbf{p}) = 0$ defined on points.

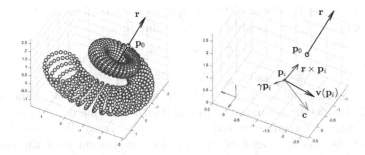

Fig. 1. (Left) Spiral-shaped surface generated by a kinematic motion with rotation axis $\mathbf{r}$ and zero velocity convergence point $\mathbf{p}_0$. (Right) Components of the velocity $\mathbf{v}(\mathbf{p}_i)$ at point $\mathbf{p}_i$ with rotation $\mathbf{r}$, translation $\mathbf{c}$, and scaling factor γ.

For the cochlea, we consider a spiral velocity field $\mathbf{v}(\mathbf{p}) = \mathbf{r} \times \mathbf{p} + \mathbf{c} + \gamma\mathbf{p}$, consisting of a rotation $\mathbf{r}$, translation $\mathbf{c}$ and scale factor γ (see Fig. 1). By choosing $\mathbf{f}(\mathbf{p}, \mathbf{n}) = \{\mathbf{p} \times \mathbf{n}, \mathbf{n}, \mathbf{p} \cdot \mathbf{n}\}$ the surface is transformed into a seven-dimensional parameter space based on extended Plücker coordinates. Then, the problem of spiral shape recognition reduces to fitting a linear subspace to $\mathbf{f}(\mathbf{p}, \mathbf{n})$ [5]. This is achieved by searching for the parameters $\mathbf{m} = \{\mathbf{r}, \mathbf{c}, \gamma\}$ such that the distance $d_i(\mathbf{m})$ between each point and the surface tangent to the velocity field $\mathbf{v}(\mathbf{p}_i)$ is minimized. By using a first order approximation of the distance (approximate maximum likelihood method [6,7]) we can write:

$$d_i(\mathbf{m}) = \frac{\mathbf{v}(\mathbf{p}_i) \cdot \mathbf{n}_i}{\sqrt{\|\mathbf{v}(\mathbf{p}_i)\|^2 + w_\mathbf{p}\|\nabla_\mathbf{p}(\mathbf{v}(\mathbf{p}_i) \cdot \mathbf{n}_i)\|^2}} \tag{1}$$

where w_p is a scalar regularizing the denominator. For a spiral velocity field, we find $\nabla_\mathbf{p}(\mathbf{v}(\mathbf{p}_i) \cdot \mathbf{n}_i) = \mathbf{n}_i \times \mathbf{r} + \gamma\mathbf{n}_i = [\mathbf{A}_\mathbf{r} + \gamma\mathbf{I}]\mathbf{n}_i$ where $\mathbf{A}_\mathbf{r}$ is the skew-symmetric matrix associated with vector $\mathbf{r}$, and $\mathbf{I}$ is the identity matrix. Then we have $\|\nabla_\mathbf{p}(\mathbf{v}(\mathbf{p}_i) \cdot \mathbf{n}_i)\|^2 = \|\mathbf{n}_i \times \mathbf{r}\|^2 + \gamma^2$ and $\|\mathbf{v}(\mathbf{p}_i)\|^2 = \|\mathbf{r} \times \mathbf{p}_i\|^2 + \gamma^2\|\mathbf{p}_i\|^2 + 2\gamma(\mathbf{p}_i \cdot \mathbf{c}) + 2[\mathbf{r}, \mathbf{p}_i, \mathbf{c}] + \|\mathbf{c}\|^2$. In a first approach, we assume a Gaussian distribution of the distance error with variance Σ, i.e., $p(d_i) = \mathcal{N}(d|0, \Sigma)$. The objective now is to determine $\mathbf{m}$ such that the log-likelihood $p(\mathcal{D}|\mathbf{m})$ is maximized:

$$\log p(\mathcal{D}|\mathbf{m}) = \log \prod_{i=1}^{n} p(d_i|\mathbf{m}) = -\frac{n}{2}\log 2\pi\Sigma - \frac{1}{2}\sum_{i=1}^{n}\frac{d_i^2}{\Sigma} = -\frac{n}{2}\log 2\pi\Sigma + \mathcal{L}(\mathbf{m}).$$

We can write $d_i^2 = \dfrac{(\mathbf{v}(\mathbf{p}_i)\cdot\mathbf{n}_i)^2}{\|\mathbf{v}(\mathbf{p}_i)\|^2 + w_p\|\nabla_p(\mathbf{v}(\mathbf{p}_i)\cdot\mathbf{n}_i)\|^2} = \dfrac{\mathbf{m}^T\mathbf{M}_i\mathbf{m}}{\mathbf{m}^T\mathbf{N}_i\mathbf{m}}$ with the 7×7 matrices $\mathbf{M}_i$, $\mathbf{N}_i$ defined as:

$$\mathbf{M}_i = \mathbf{f}(\mathbf{p}_i, \mathbf{n}_i)\mathbf{f}(\mathbf{p}_i, \mathbf{n}_i)^T, \quad \mathbf{N}_i = \begin{bmatrix} \mathbf{A}_{\mathbf{p}_i}^T\mathbf{A}_{\mathbf{p}_i} + w_p\mathbf{A}_{\mathbf{n}_i}^T\mathbf{A}_{\mathbf{n}_i} & -\mathbf{A}_{\mathbf{p}_i} & \mathbf{0} \\ -\mathbf{A}_{\mathbf{p}_i}^T & \mathbf{I} & \mathbf{p}_i \\ \mathbf{0} & \mathbf{p}_i^T & \mathbf{p}_i \cdot \mathbf{p}_i + w_p \end{bmatrix}.$$

Maximizing the log likelihood $\mathcal{L}(\mathbf{m})$ is equivalent to minimizing $\sum_{i=1}^n \dfrac{\mathbf{m}^T\mathbf{M}_i\mathbf{m}}{\mathbf{m}^T\mathbf{N}_i\mathbf{m}}$ which leads to solving the generalized eigenvalue problem [7]:

$$\mathbf{B}_m\mathbf{m} = \mathbf{C}_m\mathbf{m} \tag{2}$$

with $\mathbf{B}_m = \sum_{i=1}^n \dfrac{\mathbf{M}_i}{\mathbf{m}^T\mathbf{N}_i\mathbf{m}}$ and $\mathbf{C}_m = \sum_{i=1}^n \dfrac{\mathbf{m}^T\mathbf{M}_i\mathbf{m}}{(\mathbf{m}^T\mathbf{N}_i\mathbf{m})^2} \cdot \mathbf{N}_i$.

The non-linear problem can be tackled by iteratively computing the matrices $\mathbf{B}_m$ and $\mathbf{C}_m$ for a given estimation of $\mathbf{m}$ and then estimating $\mathbf{m}$ as the eigenvector associated with the smallest eigenvalue (closest to zero). We then define the direction of the modiolar axis as the rotation component $\mathbf{r}$ of the estimated parameters. We further need to compute the zero velocity center of the spiral motion $\mathbf{p}_0 = \frac{1}{\gamma(\mathbf{r}^2+\gamma^2)}(\gamma\mathbf{r}\times\mathbf{c} - \gamma^2\mathbf{c} - (\mathbf{r}\cdot\mathbf{c})\mathbf{r})$ to define the position of the modiolar axis.

2.2 Robust Detection

Like any least-squares fitting method, the above mentioned approach is sensitive to outliers. To increase robustness, we propose to replace the Gaussian likelihood with a Student-t distribution, which is a Gaussian Scale Mixture. More precisely, we assume $p(d_i) = \mathrm{St}(d_i|0, \Sigma, \nu) = \int_{z_i} \mathcal{N}(d_i|0, \Sigma/z_i)\,\mathrm{Ga}(z_i|\nu/2, \nu/2)dz_i$ where z_i is the variance scale variable which has a prior given by the Gamma distribution parameterized by the degrees of freedom ν. When $\nu \to +\infty$, then the Student-t is equivalent to the Gaussian distribution. Therefore, the ν variable is inversely proportional to the number of outliers. The estimation of the kinematic surface is now extended with an Expectation-Maximization scheme, where z_i is the latent variable [8]. This is equivalent to iteratively estimating ν, z_i and Σ with the following steps:

- **E-step:** Estimate z_i for each data point as $z_i = (\nu + 1)/(\nu + d_i^2/\Sigma)$. When ν is very large then z_i is close to 1, irrespective to the Mahalanobis distance d_i^2/Σ. When ν is less large then z_i is close to zero for outliers (since the Mahalanobis becomes large) and close to 1 for inliers.
- **M-Σ step:** Estimate the variance as $\Sigma = \frac{1}{n}\sum_{i=1}^n z_i d_i^2$
- **M-ν step:** Estimate ν as the solution of the non-linear problem

$$-\psi\left(\frac{\nu}{2}\right) + \log\left(\frac{\nu}{2}\right) + 1 + \psi\left(\frac{\nu+1}{2}\right) - \log\left(\frac{\nu+1}{2}\right) + \frac{1}{n}\sum_{i=1}^n(\log z_i - z_i) = 0,$$

where $\psi(x)$ denotes the digamma function.

As an output, we get the estimation of confidence z_i in each data point. To obtain a robust estimation of the parameter vector $\mathbf{m}$, we proceed as before (2) but with $\mathbf{B}_m = \sum_{i=1}^n z_i \dfrac{\mathbf{M}_i}{\mathbf{m}^T\mathbf{N}_i\mathbf{m}}$ and $\mathbf{C}_m = \sum_{i=1}^n z_i \dfrac{\mathbf{m}^T\mathbf{M}_i\mathbf{m}}{(\mathbf{m}^T\mathbf{N}_i\mathbf{m})^2}\mathbf{N}_i$.

2.3   Implementation

The detection algorithm was implemented in Matlab. It is initialized by specifying the landmarks l_1 and l_2 (Fig. 2 left) in CT to preselect a spherical segment volume approximately covering the middle and apical turns of the cochlea (radius $r_s = \|r_s\| = \|l_1 - l_2\|$ and center $c_s = (l_1 + l_2)/2$, cropped by the planes perpendicular to r_s in l_1 and l_2). This volume is chosen to minimize interference of proximal structures that may appear connected to the cochlea in clinical CT (i.e., the tympanic cavity at the round window, the internal auditory canal, and the facial nerve). The data is labelled through intensity thresholding (isovalue at 1000 HU), smoothed, and isosurfaces are generated by a marching cubes routine. The largest connected surface with the center of gravity closest to c_s is extracted. The point cloud is scaled and centered, surface normals are computed and the parameter space $f(p)$ is obtained. Kinematic surface fitting is performed by 5 iterations with $w_p = 0.001$ (Fig. 2 right).

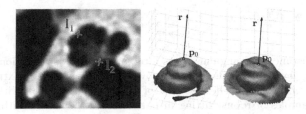

Fig. 2. (Left) CT slice with cochlear cross-section and 2 modiolar axis landmarks: the helicotrema (l_1) and the center of the modiolus in the basal turn (l_2). (Right) Examples of robust fitting in partial cochlea surfaces for modiolar axis r and zero velocity center p_0 detection. The confidence z_i of each oriented point is color-encoded from red (close to 0, outliers) to green (close to 1, high confidence). (Color figure online)

2.4   Verification in Synthetic Data

We used a polynomial cochlea model with known modiolar axis to generate a synthetic data set for algorithm verification [9]. To mimic the facial nerve located close to the cochlea and often causing segmentation artifacts, we added a tubular structure (1 mm in diameter) with constrained random alignment. In addition, point positions were perturbed with Gaussian noise (0.15 mm standard deviation). We tested the robustness of the algorithm in varying levels of surface coverage (analogous to algorithm implementation, however with different radii covering 5% to 100% of total points). For each level, 500 random cochleae were generated. For comparison, the non-robust (Gaussian) version of the detection algorithm as well as simple detection using principal component analysis (PCA) of the point cloud was applied, where the modiolar axis was selected as the component with least variance. We assessed the alignment between the estimated axis $\mathbf{r}$ and reference axis $\mathbf{r}_{ref}$ with the angular error $\Delta\theta$ and the distance error Δd defined as the closest absolute distance between the estimated axis $\mathbf{r}$ and the center point $\mathbf{p}_{ref}$ on the reference axis $\mathbf{r}_{ref}$:

$$\Delta\theta = \arcsin\frac{\|\mathbf{r}_{ref} \times \mathbf{r}\|}{\|\mathbf{r}_{ref}\|\|\mathbf{r}\|}, \qquad \Delta d = \left|(\mathbf{p}_0 - \mathbf{p}_{ref}) - \frac{\mathbf{r}\cdot(\mathbf{p}_0 - \mathbf{p}_{ref})}{\|\mathbf{r}\|}\right| \qquad (3)$$

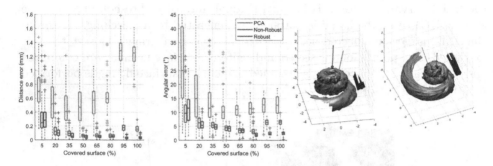

Fig. 3. (Left) Distance and angular errors after modiolar axis detection in synthetic data for varying levels of cochlea surface coverage (percentage of extracted points vs. total number of points). The coverage of the implemented algorithm is ~80%. (Right) Two examples of robust fitting in partial cochlea surfaces with facial nerve. The confidence z_i of each oriented point is color-encoded from red (close to 0, outliers) to green (close to 1, high confidence). (Color figure online)

2.5   Experimental Validation

We validated the algorithm with a data set of 23 human temporal bone specimens consisting of clinical CT (voxel size: $156 \times 156 \times 200$ µm^3) and co-registered µCT (voxel size: 60^3 µm^3) scans. Four experts manually identified 2 landmarks (see Fig. 2) for each sample in multi-planar CT reconstructions to specify the modiolar axis. The same landmarks were also used to initialize the robust detection algorithm. Again, we applied the simple PCA-based and the non-robust axis estimations for comparison. As reference, the modiolar axis and its center were determined in each specimen using high-resolution surface models from the segmented µCT data. The alignment differences were assessed with the equations shown in (3). Differences in alignment errors were estimated using (separate) linear mixed-effects models (R environment with lme4 package) [10], with a fixed effect for the detection method (categorical variable). We included random intercepts for specimens and experts to account for paired measurements. Before analysis, the data was log transformed.

3   Results

Figure 3 illustrates the verification results. With increasing surface data available, the robust algorithm converges to an angular error of 2.5° and an distance error below 0.1 mm. In contrast, the vertex-based PCA detection shows limited improvement and even yields worse distance errors with increasing cochlea surface coverage, since the basal turn vertices cause a shifting away from the modiolar axis. As expected, the non-robust (Gaussian) version of the algorithm is more sensitive to outliers (facial nerve structure).

Figure 4 summarizes the alignment error after manual landmark-based and automated modiolar axis detection in the CT data of the 23 specimens. The PCA based detection performs worse than manual selection. As measured by the linear mixed effects models, compared with the manual procedure, the robust method reduced the average distance error from 0.32 mm to 0.13 mm (improvement by 0.19 mm, 95% confidence interval [0.17 mm, 0.21 mm]) and the angular error from 9.0° to 2.4° (improvement by 6.6°, 95% confidence interval, [6.1°, 6.9°]). The non-robust version performed worse than the robust version (average distance error 0.04 mm higher and angular error 1.5° higher). The robust procedure further reduced the variability between the observers. Figure 5 visualizes an example.

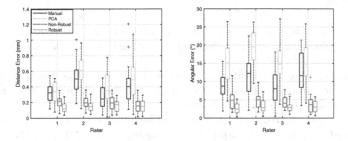

Fig. 4. Alignment errors using manual landmark-based, PCA-based, non-robust and robust kinematic modiolar axis detection in 23 specimens.

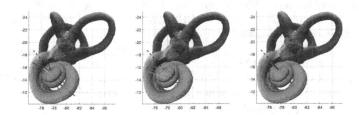

Fig. 5. Bony labyrinth visualization (μCT, specimen 11) with reference modiolar axis (dashed line). Modiolar axes after manual landmark-based (left), PCA-based (middle), and robust kinematic detection (right) in CT data are shown for comparison.

4   Conclusions

We present a novel and anatomically meaningful approach to model the spiral shape of the cochlea as a structure formed by a kinematic motion (natural growth) and extract the modiolar axis as the rotation component. This formalism enables us to detect the modiolar axis even in subsets of cochlea surfaces obtained from CT images. The approach generalizes the implicit surface representation of oriented points. The parameters $\mathbf{m} = \{\mathbf{r}, \mathbf{c}, \gamma\}$ provide a compact representation of the cochlea based on intrinsic shape properties and enable novel approaches to cochlear morphology classification. Using appropriate curves, it could be used to generate surfaces for cochlea segmentation. The approach is further applicable for kinematic surface detection of cylindrical, conical, rotational and helical motions [5]. It could be extended by improved surface extraction methods or by directly using image gradients from CT for kinematic parameter space computation. The script runs in ~3 s on a standard laptop (Intel i7).

Acknowledgments. Supported by the Swiss National Science Foundation (no. P400P2_180822) and the French government (UCA^{JEDI} - ANR-15-IDEX-01).

References

1. Verbist, B.M., et al.: Consensus panel on a cochlear coordinate system applicable in histologic, physiologic, and radiologic studies of the human cochlea. Otol. Neurotol. **31**(5), 722–730 (2010)
2. Wimmer, W., et al.: Semiautomatic cochleostomy target and insertion trajectory planning for minimally invasive cochlear implantation. Biomed. Res. Int. (2014). https://doi.org/10.1155/2014/596498
3. Demarcy, T., et al.: Automated analysis of human cochlea shape variability from seg-mented µCT images. Comput. Med. Imaging Graph. **59**, 1–12 (2017)
4. Yoo, S.K., Wang, G., Rubinstein, J.T., Vannier, M.W.: Three-dimensional geometric modeling of the cochlea using helico-spiral approximation. IEEE Trans. Biomed. Eng. **47**(10), 1392–1402 (2000)
5. Hofer, M., Odehnal, B., Pottmann, H., Steiner, T., Wallner, J.: 3D shape recognition and reconstruction based on line element geometry. In: 10th International Conference on Computer Vision, pp. 1532–1538. IEEE, Beijing (2005)
6. Andrews, J., Séquin, C.H.: Generalized, basis-independent kinematic surface fitting. Comput.-Aided Des. **45**(3), 615–620 (2013)
7. Chernov, N.: On the convergence of fitting algorithms in computer vision. J. Math. Imaging Vis. **27**, 231–239 (2007)
8. Scheffler, C.: A derivation of the EM updates for finding the maximum likelihood parameter estimates of the Student-t distribution. http://www.inference.org.uk/cs482/publications/scheffler2008derivation.pdf
9. Pietsch, M., et al.: Spiral form of the human cochlea results from spatial constraints. Sci. Rep. **7**, 7500 (2017)
10. Bates, D., Mächler, M., Bolker, B., Walker, S.: Fitting linear mixed-effects models using lme4. J. Stat. Softw. **67**(1), 1–48 (2015)

Learning to Avoid Poor Images: Towards Task-aware C-arm Cone-beam CT Trajectories

Jan-Nico Zaech[1,2,3](✉), Cong Gao[1], Bastian Bier[1,2], Russell Taylor[1],
Andreas Maier[2], Nassir Navab[1], and Mathias Unberath[1]

[1] Laboratory for Computational Sensing and Robotics,
Johns Hopkins University, Baltimore, USA
unberath@jhu.edu
[2] Pattern Recognition Lab, Friedrich-Alexander-Universität Erlangen-Nürnberg,
Erlangen, Germany
[3] Computer Vision Laboratory, Eidgenössische Technische Hochschule Zürich,
Zürich, Switzerland
jan-nico.zaech@vision.ee.ethz.ch

Abstract. Metal artifacts in computed tomography (CT) arise from a mismatch between physics of image formation and idealized assumptions during tomographic reconstruction. These artifacts are particularly strong around metal implants, inhibiting widespread adoption of 3D cone-beam CT (CBCT) despite clear opportunity for intra-operative verification of implant positioning, e.g. in spinal fusion surgery. On synthetic and real data, we demonstrate that much of the artifact can be avoided by acquiring better data for reconstruction in a task-aware and patient-specific manner, and describe the first step towards the envisioned task-aware CBCT protocol. The traditional short-scan CBCT trajectory is planar, with little room for scene-specific adjustment. We extend this trajectory by autonomously adjusting out-of-plane angulation. This enables C-arm source trajectories that are scene-specific in that they avoid acquiring "poor images", characterized by beam hardening, photon starvation, and noise. The recommendation of ideal out-of-plane angulation is performed on-the-fly using a deep convolutional neural network that regresses a detectability-rank derived from imaging physics.

Keywords: Robotic imaging · Deep reinforcement learning

1 Introduction

Background: Spinal fusion surgery is an operative therapy for chronic back pain with high economic burden [12] that is projected to further increase due to our

Electronic supplementary material The online version of this chapter (https://doi.org/10.1007/978-3-030-32254-0_2) contains supplementary material, which is available to authorized users.

D. Shen et al. (Eds.): MICCAI 2019, LNCS 11768, pp. 11–19, 2019.
https://doi.org/10.1007/978-3-030-32254-0_2

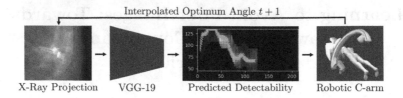

Fig. 1. High-level overview of our task-aware trajectory recommendation.

aging society and our increasingly inactive lifestyle. Despite substantial improvements in operative technique, spinal fusion surgery remains high-risk: In addition to usual complications, pedicle screws that breach cortex can result in nerve damage [5]. Surprisingly, the number of misplaced pedicle screws remains high [2,5]: Cortical breach occurs in up to 31% and 72% of the cases for freehand and fluoroscopy-guided techniques, respectively. Even when surgical navigation is employed, up to 19% of the screws are not fully contained in cortex [5]. Currently, screw placement is assessed on post-operative CT images, such that immediate repositioning of implants is not possible. Although intra-operative 3D cone-beam CT (CBCT) imaging using mobile and robotic C-arm X-ray systems is becoming widely available, it is not currently being used for spinal fusion 3D imaging, because compared to CT, C-arm CBCT images suffer from substantially stronger metal artifacts around the highly-attenuating titanium implants, which compromise the value of intra-operative CBCT for assessing cortical breach [2].

The obvious implication is that image quality must be improved, before CBCT is ready for prime-time in high-volume applications, such as spinal fusion. Most current methods that seek to lift CBCT reconstruction quality to the "clinical acceptance threshold" limit themselves to contain artifact propagation (e. g. via masking) or image-enhancement (e. g. streak reduction) [6]. These methods have in common that they try to deal with artifacts after acquisition of the CBCT short-scan is already completed, and are thus limited by the already corrupted information present in the acquired X-ray projection images.

This somewhat straight-forward realization implies that there lies huge, unexploited potential in "simply acquiring better data" to push the limits of CBCT image quality. In a more formal way, metal artifacts arise from a mismatch between the forward and inverse model, i. e. physical effects governing image formation and idealized assumptions made in the tomographic reconstruction algorithm. Sampling data that is less affected by un-explained corruption processes during reconstruction will yield a better conditioned inverse problem, and as an immediate consequence, improved image quality without any additional post-processing. The first step towards the envisioned task- and anatomy-aware CBCT imaging protocol can be realized easily. The traditional short-scan CBCT trajectory [3] is embedded in a single plane, and therefore, provides little room for scene-specific adjustment. We propose to extend this trajectory by autonomously adjusting out-of-plane angulation, which enables C-arm source trajectories that are task-aware and scene-specific in that they avoid acquiring images with substantial corruption (beam hardening and noise) as shown in

Fig. 1. The recommendation and adjustment of ideal out-of-plane angulation is performed on-the-fly using a deep convolutional neural network (ConvNet) that only relies on the current 2D X-ray projection image.

Related Work: Overall, there is little work on acquisition parameter-side image quality enhancement. Previous work on task-based trajectories [9] leveraged preoperative CT scans and optimization techniques to select optimal parameters. During application, these approaches would require registration between preoperative CT volume and intra-operative C-arm system, which cannot be achieved easily in practice. Besides this requirement, an even more important limitation is the fact that surgery will alter the patient's anatomy represented by preoperative CT in an unpredictable way. Therefore, computing task-optimality based on preoperative CT volumes can only serve as a coarse approximation of the true optimal trajectory. These assumptions become even stronger as surgical tools may still be present in the scene [9], as tools will strongly affect the optimal solution due to their high attenuation.

The prospect of altering acquisition parameters to improve image quality has recently also been recognized for magnetic resonance imaging [1], where the undersampling pattern in k-space can be optimized via end-to-end learning with respect to fully sampled image. The approach closest to ours considers finding an optimal acoustic window for cardiac ultrasound [7], where the current image is interpreted by a reinforcement learning agent that suggests an ultrasound probe displacement towards a better acoustic window. While both previous approaches have some similarity from a conceptual standpoint, they focus on image appearance rather than imaging physics and both the magnetic resonance and ultrasound acquisition protocols are substantially different from CBCT.

2 Methods

Assigning Task-optimality Rank to Projection Images: Task-based trajectory optimization relies on finding projection images that result in optimum reconstruction quality for a specific task. Therefore, the pipeline is contingent on (1) assigning a task-optimality rank to images in projection domain and (2) selecting views that are optimal in this metric. Previous work used the non-prewhitening matched filter observer derived for penalized likelihood reconstruction [9] to calculate a detectability index that correlates well with human performance in detection tasks. Calculating detectability requires the patient volume and knowledge about the task, i.e. an accurately annotated preoperative CT volume. Using the observer model, the detectability d^2 can be calculated as

$$d^2(\varphi, \theta) = \frac{\left[\int \int \int |MTF(\varphi, \theta)|^2 \, |W_{\text{task}}|^2 df_x df_y df_z \right]^2}{\int \int \int NPS(\varphi, \theta) \, |MTF(\varphi, \theta)|^2 \, |W_{\text{task}}|^2 df_x df_y df_z}, \tag{1}$$

where W_{task} is the Fourier transform of the region of interest to be imaged with highest quality. Further, MTF is the modulation transfer function and NPS is

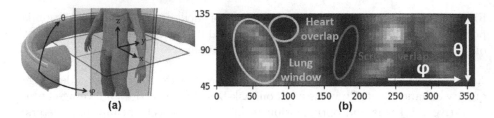

Fig. 2. (a) Diminished coordinate system for CBCT: φ describes in-plane gantry rotation (traditional short-scan) while θ is the out-of-plane angle to be adjusted in a task-aware and autonomous fashion. (b) Detectability map for test CT volume as per Eq. 1 (brighter values indicate better detectability). We also show some areas with extremal detectability that can be interpreted semantically.

the noise power spectrum (we refer to [4] for details) that both depend on the projection image, and therefore, the relative pose of the C-arm with respect to anatomy. Here we consider a diminished C-arm coordinate system (φ, θ) shown in Fig. 2(a), where φ and θ describe the in- and out-of-plane angle, respectively. It is worth mentioning that in order to compute the above detectability measure for a particular view (φ, θ), the corresponding X-ray projection image must either be simulated from the CT volume or available otherwise.

Predicting Task-Optimal Views from Live Data: If the 3D patient anatomy is perfectly known, the complete trajectory can be optimized for directly. However, this is not the case in surgical environments, where optimal view prediction may only depend on the current and previous 2D X-ray projections. Following recent work in robotics and control, we interpret the detectability index of each possible next view as the quality function and use a ConvNet to directly regress it from the current view. Then, acquiring an optimized trajectory is achieved by selecting the out-of-plane angle with the highest predicted detectability, adjusting θ as the C-arm gantry moves to the next in-plane angle φ, and acquiring the next X-ray image at this position, that is then fed back into the ConvNet. Next possible views are defined as views with an increment of 5° in sweep direction ϕ. The ConvNet predicts detectability for out-of-plane angles between ±25°, uniformly discretized in 11 steps of 5°. This definition allows generating a training dataset, where all meaningful X-ray projections together with their detectability are sampled on a uniform grid with stepsize of 5° in both φ and θ. The resulting trajectory is patient specific, as the input images used to predict the detectabilities reflect the patient's anatomy at the current point in time.

Our ConvNet is based on VGG-19 [8] with modifications to perform regression instead of classification. Initial weights are pre-trained on ImageNet and the ConvNet is subsequently retrained on our task. Due to the very short inference time of in the range of few 10^{-2} s on current GPUs, the VGG-19 network is compatible with the near real-time requirements of CBCT acquisition protocols. During application, angle increments between two views are usually below 1°, and we use linear interpolation to predict the next best angle. The complete pipeline is shown in Fig. 1, where the image from the CBCT system is fed into the ConvNet to predict the detectability of possible next views. Based on this prediction, the interpolation module provides the next out-of-plane angle to the CBCT system, that is servoed to the new position, acquires a new X-ray image, and thus, closes the loop.

Training: Training is performed on realistic digitally reconstructed radiographs (DRRs) generated from CT using the open-source tool DeepDRR [11]. The pipeline was chosen as it enables the simulation of metal artifact as well as the transfer to real data with only low degradation of prediction performance [10]. For DRR generation, five chest CT-volumes were obtained from the Cancer Imaging Archive. In every volume, six pairs of pedicle screws were annotated and simulated leading to a total of 30 different anatomical configurations, since only a single vertebral level is considered at once. Data augmentation is performed in 3D by randomly varying the C-arm isocenter, yielding a dataset of 212 "scans" with 290,016 images in total. A "scan" consists of 1368 images uniformly sampled on the truncated sphere with $\varphi \in [0°, 360°)$ and $\theta \in [45°, 135°]$, with the detectability calculated as per Eq. 1 for each image. To guarantee patient independence of training and test, splitting of data is performed on CT level, where four volumes (176 scans) are used for training and one volume (36 scans) is used for test and validation.

The images are saved both noise-free and with noise corresponding to a fluence of 20k photons emitted towards every pixel. The noise free images are used to calculate ground-truth detectability while the noisy images are used as input during training of the neural network. This approach was chosen, such that the detectability maps are the optimum learning target, while the network becomes invariant to noisy observations as they would occur in real X-ray projections.

For experiments on real data, a set of analytic phantoms (squares, cylinders, screw model) that represent the chest was implemented and a second *in silico* dataset was generated. For data generation, dimensions and location of the phantom components where randomly varied within reasonable bounds to reflect the fact that the anatomy, present during inference, is not known at training time. The dataset consists of 75 "scans", generated with the same setup as described for the synthetic data experiments, except for the photon-fluence of 500 photons per pixel, adapted to the smaller size of the phantom.

3   Experiments, Results, and Discussion

Quantitative Synthetic Data Experiments: Our trajectory optimization pipeline was tested on six different vertebral levels in the separate test volume. As direct evaluation of the training loss function would not represent the quality of the selected trajectory, two surrogate measures were defined. The angular distance of the predicted next-best action to the best action selected from the groundtruth data measures the spatial difference between the predicted and optimal trajectory. While the angular error is an intuitive and interpretable measure, it does

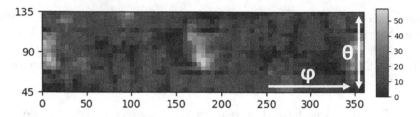

Fig. 3. Distribution of degrading detectability in % for the synthetic test set.

not fully capture the performance of the algorithm. Even if the angular distance of the selected action is high, it can still result in a close to optimal reconstruction performance, as the function of detectability values can be multimodal. Therefore, the difference in detectability between the predicted next action and the optimal next action is introduced as a better measure for reconstruction performance. On the test set, containing 36 scans across 6 different anatomical sites, these performance metrics evaluated to $8.35° \pm 11.61°$ for the angular distance error and $13.69\% \pm 18.92\%$ degradation in detectability. The spatial distribution of the average degradation of detectability in the test set is illustrated in Fig. 3.

Besides the quality of selected actions, pipeline stability w.r.t. noise is crucial for practical applications. We compare the average distance between trajectories predicted from noise-free data to noisy samples generated with 400k, 100k, and 50k photons per pixel. These measures are $0.83° \pm 1.56°$, $1.13° \pm 1.63°$, and $1.64° \pm 1.73°$ for the different noise levels, respectively.

When the C-arm is used for intra-operative imaging, no optimal alignment between the scanner and the patient's anatomy can be ensured. Therefore, robustness for different initialization angles is a major requirement, i. e. the algorithm should transition into the same or equivalent trajectory irrespective of its initialization. Theoretically this can be approached via the Markov property of the proposed prediction pipeline: The detectabilities used for optimizing the trajectory only depend on the last acquired X-ray projection, not on the history of the trajectory. Therefore, as soon as two trajectories would intersect each other, they will merge into a single trajectory.

Qualitative Synthetic Data Experiments: From a clinical perspective the quality of the reconstructions is most interesting. For the synthetic test data, representative reconstructions from a short-scan and a task-aware trajectory are shown in Fig. 4(a) and (b), respectively. Both volumes were reconstructed using iterative conjugated gradients least-squares (ASTRA Toolbox) from noise free projections. It is apparent that, for the proposed task-aware trajectory, the screw is more homogeneous, exhibits less cupping artifact, and metal artifacts (bright and dark streaks) are reduced enabling better assessment of bony anatomy in close proximity to the implant.

Real Data Experiments: Real data experiments are performed on a physical phantom consisting of two ballistic gel cylinders mounted on a wooden beam

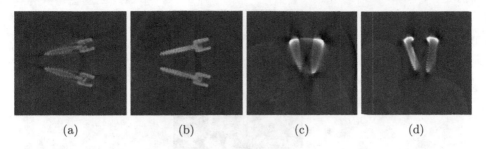

(a)   (b)   (c)   (d)

Fig. 4. Representative axial slices through reconstructed volumes for the synthetic test set at vertebral level T6 in (a,b), and for the real data set in (c,d). Slices (a,c) show images using a straight-forward short-scan, while slices (b,d) show results of a recommended task-aware trajectory.

with two iron screws, abstractly mimicking the human chest. A C-arm system (Siemens Arcadis Orbic 3D) was used to acquire five CBCT short-scans, performed with inclinations ranging from large negative ($\sim -30°$) to large positive values ($\sim 30°$). Corresponding reconstructions obtained with filtered backprojection [3] were also obtained from the system.

The detectabilities of next possible views are predicted with the ConvNet trained on our analytic phantom dataset. The resulting predictions are shown in Fig. 5. As the available C-arm geometry currently limits the reconstruction to circular trajectories, we compare the quality of the best circular scan with the conventional circular scan. The best circular scan is determined by accumulating the predicted detectability for $\Delta\Theta = 0$, which closely models the overall task. Via this approach, the scan with the highest positive tilt is selected, yielding a 19.0% increase in predicted detectability compared to the conventional scan.

In Fig. 5, we highlight the highest predicted detectability at any given time, which corresponds to the unregularized servoing commands that would be sent to the C-arm. Curves close to the centerline indicate little C-arm adjustments, while curves far from it imply our agent trying to drive the C-arm out of the central plane. We observe large out-of-plane angle commands for scans with low absolute tilt (conventional), and minimal deviation for scans with high tilt, indicating a close to optimal trajectory. This behavior is well interpretable and fits our intuition: The algorithm tries to prevent images with screw overlap, thus reducing metal artifact in the reconstruction. Slices in the screw-plane, reconstructed from the conventional and recommended trajectory are shown in Fig. 4(c) and (d), respectively. The reconstruction from the high-tilt trajectory recommended by our system exhibits a notable reduction of metal artifacts and noise, and reveals the screw thread that is completely invisible in the conventional case. We anticipate overall image quality improvements when using C-arm systems with flat-panel detectors and more brilliant X-ray sources.

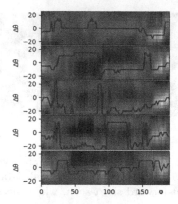

Fig. 5. Detectability maps predicted from real X-ray projection images of a simple human chest model. From top to bottom, inclination of the scan is decreasing; the midline of each map corresponds to the scan axis. The red curve indicates the optimal trajectories predicted from the map. Figure best viewed zoomed in. (Color figure online)

4 Conclusion

We present the first step towards task-aware CBCT imaging protocols. Our approach enables scene-specific source trajectories in clinical settings, where only little prior information is available. On both synthetic and real CBCT scans, in simulations with human anatomy as well as on real X-ray images of a phantom, we demonstrate that task-aware image acquisition is a promising avenue for prospectively improving image quality in CBCT reconstruction. The proposed learning-based method recommends viewing angles onto anatomy and can be combined with any (iterative) reconstruction or metal artifact reduction algorithm. In future work, we will test our system on cadaveric specimens, pedicle screws on multiple levels, and more complex tasks including soft tissue imaging.

Acknowledgement. We gratefully acknowledge support of the NVIDIA Corporation for donating GPUs, and Gerhard Kleinzig and Sebastian Vogt from SIEMENS for making an ARCADIS Orbic 3D available. JNZ was supported by a DAAD FITweltweit fellowship.

References

1. Bahadir, C.D., Dalca, A.V., Sabuncu, M.R.: Learning-based optimization of the under-sampling pattern in MRI. arXiv preprint arXiv:1901.01960 (2019)
2. Cordemans, V., Kaminski, L., Banse, X., Francq, B.G., Cartiaux, O.: Accuracy of a new intraoperative cone beam CT imaging technique compared to postoperative CT scan for assessment of pedicle screws placement and breaches detection. Eur. Spine. J. **26**(11), 2906–2916 (2017)
3. Feldkamp, L.A., Davis, L., Kress, J.W.: Practical cone-beam algorithm. Josa a **1**(6), 612–619 (1984)

4. Gang, G.J., Stayman, J.W., Zbijewski, W., Siewerdsen, J.H.: Task-baseddetectability in CT image reconstruction by filtered backprojection andpenalized likelihood estimation. Med. Phys. **41**(8), 081902 (2014)
5. Gelalis, I.D., et al.: Accuracy of pedicle screw placement: a systematic review of prospective in vivo studies comparing free hand, fluoroscopy guidance and navigation techniques. Eur. Spine J. **21**(2), 247–255 (2012)
6. Gjesteby, L., et al.: Metal artifact reduction in ct: where are we after four decades? IEEE Access **4**, 5826–5849 (2016)
7. Milletari, F., Birodkar, V., Sofka, M.: Straight to the point: reinforcement learning for user guidance in ultrasound. arXiv preprint arXiv:1903.00586 (2019)
8. Simonyan, K., Zisserman, A.: Very deep convolutional networks for large-scale image recognition. arXiv:1409.1556 [cs] (2014)
9. Stayman, J.W., Siewerdsen, J.H.: Task-based trajectories in iteratively reconstructed interventional cone-beam CT. In: Proceedings 12th International Meeting Fully 3D Image Reconstruction Radiology Nuclear Medcine, pp. 257–260 (2013)
10. Unberath, M., et al.: Enabling machine learning inx-ray-based procedures via realistic simulation of image formation. Int. J. Comput. Assist. Radiol. Surg. (2019). https://doi.org/10.1007/s11548-019-02011-2, https://doi.org/10.1007/s11548-019-02011-2
11. Unberath, M., et al.: DeepDRR – a catalyst for machine learning in fluoroscopy-guided procedures. In: Frangi, A.F., Schnabel, J.A., Davatzikos, C., Alberola-López, C., Fichtinger, G. (eds.) MICCAI 2018. LNCS, vol. 11073, pp. 98–106. Springer, Cham (2018). https://doi.org/10.1007/978-3-030-00937-3_12
12. United States Bone and Joint Initiative: The Burden of Musculoskeletal Diseases in the United States (BMUS). Third Edition edn. (2014)

Optimizing Clearance of Bézier Spline Trajectories for Minimally-Invasive Surgery

Johannes Fauser[1]([⊠]), Igor Stenin[2], Julia Kristin[2], Thomas Klenzner[2], Jörg Schipper[2], and Anirban Mukhopadhyay[1]

[1] Department of Computer Science, Technische Universität Darmstadt, 64283 Darmstadt, Germany
johannes.fauser@gris.tu-darmstadt.de
[2] Department of Oto-Rhino-Laryngology, Düsseldorf University Hospital, Düsseldorf, Germany

Abstract. Preoperative planning of nonlinear trajectories is a key element in minimally-invasive surgery. Interpolating between start and goal of an intervention while circumnavigating risk structures provides the necessary feasible solutions for such procedure. While recent research shows that Rapidly-exploring Random Trees (RRT) on Bézier Splines efficiently solve this task, access paths computed by this method do not provide optimal clearance to surrounding anatomy. We propose an approach based on sequential convex optimization that rearranges Bézier Splines computed by an RRT-connect, thereby achieving locally optimal clearance to risk structures. Experiments on real CT data of patients demonstrate the applicability of our approach on two scenarios: catheter insertion through the aorta and temporal bone surgery. We compare distances to risk structures along computed trajectories with the state of the art solution and show that our method results in clinically safer paths.

Keywords: Nonlinear trajectories · Convex optimization · RRT-connect

1 Introduction

Minimally-invasive procedures along nonlinear trajectories are an active research field targeting different applications. These new approaches, like needle insertion into soft tissue [1], drilling access canals through bone [2], ribbon design for intracavitary brachytherapy [3] or steerable guidewires [4], share a common need: accurate trajectory planning that (1) interpolates position and direction at both start and goal of the instrument's path, (2) maximizes clearance to obstacles and (3) respects the upper bound curvature of the deployed flexible tool. The first constraint allows for optimal instrument alignment for clinical requirements such as improvement of visibility [5] or optimization of implant insertion [6].

© Springer Nature Switzerland AG 2019
D. Shen et al. (Eds.): MICCAI 2019, LNCS 11768, pp. 20–28, 2019.
https://doi.org/10.1007/978-3-030-32254-0_3

The second constraint reflects the request for maximum patient safety while the third one imposes hard constraints based on the application's hardware.

Optimal solutions for linear access paths exist in many applications, e.g. at the temporal bone for linear access canals to the cochlea. Dahroug et al. [7] provided detailed comparison between existing systems for these approaches. For nonlinear trajectories on Bézier Splines and circular arcs, Fauser et al. [2] employed RRT-connects. However, due to the stochastic nature of RRTs, the computed paths exhibited characteristic random twists and did not guarantee optimal distances to risk structures. To the best of our knowledge, only few works were presented on trajectory planning for catheter insertion [8]. Azizi et al. [9] computed successive points on vessels' centerlines to find trajectories for catheters through vascular structures ignoring constraints on the curvature. Optimal trajectories are available for clinical applications in soft tissue using flexible needles [10], though. Duan et al. [11] adapted sequential convex optimization (SCO) [12] for such tools to the Special Euclidean Group $SE(3) = \mathbb{R}^3 \times SO(3)$ and its Lie-Algebra $\mathfrak{se}(3)$ to compute locally optimal solutions. However, this approach did not consider the direction at both start and goal points.

We propose a trajectory planning method featuring clearance-optimized Bézier Splines that satisfy all three constraints: An RRT-connect [2] solves for a valid initial trajectory. The result is a series of waypoints in 3D that implicitly defines a trajectory parameterized by cubic Bézier Splines. We extend SCO [12] to such trajectories. This optimization adjusts the underlying splines such that clearance to obstacles is maximized while simultaneously satisfying constraints on curvature as well as position and direction at start and goal. We evaluate our method on catheter steering through blood vessels and temporal bone surgery as two significantly diverse clinical example scenarios. Our experiments show the general applicability of our solution on the publicly available SegTHOR data set [13] and on an in-house data set of 22 CT images of the temporal bone.

2   Methods

Objective: Planning trajectories in image-guided interventions usually requires acquisition of an image, e.g. CT, of the anatomical region. Segmentation of risk structures within this data leads to a 3D representation of the anatomy (Fig. 1). Such a 3D visualization allows intuitive placement of start and goal states for the instrument by the surgeon. Motion planning algorithms use these configurations to compute feasible nonlinear trajectories through the remaining empty space. These paths interpolate between the two given states, evade obstacles and respect the maximum bend of the instrument. After all preoperative steps, a clinician navigates the respective tool along the desired trajectory.

To start the planning procedure, we require single start and goal states $q_S, q_G \in \mathbb{R}^3 \times \mathbb{S}^2$ with positions in $\mathbb{R}^3$ and directions, the instrument should point toward, in $\mathbb{S}^2$. For patient safety, an application dependent safety distance $d_{min} \in \mathbb{R}^{0+}$ is required. The trajectories also have to respect an upper bound $\kappa_{max} \in \mathbb{R}^{0+}$ on the curvature to resemble the maximum bend of the respective flexible tool. We use an RRT-connect [2] with Bézier Splines as steering function to find an initial solution that interpolates between q_S and q_G while staying away from obstacles. To extract a locally optimal solution we use the computed waypoints as optimization variables in a SCO-formulation. The convex optimization solver then rearranges these waypoints such that the implicitly defined Bézier Splines feature larger clearance to obstacles.

■ Jugular vein ■ Carotid artery ■ Facial nerve ■ Chorda tympani ■ External auditory canal ■ Internal auditory canal ■ Cochlea ■ Semicircular canals ■ Ossicles

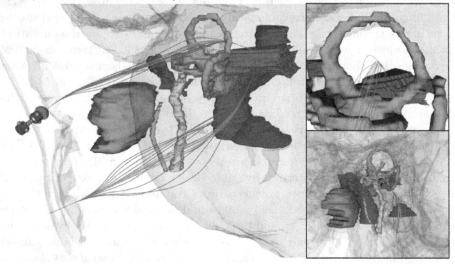

Fig. 1. A 3D surface representation of the temporal bone. Trajectories for a micro robot to the internal auditory canal via the superior semicircular canal (top) and retrolabyrinthine region (bottom). Paths locally optimized with SCO (green) achieve larger clearance to risk structures than those initially planned with RRTs (red). (Color figure online)

Bézier Spline RRT-connect: The Bézier Spline RRT-connect [2] provides fast and accurate initial solutions for curvature constrained trajectories around obstacles. A computed path consists of a series of waypoints $\mathcal{W} \equiv \{W_i\}_i \subset \mathbb{R}^3, 0 \le i \le N_{\mathcal{W}}$ (Fig. 2). Each triple $(W_{j-1}, W_j, W_{j+1}), 1 \le j \le N_{\mathcal{S}} \equiv N_{\mathcal{W}} - 1$, implicitly defines a Bézier Spline S_j, a combination of two cubic Bézier Spirals, that respects the curvature constraint κ_{max}. We refer the reader to [14] for a detailed description of the construction algorithm and proofs of smoothness and interpolation guarantees.

Clearance Optimization: We define a constrained optimization objective over the set of waypoints $\mathcal{W} \subset \mathbb{R}^3$ that minimizes a cost function f while satisfying a set of N_E equality and N_I inequality constraints h_i, g_j, i.e.

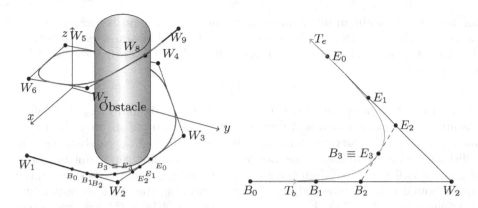

Fig. 2. *Left:* The RRT-connect is used to compute a series of waypoints $\mathcal{W} = \{W_1, \ldots, W_9\}$. Each triple of three subsequent waypoints defines a Bézier Spline (combination of one blue and one red path). *Right:* A Bézier Spline is a combination of two cubic Bézier Spirals, i.e., Bézier Curves with three colinear sample points (e.g. $B_0, \ldots, B_3$). Each spline then interpolates between the middle of subsequent waypoints, e.g. $B_0 = 1/2 \cdot (W_1 + W_2)$ and $E_0 = 1/2 \cdot (W_2 + W_3)$ on the left. (Color figure online)

$$\underset{\mathcal{W}}{\text{minimize}} \quad f(\mathcal{W})$$
$$\text{subject to} \quad h_i(\mathcal{W}) = 0, \quad i = 0, \ldots, N_E$$
$$g_j(\mathcal{W}) \leq 0, \quad j = 0, \ldots, N_I.$$

Efficient numerical solvers require each of these functions to be linear or quadratic convex functions [15]. In our case, these functions are, however, nonconvex and we thus consider an approximation rather than the original problem. By formulating adequate convex quadratic versions, convexifications, of the respective cost and constraint functions f, h_i and g_j, we derive an approximation of our original problem that is suitable for numerical solvers.

In particular, our cost function measures the quality of trajectories by a weighted sum of its length f_Γ and distance to obstacles $f_{i,O}, 0 \leq i \leq N_S$, i.e.

$$f = \alpha_\Gamma f_\Gamma + \sum_i \alpha_O f_{i,O},$$

with $\alpha_\Gamma, \alpha_O \in \mathbb{R}^{0+}$. We approximate the length as

$$f_\Gamma = \sum_{i=0}^{N_\mathcal{W}-1} \sum_{k=\{x,y,z\}} |W_{i,k} - W_{i+1,k}|^2.$$

Similar to [12], we measure distance to obstacles via linearized signed distances

$$\text{sd}_{SO}(\mathbf{x}) = \text{sd}_{SO}(\mathbf{x_0}) + \mathbf{n}(\mathbf{x_0})^\top (\mathbf{x} - \mathbf{x_0}),$$

where $\text{sd}_{SO}(\mathbf{x_0})$ is the signed distance from a spline S to the nearest obstacle O, $\mathbf{x_0} \in O$ is a point on the surface and $\mathbf{n}$ the obstacle's normal at $\mathbf{x_0}$. The point

x_0 stays fixed within an inner convex iteration sequence and is computed by a nearest neighbor search for x. The weighted convexified clearance cost functions $f_{i,O}$ then try to match a distance threshold $\theta \in \mathbb{R}^+$ on the central waypoint W_i of a spline S_i, i.e.

$$f_{i,O} = \theta - \text{sd}_{S_i O}(W_i).$$

We add constraints to guarantee the upper curvature bound κ_{max}, the safety distance d_{min} and position and direction at q_S, q_G. To ensure that the upper bound κ_{max} on the curvature and the minimal distance d_{min} to obstacles stay valid during the optimization we introduce for each spline constraint functions $g_{i,\kappa}$ and $g_{i,O}, 0 \leq i \leq N_S$. Each curvature constraint $g_{i,\kappa}$ smooths its spline, if the upper bound κ_{max} is exceeded, by slightly translating the three corresponding waypoints. With $P_i = 1/2(W_{i-1} + W_{i+1})$ and $Q_i = 1/2(W_i + P_i)$, new waypoints $\overline{W}_{i-1}, \overline{W}_i, \overline{W}_{i+1}$ are given as

$$\overline{W}_{i-1} = Q_i + (W_{i-1} - P_i),$$
$$\overline{W}_i = \frac{1}{2}(W_i + Q_i),$$
$$\overline{W}_{i+1} = Q_i + (W_{i+1} - P_i).$$

A constraint $g_{i,\kappa}$ then penalizes the difference between the original positions and these translations, i.e.

$$g_{i,\kappa} = \sum_{j=-1}^{1} \sum_{k=\{x,y,z\}} |W_{i+j,k} - \overline{W}_{i+j,k}|^2.$$

The $g_{i,O}$ are defined like the distance cost functions via signed distances. Note, that we have to set $\theta >> d_{min}$ to achieve significant improvement on clearance. Finally, we enforce that position and direction at start and goal stay the same by disallowing any changes in position of the first and last two waypoints.

We then use SCO [12] to solve for a locally optimal solution given the above costs and constraints. This iterative method repeatedly creates convexified functions based on the current solution and makes progress on this approximated objective. We refer the reader to [12] for a detailed description and show in Fig. 3 one iteration of the proposed clearance optimization method as an example.

3   Experimental Results

Data: We evaluated our method on 40 CT scans of the aorta from the publicly available SegTHOR data set [13] and 22 temporal bone CT scans of an in-house data set. C++ code of the methods will be made available at [anonymous] (available after acceptance) for the benefit of the research community.

General Procedure: For each CT image a corresponding label image with segmentations of risk structures was available. We extracted surface meshes using

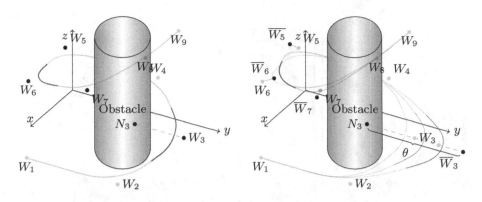

Fig. 3. One sample iteration of SCO. Spline $S_3 \equiv S_3(W_2, W_3, W_4)$ (opaque) is close enough to the obstacle such that the convexified cost function $f_{3,O}$ tries to enforce a distance of threshold θ from the nearest neighbor N_3 by translating W_3 several times. Spline S_6 violates the curvature constraint, resulting in constraint $g_{6,\kappa}$ translating corresponding waypoints W_5, W_6, W_7 to a smoother configuration $\overline{W}_5, \overline{W}_6, \overline{W}_7$.

Table 1. Quantitative comparison for Aorta-, RL- and SSC-Access.

	Aorta-access		RL-access		SSC-access	
	RRT [2]	Ours	RRT [2]	Ours	RRT [2]	Ours
Success rate	-	81.0	-	87.8	-	94.8
Mean distance	7.1	**11.2**	4.9	**5.5**	5.0	**5.2**
Aorta	1.9 ± 0.3	$\mathbf{3.0 \pm 1.6}$	-	-	-	-
Heart	8.4 ± 2.1	$\mathbf{10.3 \pm 1.7}$	-	-	-	-
Brain	-	-	1.8 ± 0.5	$\mathbf{2.0 \pm 0.6}$	2.0 ± 0.8	$\mathbf{2.1 \pm 0.8}$
Facial nerve	-	-	1.8 ± 0.7	1.8 ± 0.9	2.8 ± 0.5	$\mathbf{2.9 \pm 0.5}$
Jugular vein	-	-	3.3 ± 2.1	3.3 ± 2.1	-	-
SSC	-	-	1.5 ± 0.7	$\mathbf{1.6 \pm 0.7}$	1.0 ± 0.2	$\mathbf{1.1 \pm 0.3}$

Marching Cubes and refined those to uniformly dense meshes using approximated centroidal voronoi diagrams [16]. Single start and goal states were placed manually within these 3D environments. We then used the Bézier Spline RRT-connect to compute initial trajectories and used our sequential convex optimization approach to further optimize those.

Catheter Insertion: Initially, we planned trajectories for catheters through the aorta (Fig. 4). The start state q_S was placed at the lowest part of the descending aorta, the goal state q_g at the entrance to the left ventricle. We set the curvature constraint to $\kappa_{max} = 0.1\,\text{mm}^{-1}$ and safety distance to $d_{min} = 20.0\,\text{mm}$. The RRT-connect used a step size of $15\,\text{mm}$, resulting on average in $N_{\mathcal{W}} = 25$ waypoints for the optimization. Figure 4 shows two representative examples with distance threshold $\theta = 30\,\text{mm}$ and cost weights $\alpha_\Gamma = 0.1, \alpha_O = 10$. Running the

Aorta ▪ Heart ▪ Esophagus ▪ Trachea

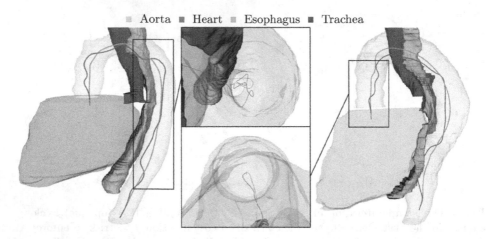

Fig. 4. Two examples of the Aorta-Access with initial (red) and corresponding optimized (green) trajectories. The weighted cost function on length and clearance to risk structures lead to smooth trajectories close to the aorta's centerline. (Color figure online)

optimization sequence took on average 1.1 s. With a success rate of 80.97% we were able to optimize the majority of trajectories, showing that the convexifications are suitable. Along the entire trajectory our clearance-optimized paths achieved a much higher mean and minimum distance to the two obstacles aorta and heart (Table 1, Aorta-Access). Such improved trajectories thus significantly reduce the risk of harming organ boundaries.

Temporal Bone Surgery: We placed a start state q_S at the surface of the lateral skull base and a goal state q_G at the internal auditory canal for two different approaches: An access via the retrolabyrinthine region (RL-Access) and an access via the superior semicircular canal (SSC-Access). Initial parameters were set to $\kappa_{max} = 0.1$ mm^{-1} and $d_{min} = 1.5$ mm and a step size of 6 mm, resulting in $N_\mathcal{W} \approx 8$ waypoints. Figure 1 shows a representative example with distance threshold $\theta = 5$ mm and cost weights $\alpha_\Gamma = 1, \alpha_O = 10$. Table 1 (RL- & SSC-Access) shows a comparison between initial and optimized planning. The high success rate highlights the valid convexification approach. As a consequence of the increase in overall mean distance, minimally-invasive approaches using our method would stay farther away from risk structures until the respective bottle necks (the SSC for SSC-Access; facial nerve, jugular vein and brain for RL-Access). Due to the very narrow passages in temporal bone surgery (Fig. 1, closeup) the differences in minimal distance at the bottlenecks were negligible.

4   Discussion and Conclusion

We introduce a clearance-optimized planning procedure for locally optimal nonlinear trajectories in minimally-invasive surgery. Our solution computes initial trajectories that satisfy the application's constraints using a Bézier Spline RRT-connect. The SCO step rearranges these splines such that clearance to obstacles is maximized. Experiments based on CT images of both aorta and temporal bone anatomy show the general applicability of this approach. Compared to initial trajectories computed from a state of the art solution, we achieve enhanced distance to risk structures and thus safer trajectories.

As convex optimization results in locally instead of globally optimal paths, incorporation of an RRT*-like stochastic optimization scheme is a promising research direction for future work. We also plan to use the clearance optimization in a framework with GUI for interactive segmentation and trajectory planning. With this system we could then analyze and improve the clinical workflow of a highly automated preoperative planning step [17] for temporal bone surgery.

References

1. Patil, S., Burgner, J., Webster, R.J., Alterovitz, R.: Needle steering in 3-d via rapid replanning. IEEE Trans. Rob. **30**(4), 853–864 (2014)
2. Fauser, J., Sakas, G., Mukhopadhyay, A.: Planning nonlinear access paths for temporal bone surgery. Int. J. Comput. Assist. Radiol. Surg. **13**(5), 637–646 (2018)
3. Patil, S., Pan, J., Abbeel, P., Goldberg, K.: Planning curvature and torsion constrained ribbons in 3d with application to intracavitary brachytherapy. IEEE Trans. Autom. Sci. Eng. **12**(4), 1332–1345 (2015)
4. Ganet, F., et al.: Development of a smart guide wire using an electrostrictive polymer: option for steerable orientation and force feedback. Sci. Rep. **5**, 18593 (2015)
5. Fichera, L., et al.: Through the eustachian tube and beyond: a new miniature robotic endoscope to see into the middle ear. IEEE Rob. Autom. Lett. **2**(3), 1488–1494 (2017)
6. Torres, R., Kazmitcheff, G., De Seta, D., Ferrary, E., Sterkers, O., Nguyen, Y.: Improvement of the insertion axis for cochlear implantation with a robot-based system. Eur. Arch. Oto-Rhino-Laryngol. **274**(2), 715–721 (2017)
7. Dahroug, B., Tamadazte, B., Weber, S., Tavernier, L., Andreff, N.: Review on otological robotic systems: Toward microrobot-assisted cholesteatoma surgery. IEEE Rev. Biomed. Eng. **11**, 125–142 (2018)
8. Burgner-Kahrs, J., Rucker, D.C., Choset, H.: Continuum robots for medical applications: a survey. IEEE Trans. Rob. **31**(6), 1261–1280 (2015)
9. Azizi, A., Tremblay, C., Martel, S.: Trajectory planning for vascular navigation from 3d angiography images and vessel centerline data. In: 2017 International Conference on Manipulation, Automation and Robotics at Small Scales (MARSS), pp. 1–6, July 2017
10. Duindam, V., Alterovitz, R., Sastry, S., Goldberg, K.: Skrew-based motion planning for bevel-tip flexible needles in 3D environments with obstacles. In: IEEE Int. Conference on Robotics and Automation, pp. 2483–2488, May 2008
11. Duan, Y., Patil, S., Schulman, J., Goldberg, K., Abbeel, P.: Planning locally optimal, curvature-constrained trajectories in 3D using sequential convex optimization. In: 2014 IEEE International Conference on Robotics and Automation, (ICRA), pp. 5889–5895, May 2014

12. Schulman, J., et al.: Motion planning with sequential convex optimization and convex collision checking. Int. J. Rob. Res. **33**(9), 1251–1270 (2014)
13. Trullo, R., Petitjean, C., Ruan, S., Dubray, B., Nie, D., Shen, D.: Segmentation of organs at risk in thoracic ct images using a sharpmask architecture and conditional random fields. In: 14th IEEE International Symposium on Biomedical Imaging, pp. 1003–1006 (2017)
14. Yang, K., Sukkarieh, S.: 3D smooth path planning for a uav in cluttered natural environments. In: 2008 IEEE/RSJ International Conference on Intelligent Robots and Systems, pp. 794–800, September 2008
15. Boyd, S., Vandenberghe, L.: Convex Optimization. Cambridge University Press, New York (2004)
16. Valette, S., Chassery, J.M.: Approximated centroidal voronoi diagrams for uniform polygonal mesh coarsening. Comput. Graph. Forum. **23**, 381–390 (2004)
17. Fauser, J., et al.: Toward an automatic preoperative pipeline for image-guided temporal bone surgery. Int. J. Computer. Assist. Radiol. Surg. (2019)

Direct Visual and Haptic Volume Rendering of Medical Data Sets for an Immersive Exploration in Virtual Reality

Balázs Faludi[1]([✉]), Esther I. Zoller[2], Nicolas Gerig[2], Azhar Zam[3], Georg Rauter[2], and Philippe C. Cattin[1]

[1] CIAN, Department of Biomedical Engineering,
University of Basel, Basel, Switzerland
`balazs.faludi@unibas.ch`

[2] BIROMED-Lab, Department of Biomedical Engineering,
University of Basel, Basel, Switzerland
`esther.zoller@unibas.ch`

[3] BLOG, Department of Biomedical Engineering,
University of Basel, Basel, Switzerland

Abstract. Visual examination of volumetric medical data sets in virtual reality offers an intuitive and immersive experience. To further increase the realism of virtual environments, haptic feedback can be added. Such systems can help students to gain anatomical knowledge or surgeons to prepare for specific interventions. In this work, we present a method for direct visual and haptic rendering of volumetric medical data sets in virtual reality. This method guarantees a continuous force field and does not rely on any mesh or surface generation. Using a transfer function, we mapped computed tomography voxel intensities to color and opacity values and then visualized the anatomical structures using a direct volume rendering approach. A continuous haptic force field was generated based on a conservative potential field computed from the voxel opacities. In a path following experiment, we showed that the deviation from a reference path on the surface of the rendered anatomical structure decreased with the added haptic feedback. This system demonstrates an immersive exploration of anatomy and is a step towards patient-specific surgical planning and simulation.

Keywords: Haptic rendering · CT · Human-robot interaction · Medical simulation · Surgical planning

---

B. Faludi and E. I. Zoller—These two authors contributed equally to this work.

Electronic supplementary material The online version of this chapter (https://doi.org/10.1007/978-3-030-32254-0_4) contains supplementary material, which is available to authorized users.

© Springer Nature Switzerland AG 2019
D. Shen et al. (Eds.): MICCAI 2019, LNCS 11768, pp. 29–37, 2019.
https://doi.org/10.1007/978-3-030-32254-0_4

1   Introduction

Visualizing medical data in virtual reality (VR) or augmented reality (AR) offers an intuitive and immersive experience. However, without being able to touch the virtual objects, the illusion is not complete. Different combinations of VR and haptic feedback have been demonstrated and successfully applied in the medical field [10]. These systems are used for virtual examination of medical volumetric data sets, such as computed tomography (CT) or magnetic resonance (MR) images, to acquire anatomical knowledge or to prepare for specific surgical interventions.

Patient-specific surgical planning systems often rely on surface models of the relevant patient anatomy. Generating these surface models requires either manual or automatic segmentation of the medical data. While manual segmentation is time-consuming, automatic segmentation cannot always provide satisfactory results [5]. Although recent work has shown promising results in fully automatic segmentation [2], most systems today use a combination of automatic segmentation with manual retopology, review, and cleanup [1]. As an alternative, direct volume rendering [7] can be used to render smooth surfaces without explicitly defining them in advance. Direct volume rendering in VR using a head-mounted display (HMD) has been reported to be beneficial to surgeons preparing for complex interventions [9].

Similarly, haptic rendering is usually implemented using meshes or surfaces to represent the objects [6], which allows the haptic forces to be computed with conventional collision detection algorithms. However, these approaches do not always guarantee a continuous force field, nor do they allow for an easy online adaptation of the force field [12]. An alternative to generating force feedback through collision detection algorithms is to compute haptic forces based on conservative potential fields. This approach has been successfully implemented to prevent users from applying excessive forces to sensitive anatomical structures in simulated surgical tasks [12], yet manual segmentation was still required. Avila and Sobierajski [3] proposed a method that derived haptic forces from the opacities of the individual voxels. However, their force field was discrete with voxel resolution, and they reported unstable haptic feedback when interacting with stiff objects.

We present a method combining VR visualization and haptic display of patient-specific anatomy that does not use any mesh or surface generation, and that guarantees a continuous force field. The medical data was visualized in VR using an HMD, thereby increasing the immersion in the virtual environment. In a pilot study, we have shown that the haptic and visual renderings coincide such that participants could accurately follow a reference path on an object's surface.

2   Methods

2.1   Visual Volume Rendering in Virtual Reality

For the visualization of volumetric medical data sets in VR, we used SpectoVR. This software is capable of loading and displaying any volumetric data that is provided in standard DICOM format. A transfer function can be defined to map voxel intensities to color and opacity values. The software uses a direct volume rendering approach that has been optimized for VR visualizations. The required refresh rate for VR is achieved using various optimization techniques, including a precomputed distance map for empty space skipping [15], early ray termination [8], a gradient map for accurate specular shading, and partially precomputed lightmaps for realistic ambient occlusion.

2.2   Haptic Volume Rendering

We only considered haptic rendering for a single point, which is comparable to touching an object with the tip of a pen. As a result, the haptic feedback was three-dimensional only, i.e., no torques were generated. The rendered haptic forces were based on a C^2-continuous, positive semi-definite, conservative potential field $\phi(\boldsymbol{q})$ surrounding the haptic device's end-effector position $\left(q_x\ q_y\ q_z\right)^{\mathsf{T}}$, similarly to the path control method described in [11]. The potential field was shaped by compactly supported radial basis functions (CSRBFs) of Wendland type [14] placed at the voxel positions $\boldsymbol{v}_i = \left(v_{i,x}\ v_{i,y}\ v_{i,z}\right)^{\mathsf{T}}$, $i = 1, ..., N$, where N is the total number of voxels:

$$\phi(\boldsymbol{q}) = \frac{\sum_{i=1}^{N}\left(\alpha_i f[r_i(\boldsymbol{q})]\right)}{\sum_{i=1}^{N} f[r_i(\boldsymbol{q})]}, \tag{1}$$

where the weights $0 \le \alpha_i \le 1$ are the voxel opacities,

$$f[r_i(\boldsymbol{q})] = \begin{cases} (1 - r_i)^4(4r_i + 1) & 0 \le r_i \le 1 \\ 0 & r_i > 1 \end{cases}, \tag{2}$$

and r_i are the distances between $\boldsymbol{q}$ and the voxel positions $\boldsymbol{v}_i$ normalized with a constant radius of influence $\left(r_x^*\ r_y^*\ r_z^*\right)^{\mathsf{T}}$ of the CSRBFs:

$$r_i(\boldsymbol{q}) = \sqrt{\left(\frac{q_x - v_{i,x}}{r_x^*}\right)^2 + \left(\frac{q_y - v_{i,y}}{r_y^*}\right)^2 + \left(\frac{q_z - v_{i,z}}{r_z^*}\right)^2}. \tag{3}$$

The voxel opacities α_i allowed shaping a landscape-like potential field $\phi(\boldsymbol{q})$. Using CSRBFs to shape the potential field has the advantage that a C^2-continuous potential field is guaranteed even though it is generated based on voxel opacities at discrete positions. In addition, the force at a certain position $\boldsymbol{q}$ only depends on a limited number of CSRBFs located at voxel positions $\boldsymbol{v}_i$ around $\boldsymbol{q}$, thus limiting the computational cost. The haptic force field was defined as

$$\boldsymbol{F}(\boldsymbol{q}) = -c\nabla\phi(\boldsymbol{q}), \tag{4}$$

i.e., the negative gradient of the potential field scaled with a constant factor c.

2.3 Combining Visual and Haptic Rendering

Apparatus. Our system consisted of an HTC Vive HMD with a Lighthouse 1.0 tracking system (HTC, New Taipei City, Taiwan) and a customized 6-DoF lambda.6 haptic input device (Force Dimension, Nyon, Switzerland) (see Fig. 1a and supplemental video). The haptic device was able to render a maximal linear force of 20 N. Both the HMD and the haptic device were controlled by the same computer (HP Z640 Workstation, Intel Xeon E5-2630 CPU @ 2.2GHz, Nvidia GTX 1080 GPU, 16 GB RAM, Windows 10).

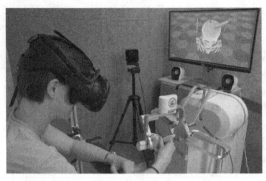
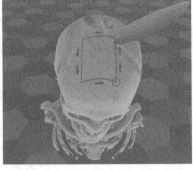

(a) System setup   (b) View of the user

Fig. 1. (a) A user operating the haptic device while wearing the head-mounted display, which is tracked by the Lighthouse system. (b) The user's view during the path following task with reference path (green) and executed path (blue). (Color figure online)

System Architecture. In human-robot collaborative systems, real-time applications, which guarantee a response within specified time constraints, are state of the art. As our virtual environment was created in Unity (Unity Technologies, San Francisco, CA, USA), which cannot provide this guarantee, we separated the haptic computation from the visualization. This separation will allow us to control the haptic device from an independent, real-time machine in future iterations. The haptic device was controlled by a custom C++ application using CHAI3D [4]. The two applications communicated over network sockets to synchronize the relevant objects between the haptic and visual scenes. To provide realistic sensory stimuli, the visual and haptic feedback were rendered at 90 Hz and 2 kHz, respectively.

Calibration. Since HMD users are effectively blind to the real world, the correct alignment of the haptic device's end-effector and its virtual representation is required for proper interaction with the real device. Due to the design of the haptic device, permanently attaching an HTC Vive Tracker 1.0 (HTC, New Taipei City, Taiwan) to the end-effector would have been impractical. Instead, we relied on the device's encoders to report the end-effector's pose in the device's coordinate system and transformed it to the virtual scene. To find the transformation between the two coordinate systems, we implemented a calibration procedure (see the supplemental document for details) that only required a temporary attachment of a tracker to the end-effector.

2.4 Experimental Validation

Data Set. To validate our implementation of direct visual and haptic rendering of medical data sets, we tested it on the CT data of a human skull. The data set consisted of $512 \times 446 \times 459$ voxels with a voxel size $s = (0.488 \; 0.488 \; 0.700)^\mathsf{T}$ mm. This resulted in a total volume size of $(250 \; 218 \; 321)^\mathsf{T}$ mm, which was rendered at $1 : 1$ scale.

Haptic Algorithm Parameters. The stiffness of the skull correlates with the chosen weight scaling factor c. To display the relatively high stiffness of bones, the weight scaling should be as high as possible without causing unstable behavior. A high influence radius r^* causes the object to feel smooth, but can also result in loss of haptic detail. A low radius provides more accurate haptic feedback but results in high gradients of the force field at the skull surface. This causes instability due to the mechanical properties of the haptic device and requires a lower weight scaling factor, which results in an unrealistically low stiffness. Reasonable values for c and r^* were found by simulating the forces along a straight line through the frontal bone. We discarded value combinations that resulted in forces or stiffnesses exceeding the capabilities of the device. The feasibility of the remaining value combinations was tested by moving the haptic device along the surface of the skull. We found $c = 11$ for the weight scaling factor and $r^* = 4s = (1.952 \; 1.952 \; 2.800)^\mathsf{T}$ mm for the influence radius to provide satisfactory results for our data set.

Path Following Experiment. We conducted a pilot study with eight healthy, right-handed participants (seven males, one female, mean age 29.1 years, range 25–37 years). We asked the participants to follow a reference path on the surface of the skull with the tip of a pen-shaped tool attached to the haptic device (see Fig. 1). The participants were instructed to follow the path as precisely as possible and to not focus on task completion time. The reference path was defined as an axis-aligned rectangle in the transverse plane that was projected onto the top of the skull by finding the first voxel with an opacity $\alpha > 0.5$ (Fig. 2a). To evaluate the impact of the haptic feedback, all participants completed the task in two conditions in randomized order. In condition "VH" the VR visualization was combined with haptic feedback, and in condition "V" the participants had to rely solely on stereo visual cues. The participants were allowed to familiarize themselves with both conditions and practice for as long as they wished before completing the task (practice times were in the range of 13–54 s).

The path following task was evaluated by computing the distance of the executed path to the reference path using dynamic time warping [13]. This distance does not provide any information about the offset direction. Therefore, we also computed the signed minimal distance of the executed path to the skull surface. To define this surface, only the voxels of the skullcap were considered, and the convex hull of all voxels with an opacity $\alpha > 0.5$ was found. A one-sided Wilcoxon signed rank test was used to test the hypotheses that with haptic feedback both the mean and variance of the distances mentioned above were smaller than without haptic feedback and that the task completion time was lower. The statistical analysis was conducted using an alpha level of .05.

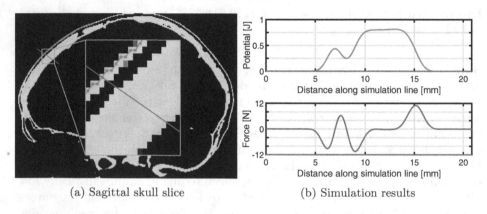

(a) Sagittal skull slice   (b) Simulation results

Fig. 2. (a) Position of one edge of the reference path on the skull surface (green) and line along which potential and force were simulated (purple). (b) Potential and force along the purple line from anterocranial (0 mm) to posterocaudal (20.9 mm). Only the component of the force parallel to the purple line is shown. (Color figure online)

3   Results

To visualize the behavior of our method, the potential and force for a straight line through the frontal bone of the skull are shown in Fig. 2b.

The data obtained from the path following experiment are displayed in Fig. 3. For all five variables of interest (mean μ_{DS} and variance σ^2_{DS} of the minimal absolute distance to the skull surface, mean μ_{DP} and variance σ^2_{DP} of the distance to the reference path, and task completion time), a one-sample Kolmogorov-Smirnov test showed that the data was not normally distributed ($p < .05$). A one-sided Wilcoxon signed rank test showed significantly lower values for μ_{DS} ($W = 31$, $p = .039$), σ^2_{DS} ($W = 36$, $p = .004$), μ_{DP} ($W = 34$, $p = .012$), σ^2_{DP} ($W = 36$, $p = .004$), and task completion time ($W = 32$, $p = .027$) with haptic feedback compared to visual feedback only. Median and range of all variables of interest are displayed in Table 1.

Table 1. Median and range for all five variables of interest with (VH) and without (V) haptic feedback. DS: minimal absolute distance to the skull surface, DP: distance to the reference path, TCT: task completion time.

	μ_{DS} [mm]		σ^2_{DS} [mm^2]		μ_{DP} [mm]		σ^2_{DP} [mm^2]		TCT [s]	
	V	VH	V	VH	V	VH	V	VH	V	VH
Median	1.281	0.394	9.475	0.025	4.550	2.112	11.801	0.301	42.624	33.630
	−0.367	0.188	1.113	0.015	1.539	1.836	0.611	0.117	23.779	24.993
Range	−	−	−	−	−	−	−	−	−	−
	19.540	0.568	211.174	0.038	23.883	2.451	221.582	0.634	67.065	67.980

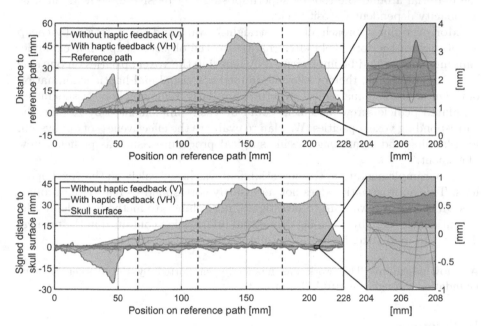

Fig. 3. The distance of the tip of the pen tool to the reference path and the skull surface. Each line corresponds to the path executed by a different participant. The areas between the bounds of each condition are shaded. The dashed vertical lines correspond to the corners of the reference path. (Color figure online)

4   Discussion and Conclusions

We showed the feasibility of a direct visual and haptic rendering approach for an immersive exploration of volumetric medical data sets in VR. Our method requires no surface definition or mesh generation and guarantees a continuous force field even when interacting with stiff objects.

The choice of the influence radius is a trade-off between accuracy and stability of the haptic rendering. Small influence radii lead to stiffnesses exceeding the capabilities of the haptic device, while large radii cause the force field to span beyond the surface of the object. This effect may be undesired where utmost accuracy is required, but could also be beneficial in situations where the user wants to feel the proximity to delicate structures without direct contact. With the settings chosen for our experiment, the haptic feedback stopped the users roughly 0.5 mm before actually colliding with the object.

In our approach, the forces were based on the gradient of a potential field. Therefore, no forces were rendered in homogeneous areas of the data set to push the tool out of the object as is common in collision-based approaches. However, it is debatable whether this is the appropriate reaction to a tool being inside an object. Our approach would allow an alternative way to provide feedback about the material around the tool by superimposing any passive force field, such as an opacity dependent viscosity field.

Moreover, our approach allows a straightforward and computationally cheap adaptation of the force field after changes to the object's shape. For example, clipping planes could be implemented by ignoring the voxel opacities on one side of the desired plane, thereby allowing immediate visual and haptic examination of the interior of an anatomical structure. Similarly, removing bone tissue during simulated pedicle screw placement could be easily implemented by zeroing the corresponding voxel opacities. We plan to evaluate the effectiveness of our system for planning and simulating specific surgical procedures, such as pedicle screw placement.

In our implementation, the potential field was based solely on the voxel opacities. This approximation does not necessarily correspond to real tissue properties. In the future, we want to investigate more elaborate methods to define the potential field, e.g., by including contextual information contained in the medical data set to map voxel intensities to material properties.

Acknowledgment. This work was financially supported by the Werner Siemens Foundation through the MIRACLE project.

References

1. Alaraj, A., et al.: Virtual reality cerebral aneurysm clipping simulation with real-time haptic feedback. Op. Neurosurg. **11**(1), 52–58 (2015)
2. Andermatt, S., Pezold, S., Cattin, P.C.: Automated segmentation of multiple sclerosis lesions using multi-dimensional gated recurrent units. In: Crimi, A., Bakas, S., Kuijf, H., Menze, B., Reyes, M. (eds.) BrainLes 2017. LNCS, vol. 10670, pp. 31–42. Springer, Cham (2018). https://doi.org/10.1007/978-3-319-75238-9_3
3. Avila, R.S., Sobierajski, L.M.: A haptic interaction method for volume visualization. In: Proceedings of Seventh Annual IEEE Visualization 1996, pp. 197–204. IEEE (1996)
4. Conti, F., et al.: The CHAI libraries. In: Proceedings of Eurohaptics 2003, Dublin, Ireland, pp. 496–500 (2003)
5. García-Lorenzo, D., Francis, S., Narayanan, S., Arnold, D.L., Collins, D.L.: Review of automatic segmentation methods of multiple sclerosis white matter lesions on conventional magnetic resonance imaging. Med. Image Anal. **17**(1), 1–18 (2013)
6. Laycock, S.D., Day, A.: A survey of haptic rendering techniques. In: Computer Graphics Forum, vol. 26, pp. 50–65. Wiley Online Library (2007)

7. Levoy, M.: Display of surfaces from volume data. IEEE Comput. Graph. Appl. **8**(3), 29–37 (1988)
8. Levoy, M.: Efficient ray tracing of volume data. ACM Trans. Graph. (TOG) **9**(3), 245–261 (1990)
9. Maloca, P.M., et al.: High-performance virtual reality volume rendering of original optical coherence tomography point-cloud data enhanced with real-time ray casting. Transl. Vis. Sci. Technol. **7**(4), 2–2 (2018)
10. Pfandler, M., Lazarovici, M., Stefan, P., Wucherer, P., Weigl, M.: Virtual reality-based simulators for spine surgery: a systematic review. Spine J. **17**(9), 1352–1363 (2017)
11. Rauter, G., Sigrist, R., Riener, R., Wolf, P.: Learning of temporal and spatial movement aspects: a comparison of four types of haptic control and concurrent visual feedback. IEEE Trans. Haptics **8**(4), 421–433 (2015)
12. Ren, J., Patel, R.V., McIsaac, K.A., Guiraudon, G., Peters, T.M.: Dynamic 3-d virtual fixtures for minimally invasive beating heart procedures. IEEE Trans. Med. Imaging **27**(8), 1061–1070 (2008)
13. Sakoe, H., Chiba, S.: Dynamic programming algorithm optimization for spoken word recognition. IEEE Trans. Acoust. Speech Signal Process. **26**(1), 43–49 (1978)
14. Wendland, H.: Piecewise polynomial, positive definite and compactly supported radial functions of minimal degree. Adv. Comput. Math. **4**(1), 389–396 (1995)
15. Yagel, R., Shi, Z.: Accelerating volume animation by space-leaping. In: Proceedings of the 4th conference on Visualization 1993, pp. 62–69. IEEE Computer Society (1993)

Triplet Feature Learning on Endoscopic Video Manifold for Online GastroIntestinal Image Retargeting

Yun Gu[1,2], Benjamin Walter[4], Jie Yang[1,2(✉)], Alexander Meining[4], and Guang-Zhong Yang[2,3(✉)]

[1] Institute of Image Processing and Pattern Recognition,
Shanghai Jiao Tong University, Shanghai, China
jieyang@sjtu.edu.cn
[2] Institute of Medical Robotics, Shanghai Jiao Tong University, Shanghai, China
gzyang@sjtu.edu.cn
[3] Hamlyn Centre for Robotic Surgery, Imperial College London, London, UK
[4] Ulm University, Ulm, Germany

Abstract. Optical biopsy is a popular technique for GastroIntestinal oncological analysis. Due to practical constraints on tissue handling, the biopsy is only limited to a few target sites. Therefore, retargeting of optical biopsy sites is fundamental in examining the GastroIntestinal tracts. As an online object tracking problem, learning the intrinsic feature is critical for robust retargeting. In this paper, we proposed an online retargeting framework for GastroIntestinal biopsy. During offline training, the endoscopic video manifold is built to mine the latent triplets to train the SiamFC tracker; In online tracking, we use both short-term and long-term template to locate the biopsy site in candidate image. To handle the out-of-view cases, reliability measurement and re-detection modules are introduced. Experiments on *in-vivo* GastroIntestinal videos demonstrate the effectiveness of the proposed method and the robustness to visual variations.

Keywords: GastroIntestinal images · Biopsy site retargeting · Siamese neural networks · Triplet mining

1 Introduction

Endoscopy is the standard technique for examining both the upper and lower GastroIntestinal (GI) tracts. To present the pathological diagnosis, the tissues are undertaken the biopsies to identify the location of tumors. Recent advances in optical biopsy have enabled real-time *in-situ* tissue characterization. Compared to previous histological analysis, the optical biopsy can be performed non-invasively *in-vivo* and *in-situ*. Despite its established benefit in non-invasive tissue characterization, retargeting of optical biopsy sites is practically challenging, even when tissue biopsy is taken using forceps immediately after the optical

© Springer Nature Switzerland AG 2019
D. Shen et al. (Eds.): MICCAI 2019, LNCS 11768, pp. 38–46, 2019.
https://doi.org/10.1007/978-3-030-32254-0_5

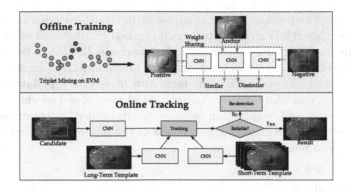

Fig. 1. The main framework of the proposed method.

biopsy. The main reason is that there is no visible markers left by optical biopsy on the surface of tissues. Furthermore, tissue deformation due to patient movement, peristalsis or respiration is another challenge to deal with in optical biopsy retargeting. For these reasons, there is a great demand clinically to develop a robust vision based technique for consistent retargeting of previously visited biopsy sites in GI endoscopic examinations.

In this work, optical biopsy retargeting is addressed as a long-term region tracking problem. For object tracking, a myriad of methods have been proposed in general computer vision [1–6]. Tracking-Learning-Detection (TLD) [1] is the representative work which integrates the PN learning and template-based detector for long-term tracking. In [2], the long-term correlation tracker (LCT) is proposed to use the Kernelized Correlation Filter (KCF) as the base tracker and random ferns classifier for long-term detection. For GI retargeting tasks, Ye et al. [7] used Haar-like random forest as feature representation and the structured support vector machine (SVM) for candidate ranking. Despite the satisfactory performance of the methods above, they all use the hand-crafted features which cannot robustly handle the appearance variations.

Recent works based on deep convolutional neural networks have shown dominate performance on tracking [6,8–10]. Among them, Siamese networks [8,9,11], which performs tracking by similarity comparison between the template and candidate, have shown promising accuracy and high efficiency for tracking. Bertinetto et al. [8] proposed a fully convolutional Siamese network (SiamFC) to estimate the feature similarity region-wise between the candidate region and the starting frame. Vamadre et al. [9] extended SiamFC with the correlation filters to enable end-to-end training of the trackers. These methods were all trained with large scale Youtube dataset with thousands of densely annotated videos. To train the siamese network, the negative and positive samples are selected via thresholding the intersection-of-union (IoU). However, the dataset in retargeting tasks is expensive to collect and annotate, particularly compared to Youtube videos.

In this paper, we proposed an online retargeting framework for gastrointestinal biopsy. As shown in Fig. 1, the proposed method is composed of two stages: During offline training, the endoscopic video manifold (EVM) is built to mine the latent triplets to train the SiamFC tracker; The online tracking step is based on SiamFC model. We use both short-term and long-term templates to locate the biopsy site in candidate images. To handle the cases of out-of-view, the reliability measurement and re-detection modules are introduced. Experiments on 20 *in-vivo* datasets demonstrate the effectiveness of the proposed method to handle appearance variations in endoscopy.

2   Methodology

2.1   Siamese Networks for Tracking

The Siamese tracker learns a similarity metric $f(x, z)$ to compare an exemplar image z to a candidate image x in the embedding space as follows:

$$f(x, z) = \phi(x) * \phi(z) + b \tag{1}$$

where $\phi(\cdot)$ is the fully convolutional neural network, $*$ denotes the cross correlation between the feature maps and b is the bias. Based on Eq. (1), the pairwise similarity is trained via the logistic loss:

$$\mathcal{L} = \sum_{x_i} \log(1 + e^{-y_i f(z, x_i)}) \tag{2}$$

where $y_i \in \{-1, +1\}$ is the groundtruth label. If z and x_i are similar, $y_i = +1$. Otherwise, $y_i = -1$. In the original SiamFC, the positive and negative pairs are determined by thresholding the IoU between the candidate and groundtruth region. However, previous works are trained with large-scale dataset, such as YoutubeBB with several thousands of videos. Moreover, there is no specific consideration on challenging cases for retargeting, e.g. illumination variation and motion blur.

2.2   Triplet Feature Learning on Endoscopic Manifold

In this section, we aim at mining the latent similar and dissimilar pairs of regions to learn the similarity metric for siamese network.

Graph Construction: Following [12], we build the endoscopic video manifold (EVM) for mining the latent similar/dissimilar pairs. Let $X = \{x_i, y_i, b_i\}, i = 1, \ldots, n$ denote the GI video where x_i denotes ith frame in video, y_i indicates whether the targeted biopsy site occurs in frame x_i and b_i is the location of bounding box. We first generate proposals as shown in Fig. 2. For frames with target as shown in Fig. 2(a), the positive proposals are generated with IoU$> \lambda_p$ while the negative proposals are with IoU$< \lambda_n$ where $\lambda_p = 0.9$ and $\lambda_n = 0.3$

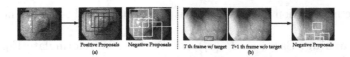

Fig. 2. The generation of proposals.

are pre-defined thresholds to control the proposals. For frames without target as shown in Fig. 2(b), the location of biopsy target in temporally-nearest positive sample is used to generate the negative proposals within the neighborhoods. Based on the proposals $\tilde{X} = \{\tilde{x}_i, i = 1, \ldots, n_p\}$ where n_p is the number of proposals, we build the semantic graph $G_S = \{V, E_S\}$ where the nodes V are proposals and edge set E_S indicates the connection between the proposals. The weight $W_S \in \mathcal{R}^{n_p \times n_p}$ is determined as follows: $W_S(x_i, x_j) = 1$ when x_i and x_j indicate the same target. Otherwise, $W_S(x_i, x_j) = 0$. Therefore, each proposal x_i is matched with the semantic positives $P_S(x_i)$ and negatives $N_S(x_i)$.

Besides the semantic graph G_S, we also build the feature graph $G_F = \{V, E_F\}$ where the nodes are also the proposals while the edge E_F is determined by the visual similarity based on the feature. For each proposal $\tilde{x}_i$, we use the pre-trained neural networks and global pooling to generate the visual representation $\tilde{f}_i$. The elements of weight matrix $W_F \in \mathcal{R}^{n_p \times n_p}$ are determined as follows: $W_F(x_i, x_j) = 1$ when x_i is within the $k-$nearest neighborhood of x_j, i.e.$x_i \in \mathcal{N}_F^k(x_j)$ based on Euclidean distance. Otherwise, $W_S(x_i, x_j) = 0$. Based on the feature graph, we calculate the geodesic distance $d(x_i, x_j)$ between x_i and x_j by Dijkstra algorithm [13]. Therefore, each proposal x_i is matched with the feature positives $P_F(x_i) = \{x \in \mathcal{N}_F^k(x_i)\}$ and feature negatives $N_F(x_i) = \{\forall x, d(x, x_i) > \theta_F\}$ where θ_F is the pre-defined threshold which is empirically set to 10.

Positive Mining: Given a proposal x_i, the task of positive mining is to generate the latent pair of $\{x_i, x_i^+\}$ where x_i^+ is similar to x_i. Due to the illumination variation and motion blur, the consecutive frames can be visually different while the target remains unchanged. Therefore, we compare the semantic positive set $P_S(x_i)$ and the feature space $N_F^k(x_i)$ to obtain the hard positive samples as follows:

$$P^*(x_i) = \{x \in P_S(x_i) \cap N_F(x_i)\} \tag{3}$$

which is the intersection between the semantic positives and feature negatives. The main idea is to abstract the samples with larger feature distance to x_i.

Negative Mining: The task of negative mining is to generate the latent pair of $\{x_i, x_i^-\}$ where x_i^- is the dissimilar to x_i. In out-of-view cases, the candidate region can be very similar to the previous tracked region while the biopsy target does not exists. Therefore, we compare the semantic negative set $N_S(x_i)$ and the feature positives $P_F^k(x_i)$ to obtain the hard negative samples as follows:

$$N^*(x_i) = \{x \in N_S(x_i) \cap P_F(x_i)\} \tag{4}$$

which is the intersection between the feature positives and semantic negatives.

Triplet Learning: Based on $P^*(x_i)$ and $N^*(x_i)$, we reformulate Eq. (2) to a triplet learning problem [11] as follows:

$$\mathcal{L} = \sum_{\substack{x_i^+ \in P^*(x_i) \\ x_i^- \in N^*(x_i)}} \log(1 + e^{-f(x_i^+, x_i) + f(x_i^-, x_i)}) \tag{5}$$

Compared to original siamese learning problem in Eq. (2), the triplet formulation in Eq. (5) aims at distinguishing the hard positive and negative samples.

2.3   Tracking Reliability and Re-Detection

The triplet learning on EVM enables the discriminative representation of endoscopic frames. However, original SiamFC only utilized the first frame as template which cannot perfectly handle the visual variations and out-of-view cases. In this section, we use the first frame as long-term template and the nearest successful frames as short-term template. The tracking problem in Eq. (1) is reformulated as follows:

$$f(x, z) = \phi(x) * (\phi(z_1) + \sum_k \phi(z_k)) + b \tag{6}$$

where z_1 is the first frame and $\{z_k\}$ is the set of tracked samples in previous N frames. In order to determine whether the tracking fails or not, we follow the strategy in [14]. Let $\hat{y}$ denote the maximum response in Eq. (6) and $\bar{y}$ is the average of maximum response in previous N successful frames. If $\hat{y} > \gamma\bar{y}$, it indicates that current tracking is successful. Otherwise, we need to reset the set of short-term template and perform re-detection. In this paper, we empirically set $\gamma = 0.8$ and $N = 20$.

The re-detection is performed based on the similarity comparison between the candidate and the long-term template. The similarity is calculate according to Eq. (1) only and the coarse-to-fine strategy with multiple scales of candidate regions is used to locate the final region. After that, we reset the short-term template set to current successful frame.

3   Experiments

Dataset and Experiment Settings: In this section, we conduct the experiments to evaluate the performance of the proposed method in retargeting. 20 *in-vivo* videos used for evaluation were collected by using Olympus NBI and Pentax i-scan endoscopes. Since the number of dataset is limited, we split the original dataset into five folds. During training, four folds of videos are randomly selected to train the siamese networks. Four attributes of visual appearances including *normal*(N), *Out-of-View* (OV), *Illumination Variation*(IV) and *Motion Blur* (MB) are presented in the dataset.

Table 1. AUC scores of four attributes: 'OV' denotes out-of-view, 'IV' denotes illumination variations, 'MB' denotes motion blur, 'N' denotes normal and 'All' denotes all frames.

Methods	OV	IV	MB	N	All
MOSSE [3]	0.254	0.263	0.415	0.164	0.274
STAPLER [4]	0.490	0.230	0.784	0.246	0.438
TLD [1]	0.237	0.145	0.301	0.442	0.231
KCF [5]	0.116	0.117	0.139	0.201	0.143
BACF [15]	0.649	0.832	0.782	0.847	0.791
LCT [2]	0.221	0.260	0.240	0.393	0.279
SiamFC [8]	0.641	0.769	0.713	0.808	0.725
ADNet [10]	0.662	0.755	0.767	0.792	0.735
ECO [6]	0.656	0.774	0.773	0.859	0.766
SiamFC-Tri [11]	0.769	0.807	0.757	0.874	0.772
Ours	0.668	0.826	0.795	0.893	0.796

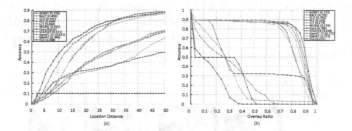

Fig. 3. Accuracy plots of the proposed method and baselines. (a) Accuracy with different location distance of center. (b) Accuracy with different overlap ratios.

The fully convolutional networks in Fig. 1 is based on convolutional layers of AlexNet [16]. We use the Adam solver (lr $= 0.001$, $\beta_1 = 0.5, \beta_2 = 0.999$) to train the model with a batch size of 1. The Pytorch framework is adopted to implement the deep convolution neural networks and the experiment platform is a workstation with Xeon E5-2630 and NVIDIA GeForce Titan Xp.

Quantitative Results: We firstly present the quantitative results of retargeting on GI dataset. The area-under-curve (AUC) of accuracy with different overlapped ratio between the groundtruth and retargeting result is reported to measure the performance of retargeting. Several baselines are adopted in this paper for comparison including MOSSE [3], STAPLER [4], TLD [1], KCF [5], BACF [15], LCT [2], SiamFC [8], SiamFC-Tri [11], ADNet [10] and ECO [6]. As illustrated in Table 1, the proposed method performs the best on multiple attributes when compared to the baselines. The favorable performance of proposed method on appearance variations (e.g. MB and IV) demonstrates the

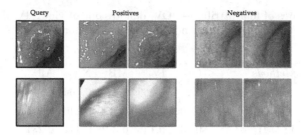

Fig. 4. Hard positive and negative samples extracted by triplet learning. Images in black boxes are query data. Images in red and green boxes are positive and negative samples respectively. (Color figure online)

effectiveness of the discriminative similarity metric based on triplet graph learning. The overall performance is evaluated in Fig. 3 based on multiple overlap ratios and location distance thresholds. The proposed method obtains the AUC scores of 0.653 and 0.796 on different evaluation metrics, indicating the superior performance compared to baseline methods. Among the baselines, SiamFC-Tri obtains competitive performance which also used the triplet feature learning based on SiamFC framework while the selection of triplet is not fully considered. The proposed method extracts the hard positive and negative samples to learn discriminative features, leading to higher accuracy.

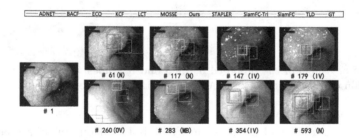

Fig. 5. Represenative frames of retargeting results.

Qualitative Results: We also present the qualitative results of triplet feature learning and typical retargeting cases. As shown in Fig. 4, two sets of hard positive and negative samples are extracted based on the query. The hard positive samples are visually different from the query while the biopsy target still exists in the ROI. In contrast, the hard negative samples without the target are more similar to the query. It demonstrates the effectiveness of the triplet mining proposed in this work. Figure 5 illustrates the representative frames with different attributes. Compared to the baselines, the proposed method obtains accurate retargeting results on appearance variations and out-of-view cases.

4   Conclusion

There is a great demand clinically to develop a robust vision based technique for consistent retargeting of previously visited biopsy sites in GI endoscopic examinations. In this paper, we proposed an online retargeting framework for gastrointestinal biopsy. During offline training, the endoscopic video manifold is built to mine the latent triplets to train the SiamFC tracker; In online tracking, we use both short-term and long-term template to locate the biopsy site in candidate image. Experiments on *in-vivo* GI videos demonstrate the two advantages of the proposed method: (1) The triplet mining on endoscopic video manifold benefits the robustness to the appearance variations. (2) The combination of long-term and short-term templates benefits the long-term retargeting for out-of-view cases. Therefore, the proposed method achieves superior AUC scores compared to baseline methods.

Acknowledgement. This research is partly supported by NSFC (No.61572315), Committee of Science and Technology, Shanghai, China (No.17JC1403000) and 973 Plan, China (No.2015CB856004).

References

1. Kalal, Z., Mikolajczyk, K., Matas, J.: Tracking-learning-detection. IEEE TPAMI **34**(7), 1409–1422 (2012)
2. Ma, C., Yang, X., Zhang, C., Yang, M.H.: Long-term correlation tracking. In: CVPR, pp. 5388–5396 (2015)
3. Bolme, D.S., Beveridge, J.R., Draper, B.A., Lui, Y.M.: Visual object tracking using adaptive correlation filters. In: CVPR, pp. 2544–2550. IEEE (2010)
4. Bertinetto, L., Valmadre, J., Golodetz, S., Miksik, O., Torr, P.H.: Staple: Complementary learners for real-time tracking. In: CVPR, pp. 1401–1409 (2016)
5. Henriques, J.F., Caseiro, R., Martins, P., Batista, J.: High-speed tracking with kernelized correlation filters. IEEE TPAMI **37**(3), 583–596 (2015)
6. Danelljan, M., Bhat, G., Shahbaz Khan, F., Felsberg, M.: Eco: efficient convolution operators for tracking. In: CVPR, pp. 6638–6646 (2017)
7. Ye, M., Giannarou, S., Meining, A., Yang, G.Z.: Online tracking and retargeting with applications to optical biopsy in gastrointestinal endoscopic examinations. Med. Image Anal. **30**, 144–157 (2016)
8. Bertinetto, L., Valmadre, J., Henriques, J.F., Vedaldi, A., Torr, P.H.S.: Fully-convolutional siamese networks for object tracking. In: Hua, G., Jégou, H. (eds.) ECCV 2016. LNCS, vol. 9914, pp. 850–865. Springer, Cham (2016). https://doi.org/10.1007/978-3-319-48881-3_56
9. Valmadre, J., Bertinetto, L., Henriques, J., Vedaldi, A., Torr, P.H.: End-to-end representation learning for correlation filter based tracking. In: CVPR, pp. 2805–2813 (2017)
10. Yun, S., Choi, J., Yoo, Y., Yun, K., Young Choi, J.: Action-decision networks for visual tracking with deep reinforcement learning. In: CVPR, pp.2711–2720 (2017)
11. Dong, X., Shen, J.: Triplet loss in siamese network for object tracking. In: ECCV, pp. 459–474 (2018)

12. Atasoy, S., Mateus, D., Meining, A., Yang, G.Z., Navab, N.: Endoscopic video manifolds for targeted optical biopsy. IEEE TMI **31**(3), 637–653 (2012)
13. Dijkstra, E.W.: A note on two problems in connexion with graphs. Numerische Mathematik **1**(1), 269–271 (1959)
14. Lee, H., Choi, S., Kim, C.: A memory model based on the siamese network for long-term tracking. In: Leal-Taixé, L., Roth, S. (eds.) ECCV 2018. LNCS, vol. 11129, pp. 100–115. Springer, Cham (2019). https://doi.org/10.1007/978-3-030-11009-3_5
15. Kiani Galoogahi, H., Fagg, A., Lucey, S.: Learning background-aware correlation filters for visual tracking. In: ICCV, pp. 1135–1143 (2017)
16. Krizhevsky, A., Sutskever, I., Hinton, G.E.: Imagenet classification with deep convolutional neural networks. In: NIPS, pp. 1097–1105 (2012)

A Novel Endoscopic Navigation System: Simultaneous Endoscope and Radial Ultrasound Probe Tracking Without External Trackers

Xiongbiao Luo[1(✉)], Hui-Qing Zeng[2], Yan-Ping Du[2], and Xiao Cheng[2]

[1] Department of Computer Science, Xiamen University, Xiamen, China
xiongbiao.luo@gmail.com
[2] Zhongshan Hospital, Xiamen University, Xiamen, China

Abstract. This paper develops a fully novel endoscopic navigation system that can simultaneously navigate a flexible endoscope and radial ultrasound miniature probe without using external tracking devices. Current navigated endoscopy (e.g., video- or electromagnetic-based navigation) usually tracks only the endoscope motion and inspects the interior of a body cavity or hollow organ and has no ability to visualize anatomical structures (e.g., pulmonary or abdominal lymph nodes) beyond the wall of the body cavity. To enhance endoscopic navigation, we introduce a radial ultrasound miniature probe that goes through the working channel of the endoscope to observe anatomical structures under the organ wall. However, the location of the ultrasound probe is difficult to determine inside the hollow organ. We propose a new navigation framework on the basis of video-volume registration, visual tracking, and ultrasound-volume alignment to simultaneously navigate the endoscope and probe in endoscopic interventions. Our framework can simultaneously and spatially synchronize pre-operative images, endoscopic video sequences, and ultrasound images to realize a fully new navigation system.

1 Endoscopic Navigation

Endoscopic navigation can continuously and accurately determine six degrees of freedom (6DoF) position and orientation of the endoscope in a preoperative image space or coordinate system. Current navigation methods have been discussed on either video-based tracking or external trackers. Video-based approaches perform 2-D/3-D image registration to track endoscope movements [1–3]. External trackers, particularly electromagnetic tracking (EMT) using an EMT position sensor attached at the endoscope tip, are widely introduced to navigate the endoscope [4–6]. Beyond visually examining the organ interior, the endoscope usually carries minimally invasive interventions, e.g., needle biopsies and tumor resection. If cancerous targets (e.g., colon polyps) were directly observed in the organ interior, navigated endoscopy can successfully execute those interventions. Unfortunately, most endoscopic interventions are

© Springer Nature Switzerland AG 2019
D. Shen et al. (Eds.): MICCAI 2019, LNCS 11768, pp. 47–55, 2019.
https://doi.org/10.1007/978-3-030-32254-0_6

performed in a *blind* way since most suspicious tumors are under organ walls; hence it is difficult for surgeons to exactly visualize tumors from 2-D video images even if they employ X-ray fluoroscopy. Navigated endoscopy remains challenging to perform endoscopic diagnosis and treatment beyond the organ walls.

The motivation of this work is to assist surgeons to perform endoscopic interventions *visually* but not *blindly* on the basis of endoscope navigation. We introduce a radial ultrasound (US) miniature probe going through the working channel of the endoscope to visually inspect anatomical structures under walls of body cavities. The miniature US probe helps to biopsy and treat pulmonary nodules that are located outside the bronchi or at the peripheral. Typically, the US and CT image fusion provides surgeons with much more useful visualization information to intraoperatively inspect pulmonary vessels that is essential to avoid and reduce surgical risk. Additionally, using miniature US probes but not fluoroscopy to locate targets or surgical tools can avoid radiation for surgeons. These aspects are also advantages (clinical motivation) of the proposed navigation system, compared to currently available navigation systems.

The main contributions of this work are clarified as follows. From the point of view of clinical applications, we construct a fully novel endoscopy navigation system. Compared to current navigation systems, the proposed navigation system, without using any external tracking devices, has several advantages: (1) the ability to visually examine anatomical structures beyond interior surfaces, (2) cost-effective and simple clinical environment setups, and (3) without any phantom-based calibration. Another new function of our system is able to automatically measure the length of the US probe. From the technical point of view, we propose a double tracker to simultaneously navigate the endoscope and US probe. Such a tracker provides purely algorithmic navigation to estimate movements of the endoscope and US probe without any external trackers.

2   Approaches

The new endoscopic navigation system contain some devices and a user interface. The system devices include: (1) a standard endoscopy system within its control unit and an endoscope integrated with one endoscopic camera (EC), (2) a radial US miniature probe (Olympus Medical, Tokyo, Japan), and (3) a host computer with a user interface display. The system user interface consists of five subwindows: (1) EC sequences, (2) US images, (3) axial view of CT slices, (4) CT-based virtual rendering images that correspond to EC and US images, and (5) US probe location visualization by overlapping US images on the anatomical model that is segmented from CT images. We propose a new navigation concept to fuse CT, EC, and US images without using any additional external tracking devices.

Our navigation framework consists of several main steps: (1) camera-channel calibration, (2) video-volume registration, (3) ultrasonic vibrator visual tracking, and (4) ultrasound-volume alignment. The first step is only performed once to calibrate the EC and working channel of the endoscope. The second step seeks to estimate the current endoscope motion pose of 6DoF position and orientation in the CT volume. The next step is to track the ultrasonic vibrator center position at the US probe from endoscopic video images. Based on camera geometry analysis and the center position of the ultrasonic vibrator on the current video image, we align the current 6DoF motion pose of the US probe to the segmented CT volume and can compute the insertion length of the US probe.

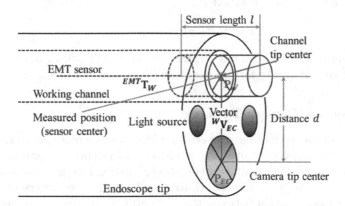

Fig. 1. Camera-channel calibration to compute vector $^W\mathbf{V}_{EC}$ to determine the relationship of endoscopic camera center $\mathbf{P}_{EC}$ and working channel center $\mathbf{P}_W$.

2.1 Camera-Channel Calibration

The relationship between the endoscopic camera and working channel centers needs to be determined, i.e., center position $\mathbf{P}_W$ of the working channel relative to center position $\mathbf{P}_{EC}$ of the endoscopic camera is necessarily calculated (Fig. 1). We use an EMT system and patten chart to perform hand-eye calibration to obtain such a relationship $^W\mathbf{T}_{EC}$. We fix an EMT sensor at the working channel center of the endoscope, move the endoscope tip at different locations, and obtain a sequence of sensor measurements and pattern images. Transformation $^W\mathbf{T}_{EC}$ can be determined by solving the following equations:

$$\begin{cases} \Delta^W\mathbf{T}^{ij} \cdot {}^W\mathbf{T}_{EC} = {}^W\mathbf{T}_{EC} \cdot \Delta^{EC}\mathbf{T}^{ij} \\ \Delta^W\mathbf{T}^{ij} = {}^W\mathbf{T}^i_{EMT} \cdot {}^{EMT}\mathbf{T}^j_W \\ \Delta^{EC}\mathbf{T}^{ij} = {}^{EC}\mathbf{T}^i_P \cdot {}^P\mathbf{T}^j_{EC} \end{cases}, \qquad (1)$$

where $\Delta^W\mathbf{T}^{ij}$ is the relative motion measured by the EMT sensor and $\Delta^{EC}\mathbf{T}^{ij}$ is the camera movement relative to the calibration pattern frame for the endoscope moving from i-th pose to j-th pose. Endoscopic camera pose $^{EC}\mathbf{T}^i_P$ is computed by performing the camera calibration. We also use the camera calibration to estimate the endoscopic camera intrinsic matrix (or parameters) $\mathbf{K}$.

After obtaining $^W\mathbf{T}_{EC}$, we can compute vector $^W\mathbf{V}_{EC}$ from the EC center to the working channel center of the endoscope (Fig. 1):

$$^W\mathbf{V}_{EC} = \frac{^W\mathbf{T}_{EC} \cdot \mathbf{P}_{EC} - \mathbf{P}_{EC}}{\|^W\mathbf{T}_{EC} \cdot \mathbf{P}_{EC} - \mathbf{P}_{EC}\|}. \tag{2}$$

Based on vector $^W\mathbf{V}_{EC}$ and distance d between the EC and the working channel centers, we can determine position $\mathbf{P}_W$ in the EC coordinate system:

$$\mathbf{P}_W = \mathbf{P}_{EC} + {}^W\mathbf{V}_{EC} \cdot d. \tag{3}$$

After the camera-channel calibration, we take the EMT sensor out the working channel and keep it empty for inserting the US probe in navigation.

2.2 Endoscopic Camera Tracking

To track the endoscope motion, we perform video-volume registration to estimate the current endoscope pose of 6DoF position and orientation parameters that establish the spatial alignment between the EC and CT coordinate systems.

Similar to [1], we perform an optimization procedure to determine the current spatial transformation between the EC and CT coordinate systems to continuously navigate the endoscope during interventions. Such a procedure that searches for the optimal spatial transformation $^{CT}\mathbf{Q}_{EC}^k$ with 6DoF position and orientation parameters to maximize the similarity between the current endoscopic video and virtual rendering images can be formulated by

$$^{CT}\tilde{\mathbf{Q}}_{EC}^k = \arg \max_{^{CT}\mathbf{Q}_{EC}^k} DSSM\left(\mathbf{I}_k, \mathbf{I}_{CT}(^{CT}\mathbf{Q}_{EC}^k)\right), \tag{4}$$

where $^{CT}\mathbf{Q}_{EC}^k$ is the spatial alignment or transformation matrix with position $^{CT}\mathbf{t}_{EC}^k$ and rotation matrix $^{CT}\mathbf{R}_{EC}^k$ from the endoscopic camera to CT coordinate systems at time k, and $DSSM(\mathbf{I}_k, \mathbf{I}_{CT})$ is the cost function to characterize the similarity between the endoscopic video image $\mathbf{I}_k$ and virtual rendering image $\mathbf{I}_{CT}(^{CT}\mathbf{Q}_{EC}^k)$ generated from pose parameters $^{CT}\mathbf{Q}_{EC}^k$.

2.3 Ultrasonic Vibrator Visual Tracking

The visual tracking step seeks to estimate the ultrasonic vibrator center position on the current endoscopic video image. We use a kernel-based visual tracking method – mean shift (MS) to estimate the ultrasonic vibrator center [7].

The MS algorithm to track the ultrasonic vibrator involves two main steps of vibrator representation and mean shift tracking, as discussed as follows.

Vibrator Representation. In visual tracking, targets or objects are widely represented by color histograms that are independent from scaling, rotation, and adaptive to partial occlusion [7]. We define the ultrasonic vibrator as its normalized color histogram, $\mathcal{H} = \{H_\pi\}_{\pi=1}^n$ (n is the number of bins). The normalized color distribution of an ultrasonic vibrator candidate $\mathcal{H}(\mathbf{p}_c) = \{H_\pi(\mathbf{p}_c)\}_{\pi=1}^n$ centered at pixel $\mathbf{p}_c$ in current endoscope video image $\mathbf{I}_k$ can be computed by:

$$H_\pi(\mathbf{p}_c) = \mathcal{N}_F \sum_{i=1}^N \mathcal{K}\left(\left\|\frac{\mathbf{p}_c - \mathbf{p}_i}{F}\right\|^2\right) \delta(b(\mathbf{p}_i) - \pi), \tag{5}$$

where $\mathcal{N}_F$ is a normalization function, $\mathcal{K}(\cdot)$ is the kernel profile with bandwidth F, $\mathbf{p}_i$ is one pixel in the candidate region with N locations, $\delta(\cdot)$ is the Kronecker function, and $b(\mathbf{p}_i)$ relatives pixel $\mathbf{p}_i$ to the histogram bin. Before tracking, Eq. 5 is also used to obtain the ultrasonic vibrator model $\mathcal{G} = \{G_\pi\}_{\pi=1}^n$.

A similarity function to measure a distance between the model and the candidate for calculating the probability of the candidate is defined as:

$$d(\mathcal{H}(\mathbf{p}_c), \mathcal{G}) = \sqrt{1 - \psi(\mathcal{H}(\mathbf{p}_c), \mathcal{G})} = \sqrt{1 - \sum_{\pi=1}^n \sqrt{H_\pi(\mathbf{p}_c)G_\pi}}, \tag{6}$$

where $\psi(\cdot)$ is the Bhattacharyya coefficient to measure distance $d(\mathcal{H}(\mathbf{p}_c), \mathcal{G})$.

Mean Shift Tracking. The MS tracking algorithm is to iteratively minimize distance $d(\mathcal{H}(\mathbf{p}_c), \mathcal{G})$ (Eq. 6), given previous center position $\mathbf{p}_{UV}^{k-1}$ of the ultrasonic vibrator at previous video image $\mathbf{I}_{k-1}$. Based on Taylor expansion, the Bhattacharyya coefficient around the initial position $\mathbf{p}_{UV}^{k-1}$ can be calculated by:

$$\psi(\mathcal{H}(\mathbf{p}_c), \mathcal{G}) \approx \frac{1}{2} \sum_{\pi=1}^n \sqrt{H_\pi(\mathbf{p}_{UV}^{k-1})G_\pi} + \frac{\mathcal{N}_F}{2} \sum_{i=1}^N \mu_i \mathcal{K}\left(\left\|\frac{\mathbf{p}_c - \mathbf{p}_i}{F}\right\|^2\right), \tag{7}$$

where

$$\mu_i = \sum_{i=1}^N \sqrt{\frac{G_\pi}{H_\pi(\mathbf{p}_{UV}^{k-1})}} \delta(b(\mathbf{p}_i) - \pi). \tag{8}$$

Optimizing Eq. 6 also means minimizing the second term of Eq. 7. Hence, at each iteration, current center position $\mathbf{p}_{UV}^k$ of the ultrasonic vibrator is updated from previous center position $\mathbf{p}_{UV}^{k-1}$ by the following:

$$\mathbf{p}_{UV}^k = \frac{\sum_{i=1}^N \mathbf{p}_i \mu_i \mathcal{A}\left(\left\|\frac{\mathbf{p}_{UV}^{k-1} - \mathbf{p}_i}{F}\right\|^2\right)}{\sum_{i=1}^N \mu_i \mathcal{A}\left(\left\|\frac{\mathbf{p}_{UV}^{k-1} - \mathbf{p}_i}{F}\right\|^2\right)}. \tag{9}$$

If $\mathcal{A}(\cdot) = -\mathcal{K}'(\cdot)$, then $\mathbf{p}_{UV}^{k-1} - \mathbf{p}_i$ is in the gradient direction. When the minimization stops at $\|\mathbf{p}_{UV}^{k-1} - \mathbf{p}_i\| < \sigma$ (usually $\sigma = 1$ pixel), we obtain center position $\mathbf{p}_{UV}^k = (p_{UV}^{k,x}, p_{UV}^{k,y}, 1)^T$ of the ultrasonic vibrator on current image $\mathbf{I}_k$.

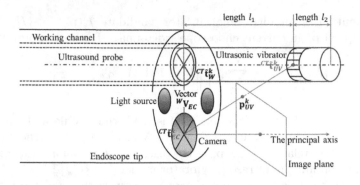

Fig. 2. Determine the ultrasonic vibrator position $^{CT}\tilde{\mathbf{t}}_{US}^k$ in the CT volume in terms of camera-channel calibration $^W\mathbf{T}_{EC}$ and camera geometry analysis.

2.4   Ultrasound-Volume Alignment

The section estimates spatial transformation $^{CT}\tilde{\mathbf{M}}_{US}^k$ with position $^{CT}\tilde{\mathbf{t}}_{US}^k$ and orientation matrix $^{CT}\tilde{\mathbf{R}}_{US}^k$ from the US probe to CT coordinate systems.

In the endoscopic camera tracking, we obtain the EC pose $^{CT}\tilde{\mathbf{Q}}_{EC}^k$ and endoscope position $^{CT}\tilde{\mathbf{t}}_{EC}^k$ in the CT volume.

In the camera-channel calibration (Eq. 3), position $^{CT}\tilde{\mathbf{t}}_W^k$ of the working channel in CT is computed by:

$$^{CT}\tilde{\mathbf{t}}_W^k = {}^{CT}\tilde{\mathbf{t}}_{EC}^k + {}^W\mathbf{V}_{EC} \cdot d. \tag{10}$$

In the MS visual tracking, distorted pixel position $\mathbf{p}_{UV}^k$ of the ultrasonic vibrator can be obtain. By applying the calibrated camera intrinsic matrix $\mathbf{K}$ to $\mathbf{p}_{UV}^k$, we corrected pixel position $\tilde{\mathbf{p}}_{UV}^k = (\tilde{p}_{UV}^{k,x},\ \tilde{p}_{UV}^{k,y},\ 1)^T$. Based on camera geometry, the position $^{CT}\tilde{\mathbf{t}}_{US}^k = ({}^{CT}\tilde{t}_{UV}^{k,x},\ {}^{CT}\tilde{t}_{UV}^{k,y},\ {}^{CT}\tilde{t}_{UV}^{k,z},\ 1)^T$ of the ultrasonic vibrator in the CT volume and the corrected position $\tilde{\mathbf{p}}_{UV}^k$ satisfies the equation (Fig. 2):

$$\tilde{\mathbf{p}}_{UV}^k = \mathbf{K} \cdot {}^{CT}\tilde{\mathbf{Q}}_{EC}^k \cdot {}^{CT}\tilde{\mathbf{t}}_{US}^k. \tag{11}$$

By solving Eq. 11, we can obtain the ultrasonic vibrator position $^{CT}\tilde{\mathbf{t}}_{US}^k$ in the CT volume. Orientation matrix $^{CT}\tilde{\mathbf{R}}_{US}^k$ with three directions $^{CT}\tilde{\mathbf{R}}_{US}^{k,x}$, $^{CT}\tilde{\mathbf{R}}_{US}^{k,y}$, and $^{CT}\tilde{\mathbf{R}}_{US}^{k,z}$ of the ultrasonic vibrator can be defined as:

$$^{CT}\tilde{\mathbf{R}}_{US}^{k,z} = \frac{{}^{CT}\tilde{\mathbf{t}}_{US}^k - {}^{CT}\tilde{\mathbf{t}}_W^k}{\left\|{}^{CT}\tilde{\mathbf{t}}_{US}^k - {}^{CT}\tilde{\mathbf{t}}_W^k\right\|}, \quad {}^{CT}\tilde{\mathbf{R}}_{US}^{k,y} = {}^W\mathbf{V}_{EC} = \frac{{}^{CT}\tilde{\mathbf{t}}_W^k - {}^{CT}\tilde{\mathbf{t}}_{ES}^k}{\left\|{}^{CT}\tilde{\mathbf{t}}_W^k - {}^{CT}\tilde{\mathbf{t}}_{ES}^k\right\|}, \tag{12}$$

$$^{CT}\tilde{\mathbf{R}}_{US}^{k,x} = {}^{CT}\tilde{\mathbf{R}}_{US}^{k,y} \times {}^{CT}\tilde{\mathbf{R}}_{US}^{k,z}, \tag{13}$$

where $\times$ denotes the cross product. Eventually, spatial alignment $^{CT}\tilde{\mathbf{M}}_{US}^k$ from the ultrasonic vibrator to the CT volume is presented by:

$$^{CT}\tilde{\mathbf{M}}_{US}^k = \begin{pmatrix} {}^{CT}\tilde{\mathbf{R}}_{US}^{k,x} & {}^{CT}\tilde{\mathbf{R}}_{US}^{k,y} & {}^{CT}\tilde{\mathbf{R}}_{US}^{k,z} & {}^{CT}\tilde{\mathbf{t}}_{US}^k \\ 0 & 0 & 0 & 1 \end{pmatrix}. \tag{14}$$

During endoscopic interventions, physicians expect to know how far the US probe is inserted into the body. Based on the analysis above, the total insertion length L (from the endoscope tip to the target) of the US probe can be calculated by (Fig. 2):

$$L = l_0 + l_1 + l_2 = l_0 + \left\| {}^{CT}\tilde{\mathbf{t}}^k_{US} - {}^{CT}\tilde{\mathbf{t}}^k_W \right\| + l_2, \tag{15}$$

where l_0 denotes the length of the working channel and l_2 is the distance from the ultrasonic vibrator to the US probe distal tip.

3   Validation Results

In our validation, we used a 3-D Guidance medSAFE tracker (Ascension Technology Corporation, USA) as our EM system with an electromagnetic field generator and sensors (1.5 mm, 6DoF) for camera-channel calibration. An endoscope (BF Type 200, Olympus, Tokyo) and US probe (UM-S20-17S, Olympus, Tokyo) were used in our navigation system. The tip diameter of the endoscope and the US probe was 5.7 and 1.7 mm. The diameter of the working channel of the endoscope was 2.0 mm. We constructed a phantom in our experiments. Its CT space parameters were $512 \times 512 \times 611$ voxels and $0.892 \times 0.892 \times 0.5$ mm^3.

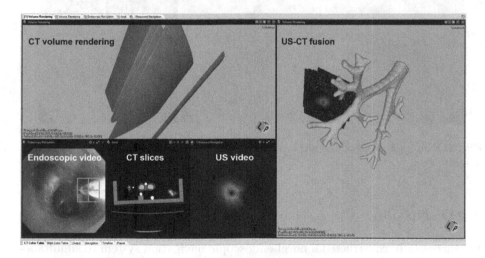

Fig. 3. Our developed navigation system with five subwindows to visualize different images and tool location information during endoscopic interventions.

Figure 3 shows the interface of the novel navigation system with different visualization information. The right side of the interface displays the fusion of the US and CT volume after the ultrasound-volume alignment. While the camera-channel calibration error was about 0.5 mm, Table 1 summarizes the endoscopic camera tracking error ϵ_r, ultrasonic vibrator visual tracking error ϵ_t, and ultrasound-volume alignment error ϵ_a on the basis of ground truth data manually generated by three experts. Figure 4 illustrates several images with the tracked ultrasound probe. In addition, the computational time was about 0.1 second per frame.

Table 1. Quantitative errors in our navigation approaches (unit: mm)

Datasets	Error ϵ_r	Error ϵ_t	Error ϵ_a
1	1.2 ± 0.3	1.2 ± 1.4	2.2 ± 1.2
2	1.6 ± 0.6	2.1 ± 1.7	2.9 ± 1.1
3	1.4 ± 0.2	1.7 ± 1.1	2.6 ± 1.7
4	2.3 ± 0.5	2.9 ± 1.5	3.2 ± 1.4
5	2.7 ± 0.8	3.4 ± 1.2	4.1 ± 1.3
Average	1.8 ± 0.5	2.2 ± 1.4	3.0 ± 1.3

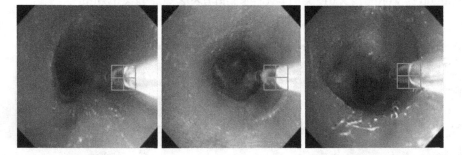

Fig. 4. Examples of MS-based ultrasonic vibrator tracking (*green square*) (Color figure online)

4   Discussion

We successfully constructed a novel endoscopic navigation system to simultaneously track two surgical tools of the endoscope and radial US miniature probe. Such a navigation system employs video-volume registration, MS visual tracking, and 3-D camera geometry analysis to fuse multimodal information. In particular, our system provides a promising and effective strategy to navigate endoscopes and US probes without using any additional external tracking systems.

Although our navigation method works well, it was only evaluated on the phantom model with several limitations. Patient movement such as coughing and respiratory motion deteriorates the navigation accuracy of our system. Moreover, patient endoscopic video images with low quality or artifacts increase the error of endoscopic camera tracking. This is still an open issue. On the other hand, targets such as tumor and vessels in 2-D ultrasound sequences will be segmented and reconstructed in 3-D visualization fused with CT-based anatomical models. The fusion accuracy should be improved. In addition, animal study will be conducted to further demonstrate the effectiveness of our navigation system.

In summary, this work develops a new endoscopy guidance system that can simultaneously navigate an endoscope and radial US miniature probe without using external trackers. Compared to current navigated endoscopy systems, the developed system is promising to visually inspect and biopsy the suspicious structures beyond the walls of hollow organs without using X-ray fluoroscopy.

Acknowledgment. This work was partly supported by the Fundamental Research Funds for the Central Universities (No. 20720180062) and National Natural Science Foundation of China (No. 61971367).

References

1. Luo, X., Mori, K.: A discriminative structural similarity measure and its application to video-volume registration for endoscope three-dimensional motion tracking. IEEE TMI **33**(6), 1248–1261 (2014)
2. Shen, M., Giannarou, S., Yang, G.-Z.: Robust camera localisation with depth reconstruction for bronchoscopic navigation. IJCARS **10**(6), 801–813 (2015)
3. Shen, M., Giannarou, S., Shah, P.L., Yang, G.-Z.: BRANCH: bifurcation recognition for airway navigation based on struCtural cHaracteristics. In: Descoteaux, M., Maier-Hein, L., Franz, A., Jannin, P., Collins, D.L., Duchesne, S. (eds.) MICCAI 2017. LNCS, vol. 10434, pp. 182–189. Springer, Cham (2017). https://doi.org/10.1007/978-3-319-66185-8_21
4. Luo, X., Wan, Y., He, X., Mori, K.: Observation-driven adaptive differential evolution and its application to accurate and smooth bronchoscope three-dimensional motion tracking. MedIA **24**(1), 282–296 (2015)
5. Sorger, H., Hofstad, E.F., Amundsen, T., Lango, T., Leira, H.O.: A novel platform for electromagnetic navigated ultrasound bronchoscopy (EBUS). IJCARS **11**(8), 1431–1443 (2016)
6. Hofstad, E.F., et al.: Intraoperative localized constrained registration in navigated bronchoscopy. Med. Phys. **44**(8), 4204–4212 (2017)
7. Comaniciu, D., Ramesh, V., Meer, P.: Kernel-based object tracking. IEEE TPAMI **25**(5), 564–577 (2003)

An Extremely Fast and Precise Convolutional Neural Network for Recognition and Localization of Cataract Surgical Tools

Dongqing Zang, Gui-Bin Bian[✉], Yunlai Wang, and Zhen Li

Institute of Automation, Chinese Academy of Sciences, Beijing, China
guibin.bian@ia.ac.cn

Abstract. Recognition and localization of surgical tools is a crucial requirement to provide safe tool-tissue interaction in various computer-assisted interventions (CAI). Unfortunately, most state-of-the-art approaches are committed to improving detection precision regardless of the real-time performance, which leads to poor prediction for these methods in intraoperative detection task. In this paper, we propose an extremely fast and precise network (EF-PNet) for tool detection that performs well both in intraoperative tracking and postoperative skill evaluation. The proposed approach takes a single sweep of the single network to achieve rapid tool detection during intraoperative tasks, and also integrates densely connected constraint to guarantee a comparable precision for skill assessment. We demonstrate the superiority of our method on a newly built dataset: cataract surgical tool location (CaSToL). Experimental results with a mean inference time of 3.7 ms per test frame detection (i.e. 270 fps) and a mean average precision (mAP) of 93%, demonstrate the effectiveness of the proposed architecture, and also indicate that our study is far superior to recent region-based methods for tool detection in terms of detection speed, surely with a comparable precision.

1 Introduction

Real-time recognition and localization for surgical tools plays a fundamental role in computer-assisted interventions (CAI) to improve the quality of surgical intervention, reduce surgical trauma and facilitate surgical training [1], which however has long been regarded as a challenging task due to the inherent contradiction between precision and computation and the great variability in the appearance of surgical tools caused by blurring and occlusion [2]. Conventional methods based on color or shape features in [3–5] and temple matching in [6–8] cannot

Electronic supplementary material The online version of this chapter (https://doi.org/10.1007/978-3-030-32254-0_7) contains supplementary material, which is available to authorized users.

© Springer Nature Switzerland AG 2019
D. Shen et al. (Eds.): MICCAI 2019, LNCS 11768, pp. 56–64, 2019.
https://doi.org/10.1007/978-3-030-32254-0_7

handle all above challenges due to the lack of generality and the restriction of traditional algorithms. Andru et al. [9,10] made massive leaps in the generality of tool detection algorithms by using CNNs. Nevertheless there is no localization information for detected tools in that studies. Amy et al. [11] and Sarikaya et al. [12] presented a region based deep learning approach for tool detection and localization, achieving benefit in accuracy. These studies, however, to our best knowledge, cannot perform detection in one framework, and usually leverage two sub structures to implement the task, making detection both computationally inefficient and time consuming.

In this paper, to tackle these challenges, we propose an extremely fast and precise network (EF-PNet) for tool detection which regresses multiple tool locations and categories within a single network instead of two sub models for achieving high real-time performance. To demonstrate the proposed architecture, a new large dataset: CaSToL, is introduced, where every frame is labeled with spatial locations and class annotations. For learning suitable features, we integrate a densely connected mechanism into the model and train it with an optimized loss function. The experimental results reach a mean Average Precision (mAP) of 93% with a fairly short inference time of 3 ms per test frame detection that is 30 times faster than [12] and 50 times faster than [9,11]. In addition, the comparison results with the original convolutional stacked method also confirm the effectiveness of the proposed architecture.

In summary, the contributions of this work are as follows: (1) We construct an extremely fast and precise CNN architecture: EF-PNet for tool tracking and localization, which to our best knowledge, is the first study to perform tool detection in such a fast inference speed with a comparable precision. (2) We build a new large dataset named CaSToL with location and category annotations of real-world cataract surgery tools to demonstrate the performance of the approach, also to improve over existing datasets in size and diversity. (3) For discriminative features, the proposed model is integrated with the densely connected mechanism and an optimized loss function.

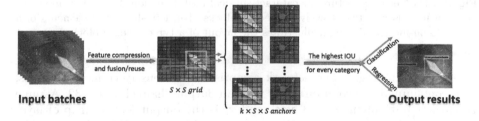

Fig. 1. Overview of the proposed framework.

2   Approach

The overview of the proposed framework:EF-PNet is shown in Fig. 1 which draws inspiration from YOLOv2 detection algorithm [13]. EF-PNet divides the input image into a grid of size $S * S$ cells. Then we predict $k = 5$ sets of anchor boxes, confidence scores and class probabilities on each cell location. Finally, the anchor which gets the highest intersection over union (IoU) with the ground truth of an object, becomes responsible for detecting that object. Unlike commonly used region-based networks, our model reasons the presence of tools with a single sweep of a single network to improve the real-time performance in tool detection.

2.1   Proposed EF-PNet Architecture

Distinct from generalizations in YOLO series, we do not adopt a stack of convolution and pooling layers for feature extraction. Because there is either some rough characteristics for a shallow stack, or a complex computation for a deep stack. Instead, our model extracts features leveraging a shallow stack of five compression models and two narrow densely connected blocks, aiming for better accuracy speed trade-offs. The integrated structure is shown in Fig. 2.

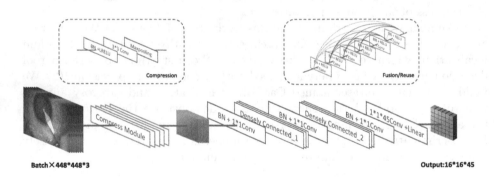

Fig. 2. EF-PNet architecture for cataract surgical tool detection. It consists of 5 compression models and two densely connected blocks. Top left shows the elements of a compression model. Top right illustrates the layout of a typical dense block.

As shown in Fig. 2, our network comprises of 2 densely connected blocks, each containing 6 convolution layers with an output channel of $g = 32$. Assume x_0 is the input volume of the block and x_l is the output feature map of layer l. Each layer implements a non-linear transformation $H_l(.)$. With dense connections, each layer receives a concatenation of all previous layers' feature maps as input:$x_i = H_l([x_0, x_1, ..., x_{l-1}])$, where $[x_0, x_1, ..., x_{l-1}]$ refers to concatenation operation of all previous layers' feature maps. This strategy strengthens feature propagation and enables the reuse of features among layers. Another advantage of these blocks is the fewer parameters than traditional network even with an increased depth.

2.2   Multiple Loss Function

The EF-PNet model introduces an optimized joint loss function to evaluate loss values between the predicted labels and ground truths. Unlike most widely used coordinate errors in bounding box detection, we train our model weighting the loss of center point coordinates (x, y) approximately double that of width (w) and height (h) of bounding boxes, to alleviate the influence of errors made by manual labeling. We also set adjustable coefficients: λ_{box} and λ_{cls} for better results. The final loss function used to train the network can be expressed as $L_{final} = \lambda_{box}L_{box}(X, Y) + L_{conf} + \lambda_{cls}L_{cls}$, where

$$L_{box}(X, Y) = \sum_{i}^{S*S} \sum_{j}^{k} (\omega_1\|X_{ij} - \widehat{X}_{ij}\|_2^2 + \omega_2\|\sqrt{W_{ij}} - \sqrt{\widehat{W}_{ij}}\|_2^2) \qquad (1)$$

Here, X and Y indicate center point vector (x, y) and size vector (w, h) of the box respectively. ω_1 and ω_2 are the improved weight coefficients for better learning and convergence. Figure 3 shows the training results with the final loss function.

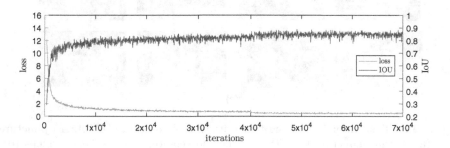

Fig. 3. Loss and average IoU for different iterations during training. The IoU consistently increases as the training loss goes down, demonstrating that the model is distinctly convergent with our CaSToL dataset.

3   CaSToL Dataset

We construct a new large and spatially annotated dataset: cataract surgery tool labeling (CaSToL)[1] to demonstrate the performance of the proposed network, and to improve over existing datasets in size and diversity. CaSToL covers 52 real-world cataract surgical sequences totaling 5010 frames labeled with class and spatial location annotations as shown in Fig. 4. To reduce redundancy, the original sequences are downsampled from 30 fps to 1.7 fps by taking the first frame per 20 frames. To be more effective and efficient, detected objects are constrained to tools which are present before the phacoemulsific stage. Because

---

[1] http://www.sklmccs.ia.ac.cn/dataset/CaSToL.html.

for the selected tools, additional attention or constraint is indispensable during the operation whether for human-in-the-loop control or CAI safety control.

The CaSToL dataset was divided into two subsets for training and testing respectively. The first one contains 45 sequences, 6119 annotated bounding boxes that are utilized to train the proposed model. The other one, including the rest of 7 sequences totaling 1268 annotations, is used to test or validate the model for both category and location detection. These two sub sets are independent of each other, and there is no one frame extracted from the same video for both training and testing. Figure 5 shows the statistics of the entire annotations in detail.

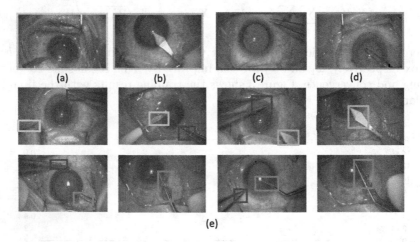

Fig. 4. The first line: List of the four critical tools used in CaSToL: 15 puncture knife (a), 3.2 mm puncture knife (b), toothed forceps (c), capsulorhexis forceps (d). **The rest:** Example frames with their category and location annotations. The detected tools vary in pose and appearance as shown in (e).

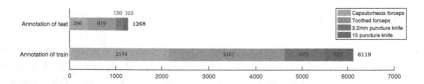

Fig. 5. Statistical table of annotations for each class both in training and testing. Since the capsulorhexis and toothed forceps appear more often than other two tools, their annotations get a more sufficient number likewise.

4   Experiment Setup and Results

In this section, we evaluate our architecture on the new large CaSToL dataset. We use inference time per test frame detection and PASCAL VOC evaluation to evaluate the performance of our detection. And in order to secure the stability of the results, we do five experiments repeatedly for every attempt. We also present a wide range of comparisons between our method and other existing approaches to demonstrate the effectiveness of the proposed method.

4.1   Implementation Details

The proposed model initialized with YOLOv2-tiny weights pre-trained on ImageNet. All newly added layers are initialized randomly. All input images are resized to 448 ∗ 448 pixels and augmented during training with random scaling and cropping. We implement our model with stochastic gradient descent for 70k iterations on our new CaSToL dataset. All training steps used mini-batches of 32 samples. The learning rate, weight decay and momentum of the proposed model were set as 0.001, 0.005 and 0.9 respectively, where the learning rate was reduced by a factor of 10 at 40k and 45k iterations for better convergence. Total training time was approximately half day time on an NVIDIA Titan XP GPU.

4.2   Results

State of the Art Performance. Our experimental results reach a mean Average Precision (mAP) of 92.85% with a fairly short inference time of 3 ms per test frame that is greatly faster than the 103 ms in [12], and the 200 ms in [9,11]. Detail results for our tool detection task are shown in Table 1. We can find that 15 puncture knife is the highest performing tool, mainly owed to its simple fixed appearance throughout the operation. Capsulorhexis forceps, however, is difficult mainly due to its diversity in posture and the inevitable manual labeling errors.

Table 1. Evaluation results for each class on CaSToL. 15 puncture knife achieves the highest performance, mainly owed to its simple fixed appearance throughout the operation. Capsulorhexis forceps, however, is difficult mainly due to its diversity in posture and the influence of occlusion or blurring during operation.

Categories	AP (%)	Rec (%)	Pre (%)
3.2 mm puncture knife	95.90	96.00	96.00
Toothed forceps	93.51	94.67	91.41
Capsulorhexis forceps	84.44	89.39	90.31
15 puncture knife	97.56	98.58	90.18
Mean	92.85	94.53	91.98

Example detection results of test frames are provided in Fig. 6. Row (a) displays frames with the order of tools present during surgical operation. Rows (b) and (c) are selected examples to show the diversity of detected tools. We have reason to believe that our model is able to successfully recognize, localize and classify surgical instruments despite varying tool attitudes and angles, as shown in row (b), and despite some parts of the tools being occluded, as shown in row (c).

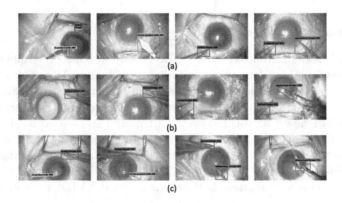

Fig. 6. Example frames of spatial detection results. Bounding box color corresponds to predicted tool identity. Row (a) displays frames with the order of tools present during surgical operation. EF-PNet is able to successfully classify and localize surgical instruments despite varing tool postures and angles as shown in row (b), and despite some parts of the tools being occluded as shown in row (c).

Performance Analysis. Since EF-PNet is inspired by YOLO series, we use YOLOs as the benchmark to analyze the performance of our method. Figure 7 shows the detection results of ours and YOLO series. We found that EF-PNet

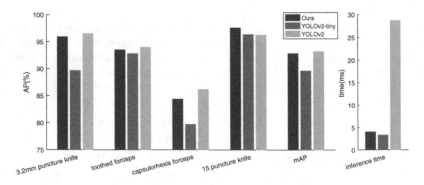

Fig. 7. Comparisons between EF-PNet and YOLO series for tool detection on CaSToL. By leveraging compression models and densely connected mechanism, the EF-PNet performs better in accuracy than YOLOv2-tiny and better in speed than YOLOv2.

exceeds YOLOv2-tiny by 3.2% in mAP (a 4.7% improvement for capsulorhexis forceps class) with a reasonable increase of 0.7 ms in inference time. This suggests the proposed EF-PNet is effective in accuracy. Although there is a few 0.4% descent in mAP relative to YOLOv2, our architecture is 8 faster than YOLOv2 during inference. This indicates the EF-PNet is also effective in detection speed. Therefore, we have reason to believe that our model achieves both comparable mAP to YOLOv2 and high real-time performance to YOLOv2-tiny.

5   Conclusion

In this work, we propose a novel end-to-end architecture: EF-PNet, leveraging simple convolutional stacked and densely connected mechanism for tool recognition and localization in real-world cataract surgery videos, which to our best knowledge, is the first study to perform tool detection in such a fast inference speed, while maintaining a high precision. Distinct from region-based series algorithms [9,11,12], we use one neural network to predict bounding boxes and class probabilities directly from the whole image for better real-time performance. To demonstrate the proposed architecture, we construct a large new dataset: CaSToL containing 52 videos of cataract surgery, totaling 5010 frames annotated with spatial locations and categories of tools. We run k-mean algorithm on CaSToL annotations to give better prior and optimize loss function for better convergence. Our experimental results reach a mean Average Precision (mAP) of 93% with a fairly short inference time of 3.7 ms per test frame detection that is greatly faster than the 103 ms in [12], and the 200 ms in [9,11]. The results of comparison with the original convolutional stacked methods also confirm the effectiveness of the proposed EF-PNet model.

Acknowledgements. This research was supported by the National Key Research and Development Program of China (Grant 2017YFB1302704), the National Natural Science Foundation of China (Grant U1713220) and Youth Innovation Promotion Association of the Chinese Academy of Sciences (Grant 2018165).

References

1. Bouget, D., Allan, M., Stoyanov, D., Jannin, P.: Vision-based and marker-less surgical tool detection and tracking: a review of the literature. Med. Image Anal. **35**, 633–654 (2017)
2. Mishra, K., Sathish, R., Sheet, D.: Tracking of retinal microsurgery tools using late fusion of responses from convolutional neural network over pyramidally decomposed frames. In: Mukherjee, S., et al. (eds.) ICVGIP 2016. LNCS, vol. 10481, pp. 358–366. Springer, Cham (2017). https://doi.org/10.1007/978-3-319-68124-5_31
3. Dewan, M., Marayong, P., Okamura, A.M., Hager, G.D.: Vision-based assistance for ophthalmic micro-surgery. In: Barillot, C., Haynor, D.R., Hellier, P. (eds.) MICCAI 2004. LNCS, vol. 3217, pp. 49–57. Springer, Heidelberg (2004). https://doi.org/10.1007/978-3-540-30136-3_7

4. Ko, S.Y., Kim, J., Kwon, D.S., Lee, W.J.: Intelligent interaction between surgeon and laparoscopic assistant robot system. In: IEEE International Workshop on Robot & Human Interactive Communication (2005)
5. Tonet, O., Thoranaghatte, R.U., Megali, G., Dario, P.: Tracking endoscopic instruments without a localizer: a shape-analysis-based approach. Stud. Health Technol. Inform. **119**(1), 544 (2006)
6. Raphael, S., Karim, A., Rogério, R., Taylor, R.H., Hager, G.D., Pascal, F.: Data-driven visual tracking in retinal microsurgery. Med. Image Comput. Comput. Assist. Interv. **15**(2), 568–575 (2012)
7. Ye, M., Zhang, L., Giannarou, S., Yang, G.-Z.: Real-time 3D tracking of articulated tools for robotic surgery. In: Ourselin, S., Joskowicz, L., Sabuncu, M.R., Unal, G., Wells, W. (eds.) MICCAI 2016. LNCS, vol. 9900, pp. 386–394. Springer, Cham (2016). https://doi.org/10.1007/978-3-319-46720-7_45
8. Li, Y., Chen, C., Huang, X., Huang, J.: Instrument tracking via online learning in retinal microsurgery. In: Golland, P., Hata, N., Barillot, C., Hornegger, J., Howe, R. (eds.) MICCAI 2014. LNCS, vol. 8673, pp. 464–471. Springer, Cham (2014). https://doi.org/10.1007/978-3-319-10404-1_58
9. Twinanda, A.P., Shehata, S., Mutter, D., Marescaux, J., De Mathelin, M., Padoy, N.: EndoNet: a deep architecture for recognition tasks on laparoscopic videos. IEEE Trans. Med. Imaging **36**(1), 86–97 (2017)
10. Twinanda, A.P., Mutter, D., Marescaux, J., de Mathelin, M., Padoy, N.: Single- and multi-task architectures for tool presence detection challenge at M2CAI 2016. arXiv preprint arXiv:1610.08851 (2016)
11. Jin, A., et al.: Tool detection and operative skill assessment in surgical videos using region-based convolutional neural networks. In: 2018 IEEE Winter Conference on Applications of Computer Vision (WACV), pp. 691–699. IEEE (2018)
12. Sarikaya, D., Corso, J.J., Guru, K.A.: Detection and localization of robotic tools in robot-assisted surgery videos using deep neural networks for region proposal and detection. IEEE Trans. Med. Imaging **36**(7), 1542–1549 (2017)
13. Redmon, J., Farhadi, A.: YOLO9000: better, faster, stronger. In: Proceedings of the IEEE Conference on Computer Vision and Pattern Recognition, pp. 7263–7271 (2017)

Semi-autonomous Robotic Anastomoses of Vaginal Cuffs Using Marker Enhanced 3D Imaging and Path Planning

M. Kam[1(✉)], H. Saeidi[1], S. Wei[2], J. D. Opfermann[3], S. Leonard[2], M. H. Hsieh[3], J. U. Kang[2], and A. Krieger[1]

[1] Department of Mechanical Engineering, University of Maryland, College Park, MD 20742, USA
{mkam,hsaeidi,axel}@umd.edu
[2] Electrical and Computer Science Engineering Department, Johns Hopkins University, Baltimore, MD 21211, USA
{swei14,sleonard,jkang}@jhu.edu
[3] Sheikh Zayed Institute for Pediatric Surgical Innovation, Children's National Health System, 111 Michigan Avenue N.W., Washington, DC 20010, USA
{jopferma,mhsieh}@childrensnational.org

Abstract. Autonomous robotic anastomosis has the potential to improve surgical outcomes by performing more consistent suture spacing and bite size compared to manual anastomosis. However, due to soft tissue's irregular shape and unpredictable deformation, performing autonomous robotic anastomosis without continuous tissue detection and three-dimensional path planning strategies remains a challenging task. In this paper, we present a novel three-dimensional path planning algorithm for Smart Tissue Autonomous Robot (STAR) to enable semi-autonomous robotic anastomosis on deformable tissue. The algorithm incorporates (i) continuous detection of 3D near infrared (NIR) markers manually placed on deformable tissue before the procedure, (ii) generating a uniform and consistent suture placement plan using 3D path planning methods based on the locations of the NIR markers, and (iii) updating the remaining suture plan after each completed stitch using a non-rigid registration technique to account for tissue deformation during anastomosis. We evaluate the path planning algorithm for accuracy and consistency by comparing the anastomosis of synthetic vaginal cuff tissue completed by STAR and a surgeon. Our test results indicate that STAR using the proposed method achieves 2.6 times better consistency in suture spacing and 2.4 times better consistency in suture bite sizes than the manual anastomosis.

Research reported in this paper was supported by the National Institutes of Health under award numbers 1R01EB020610 and R21EB024707. The content is solely the responsibility of the authors and does not necessarily represent the official views of the National Institutes of Health.

D. Shen et al. (Eds.): MICCAI 2019, LNCS 11768, pp. 65–73, 2019.
https://doi.org/10.1007/978-3-030-32254-0_8

Keywords: Medical robotics · Image-guided surgery · 3D path planning

1 Introduction

Minimally invasive surgery (MIS) has advantages over open surgery which include smaller incisions, tissue sparing techniques, shorter hospital stay, and quicker recovery times. However, MIS remains challenging for new and experienced surgeons because complex surgical tasks are completed with surgical instruments that have limited dexterity [2]. These challenges are mitigated with assistance from Robot-assisted surgery (RAS), whereby a surgeon controls dexterous surgical instruments to perform MIS procedures more efficiently. However, functional outcomes of the above-mentioned paradigm depend on the surgeon's proficiency and training, which varies between individuals. Such performance variations tend to increase complication rates in general surgeries [8]. Autonomous RAS is one emerging solution with the potential to minimize inconsistency between surgeons, and reduce procedure complications [12].

Thus far, autonomous RAS research has mostly focused on automating surgical tasks on static anatomy via pre-planning methods and without considering *in situ* tissue deformation and motion [6,11]. Implementing a similar workflow in deformable tissue surgery would be risky, as interactions with the tissue induce unpredictable changes in position, orientation, and deformation during surgery. An ideal autonomous robotic system needs to identify these changes, and regularly update the surgical path to complete the task. Since changes in deformable tissue are unpredictable, implementing accurate path planning remains challenging. Several path planning strategies have been proposed for deformable tissue in autonomous robotic surgery. Schulman et al. implemented a non-rigid transformation that updates motion trajectories for autonomous suturing on a deformable target [10]. Yet, the proposed method did not involve initial planning for placing suture points on the target. Moreover, Shademan et al. demonstrated an *in vivo* supervised autonomous suture routine for deformable tissue [12] based on tracking and linear suture path planning between biocompatible near-infrared (NIR) markers placed on the tissue. This strategy breaks down if the contour of the tissue surface is not a linear shape (Fig. 1e), since 3D information from the tissue edge is not considered. To plan a path using surface features, Le et al. implemented a 3D shortest path planning method into an autonomous robotic system to achieve 3D tumor resection [3]. Nevertheless, the method was not fully automated and repeating such paradigm to plan a 3D path is time consuming.

To address the drawbacks mentioned above, we present a novel 3D path planning algorithm using bio-compatible NIR markers and a non-rigid registration technique. NIR markers have strong signal penetration, and are suitable for intra-operative robot guidance since their high signal to noise ratio (SNR) allows them to be readily detected when obstructed by blood and tissue [1]. The proposed algorithm first utilizes locations of the NIR markers to calculate and place planned suture points on the edge of a vaginal cuff. Since the planned suture

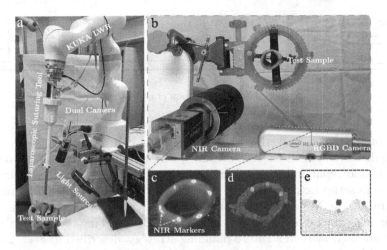

Fig. 1. (a) Experimental testbed, (b) dual camera system, (c) NIR camera image of the vaginal cuff phantom, (d) overlayed marker positions on the point cloud, and (e) comparison between linear (i.e. blue box) and 3D path planning (i.e. green point) on an uneven surface. (Color figure online)

points are placed virtually and can not be tracked after the tissue is deformed, a non-rigid registration technique is used to update the new suture plan. More specifically, the algorithm incorporates (i) continuous 3D location detection of NIR markers placed on deformable tissue before the procedure, (ii) generating a uniform and consistent suture placement plan using 3D path planning based on locations of the NIR markers, and (iii) updating the remaining suture plan after each completed stitch using a non-rigid registration technique to account for tissue deformation during anastomosis. We implement this novel path planning algorithm with the Smart Tissue Autonomous Robot (STAR) to perform semi-autonomous anastomosis on synthetic vaginal cuff phantoms. We experimentally demonstrate the accuracy and consistency, and compare the results against manual laparoscopic suturing performed by an experienced surgeon.

2 Methods

2.1 Testbed

The experimental testbed is shown in Fig. 1a. The testbed includes a robotic laparoscopic suturing tool mounted on a 7-DOF KUKA Med lightweight arm (KUKA AG, Augsburg Germany), and a dual camera system to provide visual feedback. The dual camera imaging system (Fig. 1b) consists of a Realsense D415 RGBD camera (Intel Corp., Santa Clara, California) to detect 3D tissue surface information and a 845 nm ± 55 nm 2D NIR camera (Basler Inc., Exton, PA) for detecting the NIR markers. Both camera coordinate systems are registered onto the robot coordinate systems using standard hand-eye calibration with a

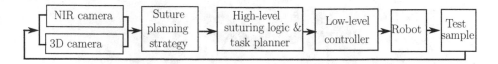

Fig. 2. The autonomous control loop.

calibration rod and a checkerboard. A light source with 760 nm high power light-emitting diode (North Coast Technical Inc., Chesterland, OH) was used to excite the fluorophore, enabling the markers to be visualized with the NIR camera. The dual camera setup extracts the 3D position of the biocompatible NIR markers by ray tracing the NIR marker positions (Fig. 1b) via a co-registered point cloud from the 3D camera (as shown in Fig. 1c and d) [1]. The 3D location of the markers are used later in a suture planning strategy, described in Sect. 2.3.

A multi-axis suturing tool was used by STAR to perform the semi-autonomous suturing tasks in this study (Fig. 1a). The structure and mechanism of the tool is detailed in Section III [7]. The tool is modified from the commercial Proxisure suturing device (Ethicon Inc. Somerville, NJ, United States) and incorporates a multi axis motor pack to independently control the motions of the tool (e.g., pitch, roll, and needle drive). Each motor includes an encoder for precise positioning using EPOS2 controllers (Maxon Motors, Sachseln, Switzerland), and are integrated using a controller area network (CAN). 2-0 polyester Ethibond suture was used with the suturing tool for this experiment.

2.2 Surgical Task and Evaluation Criteria

An expert surgeon and STAR were asked to perform anastomosis consisting of a knot and running stitches in synthetic vaginal cuff tissue (3-Dmed, Ohio, United States). Synthetic tissue, with 5 cm diameter and 5 mm wall thickness, was chosen because it is specifically designed for anastomosis training in vaginal cuff closure, is easier to maintain and analyze than *ex vivo* tissue, and is reproducible. The test sample was secured within a surgical ring using two stay sutures from the side and two alligator clips from the bottom to simulate attachment of the vaginal cuff to surrounding tissue. NIR markers were manually placed on the surface of the tissue edge using a syringe, prior to starting the semi-autonomous robotic anastomosis. Both manual and semi-autonomous robotic anastomoses were compared on (i) task completion time, (ii) suture spacing (i.e. the distance between consecutive stitches), and (iii) bite size (i.e. distance between where a stitch enters into tissue and the tissue edge). The latter two measures are related to post surgical complications including dehiscence and infection [5]. T-test and Levene's test statistic were used to compare the equality of averages and variances, respectively, in suture spacing and bite size across modalities.

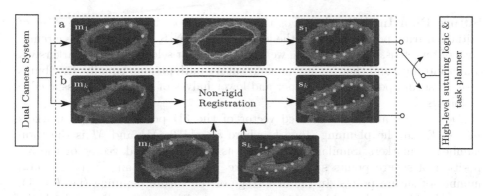

Fig. 3. The pipeline for suturing planning strategies. (a) Suture plan initialization: determines equally spaced suture points s_1 using 3D path planning with NIR markers m_1 on circular tissue edge, and (b) suture plan update strategy: updates a new suture plan s_k based on the previous suture plan s_{k-1}, current markers m_k, and previous markers m_{k-1} via non-rigid registration technique.

2.3   Control System

The block diagram of the autonomous robot controller is shown in Fig. 2. In the control loop, a dual camera system obtains the point cloud and the 3D coordinates of the NIR markers in real-time via a ray tracing technique detailed in [1]. The suture planning strategy, developed in this paper, utilizes the locations of NIR markers and performs 3D path planning via non-rigid registration to update suture points (later described in Sect. 2.3). The suture points are used in a high-level suturing logic and task planner that plans a sequence of robot motions to complete suturing sub-steps such as knot and running stitches on the planned points. The high-level suturing logic and task planner is similar to the algorithms developed and tested in [4,7] and hence details are not repeated here. A low-level controller based on Fast Research Interface (FRI) [9] and Kinematics and Dynamics Library (KDL) in Open Robot Control Systems (OROCOS) [13] guarantees the motion control of the robot to perform each subtask. More specifically, the low-level controller solves the inverse kinematics of the robot motion to perform subtasks, such as reaching the target suturing point and tensioning the suture, and also generates smooth task-space and joints-space motion trajectories for the robot to follow.

Suture Planning Strategies. The pipeline of suture planning strategies developed in this paper is shown in Fig. 3 which includes (i) a suture plan initialization strategy (i.e. Fig. 3a), and (ii) a suture plan update strategy (i.e. Fig. 3b). The initialization strategy determines the location of suture points before placing any stitch on the test sample while the suture plan update strategy updates the suture point after placing each stitch and repeats it until the end of the suturing task. The two planning strategies are detailed in the following.

Suture Plan Initialization: For this step, the goal is to determine a set of initial suturing points based on the location of the NIR markers on the circular edge of target tissue. To this aim, we let the operator select the NIR markers via a user interface and then an autonomous suture path planner equally distributes a set of suture points on the upper and lower halves of the circular tissue edge as follows.

Denote $\mathbf{m}_k$ as the augmented vector of the 3D position of NIR markers $\mathbf{m}_{i_k} \in \mathcal{R}^3$ at the planning stage k, where $i \in \{1, 2...M\}$ and M is the total number of markers. Similarly, denote $\mathbf{s}_k$ as the augmented vector of the 3D position of suture points $\mathbf{s}_{j_k} \in \mathcal{R}^3$, where $j \in \{1, 2...N\}$ and N is the total number of suture points. In the first stage of the suture planning (i.e. $k = 1$), the path planner places identical suture points with even spacing on both the upper and lower halves of the circular tissue edge (Fig. 3a). A human operator first selects NIR markers via mouse clicks (Fig. 1c), and the dual camera system extracts the 3D position of the selected markers $\mathbf{m}_1$ in Fig. 3a using the method detailed in [1]. Next, the path planner utilizes a 3D path planning method to calculate a 3D path between the NIR markers on the tissue edge. The 3D path planning method used in this paper is based on the 3D path planning that finds a shortest 3D path between two different positions on a point cloud [3]. The calculated 3D paths are grouped, to represent the upper and lower paths on the tissue edge (i.e. green lines in Fig. 3a). Suture points $\mathbf{s}_1$ are then distributed with equal spacing using the total length l of each grouped path (i.e. breaking l into $n + 1$ equal sections). We determine the positions of $\mathbf{s}_{1_j}$ as a point on the path that is the closest point to the location $\frac{j}{n+1}l$ from the start point of the 3D path (e.g. at $\frac{1}{4}l$, $\frac{2}{4}l$, and $\frac{3}{4}l$ for $n = 3$). In our experiment, six suture points (i.e. $n = 6$) were placed on each of the tissue edges (i.e. pink points in Fig. 3a), and the 3D position of the suture points $\mathbf{s}_k$ were passed to the high-level suturing logic and task planner to perform the corresponding suturing sub-tasks (e.g. reaching the tissue, firing a stitch, tensioning the suture, etc.).

Suture Plan Update Strategy: The goal of this step is to estimate the new position of the initial planned suture points after each completed stitch (Fig. 3b). We use the 3D position of NIR markers as landmarks after the tissue deformation, resulting from the placement of stitch and the tensioning of tissue, with the thin-plate spline robust point matching (TPS-RPM) algorithm [10] to obtain an updated position of the suturing points according to what follows.

At the planning stage k (i.e. planning for the kth suture, $k > 1$), the planner uses the TPS-RPM algorithm to find a warping function f that estimates a non-rigid transformation between the current NIR marker positions (i.e. $\mathbf{m}_k$) and their corresponding positions at the previous planning stage (i.e. $\mathbf{m}_{k-1}$). To this aim, the algorithm iteratively solves the following least-square problem

$$\min_f \sum_{i=1}^{M} \|\mathbf{y}_{i_k} - f(\mathbf{m}_{i_{k-1}})\|^2 + \lambda T \|Lf\|^2 \tag{1}$$

where f is a non-rigid transformation that maps $\mathbf{m}_{k-1}$ to $\mathbf{y}_k$. More specifically, $\mathbf{y}_k$ is encoded with a correspondence matrix and $\mathbf{m}_k$, and is the augmented vector of newly estimated positions $\mathbf{y}_{i_k} \in \mathcal{R}^3$ at the planning stage k, where $i \in \{1, 2...M\}$. In (1), $\|Lf\|^2$ is a TPS smoothness constraint preventing arbitrary mappings, λ controls the weighting of the smoothness constraint, and T is a annealing parameter that reduces gradually every iteration. The algorithm iterates to solve for (1), as $\mathbf{y}_k$ become closer to $\mathbf{m}_k$, and update the warping function f until T reaches T_{final} and terminates the algorithm. Once the iteration is terminated, the planner utilizes f to transform $\mathbf{s}_{k-1}$ to $\mathbf{s}_k$. Finally, the suture points $\mathbf{s}_k$ are passed to the high-level suturing logic and task planner.

Table 1. Comparison of the results.

Modality	Total time (sec)	Time per knot(sec)	Time per stitch (sec)	Suture spacing (mm)	Bite size (mm)
STAR	718.5 ± 53.5	149 ± 4	54.7 ± 6.17	7.92 ± 0.79	7.94 ± 0.98
Manual	419.5 ± 12.5	205 ± 16	19.5 ± 3.818	9.19 ± 2.08	4.96 ± 2.39

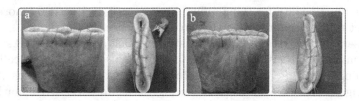

Fig. 4. Results of anastomosis. (a) Semi-autonomous, and (b) manual.

3 Experiment and Result

Using the vaginal cuff phantom, four experiments were conducted for the manual suturing method and two experiments for the semi-autonomous robotic suturing. The manual suturing experiments were completed by an expert surgeon using a laparoscopic trainer. For the semi-autonomous suturing, the control and planning algorithm detailed earlier in Sect. 2.3 were implemented via the testbed in Fig. 1a. During the semi-autonomous suturing, since the robotic suturing is performed by a single robotic arm, a surgical assistant uses a laparoscopic needle driver to manage the excess length of the suture thread. The experiment data detailed in Sect. 2.2 were recorded and evaluated.

The results of the manual and robotic anastomoses are summarized in Table 1. Representative results through semi-autonomous and manual suturing are shown in Fig. 4. In Table 1, the average task completion time for the semi-autonomous method is 299.0 s longer than manual method. More specific, STAR performed slower in completing both knot and stitch than the surgeon (i.e. 56 s longer in the knot, and 35.2 s longer in per stitch, $p < 0.001$). The average suturing spacing obtained by STAR is statistically 1.27 mm smaller than the manual, $p < 0.05$. Moreover, variance of suture spacing is statistically less for STAR than human ($p < 0.05$) which indicates that STAR placed the running stitches more uniformly (2.6 times better) compared to the human surgeon. Regarding the bite size, STAR produced statistically 2.98 mm larger average bite size than manual, $p < 0.001$. The variance of the bite size of STAR is statistically smaller than human ($p < 0.05$), which means STAR is more consistent in bite depth (2.4 times better) compared to manual surgery.

4   Discussion and Conclusions

The results indicate that the STAR was more consistent in bite depth and suturing spacing. However, in terms of the closure completeness, shown in Fig. 4, manual anastomosis was better than semi-autonomous anastomosis. Two possible causes lead to such a difference. First, two knots, a first and final knot, were tied for manual anastomosis but only a first knot was tied for semi-autonomous anastomosis. Second, lack of experience on handling the suture thread on tying a knot affects the closure completeness in semi-autonomous anastomosis. We will incorporate functionality for tying a final knot as well as practicing more on the task of knot tying to improve the closure completeness in the future.

We present a novel suturing planning strategy that advances STAR system to perform semi-autonomous anastomosis on deformable tissue. Specifically, a 3D path planning algorithm and a non-rigid registration algorithm are used during the planning process to achieve the suturing task. Moreover, NIR markers are placed on test sample as tracking landmarks with using our imaging system to function suture planning strategies. The experiments demonstrate that our proposed strategy can achieve a better consistency in suture spacing and bite size compared to the manual laparoscopic method. Future work will include improving the speed of the suturing procedures, evaluating proposed planning strategy on actual tissue, and integrating laparoscopic constrains to proceed to *in vivo* anastomoses tests.

References

1. Decker, R.S., Shademan, A., Opfermann, J.D., Leonard, S., Kim, P.C., Krieger, A.: Biocompatible near-infrared three-dimensional tracking system. IEEE Trans. Bio-Med. Eng. **64**(3), 549–556 (2017)
2. Fullum, T.M., Ladapo, J.A., Borah, B.J., Gunnarsson, C.L.: Comparison of the clinical and economic outcomes between open and minimally invasive appendectomy and colectomy: evidence from a large commercial payer database. Surg. Endosc. **24**(4), 845–853 (2010)
3. Le, H.N.D., et al.: Semi-autonomous laparoscopic robotic electro-surgery with a novel 3D endoscope. In: 2018 IEEE International Conference on Robotics and Automation (ICRA). pp. 6637–6644, May 2018

4. Leonard, S., Wu, K.L., Kim, Y., Krieger, A., Kim, P.C.: Smart tissue anastomosis robot (STAR): a vision-guided robotics system for laparoscopic suturing. IEEE Trans. Biomed. Eng. **61**(4), 1305–1317 (2014)
5. Millbourn, D., Cengiz, Y., Israelsson, L.A.: Effect of stitch length on wound complications after closure of midline incisions: a randomized controlled trial. Arch. Surg. **144**(11), 1056–1059 (2009)
6. Pedram, S.A., Ferguson, P., Ma, J., Dutson, E., Rosen, J.: Autonomous suturing via surgical robot: an algorithm for optimal selection of needle diameter, shape, and path. In: 2017 IEEE International Conference on Robotics and Automation (ICRA), pp. 2391–2398, May 2017
7. Saeidi, H., et al.: Autonomous laparoscopic robotic suturing with a novel actuated suturing tool and 3D endoscope. In: IEEE International Conference on Robotics and Automation (ICRA) (2019). Accepted for publication
8. Salman, M., Bell, T., Martin, J., Bhuva, K., Grim, R., Ahuja, V.: Use, cost, complications, and mortality of robotic versus nonrobotic general surgery procedures based on a nationwide database. Am. Surg. **79**(6), 553–560 (2013)
9. Schreiber, G., Stemmer, A., Bischoff, R.: The fast research interface for the KUKA lightweight robot. In: IEEE Workshop on Innovative Robot Control Architectures for Demanding (Research) Applications How to Modify and Enhance Commercial Controllers (ICRA 2010), pp. 15–21. Citeseer (2010)
10. Schulman, J., Gupta, A., Venkatesan, S., Tayson-Frederick, M., Abbeel, P.: A case study of trajectory transfer through non-rigid registration for a simplified suturing scenario. In: 2013 IEEE/RSJ International Conference on Intelligent Robots and Systems, pp. 4111–4117, November 2013
11. Sen, S., Garg, A., Gealy, D.V., McKinley, S., Jen, Y., Goldberg, K.: Automating multi-throw multilateral surgical suturing with a mechanical needle guide and sequential convex optimization. In: 2016 IEEE International Conference on Robotics and Automation (ICRA), pp. 4178–4185, May 2016
12. Shademan, A., Decker, R.S., Opfermann, J.D., Leonard, S., Krieger, A., Kim, P.C.W.: Supervised autonomous robotic soft tissue surgery. Sci. Transl. Med. **8**(337), 337ra64 (2016)
13. Smits, R.: KDL: Kinematics and Dynamics Library. http://www.orocos.org/kdl

ARAMIS: Augmented Reality Assistance for Minimally Invasive Surgery Using a Head-Mounted Display

Long Qian$^{(\boxtimes)}$, Xiran Zhang, Anton Deguet, and Peter Kazanzides

Laboratory for Computational Sensing and Robotics, Johns Hopkins University,
Baltimore, MD 21218, USA
{long.qian,zhangxiran,anton.deguet,pkaz}@jhu.edu

Abstract. We propose *ARAMIS*, a solution to provide real-time "x-ray see-through vision" of a patient's internal structure to the surgeon, via an optical see-through head-mounted display (OST-HMD), in minimally invasive laparoscopic surgery. *ARAMIS* takes input imaging from a binocular endoscope, reconstructs a dense point cloud with a GPU-accelerated semi-global matching algorithm on a per-frame basis, and then wirelessly streams the point cloud to an untethered OST-HMD (currently, Microsoft HoloLens) for visualization. The OST-HMD localizes the endoscope distal tip by fusing fiducial-based tracking and self-localization. The point cloud is rendered on the OST-HMD with a custom shader supporting our data-efficient point cloud representation. *ARAMIS* is able to visualize the reconstructed point cloud ($184k$ points) at 41.27 Hz with an end-to-end latency of 178.3 ms. A user study with 25 subjects, including 2 experienced users, compared *ARAMIS* to conventional laparoscopy during a peg transfer task on a deformable phantom. Results showed no significant difference in task completion time, but users generally preferred *ARAMIS* and reported improved intuitiveness, hand-eye coordination and depth perception. Inexperienced users showed a stronger preference for *ARAMIS* and achieved higher task success rates with the system, whereas the two experienced users indicated a slight preference for *ARAMIS* and succeeded in all tasks with and without assistance.

Keywords: Augmented Reality · Minimally invasive surgery · Laparoscopic surgery · Head-mounted display · Microsoft hololens

1 Introduction

Laparoscopic surgery, also known as minimally invasive surgery (MIS) in the abdomen, has numerous advantages over the traditional open surgery, including smaller abdominal incision, reduced trauma, and preventing undue blood

Electronic supplementary material The online version of this chapter (https://doi.org/10.1007/978-3-030-32254-0_9) contains supplementary material, which is available to authorized users.

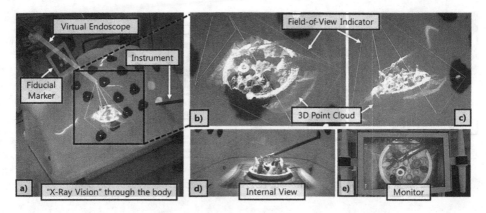

Fig. 1. (a) The "x-ray vision" provided by *ARAMIS*, captured using a camera behind HoloLens. (b, c) Closer views of the 3D point cloud overlay. (d) An alternative view inside the body phantom. (e) Traditional monitor for laparoscopy.

loss [3]. In laparoscopic surgery, a laparoscope or endoscope is inserted through a keyhole on the patient's abdominal wall. The real-time image captured by the endoscope is displayed on a monitor, and based on the visual guidance, the surgeon manipulates laparoscopic instruments, such as graspers and scissors, to perform the procedure. Although laparoscopic surgery has become the preferred approach for various procedures, it impairs the ergonomics and perception of the surgeon due to: (i) the fulcrum effect, (ii) the mislocation and misorientation of the endoscope display [2], and (iii) poor depth visualization [1].

Robotic-assisted surgery and AR-assisted surgery provide two solutions to address the ergonomic issues of laparoscopic surgery. Although robotic surgery has achieved great success, it requires extra training of the entire surgical team and has been considered more expensive [14]. AR is able to provide "x-ray vision" to the surgeon, where the real-time imaging of the anatomy is displayed at the correct position and depth, superimposed on the surgeon's normal vision, regardless of the viewing perspective of the surgeon. Fuchs et al. first proposed to use a video see-through head-mounted display (VST-HMD) to achieve "x-ray vision" in laparoscopic surgery [4]. The surgery scene is reconstructed by structured-light methods, which introduces a considerable amount of latency. Moreover, using VST-HMD is not fail-safe in contrast to OST-HMD [11], where the surgeon can always look at the normal laparoscopic monitor. The resolution of the system was also limited by the capability of hardware in the 1990s. Since then, the literature has focused more on in-situ visualization of pre-operative models with different types of AR media, e.g., integral videography [6]. More recently, we proposed to visualize the instruments and endoscopic video inside the patient body in a robotic surgery, but rendering the laparoscopy as a 2D plane does not fully restore the depth perception [10]. There are many challenges towards achieving "x-ray vision" in laparoscopic surgery, for example:

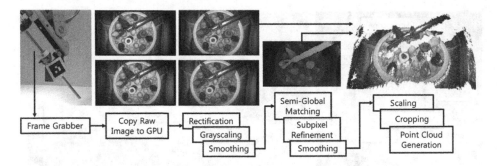

Fig. 2. Image processing pipeline in *ARAMIS* to generate real-time point cloud

- the surgery scene is highly deformable and dynamic
- the surgeon's motion and viewing perspective are unrestricted
- the rendering should be real time and high quality as visual feedback
- the augmented reality system needs to be fail-safe.

In this paper, we propose *ARAMIS*, an augmented reality system providing real-time "x-ray vision" in laparoscopic surgery based on an OST-HMD, as shown in Fig. 1, which addresses all the above technical challenges. We describe the system components and key contributions of *ARAMIS* in Sect. 2, evaluate the system performance in Sect. 3, then report the preliminary user study in Sect. 4, followed by a discussion of conclusions and future work in Sect. 5.

2 Materials and Methods

2.1 System Overview

We used the da Vinci Si binocular endoscope (calibrated as a stereo camera) and Microsoft HoloLens for the current implementation. The endoscope is configured to output a stereo $720P$ image at $60\,$Hz, which is captured with a Blackmagic Duo 2 frame grabber. The images are immediately copied to an Nvidia Titan GPU where further processing takes place. An overview of the image processing pipeline is shown in Fig. 2. The method for point cloud representation, streaming and rendering in *ARAMIS* is shown in Fig. 3.

2.2 GPU-Accelerated Semi-global Matching

Stereo matching is the technique to find the corresponding points in a stereo image pair (I_L, I_R). The image pair is first rectified using the stereo camera calibration (I'_L, I'_R), so that the corresponding points of the left and right images are aligned horizontally. The rectification limits the corresponding point search region from $2D$ to $1D$ (horizontal). After that, the rectified image pair is smoothed using a Gaussian kernel, and converted to grayscale.

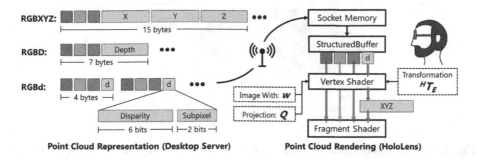

Fig. 3. The point cloud representation, streaming and rendering in *ARAMIS*

For each point on the rectified left image $I'_L(i,j)$, we compare the point on the rectified right image in the same row, with a maximum search range of 64 pixels $I'_R(i-c-d,j)$, $d < 64$. The number c is a constant offset that we applied to adjust the minimum disparity value to search for. Census transform is used as a similarity metric when comparing two pixels. As an important concept of semi-global matching, the disparity value of nearby pixels should be similar, and a common approach to achieve this is to include a penalization term aggregating the cost along multiple paths towards the target pixel [5]. With a pre-computed table of similarity scores, the cost aggregation of each path direction can be performed asynchronously with GPU computation. A post-processing sub-pixel refinement is performed to interpolate the integer-valued disparity map D (0–64) to increase precision. The resulting point cloud can be scaled down before being packed into a data buffer. The edges of the point cloud are discarded because the pixels at the border are noisy and unstable.

2.3   Dense Point Cloud Representation, Streaming and Rendering

The $3D$ position of a point (i,j) in the disparity map D, with respect to the camera coordinate system, can be calculated with a projection matrix Q:

$$\begin{bmatrix} p_x \\ p_y \\ p_z \\ p_w \end{bmatrix} = \begin{bmatrix} 1 & 0 & 0 & -c_x \\ 0 & 1 & 0 & -c_y \\ 0 & 0 & 0 & f \\ 0 & 0 & 1/b & 0 \end{bmatrix} \begin{bmatrix} i \\ j \\ D(i,j) \\ 1 \end{bmatrix} \tag{1}$$

where (i,j) is the pixel coordinates of the target point, c_x, c_y, f are the left camera principle point and focal length, and b is the baseline distance of the stereo camera. The result is represented in homogeneous coordinates.

Conventionally, each point in the point cloud is stored in $RGBXYZ$ or $RGBD$ format. $RGBXYZ$ requires 15 bytes per pixel: a 3-byte color component and 3 floating point numbers for position. For $RGBD$, the depth value of each pixel is calculated with p_z/p_w of Eq. 1, requiring a total of 7 bytes per pixel. In contrast, we store the point cloud in a flattened $RGBd$ array, where d

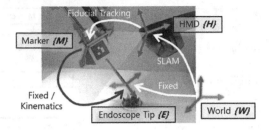

Fig. 4. The transformation between each component in $ARAMIS$, $^{H}T_{E}$ is necessary for real-time point cloud rendering

refers to disparity instead of depth. We use 1 byte for the disparity value, with 6 bits contributed by the semi-global matching algorithm and 2 bits from the sub-pixel refinement. $RGBd$ is a more compact representation that preserves the precision of the disparity value. Prior to the streaming of point cloud data, the image width w and the projection matrix Q are sent to the HoloLens in order to compute the position of each pixel from the disparity value.

Upon receiving a complete buffer containing point cloud data on HoloLens, the data is uploaded to a pre-allocated StructuredBuffer on the GPU. We implement a custom shader to render the received data packet. We choose point as a render primitive. For each $RGBd$ datum, Eq. 1 is performed in the vertex shader with parameters w, Q, disparity value d, and the current transformation between the HMD and the endoscope tip $^{H}T_{E}$. The RGB component is parsed in the fragment shading stage. The rendering pipeline is shown in Fig. 3.

2.4   Localizing the Endoscope Tip

We attach a fiducial marker to the endoscope, outside of the cannula. We denote the coordinate system of the HMD as $\{H\}$, fiducial marker as $\{M\}$, endoscope tip as $\{E\}$, and the world as $\{W\}$, as shown in Fig. 4.

In order to render the point cloud with the correct pose while allowing the surgeon to freely walk around, the transformation $^{H}T_{E}$ (between endoscope tip and HMD) is required at every frame of rendering. $^{H}T_{E}$ can be determined in two ways (via SLAM or via fiducial tracking):

$$^{H}T_{E} = {}^{H}T_{W}\,{}^{W}T_{E} \quad (2) \quad or \quad {}^{H}T_{E} = {}^{H}T_{M}\,{}^{M}T_{E} \quad (3)$$

where $^{M}T_{E}$ is known either by a pivot calibration or by kinematics if the endoscope is in a mechanical linkage. We apply a priority-based sensor fusion technique to combine both tracking methods [12]. When the fiducial marker is in the tracking volume of HoloLens, Eq. 2 is used for localizing the endoscope tip and we can also estimate the pose of the endoscope tip in world coordinate system $^{W}T_{E}$ by equating Eqs. 2 and 3. When the fiducial marker is not visible for the HoloLens or $^{H}T_{M}$ is not reliable enough, we use Eq. 3 with the most recent estimation of $^{W}T_{E}$. The $^{H}T_{E}$ is used by the vertex shading stage on HoloLens, as shown in Fig. 3. The relative position between each point of the point cloud and the endoscope tip is obtained from Sects. 2.2 and 2.3.

Apart from the localization of the endoscope tip, a display calibration procedure is also required in order to properly align the virtual scene space with the human vision via the OST-HMD [9].

3 System Evaluation

3.1 Overlay Accuracy

We position a smartphone, showing a white crosshair, under the binocular endoscope. With *ARAMIS*, a point cloud of the crosshair is displayed on the HMD as well. We capture the see-through view using a camera (Fig. 5a). The centers of the crosshairs are represented as C_1 and C_2 in the image space. We back-project the two crosshair centers to two rays ($\overrightarrow{r_1}$ and $\overrightarrow{r_2}$) intersecting with the camera center, and then calculate the visual angular error as the angle between the two rays: $\theta = arccos((\overrightarrow{r_1} \cdot \overrightarrow{r_2})/(\|\overrightarrow{r_1}\| \cdot \|\overrightarrow{r_2}\|))$.

We captured 32 overlay images from different poses ($^H T_E$), and the visual angular error is calculated to be 0.53°, with a standard deviation of 0.15°. At a distance of 0.5 m, which is a typical working range of a laparoscopic surgeon, the visual error will be 4.6 mm. It is noticeable that the error reported is the absolute error between the point cloud and the real object. Relative error between multiple objects, for example, between the laparoscopic instrument and the surgery scene in the point cloud, is much smaller. The overlay accuracy result is similar to the reprojection error reported by the display calibration method of HoloLens [9].

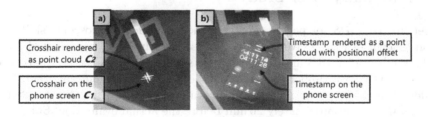

Fig. 5. The setup for evaluating overlay accuracy (a) and end-to-end latency (b). A positional offset is applied in (b) so that both timestamps can be seen clearly.

3.2 End-to-End Latency

A timestamp is displayed on the smartphone screen and therefore visualized on the point cloud on the HoloLens. The difference between the two timestamps reveals the end-to-end latency T. We measure the latency for multiple levels of point cloud scaling. As shown in Fig. 6, the end-to-end latency is 337.2 ± 31.7 ms for 1080×680 points, 256.7 ± 30.8 ms for 810×510 points, 223.0 ± 24.7 ms for 648×408 points, 178.3 ± 21.0 ms for 540×340 points, and 158.7 ± 19.0 ms for

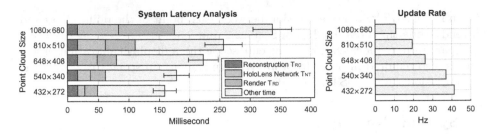

Fig. 6. The end-to-end latency T and its decomposition, and update rate R with respect to different point cloud sizes (number of points) in $ARAMIS$

432×272 points. With the largest point cloud, the update rate is 10.91 Hz. The update rate increases when the point cloud is scaled down. $ARAMIS$ is able to achieve a 26.16 Hz update rate when the point count is 648×408, 36.98 Hz with 540×340 points, and 41.27 Hz with 432×272 points.

We further decompose the time that is spent on point cloud reconstruction T_{RC}, client-side networking[1] T_{NT}, and rendering T_{RD}, as shown in Fig. 6. The time for reconstruction on the desktop server is almost constant for different numbers of points in the point cloud because the scaling is a post-processing procedure. On the contrary, the time for streaming the point cloud and rendering increases significantly with the size of the point cloud. "Other time" is calculated by $T - T_{RC} - T_{NT} - T_{RD}$, which includes the time spent by the endoscopic imaging (exposure), the frame grabber and system overhead.

4   Preliminary User Study

We set up $ARAMIS$ for peg transfer, a typical task for laparoscopic skill evaluation (shown in Fig. 7). We recruited 25 users, including 2 experienced users, for the study under IRB approval. The users were asked to use a laparoscopic grasper to transfer a rubber ring from one deformable spike onto another, from 3 different incision ports, repeating twice at each port. They are trained to use $ARAMIS$ for approximately 20 min before the actual evaluation. Subjective feedback is collected after the experiments via questionnaires.

Of the 150 trials (25 subjects × 3 ports × 2 setups), there were 11 failure cases of peg transfer with the traditional laparoscopic setup (LAP) and 5 failure cases with $ARAMIS$. Both experienced users succeeded in all tasks. Excluding failure cases, average task time was 22.02 ± 18.06 s with LAP and 20.08 ± 15.02 s with $ARAMIS$. The ANOVA test does not show statistical significance for task time ($p = 0.3$). Experienced users spent 11.16 ± 7.06 s with $ARAMIS$, and 11.24 ± 4.99 s without it. Subjective ratings (0–5 scale) significantly prefer $ARAMIS$ in terms of hand-eye coordination (2.0 for LAP and 4.2 for $ARAMIS$, $p =$

---

[1] The client-side networking T_{NT} starts when the HoloLens starts receiving the point cloud, instead of when the server starts sending, because the latter would require precise synchronization of clocks on both systems.

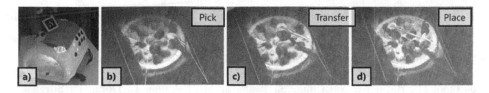

Fig. 7. (a) The preliminary user study setup; (b, c, d) sample visualization of *ARAMIS* during peg transfer on a deformable phantom

4.1e−8). In average, experienced users slightly preferred *ARAMIS* for hand-eye coordination as well (3 for LAP and 4 for *ARAMIS*). Experienced user 1 reported that the depth perception of *ARAMIS* was better, and *ARAMIS* could also potentially benefit the bedside assistant in a robotic surgery. Experienced user 2 reported that the in-situ visualization made the insertion of the instrument more intuitive. This user also suggested to enlarge the displayed point cloud in order to observe details more easily. Since the point cloud reveals the real-world scale of the scene, it is relatively small compared to the magnified monitor view. From the preliminary user study, we can conclude that it is possible to perform certain laparoscopic tasks with the guidance of *ARAMIS*, and the user performance is similar to the traditional setup in terms of the completion time.

5   Conclusions and Future Work

In this paper, we propose and implement *ARAMIS*: an AR system to achieve "x-ray vision" in laparoscopic surgery which is real-time, model-free, fail-safe, and does not restrict the viewpoint of the user. We evaluate the system performance and a preliminary user study shows improved hand-eye coordination and similar completion time for peg transfer with the guidance of *ARAMIS*.

Our future work includes a clinical study with experienced users. The fidelity of point cloud rendering can be further improved with techniques such as super-pixel segmentation [8] and instrument tracking [13]. The current implementation of *ARAMIS* uses a binocular endoscope, but could also be integrated with a monocular endoscope, using deep-learning-based reconstruction methods [7].

References

1. Bogdanova, R., Boulanger, P., Zheng, B.: Depth perception of surgeons in minimally invasive surgery. Surg. Innov. **23**(5), 515–524 (2016)
2. Breedveld, P., Wentink, M.: Eye-hand coordination in laparoscopy-an overview of experiments and supporting aids. Minim. Invasive Ther. Allied Technol. **10**(3), 155–162 (2001)
3. Colon Cancer Laparoscopic or Open Resection Study Group: Laparoscopic surgery versus open surgery for colon cancer: short-term outcomes of a randomised trial. Lancet Oncol. **6**(7), 477–484 (2005)

4. Fuchs, H.: Augmented reality visualization for laparoscopic surgery. In: Wells, W.M., Colchester, A., Delp, S. (eds.) MICCAI 1998. LNCS, vol. 1496, pp. 934–943. Springer, Heidelberg (1998). https://doi.org/10.1007/BFb0056282
5. Hirschmuller, H.: Stereo processing by semiglobal matching and mutual information. IEEE TPAMI **30**(2), 328–341 (2008)
6. Liao, H., Hata, N., Nakajima, S., Iwahara, M., Sakuma, I., Dohi, T.: Surgical navigation by autostereoscopic image overlay of integral videography. IEEE Trans. Inf Technol. Biomed. **8**(2), 114–121 (2004)
7. Liu, X., et al.: Self-supervised learning for dense depth estimation in monocular endoscopy. In: Stoyanov, D., et al. (eds.) CARE/CLIP/OR 2.0/ISIC -2018. LNCS, vol. 11041, pp. 128–138. Springer, Cham (2018). https://doi.org/10.1007/978-3-030-01201-4_15
8. Penza, V., Ortiz, J., Mattos, L.S., Forgione, A., De Momi, E.: Dense soft tissue 3D reconstruction refined with super-pixel segmentation for robotic abdominal surgery. Int. J. Comput. Assist. Radiol. Surg. **11**(2), 197–206 (2016)
9. Qian, L., Azimi, E., Kazanzides, P., Navab, N.: Comprehensive tracker based display calibration for holographic optical see-through head-mounted display. arXiv preprint arXiv:1703.05834 (2017)
10. Qian, L., Deguet, A., Kazanzides, P.: ARssist: augmented reality on a head-mounted display for the first assistant in robotic surgery. Healthc. Technol. Lett. **5**(5), 194–200 (2018)
11. Rolland, J.P., Fuchs, H.: Optical versus video see-through head-mounted displays in medical visualization. Presence: Teleoperators Virtual Environ. **9**(3), 287–309 (2000)
12. Wang, J., Qian, L., Azimi, E., Kazanzides, P.: Prioritization and static error compensation for multi-camera collaborative tracking in augmented reality. In: IEEE Virtual Reality (VR), pp. 335–336. IEEE (2017)
13. Wang, Z., et al.: Image-based trajectory tracking control of 4-DoF laparoscopic instruments using a rotation distinguishing marker. EEE Robot. Autom. Lett. **2**(3), 1586–1592 (2017)
14. Wilensky, G.R.: Robotic surgery: an example of when newer is not always better but clearly more expensive. Milbank Q. **94**(1), 43 (2016)

Interactive Endoscopy: A Next-Generation, Streamlined User Interface for Lung Surgery Navigation

Paul Thienphrapa[1]([✉]), Torre Bydlon[1], Alvin Chen[1], Prasad Vagdargi[2], Nicole Varble[1], Douglas Stanton[1], and Aleksandra Popovic[1]

[1] Philips Research North America, Cambridge, MA, USA
paul.thienphrapa@philips.com
[2] I-STAR Lab, Johns Hopkins University, Baltimore, MD, USA

Abstract. Computer generated graphics are superimposed onto live video emanating from an endoscope, offering the surgeon visual information that is hiding in the native scene—this describes the classical scenario of augmented reality in minimally invasive surgery. Research efforts have, over the past few decades, pressed considerably against the challenges of infusing a priori knowledge into endoscopic streams. As framed, these contributions *emulate perception* at the level of the surgeon expert, perpetuating debates on the technical, clinical, and societal viability of the proposition.

We herein introduce *interactive endoscopy*, transforming passive visualization into an interface that allows the surgeon to label noteworthy anatomical features found in the endoscopic video, and have the virtual annotations remember their tissue locations during surgical manipulation. The streamlined interface combines vision-based tool tracking and speech recognition to enable interactive selection and labeling, followed by tissue tracking and optical flow for label persistence. These discrete capabilities have matured rapidly in recent years, promising technical viability of the system; it can help clinicians offload the cognitive demands of visually deciphering soft tissues; and supports societal viability by engaging, rather than emulating, surgeon expertise. Through a video-assisted thoracotomy use case, we develop a proof-of-concept to improve workflow by tracking surgical tools and visualizing tissue, while serving as a bridge to the classical promise of augmented reality in surgery.

Keywords: Interactive endoscopy · Lung surgery · VATS · Augmented reality · Human-computer interaction

1 Introduction and Motivation

Lung cancer is the deadliest form of cancer worldwide, with 1.6 million new diagnoses and 1.4 million deaths each year, more than cancers of the breast, prostate,

© Springer Nature Switzerland AG 2019
D. Shen et al. (Eds.): MICCAI 2019, LNCS 11768, pp. 83–91, 2019.
https://doi.org/10.1007/978-3-030-32254-0_10

and colon—the three next most prevalent cancers—combined. In response to this epidemic, major screening trials have been enacted including the Dutch/Belgian NELSON trial, the US NLST, and Danish trials. These studies found that proactive screening using low dose computed tomography (CT) can detect lung cancer at an earlier, treatable stage at a rate of 71%, leading to a 20% reduction in mortality [2]. This prompted Medicare to reimburse lung cancer screening in 2015 and with that, the number of patients presenting with smaller, treatable tumors was expected to rise dramatically. The projected increase was observed within the Veterans Health Administration [17], and while this population bears a heightened incidence of lung cancer due to occupational hazards, the need to optimize patient care was foretold.

Surgical resection is the preferred curative therapy due to the ability to remove units of anatomy that sustain the tumor, as well as lymph nodes for staging. Most of the 100,000 surgical resections performed in the US annually are minimally invasive, with 57% as video-assisted thoracoscopic surgery (VATS) and 7% as robotic surgery [1]. Anatomically, the lung follows a tree structure with airways that root at the trachea and narrow as they branch towards the ribcage; blood vessels hug the airways and join them at the alveoli, or air sacs, where oxygen and carbon dioxide interchange. Removing a tumor naturally detaches downstream airways, vessels, and connective lung tissue, so tumor location and size prescribe the type of resection performed. Large or central tumors are removed via pneumonectomy (full lung) or lobectomy (full lobe), while small or peripheral tumors may be "wedged" out. Segmentectomy, or removal of a sub-lobar segment, is gaining currency because the procedure balances disease removal with tissue preservation; and because the trend towards smaller, peripheral tumors supports it.

2   Background

In an archetypal VATS procedure, the surgeon examines a preoperative CT; here the lung is inflated. They note the location of the tumor, relative to adjacent structures. Now under the thoracoscope, the lung is collapsed, the tumor invisible. The surgeon roughly estimates the tumor location. They look for known structures; move the scope; manipulate the tissue; reveal a structure; remember it. They carefully dissect around critical structures [14]; discover another; remember it. A few iterations and their familiarity grows. They mentally align new visuals with their knowledge, experience, and the CT. Thusly, they converge on an inference of the true tumor location.

The foregoing exercise is cognitively strenuous, time consuming, yet merely a precursor to the primary task of tumor resection. It is emblematic of endoscopic surgery in general and of segmentectomy in particular, as the surgeon continues to mind critical structures under a limited visual field [18]. Consequently, endoscopic scenes are difficult to contextualize in isolation, thereby turning the lung into a jigsaw puzzle in which the pieces may deform, and must be memorized. Indeed, surgeons routinely retract the scope or zoom out to construct associations and context. Moreover, the lung appearance may not be visually distinctive nor instantly informative, further intensifying the challenges, and thus the inefficiencies, of minimally invasive lung surgery.

The research community has responded vigorously, imbuing greater context into endoscopy using augmented reality [5,24] by registering coherent anatomical models onto disjoint endoscopic snapshots. For example, Puerto-Souza et al. [25] maintain registration of preoperative images to endoscopy by managing tissue anchors amidst surgical activity. Du et al. [11] combine features with lighting, and Collins et al. [9], texture with boundaries, to track surfaces in 3D. Lin et al. [19] achieve surface reconstruction using hyperspectral imaging and structured light. Simultaneous localization and mapping (SLAM) approaches have been extended to handle tissue motion [23] and imaging conditions [21] found in endoscopy. Stereo endoscopes are used to reconstruct tissue surfaces with high fidelity, and have the potential to render overlays in 3D or guide surgical robots [29,32]. Ref. [22] reviews the optical techniques that have been developed for tissue surface reconstruction.

In recent clinical experiments, Chauvet et al. [8] project tumor margins onto the surfaces of *ex vivo* porcine kidneys for partial nephrectomy. Liu et al. [20] develop augmented reality for robotic VATS and robotic transoral surgery, performing preclinical evaluations on ovine and porcine models, respectively, in elevating the state of the art. These studies uncovered insights on registering models to endoscopy and portraying these models faithfully. However, whether pursuing a clinical application or technical specialty, researchers have faced a timeless obstacle: tissue deformation. Modeling deformation is an ill-posed problem, and this coinciding domain has likewise undergone extensive investigation [28]. In the next section, we introduce an alternative technology for endoscopy that circumvents the challenges of deformable modeling.

3   Interactive Endoscopy

3.1   Contributions

The surgeon begins a VATS procedure as usual, examining the CT, placing surgical ports, and estimating the tumor location under thoracoscopy. They adjust both scope and lung in search of known landmarks, the pulmonary artery for instance. Upon discovery, now under the proposed interactive endoscopy system (Fig. 1, from a full *ex vivo* demo), they point their forceps at the target and verbally instruct, "Mark the pulmonary artery". An audible chime acknowledges, and a miniature yet distinctive icon appears in the live video at the forceps tip, accompanied by the semantic label. The surgeon continues to label the anatomy and as they move the scope or tissue, the virtual annotations follow.

The combination of a limited visual field and amorphous free-form tissue induces the surgeon to perform motions that are, in technical parlance, computationally intractable—it is the practice of surgery itself that postpones surgical augmented reality ever farther into the future. In that future, critical debates on validation and psychophysical effects await, yet the ongoing challenges of endoscopic surgery have persisted for decades. The present contribution transforms

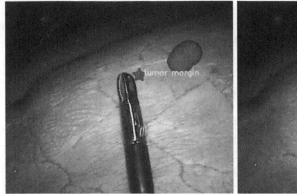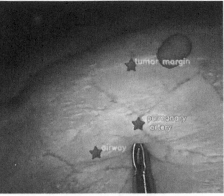

Fig. 1. Interactive endoscopy annotation system on an *ex vivo* porcine lung; the red simulated tumor is part of the live demonstration. (*Left*) The surgeon points a tool at a feature of interest then speaks the desired label, "tumor margin". (*Right*) Multiple labels are tracked as the surgeon manipulates the tissue. Note that the system is non-disruptive to existing workflows and requires no setup. (Color figure online)

endoscopy from a passive visualization tool to an interactive interface for labeling live video. We recast static preoperative interactivity from Kim et al. [16] into an intraoperative scheme; and repurpose OCT review interactivity from Balicki et al. [4] to provide live spatial storage for the expert's knowledge. We show how the system can help surgeons through a cognitively strenuous and irreproducible exploration routine, examine circumstances that would enable clinical viability, and discuss how the approach both complements and enables augmented reality in surgery, as envisioned a generation ago (Fuchs et al. [15]).

3.2   Key Components

For the proposed interactive endoscopy system, the experimental setup and usage scenario are pictured in Fig. 2. Its key components include (1) vision-based tool tracking, (2) a speech interface, and (3) persistent tissue tracking. While these discrete capabilities have been historically available, they have undergone marked improvement in recent years due to the emergence of graphical processing units (GPUs), online storage infrastructure, and machine learning. A system capitalizing on these developments has the potential to reach clinical reliability in the near future. While these technologies continue to evolve rapidly, we construct a proof-of-concept integration of agnostic building blocks as a means of assessing baseline performance.

Tool Tracking. Upon discovering each landmark, the surgeon points out its location to the system. A workflow-compatible pointer can be repurposed from a tool already in use, such as a forceps, by tracking it in the endoscope. We use a hierarchical heuristic method (Fig. 3) with similar assumptions as in [10] that

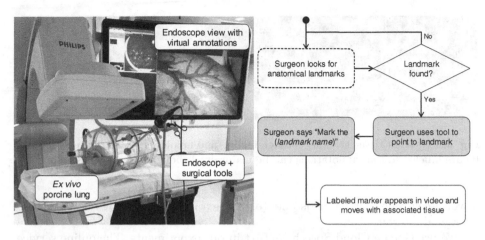

Fig. 2. (*Left*) Experimental setup. Minimal instrumentation beyond that of standard VATS is required, primarily a microphone and a computer (the C-arm is presently unused). (*Right*) Workflow for applying a label. Pointing and verbal annotation (yellow) are likewise minimal steps. (Color figure online)

thoracic tools are rigid, straight, and of a certain hue. The low-risk demands of the pointing task motivates our simple approach: 2D tool tracking can reliably map 3D surface anatomy due to the projective nature of endoscopic views. Our *ex vivo* tests indicate 2D tip localization to within 1.0 mm 92% of the time that the tool points to a new location, and more advanced methods [6,27] suggest that clinical-grade tool tracking is well within reach.

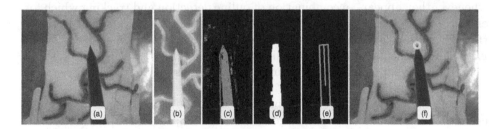

Fig. 3. Tool tracking pipeline: (a) Original (b) HSV threshold (c) Foreground learning using MoG (d) Foreground mask (e) Contour detection (f) Tip detection.

Speech Interface. Pointing the forceps at a landmark, the surgeon uses speech to generate a corresponding label. This natural, hands-free interface is conducive to workflow and sterility, as previously acknowledged in the voice-controlled AESOP endoscope robot [3]. Recognition latency and accuracy were at the time prohibitive, but modern advances have driven widespread use. The proliferation

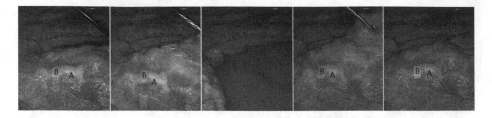

Fig. 4. Persistent tissue tracking through folding and unfolding. SURF features (A and B) are labeled so that annotations can be maintained though surgical manipulation.

of voice-controlled virtual assistants (e.g., Alexa) obliges us to revisit speech as a surgical interface.

We use Google Cloud Speech-to-Text in our experiments. The online service allows the surgeon to apply arbitrary semantic labels; offline tools or preset vocabularies may be preferred in resource-constrained settings. Qualitatively, we observed satisfactory recognition during demos using a commodity wireless speaker-microphone, and this performance was retained in a noisy exhibition room by switching to a wireless headset, suggesting that the clinical benefits of speech interfaces may soon be realizable.

Persistent Tissue Tracking. After the surgeon creates a label, the system maintains its adherence by encoding the underlying tissue and tracking it as the lung moves, deforms, or reappears in view following an exit or occlusion. This provides an intuition of the lung state, with similar issues faced in liver surgery. The labeling task asks that arbitrary patches of tissue be persistently identified whenever they appear—a combination of online detection and tracking which for endoscopy is well served by SURF and optical flow [12]. SURF can identify tissue through motion and stretching 83% and 99% of the time respectively [30].In *ex vivo* experiments, uniquely identified features could be recovered successfully upon returning into view so long as imaging conditions remain reasonably stable, as illustrated in Fig. 4.

Labels should be displayed, at minimum, when the tissue is at rest, and modern techniques in matching sub-image elements [13,33] show promise in overcoming the challenges of biomedical images [26]. Approaches such as FlowNet can then be used to track moving tissue and enhance the realism of virtual label adherence. In short, there is a new set of tools to address traditional computer vision problems in endoscopy.

3.3 Capturing Surgeon Expertise

Interactive endoscopy ties maturing technologies together into a novel application with forgiving performance requirements, paving the way to the level of robustness needed for clinical use. The simplicity of the concept belies its potential to alleviate cognitive load, which can impact both judgment and motor skills [7]. When the surgeon exerts mental energy in parsing what they see, the system lets them translate that expertise directly onto the virtual surgical field. This mitigates redundant exploration, and the visibility of labels can help them infer context more readily.

In fact, many surgeons already use radiopaque, tethered (iVATS), dye [31], and ad hoc electrocautery markers to aid localization prior to or during surgery. These varied practices introduce risk and overhead, whereas virtual markers are easy to use and provide a reason for use, potentially bridging gaps between clinical practices and supporting technology. Moreover, surgeon engagement with technology has a broader implication: digitization of the innards of surgery, which has been a black box. Digital labels offer a chance to capture semantic, positional, temporal, visual, and procedural elements of surgery, forming a statistical basis for understanding—and anticipating—surgical acts at multiple scales. This, in turn, can help make augmented reality a clinical reality.

4 Conclusions

The promise of augmented reality in surgery has been tempered by challenges such as soft tissue deformation, and efforts to overcome this timeless adversary has inadvertently suspended critical debates on the role of augmented perception in medicine altogether. We present, as a technological bridge, a streamlined user interface that allows surgeons to tag the disjoint views that comprise endoscopic surgery. These virtual labels persist as the organ moves, so surgeons can potentially manage unfamiliar tissue more deterministically. This approach embraces the finiteness of human cognition and alleviates reliance on cognitive state, capturing expert perception and judgment without attempting to emulate it. We design a minimal feature set and a choice architecture with symmetric freedom to use or not, respecting differences between surgeons. Our baseline system demonstrates promising performance in a lab setting, while rapid ongoing developments in the constituent technologies offer a path towards clinical robustness. These circumstances present the opportunity for surgeons to change surgery, without being compelled to change.

References

1. Healthcare Cost and Utilization Project. https://hcupnet.ahrq.gov/#setup
2. Reduced lung-cancer mortality with low-dose computed tomographic screening. New Engl. J. Med. **365**(5), 395–409 (2011)
3. Allaf, M.E., et al.: Laparoscopic visual field. Surg. Endosc. **12**(12), 1415–1418 (1998)
4. Balicki, M., et al.: Interactive OCT annotation and visualization for vitreoretinal surgery. In: Linte, C.A., Chen, E.C.S., Berger, M.-O., Moore, J.T., Holmes, D.R. (eds.) AE-CAI 2012. LNCS, vol. 7815, pp. 142–152. Springer, Heidelberg (2013). https://doi.org/10.1007/978-3-642-38085-3_14
5. Bernhardt, S., Nicolau, S.A., Soler, L., Doignon, C.: The status of augmented reality in laparoscopic surgery as of 2016. Med. Image Anal. **37**, 66–90 (2017)

6. Bodenstedt, S., et al.: Comparative evaluation of instrument segmentation and tracking methods in minimally invasive surgery (2018)

7. Carswell, C.M., Clarke, D., Seales, W.B.: Assessing mental workload during laparoscopic surgery. Surg. Innov. **12**(1), 80–90 (2005)

8. Chauvet, P., et al.: Augmented reality in a tumor resection model. Surg. Endosc. **32**(3), 1192–1201 (2018)

9. Collins, T., Bartoli, A., Bourdel, N., Canis, M.: Robust, real-time, dense and deformable 3D organ tracking in laparoscopic videos. In: Ourselin, S., Joskowicz, L., Sabuncu, M.R., Unal, G., Wells, W. (eds.) MICCAI 2016. LNCS, vol. 9900, pp. 404–412. Springer, Cham (2016). https://doi.org/10.1007/978-3-319-46720-7_47

10. Doignon, C., Nageotte, F., de Mathelin, M.: Segmentation and guidance of multiple rigid objects for intra-operative endoscopic vision. In: Vidal, R., Heyden, A., Ma, Y. (eds.) WDV 2005-2006. LNCS, vol. 4358, pp. 314–327. Springer, Heidelberg (2007). https://doi.org/10.1007/978-3-540-70932-9_24

11. Du, X., et al.: Robust surface tracking combining features, intensity and illumination compensation. Int. J. Comput. Assist. Radiol. Surg. **10**(12), 1915–1926 (2015)

12. Elhawary, H., Popovic, A.: Robust feature tracking on the beating heart for a robotic-guided endoscope. Int. J. Med. Robot. Comput. Assist. Surg. **7**(4), 459–468 (2011)

13. Fischer, P., Dosovitskiy, A., Brox, T.: Descriptor matching with convolutional neural networks: a comparison to SIFT (2014)

14. Flores, R.M., et al.: Video-assisted thoracoscopic surgery (VATS) lobectomy: catastrophic intraoperative complications. J. Thorac. Cardiovasc. Surg. **142**(6), 1412–1417 (2011)

15. Fuchs, H., et al.: Augmented reality visualization for laparoscopic surgery. In: Wells, W.M., Colchester, A., Delp, S. (eds.) MICCAI 1998. LNCS, vol. 1496, pp. 934–943. Springer, Heidelberg (1998). https://doi.org/10.1007/BFb0056282

16. Kim, J.-H., Bartoli, A., Collins, T., Hartley, R.: Tracking by detection for interactive image augmentation in laparoscopy. In: Dawant, B.M., Christensen, G.E., Fitzpatrick, J.M., Rueckert, D. (eds.) WBIR 2012. LNCS, vol. 7359, pp. 246–255. Springer, Heidelberg (2012). https://doi.org/10.1007/978-3-642-31340-0_26

17. Kinsinger, L.S., et al.: Implementation of lung cancer screening in the Veterans Health Administration. JAMA Intern. Med. **177**(3), 399–406 (2017)

18. Lee, C.Y., et al.: Novel thoracoscopic navigation system with augmented real-time image guidance for chest wall tumors. Ann. Thorac. Surg. **106**(5), 1468–1475 (2018)

19. Lin, J., et al.: Dual-modality endoscopic probe for tissue surface shape reconstruction and hyperspectral imaging enabled by deep neural networks. Med. Image Anal. **48**, 162–176 (2018)

20. Liu, W.P., Richmon, J.D., Sorger, J.M., Azizian, M., Taylor, R.H.: Augmented reality and CBCT guidance for transoral robotic surgery. J. Robot. Surg. **9**(3), 223–233 (2015)

21. Mahmoud, N., Collins, T., Hostettler, A., Soler, L., Doignon, C., Montiel, J.M.M.: Live tracking and dense reconstruction for handheld monocular endoscopy. IEEE Trans. Med. Imaging **38**(1), 79–89 (2019)

22. Maier-Hein, L., et al.: Optical techniques for 3D surface reconstruction in computer-assisted laparoscopic surgery. Med. Image Anal. **17**(8), 974–996 (2013)

23. Mountney, P., Yang, G.-Z.: Motion compensated SLAM for image guided surgery. In: Jiang, T., Navab, N., Pluim, J.P.W., Viergever, M.A. (eds.) MICCAI 2010. LNCS, vol. 6362, pp. 496–504. Springer, Heidelberg (2010). https://doi.org/10.1007/978-3-642-15745-5_61

24. Nicolau, S., Soler, L., Mutter, D., Marescaux, J.: Augmented reality in laparoscopic surgical oncology. Surg. Oncol. **20**(3), 189–201 (2011)
25. Puerto-Souza, G.A., Cadeddu, J.A., Mariottini, G.L.: Toward long-term and accurate augmented-reality for monocular endoscopic videos. IEEE Trans. Biomed. Eng. **61**(10), 2609–2620 (2014)
26. Ronneberger, O., Fischer, P., Brox, T.: U-net: convolutional networks for biomedical image segmentation. In: Navab, N., Hornegger, J., Wells, W.M., Frangi, A.F. (eds.) MICCAI 2015. LNCS, vol. 9351, pp. 234–241. Springer, Cham (2015). https://doi.org/10.1007/978-3-319-24574-4_28
27. Shvets, A.A., Rakhlin, A., Kalinin, A.A., Iglovikov, V.I.: Automatic instrument segmentation in robot-assisted surgery using deep learning. In: IEEE International Conference on Machine Learning and Applications (ICMLA), pp. 624–628 (2018)
28. Sotiras, A., Davatzikos, C., Paragios, N.: Deformable medical image registration: a survey. IEEE Trans. Med. Imaging **32**(7), 1153–1190 (2013)
29. Stoyanov, D., Scarzanella, M.V., Pratt, P., Yang, G.-Z.: Real-time stereo reconstruction in robotically assisted minimally invasive surgery. In: Jiang, T., Navab, N., Pluim, J.P.W., Viergever, M.A. (eds.) MICCAI 2010. LNCS, vol. 6361, pp. 275–282. Springer, Heidelberg (2010). https://doi.org/10.1007/978-3-642-15705-9_34
30. Thienphrapa, P., Bydlon, T., Chen, A., Popovic, A.: Evaluation of surface feature persistence during lung surgery. In: BMES Annual Meeting, Atlanta, GA (2018)
31. Willekes, L., Boutros, C., Goldfarb, M.A.: VATS intraoperative tattooing to facilitate solitary pulmonary nodule resection. J. Cardiothorac. Surg. **3**(1), 13 (2008)
32. Yip, M.C., Lowe, D.G., Salcudean, S.E., Rohling, R.N., Nguan, C.Y.: Tissue tracking and registration for image-guided surgery. IEEE Trans. Med. Imaging **31**(11), 2169–2182 (2012)
33. Zagoruyko, S., Komodakis, N.: Learning to compare image patches via CNNs. In: IEEE Conference on Computer Vision and Pattern Recognition, pp. 4353–4361 (2015)

Non-invasive Assessment of in Vivo Auricular Cartilage by Ultra-short Echo Time (UTE) T_2^* Mapping

Xue Li, Cheng Zhao, and Weiwei Zhang[✉]

Institute of Basic Medical Sciences,
Chinese Academy of Medical Sciences and Peking Union Medical Collage,
Beijing, China
weiwei.zhang@ibms.pumc.edu.cn

Abstract. In this paper, Ultra-short Echo Time (UTE) T_2^* mapping is proposed to non-invasively evaluate auricular cartilages from volunteers and donated bodies. The mono- and bi-exponential models were used for mono- and bi-component analysis (short component T_2^* and long component T_2^*) respectively. The external ears were manually segmented from images and then reconstructed into 3D T_2^* mappings. In the mono-component analysis, the mean T_2^* value for 3 volunteers was 34.987 ± 2.266 ms. As for results from the bi-component analysis, the mean values for 3 volunteers were 8.992 ± 0.466 ms and 53.648 ± 1.961 ms for short component T_2^* and long component T_2^* respectively, with the ratio of bound water to free water of 0.464 ± 0.020. The bi-exponential fitting model performed better than the mono-exponential fitting model on the curve fitting in volunteers, with $R^2[\text{bi}] = 0.999 \pm 0.131$ vs. $R^2[\text{mono}] = 0.972 \pm 0.144$. According to the bi-component analysis from donated specimens of auricular cartilage, the ratio of bound water to free water was 0.023 ± 0.018, which was significantly different from that of volunteers (p < 0.01), but the fitting curves of specimens showed similar findings with volunteers, with $R^2[\text{bi}] = 0.999 \pm 0.001$ vs. $R^2[\text{mono}] = 0.903 \pm 0.005$. Our preliminary results demonstrated that the proposed UTE T_2^* mapping is a feasible non-invasive means for evaluating the development of auricular cartilage scaffold with bio-inks in reconstructive surgery using 3D bioprinting technique.

Keywords: Auricular cartilage · Non-invasive assessment · Ultra-short echo time T_2^* · Component analysis

1 Introduction

Microtia is a congenital deformity where the pinna is underdeveloped, with an incidence of 1 to 10 per 10000 births [1]. Currently, reconstruction with autologous costochondral cartilage is one of the mainstays of surgical management of congenital microtia [2]. However, such surgery brings an extra incision to harvest

© Springer Nature Switzerland AG 2019
D. Shen et al. (Eds.): MICCAI 2019, LNCS 11768, pp. 92–100, 2019.
https://doi.org/10.1007/978-3-030-32254-0_11

the costal cartilage, and the aesthetic outcomes of the surgery highly depend on the experience of the surgeon [3]. In addition to current clinical approaches, the innovative techniques of tissue engineering and 3D bioprinting are becoming parts of the routine clinical practice for microtia [3]. The tissue-engineered cartilage reconstruction has been extensively studied in animal models [4–6], and the 3D bioprinting technique can provide the complex patient-specific ear shapes by depositing biomaterials layer-by-layer in a controllable manner [7]. But there are still many challenges in applying these techniques to clinical practice, such as sourcing the suitable stem cells and fabricating a 3D scaffold onto which cartilage cells can anchor and subsequently grow [8]. Moreover, after the implantation of the complex of tissue-engineered or bio-printed scaffold with cartilage cells, assessing the development of auricular cartilage and the degradation of the scaffold in a non-invasive way is of great importance.

Considering that the follow-up assessment of the reconstructive complex may continue for years, a non-invasive and ALARA (as low as reasonably achievable)-principled means of imaging is highly expected for young microtia patients. Due to the known characteristics of safety, diverse imaging sequences, and excellent soft-tissue contrast in magnetic resonance imaging (MRI), it has been widely used to monitor the changes that occur during biomaterial resorption and neo-tissue remodeling [9]. However, conventional MRI sequences designed with relatively long echo times (TEs), such as rapid acquisition with relaxation enhancement (RARE) and gradient-recalled echo (GRE), are not suited to encode the decaying signal of tissues with ultra-short and short transverse relaxation times (T_2/T_2^*) like cartilage. In general, therefore, it is difficult to quantify longitudinal T_1 or T_2^* [10]. In this paper, we propose a method of utilizing an ultra-short echo time (UTE) sequence with multiple echoes (as short as 0.401 ms) to obtain the short signal of auricular cartilage and a quantitative assessment by using mono- and bi-component analyses to generate 3D T_2^* mappings and curve fittings to distinguish auricular cartilage from surrounding tissues.

2 Method

2.1 UTE and T_2^* Mapping Technique

The UTE sequence uses a short radio frequency (RF) pulse and acquires signals as soon as possible after excitation finishes, so it is possible to obtain signals from the tissue with ultra-short and short T_2^* [10]. UTE sequences can allow for quantitative evaluation, such as evaluation of bi-component fraction of tendon [11]. Measuring T_2^* values is made possible with the acquisition of a series of images with constant repetition time (TR) and variable TE, in which tissue with short T_2^* can be quantified with the UTE sequence [10]. T_2^* values can be used to measure cartilage degeneration with a mono- or bi-exponential decay model due to their dependence on water and collagen contents as well as properties of the extracellular matrix [12].

2.2 Study Subjects and Image Acquisition

All subjects signed informed consent prior to their participation in this study. The study group consisted of 3 healthy volunteers and 3 pairs of auricular cartilage from donated bodies, as summarized in Table 1.

Table 1. Basic information of volunteers and specimens.

Volunteers		Specimens	
Male: female	Average age	Male: female	Average age
2:1	27.3	2:1	79

All images were collected on a 3T MRI scanner (Philips Achieva, Best, The Netherlands, 32 channel coil). For the quantitative T_2^* assessment, a variable echo time sequence was obtained, with sequentially shifted six echo times: TE = $\{0.401, 2.693, 4.986, 7.278, 9.570, 11.863\}$ ms. Other parameters were set as: TR 80 ms, field of view 100 × 100 mm, slice thickness 2 mm, 15° flip angle, and 543 Hz/pixel bandwidth.

2.3 Image Processing

All images were registered to the first echo time image in the sequence using a rigid registration method implemented in MATLAB (v. 2018a, MathWorks, Natick, MA) to correct for intra-subject motions during scanning [11]. After registration, the images were manually segmented by an experienced research assistant. Mono- and bi-component fitting procedures were performed on all datasets. For the mono-component fitting, the signal intensity fitting function was

$$S_m = A_0 \times exp(-TE/A_1) + A_2 \tag{1}$$

where A_0 is the signal intensity at a TE < 1 ms; A_1 corresponds to the actual T_2^*; A_2 is the baseline (mostly the noise). The same datasets were also processed by the bi-component analysis, using the function

$$S_b = B_0 \times exp(-TE/B_1) + B_2 \times exp(-TE/B_3) + B_4 \tag{2}$$

where B_1 corresponds to the short component of T_2^*; B_3 corresponds to the long component of T_2^*; B_0 and B_2 are the component ratios expressed further as a percentage value of $B_0 + B_2$: fraction of short component (F_s) = 100 × B_0 / ($B_0 + B_2$) and fraction of long component (F_l) = 100 × B_2 / ($B_0 + B_2$); B_4 is the offset given primarily by noise [13].

2.4   UTE T_2^* Mapping

We used mono- and bi-component analysis in both volunteer and specimen images. In the mono-component analysis, two different methods were implemented to get the T_2^* mapping image. For the method based on ROI with weighted factors, MRI images in different echo times were respectively calculated with Eq. (1); then, each provided ROI (segmented external ear) was represented by the weighted mean value calculated using an R^2 correction algorithm to get the T_2^* mapping image [13]. The other one, based on voxels (voxel-by-voxel) within ROI, was to utilize voxels with provided ROI of the same coordinates in different images of echo times to generate the T_2^* mapping image, and the T_2^* value of each voxel in the images was calculated with Eq. (1). The second method for computing T_2^* mapping images was applied to the bi-component analysis but with Eq. (2).

The program allowed for ROIs placed on the first image of the series, and these ROIs were then copied to each subsequent echo image. The mean intensity within each ROI was used for curve fitting. To further improve the accuracy of fitting, the formulae of the noise-corrected model were derived and provided to the lsqcurvefit algorithm in MATLAB [14]. For statistical analysis, we expressed continuous variables as mean standard deviation (SD) and categorical data as numbers (percentages), and the regression analysis was used to evaluate the mono- and bi-component analyses. All statistical analyses were performed using SPSS (v.24, IBM Corporation 2016), in which results were considered significant when the probability of making a type I error was less than 5% ($p < 0.05$).

3   Results

As for results from the mono-component analysis, in volunteers, the mean T_2^* value was 34.987 ± 2.266 ms. In the bi-component analysis for volunteers, the mean short component T_2^* was 8.992 ± 0.466 ms; the mean long component T_2^* was 53.648 ± 1.961 ms; the ratio of bound water to free water was 0.464 ± 0.020. The mean T_2^* value from mono-component analysis for specimens was 90.536 ± 3.745 ms. In the bi-component analysis for specimens, the mean short component T_2^* was 19.454 ± 0.446 ms; the mean long component T_2^* was 97.711 ± 1.869 ms; the ratio of bound water to free water was 0.023 ± 0.018 (summarized in Table 2). The ratio of bound water to free water was represented by F_s that was calculated with Eq. (2).

All computed T_2^* values (including the T_2^* value in mono-component analysis, the short component T_2^*, and long component T_2^* values in bi-component analysis) were significantly different between volunteer and specimen ($p < 0.01$). The model with the bi-exponential fitting function computed the values with slightly higher precision than that with a mono-exponential fitting function both in volunteers ($R^2[\text{bi}] = 0.999 \pm 0.131$ vs. $R^2[\text{mono}] = 0.972 \pm 0.144$) and specimens ($R^2[\text{bi}] = 0.999 \pm 0.001$ vs. $R^2[\text{mono}] = 0.903 \pm 0.005$) (summarized in Table 3). The data with the corresponding mono- and bi-exponential curve fittings are plotted in Fig. 1.

Table 2. T_2^* values of volunteers and specimens.

	$T_2^*{}_{mono}$ (ms)	$T_2^*{}_{bi-s}$ (ms)	$T_2^*{}_{bi-l}$ (ms)	Ratio (F_s)
Volunteer 1	32.779	8.540	51.744	0.483
Volunteer 2	34.874	8.966	53.538	0.465
Volunteer 3	37.307	9.470	55.662	0.443
Specimen 1	94.406	19.135	96.393	0.036
Specimen 2	90.272	19.964	99.850	0.002
Specimen 3	86.929	19.263	96.890	0.031
Mean ± SD for Volunteers	34.987 ± 2.266	8.992 ± 0.466	53.648 ± 1.961	0.464 ± 0.020
Mean ± SD for Specimens	90.536 ± 3.745	19.454 ± 0.446	97.711 ± 1.869	0.023 ± 0.018

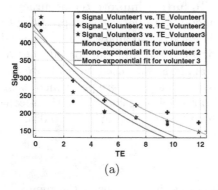

(a)

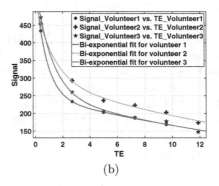

(b)

Fig. 1. (a) The plotted mono-exponential curve fitting of the mean intensity value from 3 volunteers with mean T_2^* value of 34.987 ms ± 2.266 ms and R^2 of 0.972 ± 0.144. (b) The plotted bi-exponential curve fitting of the mean intensity value from 3 volunteers with the mean short component T_2^* of 8.992 ms ± 0.466 ms, the mean long component T_2^* of 53.648 ms ± 1.961 ms, and R^2 of 0.999 ± 0.131.

Table 3. Precision analysis of different fitting models for volunteers and specimens.

	Mono-exponential			Bi-exponential		
	SSE	R-square	RMSE	SSE	R-square	RMSE
Volunteer 1	294.914	0.972	8.587	6.168	0.999	1.756
Volunteer 2	68.019	0.982	4.762	0.018	1	0.137
Volunteer 3	287.199	0.982	8.474	1.763	0.999	0.939
Specimen 1	29.686	0.905	3.146	0.019	0.999	0.137
Specimen 2	43.496	0.904	3.808	0.021	1	0.146
Specimen 3	40.648	0.908	3.681	0.014	1	0.116

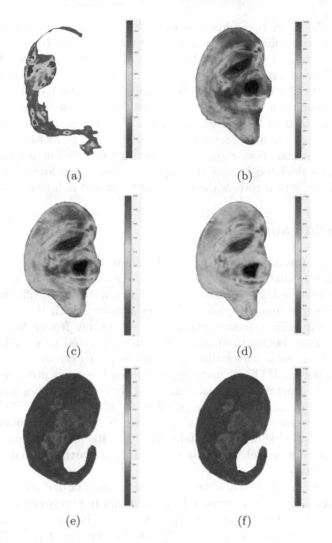

Fig. 2. (a) T_2^* mapping calculated by provided ROI with weighted factors in the mono-component analysis for volunteer 1. The selected slice shows broken structures around helix found in generated 3D T_2^* mapping. (b) T_2^* mapping calculated by using voxel-by-voxel within ROI in the mono-component analysis for volunteer 1. (c) T_2^* mapping of short component calculated by the bi-component analysis for volunteer 1. (d) T_2^* mapping of long component calculated by the bi-component analysis for volunteer 1. (e) T_2^* mapping calculated by using voxel-by-voxel within ROI in the mono-component analysis for specimen 1. (f) T_2^* mapping of short component calculated by the bi-component analysis for specimen 1.

In Fig. 2(a) and (b) showed the mappings of volunteer 1 calculated by the method based on ROI with weighted factors and the method based on voxels (voxel-by-voxel) within ROI (described in 2.4) in the mono-component analysis respectively. The T_2^* mapping image in Fig. 2(b) was visually better than that in Fig. 2(a) due to the difference of manipulating voxels within ROI between methods. From the method using voxel-by-voxel within ROI, T_2^* value of auricular cartilage exhibits in a range of 35 to 65 ms, and it is considered to be fairly long, compared to articular cartilage in several published studies [10,11].

In the bi-component analysis for volunteers, the T_2^* value of short component was in a range of 0 to 20 ms, which implies that the signal of the auricular cartilage may occur at 4 to 13 ms as the elastic cartilage has large amount of bound water that can decay rapidly with short T_2^* signal. The mapping of long component T_2^* calculated by the bi-component model was longer than that of short component, which reveals the biological tissues of rich free water.

4 Discussion and Conclusions

The experimental results showed that images from the multi-echo time sequence are suitable for T_2^* analysis of the auricular cartilage in vivo. In our study, the shortest echo time of UTE sequences is 0.401 ms, which is significantly shorter than that of conventional sequences. Images acquired with dense intervals of echo times in the UTE sequence, particularly echo times from 0 to 10 ms when cartilaginous tissue begins to appear, are highly expected to visualize detailed information about auricular cartilage and reduce fitting errors.

Mono-component UTE T_2^* mapping technique has been previously used to detect tendon degeneration with advantages of shorter scan times and less complex reconstruction algorithms, compared with bi-component UTE T_2^* mapping [11]. However, our study has demonstrated that the bi-component analysis model is able to provide improved quality of curve fitting better than the mono-component analysis model for evaluating auricular cartilage images acquired with high resolution.

From a biochemical point of view, there is the existence of distinct water compartments with different transverse relaxation times in highly organized biological tissues [15]. The short component T_2^* is related to bound water and the long component T_2^* is related to free water [16]. The bi-component UTE T_2^* mapping analysis is useful for monitoring disease- and treatment-related changes in articular cartilage composition and structure with the ability of computing the fraction of bound water which can be used to detect changes in the collagen and bound water content of cartilage [11,13]. Short component T_2^* and long component T_2^* are useful for detecting changes in collagen organization at micro-structural and macro-structural levels [11].

In Table 2, the experimental results have showed that the donated specimens of auricular cartilage contain mainly free water with F_s of more than 90%. The reason is that the postmortem collagen type II fibrils and other proteins degrade so that the bound water is released and then become free water. The results of T_2^* mapping images in donated auricular cartilages have showed that the type of water is significantly different from that in vivo, which reinforced that UTE T_2^* mapping technique is able to distinguish different components of water.

There are two major limitations in the proposed method. One is the small sample size used. In this early experiment phase, we used very small size samples to complete a preliminary study for verifying the feasibility of the method of component analysis. The other one is that the multi-echo UTE imaging protocol requires a scan time of around 18 min. The involuntary movements during scanning can not be avoided and thus arise the problem of intra-subject registration. If large mismatch is found, it is challenging for curve fitting.

In conclusion, the imaging sequence with multi-short echo times is capable of assessing the auricular cartilage in vivo by T_2^* mapping with component analysis. The short component T_2^* can be considered as an imaging marker that reflects the bound water component of the auricular cartilage. Based on these preliminary findings from healthy volunteers, this UTE T_2^* mapping method is expected to be a non-invasive means of dynamically monitoring the development of 3D bio-printed auricular cartilage and evaluating the reconstructive surgery for microtia patients.

Acknowledgement. This work is supported by CAMS Innovation Fund for Medical Sciences (CIFMS) (2017-I2M-1-007). The donated specimens of auricular cartilage were provided by Human Tissue Bank, Neuroscience Center, Chinese Academy of Medical Sciences and Peking Union Medical College. Authors would like to thank Chao Ma, Naili Wang from the above center, and Rui Li, Le He, Yandong Zhu from Center for Biomedical Imaging Research Department of Biomedical Engineering School of Medicine, Tsinghua University, for their supports.

References

1. Bly, R.A., Bhrany, A.D., Murakami, C.S., et al.: Microtia reconstruction. Facial Plast. Surg. Clin. North Am. **24**(4), 577–591 (2016)
2. Patel, R.S., Katzen, B.T.: Autologous costochondral microtia reconstruction. Facial Plast. Surg. **32**(2), 188–198 (2016)
3. Mussi, E., Furferi, R., et al.: Ear reconstruction simulation: from handcrafting to 3D printing. Bioengineering **6**(1), 14 (2019)
4. Reiffel, A.J., Concepcion, K., Hernandez, K.A., et al.: High-fidelity tissue engineering of patient-specific auricles for reconstruction of pediatric microtia and other auricular deformities. PLoS One **8**(2), e56506 (2013)
5. Schroeder, M.J., Lloyd, M.S.: Tissue engineering strategies for auricular reconstruction. J. Craniofac. Surg. **28**(8), 2007–2011 (2017)
6. Cohen, P., Bernstein, J.L., et al.: Tissue engineering the human auricle by auricular chondrocyte-mesenchymal stem cell co-implantation. PLoS One **13**(10), e0202356 (2018)
7. Otto, I.A., Melchels, F.P.W., Zhao, X., et al.: Auricular reconstruction using biofabrication-based tissue engineering strategies. Biofabrication **7**(3), 032001 (2015)
8. Wilkes, G.H., Wong, J., Guilfoyle, R.: Microtia reconstruction. Plast. Reconstr. Surg. **134**(3), 464e–479e (2014)
9. Chen, Z., Yan, C., Yan, S.: Non-invasive monitoring of in vivo hydrogel degradation and cartilage regeneration by multiparametric MR imaging. Theranostics **8**(4), 1146–1158 (2018)

10. Chang, E.Y., Du, J., Chung, C.B.: UTE imaging in the musculoskeletal system. J. Magn. Reson. Imaging **41**(4), 870–883 (2015)
11. Kijowski, R., Wilson, J.J., Liu, F.: Bicomponent ultrashort echo time T_2^* analysis for assessment of patients with patellar tendinopathy: ultrashort TE T_2^* Analysis of Tendinopathy. J. Magn. Reson. Imaging **46**(5), 1441–1447 (2017)
12. Link, T.M., Neumann, J., Li, X.: Prestructural cartilage assessment using MRI. J. Magn. Reson. Imaging **45**(4), 949–965 (2017)
13. Juras, V., Apprich, S., Szomolanyi, P., et al.: Bi-exponential T_2^* analysis of healthy and diseased Achilles tendons: an in vivo preliminary magnetic resonance study and correlation with clinical score. Eur. Radiol. **23**(10), 2814–2822 (2013)
14. Diaz, E., Chung, C.B., Bae, W.C., et al.: Ultrashort echo time spectroscopic imaging (UTESI): an efficient method for quantifying bound and free water. NMR Biomed. **25**(1), 161–168 (2012)
15. Cameron, I.L., Short, N.J., Fullerton, G.D., et al.: Verification of simple hydration/dehydration methods to characterize multiple water compartments on tendon type 1 collagen. Cell Biol. Int. **31**(6), 531–539 (2007)
16. Du, J., Diaz, E., Carl, M., et al.: Ultrashort echo time imaging with bicomponent analysis. Magn. Reson. Med. **67**(3), 645–649 (2012)

INN: Inflated Neural Networks
for IPMN Diagnosis

Rodney LaLonde[1], Irene Tanner[1], Katerina Nikiforaki[2],
Georgios Z. Papadakis[2], Pujan Kandel[3], Candice W. Bolan[3],
Michael B. Wallace[3], and Ulas Bagci[1(✉)]

[1] University of Central Florida (UCF), Orlando, FL, USA
bagci@ucf.edu
[2] Foundation for Research and Technology Hellas (FORTH), Heraklion, Crete, Greece
[3] Mayo Clinic, Jacksonville, FL, USA

Abstract. Intraductal papillary mucinous neoplasm (IPMN) is a precursor to pancreatic ductal adenocarcinoma. While over half of patients
are diagnosed with pancreatic cancer at a distant stage, patients who are
diagnosed early enjoy a much higher 5-year survival rate of 34% compared to 3% in the former; hence, early diagnosis is key. Unique challenges
in the medical imaging domain such as extremely limited annotated data
sets and typically large 3D volumetric data have made it difficult for deep
learning to secure a strong foothold. In this work, we construct two novel
"inflated" deep network architectures, *InceptINN* and *DenseINN*, for the
task of diagnosing IPMN from multisequence (T1 and T2) MRI. These
networks inflate their 2D layers to 3D and bootstrap weights from their
2D counterparts (Inceptionv3 and DenseNet121 respectively) trained on
ImageNet to the new 3D kernels. We also extend the inflation process by
further expanding the pre-trained kernels to handle any number of input
modalities and different fusion strategies. This is one of the first studies to
train an end-to-end deep network on multisequence MRI for IPMN diagnosis, and shows that our proposed novel inflated network architectures
are able to handle the extremely limited training data (139 MRI scans),
while providing an absolute improvement of **8.76%** in accuracy for diagnosing IPMN over the current state-of-the-art. Code is publicly available
at https://github.com/lalonderodney/INN-Inflated-Neural-Nets.

Keywords: IPMN · Pancreatic cancer · Inflated networks · MRI ·
CAD

1 Introduction

Pancreatic cancer is currently the fourth leading cause of cancer-related death
in the United States in both men and women, behind Lung & Bronchus, Breast
(women)/Prostate (men), and Colon & Rectum. These latter four forms of cancer have all seen massive declines in mortality over the past decades; however,
the same cannot be said for pancreatic cancer, which has seen an increase in

© Springer Nature Switzerland AG 2019
D. Shen et al. (Eds.): MICCAI 2019, LNCS 11768, pp. 101–109, 2019.
https://doi.org/10.1007/978-3-030-32254-0_12

both occurrence and mortality from 2006 to 2017. Worse still, pancreatic cancer continues to carry one of the poorest prognoses of any form of cancer at a grim 9% 5-year survival rate [1]. Because the cancer has usually spread beyond the pancreas by the time it is diagnosed, less than 20% of patients are candidates for surgery. However, for cases in which diagnosis occurs while the disease is still local, which is true for approximately 10% of patients, the 5-year survival rate has been steadily increasing from 29% to 32% to 34% from 2017 to 2019 [1]. For these reasons, early diagnosis will be vital to increase the five-year survival rate of pancreatic cancer and make surgery a viable option for more patients.

Diagnosing Intraductal Papillary Mucinous Neoplasm

Intraductal papillary mucinous neoplasm (IPMN) is a radiographically detectable neoplasm that is found in the main and branch pancreatic ducts and is often a precursor to pancreatic ductal adenocarcinoma. IPMN has the potential to progress into invasive carcinoma, as a large proportion of main duct-IPMN exhibits malignant progression. Example magnetic resonance imaging (MRI) scans with the associated grade of IPMN are shown in Fig. 1, where the scans are cropped to a regions of interest (ROI) surrounding the pancreas. In this study, the cases of IPMN were graded in a pathology report after surgery: (0) normal, (1) low-grade IPMN, (2) high-grade IPMN, and (3) invasive carcinoma. Being able to accurately detect IPMN early may help diagnose pancreatic cancer sooner and, in turn, increase the abysmally low 5-year survival rates. While progress has been made in diagnosing and managing IPMN preoperatively using the radiographic criteria and international consensus guidelines, automated computer-aided diagnosis (CAD) systems are a strong candidate for helping with this task. CAD systems could be used to distinguish IPMN in the pancreas and differentiate between grades potentially more efficiently and effectively than current standards.

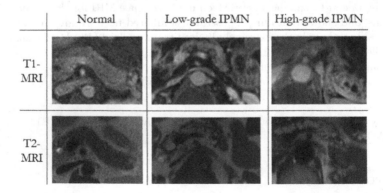

Fig. 1. Pancreas-ROIs from T1 & T2-weighted MRI scans with the associated grades of IPMN from the post-surgery pathology report.

Literature on Classification of Pancreatic Cysts

There are very few studies attempting to diagnose IPMN from MRI scans, and the presented work in this study is one of the first in literature to diagnose IPMN in MRI scans using deep learning. Hussein et al. [8] introduced an architecture for automatic IPMN classification using a pre-trained 3D convolutional neural network (CNN) to perform feature extraction with canonical correlation analysis and feature fusion. Unlike [8], our proposed approach allows for novel 3D network structures, intermediate fusion strategies, and end-to-end training.

Although the goal is not related to IPMN diagnosis, Chen et al. [3] proposed PCN-Net, a study which can be considered a relevant work to ours because PCN-Net aims to classify pancreatic cystic neoplasms (PCNs). Briefly, the proposed network structure uses the 2D Inceptionv3 [11] as a backbone, pre-trained on ImageNet [10] and fine-tuned on optical coherence tomography images. MRI sequences are aligned with a Z-Continuity Filter and combined using a late fusion strategy. Unlike [3], our proposed approach utilizes 3D networks, again allows for intermediate fusion strategies, and does not require additional costly pre-training on external medical datasets. Furthermore, we focus on a relatively more challenging problem of IPMN diagnosis, not PCNs. Other studies in literature have focused on the use of pre-deep learning strategies such as conventional radiomics measurements (texture, intensity, and component enhancing features) to classify IPMNs. Not only is the success of these features fundamentally limited compared to deep learning-based approaches, but also these studies have focused on using CT images and require a priori segmentation of the pancreas [4,6], which itself is a challenging process.

Proposed Solution: Multimodal Inflated Neural Networks

While newer and more powerful deep network architectures continue to emerge, a difficulty arises when the new architecture differs in structure, preventing efficient weight transfer from pre-trained models. This is especially an issue in the medical imaging domain where annotated data is extremely limited and utilizing pre-trained deep networks often leads to dramatic performance increases. Additionally, due to the 3D nature of most medical imaging modalities, 3D networks tend to outperform their 2D counterparts, but most pre-trained networks exist only in 2D versions. There currently exists two solutions to this challenging problem. First, researchers can take their novel architecture and train on existing large datasets (e.g. ImageNet). This solution, however, is impractical and prohibitively expensive for many researchers. While some recent works in the literature have been proposed for shortening the typically multi-week process of training on ImageNet [5], these approaches typically require large clusters of GPUs for processing.

The other solution is to cannibalize existing pre-trained networks and transfer weights in a process often referred to as "network surgery". Carreira and Zisserman [2] used this strategy to great effect in a process they called "network inflation" to inflate the Inceptionv1 network for the task of action recognition. The network inflation process swaps out all 2D convolutional kernels and pooling operations for their 3D counterparts and replicates the kernels along the third dimension, while dividing the value of the weights by the number of replications to preserve relatively similar activation values. Liu et al. [9] proposed AH-Net, which inflated part of its architecture from 2D for lesion segmentation. In this work, we follow a similar strategy of network inflation to inflate deeper, more advanced, and more complicatedly-connected networks while also tackling the issue of transferring weights when we have multiple imaging modalities.

Several different fusion strategies exist for combining imaging modalities: early (pixel-level) fusion, intermediate fusion, and late fusion. In early fusion, images from different modalities are simply concatenated at the pixel level before being input to the network. In late fusion, inputs are fed to the network separately and the final embeddings are concatenated and fed to the final classification layers. Intermediate fusion is between early and late fusion, where information from multiple modalities are combined somewhere in the network. Which of these strategies is best depends on how similar the information is in each modality. Working with multiple modalities as input to a neural network adds an additional challenge for transferring weights from pre-trained networks, which typically accept only three-channel images as input. Transferring the weights of these earliest layers is critical for transfer learning, as these lowest-level layers have been found to share filters across virtually any imaging data, while higher-level layers become more specialized to the specific training data.

Summary of Our Contributions
(1) In this work, we construct two novel inflated deep network architectures, *InceptINN* and *DenseINN*, transferring weights from their 2D counterparts (Inceptionv3 [11] and DenseNet121 [7] respectively) trained on ImageNet to the new 3D kernels. (2) We extend the inflation process by further expanding the pre-trained kernels to handle any number of input modalities and different fusion strategies. In general, this modification is the key component for any image-based diagnosis system accepting multiple image modalities as input. Particularly for our study, since T1- and T2-weighted MRI scans are the modality of choice for IPMN diagnosis, there is a strong need to combine the complementary information of both imaging modalities. The proposed network architecture provides the needed flexibility both at the input and fusion levels. (3) We investigate both early fusion as well as a version of intermediate fusion in greater detail and perform image-based diagnosis experiments at both the whole-MRI and pancreas-ROI levels for comprehensive evaluations, which have never been done in the literature before. (4) To our best of knowledge, our study is also the first one to train an end-to-end deep network on multisequence MRI for IPMN diagnosis. (5) Finally, we demonstrate that our newly designed inflated network architectures have a major advantage over the state-of-the-art by utilizing the extremely limited training data (139 MRI scans) while still obtaining an absolute improvement in accuracy for diagnosing IPMN of **8.76%**.

2   Methods

The overview of our proposed framework is shown in Fig. 2. During training and testing, k slices from either whole MRI scans or cropped pancreas-ROIs are used

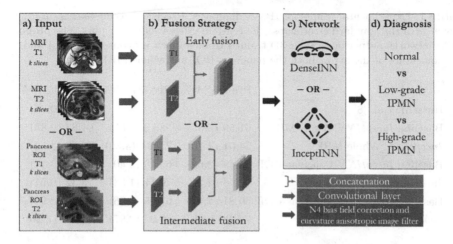

Fig. 2. Proposed network inflation framework overview.

as input to one of our deep networks. Prior to entering the network, MRI scans are preprocessed by first aligning the T1 scans to the T2 scans using b-spline registration, then performing N4 bias field correction and applying a curvature anisotropic image filter. Following this, the k slices of each modality are either concatenated along the channel axis ($height \times width \times slices \times channels$) and input to the network or are input separately, depending on if the early or intermediate fusion strategy is being followed. If intermediate fusion is chosen, each modality is passed through its own convolutional layer before being concatenated and passed through the remainder or the network. At the end of the network, either *InceptINN* or *DenseINN*, a softmax output over three values is obtained, representing the probability of our three possible grades of IPMN.

INN: Inflating Neural Networks

INN is a relatively straightforward two-step process. A 2D network is chosen for which pre-trained weights are available without needing major modifications to the overall network architecture that cannot be corrected with basic network surgery. The first step simply requires changing all 2D layers to their corresponding 3D counterparts (e.g. 2D convolution becomes 3D convolution, 2D pooling becomes 3D pooling). The choice of convolutional kernel size, pooling size, or stride length in this new third dimension is somewhat application dependant. For example, if training on a 30 fps video, one can afford larger kernels, strides, and pooling in the third dimension. For the application of IPMN diagnosis in MRI, since the pancreas typically only occupies a relatively small number of slices, we chose to favor strides of one in this new third dimension. For square kernels, we chose to extend these to cubes; however, for the $h \times 1$ or $1 \times w$ kernels, we chose to extend the third dimension to be $h \times 1 \times 1$ or $1 \times w \times 1$.

The second step is to transfer the weights from the 2D kernels to the 3D kernels by bootstrapping them along the third dimension. This is accomplished by tiling the weights along the new dimension, then dividing all of the values

Table 1. Experimental results for IPMN diagnosis. Precision, recall, and accuracy are shown with the standard error across the ten-fold cross-validation splits. The proposed *INN* networks outperforms their 3D trained from scratch versions (baselines) and the previous state-of-the-art at both the pancreas-ROI and whole-MRI levels.

Method	Pre (SEM)%	Rec (SEM)%	Acc (SEM)%
Hussein et al. [8]	–	–	64.67 (0.83)
Baseline *InceptINN* Whole-MRI	61.59 (5.83)	58.18 (4.05)	61.87 (2.83)
InceptINN Whole-MRI	74.51 (4.70)	**71.24** (4.39)	73.38 (3.52)
Baseline *InceptINN* Pancreas-ROI	68.49 (2.63)	69.18 (3.40)	69.37 (3.11)
InceptINN Pancreas-ROI	71.68 (2.25)	70.11 (1.33)	72.32 (0.97)
Baseline *DenseINN* Pancreas-ROI	66.81 (4.51)	67.05 (3.06)	67.16 (2.93)
DenseINN Pancreas-ROI	**78.20** (4.17)	69.09 (2.97)	**73.43** (2.26)

of the kernel by the new depth of the kernel. This division is important to keep the network activations approximately the same from layer to layer. It may be straightforward when working with RGB images, but it can quickly become complicated with non-three-channel images and multiple imaging modalities.

Handling Multiple Imaging Modalities

There is a critical limitation of not having the proper number of kernels in the first convolutional layer when using a 2D network pre-trained on ImageNet with non-RGB images. This becomes even more worrisome when you want to extend to multiple imaging modalities. In this work, we introduce the following strategies for handling multiple modalities while still allowing for the transfer of pre-trained weights. First, since the majority of medical imaging modalities (e.g. MRI, computed tomography) are single-channel, we tile the images to create three-channel images. This would be sufficient for a single modality input, but not for multiple modalities. If we are following the early fusion strategy, these three-channel images are concatenated prior to input into the network. Therefore, for each modality M, we create a copy of the first layer's kernels not only along the third dimension during the inflation process, but also along the input channel axis for the number of modalities given ($kern_h \times kern_w \times kern_d * 1 \times |M| * channels$). This also increases the amount we divide the kernel values by a factor of $|M|$.

If we are following the intermediate fusion strategy, the original first convolutional layer simply transfers copies of its weights (now also tiled along the new third dimension) to each modalities' individual convolution layer. These initial layer kernels are only divided by the length of the new third dimension. After these layers, the results are all concatenated and fed into the remainder of the network. The first layer after concatenation is now the one which must have M copies made of its kernels along the input channel dimension and its values divided by $|M|$. *DenseINN* adds some further complications due to the addition of concatenation layers starting from the second layer, but careful bookkeeping avoids any confusion.

Table 2. Examining the role of different fusion strategies. Precision, recall, and accuracy are shown comparing early versus intermediate fusion on a single training fold.

Method	Early fusion			Intermediate fusion		
	Pre %	Rec %	Acc %	Pre %	Rec %	Acc %
InceptINN Whole-MRI	69.44	66.35	73.33	66.67	59.68	66.67
InceptINN Pancreas-ROI	79.29	**80.48**	78.57	70.77	69.66	75.00
DenseINN Pancreas-ROI	73.08	73.08	75.00	**88.10**	75.21	**82.14**

3   Experiments and Results

Images were split across three categories: normal (i.e. no IPMN was present), low-grade IPMN, and high-grade IPMN/invasive carcinoma. Whole-MRI experiments used 139 scans, of which 29 were normal, 45 were low-grade, and 65 were high-grade. Due to the challenging nature of cropping the pancreas-ROI, two sets of crops were extracted by two experts. In cases where an expert could not confidently extract a pancreas-ROI, this scan was skipped, yielding 271 pancreas-ROIs. Experiments were carried out corresponding to each of the '-or-'s in our framework overview shown in Fig. 2. The results are summarized in Table 1 for the intermediate fusion strategy. For all experiments, slices is set to $k = 5$, excluding the experiments specifically examining the effect of k shown in Table 3. Unless otherwise specified, all experiments were conducted with stratified 10-fold cross-validation. Although the main focus of this work is on inflated networks and not modality fusion strategies, a set of experiments was conducted across one training fold to determine the relative performance of the two fusion strategies, with results shown in Table 2. Note, experiments were not performed with *DenseINN* for whole-MRI due to memory constraints. Whole-MRI images are resized in-plane to 256×256 and pancreas-ROIs are resized to 128×128.

All training and testing was performed using Keras with TensorFlow on a single Titan-X GPU with 12G memory. The Adam optimizer was used with its default parameters, early stopping, and learning rate reduction by 0.05 on loss plateau. At training, input batches are formed by first sliding through each set of k slices containing the pancreas in a given scan, before moving on to the next scan. At testing, k slices are chosen around a central slice, where this slice is determined as the one in which the pancreas appears the largest. For pancreas-ROI images, a batch size of 32 was used for both networks. Due to memory limitations, *InceptINN* used a batch size of 16 when using the whole-MRI. The average test time for InceptINN per patient on a single Titan X GPU is 0.2 sec for whole-slide MRI and 0.05 seconds for pancreas-ROI of MRI.

4   Discussion and Concluding Remarks

In this work, we demonstrate the effectiveness of inflating deep CNNs for the task of IPMN diagnosis, and train two different end-to-end, novel network architectures on the extremely limited multisequence MRI data set. Our proposed

Table 3. Examining the role of 3D context information. Precision, recall, and accuracy are shown for *InceptINN* on a single training fold on both whole-MRI and pancreas-ROI inputs. Note: the whole-MRI level at $k = 7$ slices is unable to fit into GPU memory, even at a reduced batch size, and thus was not included in experiments.

k slices	Whole-MRI			Pancreas-ROI		
	Pre%	Rec%	Acc%	Pre%	Rec%	Acc%
$k = 3$	57.22	56.83	60.00	82.83	**83.76**	**85.71**
$k = 5$	**66.67**	**59.68**	**66.67**	70.77	69.66	75.00
$k = 7$	–	–	–	**85.45**	81.91	82.14

networks, *InceptINN* and *DenseINN*, outperform the previous state-of-the-art by over 8% when operating either on a cropped bounding box around the pancreas or when using the entire MRI. One fundamental advantage of the proposed approach is that it is flexible enough to adapt almost any network structures to volumetric data while any number of input modalities can be handled. We have also showed that while *InceptINN* tended to favor the early fusion approach, *DenseINN* favored the intermediate fusion approach instead. Although our observations were empirical, full cross validation experiments can be performed as an extension of this study to determine if this is a data driven or network structure driven preference.

References

1. American Cancer Society: Cancer Facts & Figures 2019. American Cancer Society, Atlanta (2019)
2. Carreira, J., Zisserman, A.: Quo vadis, action recognition? A new model and the kinetics dataset. In: proceedings of the IEEE Conference on Computer Vision and Pattern Recognition, pp. 6299–6308 (2017)
3. Chen, W., et al.: Classification of pancreatic cystic neoplasms based on multi-modality images. In: Shi, Y., Suk, H.-I., Liu, M. (eds.) MLMI 2018. LNCS, vol. 11046, pp. 161–169. Springer, Cham (2018). https://doi.org/10.1007/978-3-030-00919-9_19
4. Gazit, L., et al.: Quantification of CT images for the classification of high-and low-risk pancreatic cysts. In: SPIE Medical Imaging International Society for Optics and Photonics, p. 101340X (2017)
5. Goyal, P., et al.: Accurate, large minibatch SGD: training imagenet in 1 hour. arXiv preprint arXiv:1706.02677 (2017)
6. Hanania, A., et al.: Quantitative imaging to evaluate malignant potential of IPMNs. Oncotarget **7**(52), 85776 (2016)
7. Huang, G., Liu, Z., Van Der Maaten, L., Weinberger, K.Q.: Densely connected convolutional networks. In: Proceedings of the IEEE Conference on Computer Vision and Pattern Recognition, pp. 4700–4708 (2017)
8. Hussein, S., Kandel, P., Corral, J., Bolan, C., Wallace, M., Bagci, U.: Deep multi-modal classification of intraductal papillary mucinous neoplasms (IPMN) with canonical correlation analysis. In: IEEE International Symposium on Biomedical Imaging (2018)

9. Liu, S., et al.: 3D anisotropic hybrid network: transferring convolutional features from 2D images to 3D anisotropic volumes. In: Frangi, A.F., Schnabel, J.A., Davatzikos, C., Alberola-López, C., Fichtinger, G. (eds.) MICCAI 2018. LNCS, vol. 11071, pp. 851–858. Springer, Cham (2018). https://doi.org/10.1007/978-3-030-00934-2_94

10. Russakovsky, O., et al.: ImageNet large scale visual recognition challenge. IJCV **115**, 211–252 (2015)

11. Szegedy, C., Vanhoucke, V., Ioffe, S., Shlens, J., Wojna, Z.: Rethinking the inception architecture for computer vision. In: Proceedings of the IEEE Conference on Computer Vision and Pattern Recognition, pp. 2818–2826 (2016)

Development of a Multi-objective Optimized Planning Method for Microwave Liver Tumor Ablation

Libin Liang[1,2], Derek Cool[3], Nirmal Kakani[4], Guangzhi Wang[1(✉)], Hui Ding[1], and Aaron Fenster[2,3]

[1] Department of Biomedical Engineering, Tsinghua University, Beijing, China
wgz-dea@tsinghua.edu.cn
[2] Robarts Research Institute, Western University, London, ON, Canada
[3] Department of Medical Imaging, Western University, London, ON, Canada
[4] Department of Radiology, Manchester Royal Infirmary, Manchester, UK

Abstract. Microwave ablation (MWA) is an effective minimal invasive therapy of hepatic cancer. Preoperative treatment planning is key to successful ablation, which aims to find a plan with the minimum number of electrode trajectories, least damage to surrounding tissues, while satisfying multiple clinical constraints. However, this is a multiple objective optimization problem, making it very challenging to find an optimized plan while achieving all the above goals, especially for larger tumors. In this paper, we present a set cover-based method, which can provide Pareto optimal solutions for MWA planning. Evaluation has been performed on 6 tumors with varied sizes selected by interventionalists. Results show that all the generated plans satisfied the clinical constraints and the Pareto optimal solutions are useful to find a suitable trade-off between the number of electrode trajectories and damage to normal tissues.

Keywords: Treatment planning · Microwave ablation · Set cover · Liver cancer · Pareto optimization

1 Introduction

Microwave ablation (MWA) is an effective local thermal therapy for hepatic cancer, which is used widely clinically. The procedure involves percutaneous insertion of one or more electrodes into a liver tumor, ablating it by thermal heating using microwave energy [1]. To completely destroy the tumor with a low rate of complications, preoperative planning of the MWA electrode trajectories and locations in the tumor is required. Conventional manual planning is based on the patient's CT images, which does not guarantee an optimal plan, possibly leading to incomplete tumor ablation and unnecessary excessive amount of ablated normal liver tissue. Therefore, computer assisted planning methods are needed to improve the planning process.

Electronic supplementary material The online version of this chapter (https://doi.org/10.1007/978-3-030-32254-0_13) contains supplementary material, which is available to authorized users.

Several related planning methods have been developed for radio-frequency ablation (RFA) [2–6], which are also applicable to MWA. These methods focused on electrode trajectories optimization and aimed to find the optimal trajectories satisfying multiple clinical constraints. Only a few methods were proposed specifically for MWA. These studies focused on simulation of the necrosis area [7] and visualization of the treatment plan [8].

Since the MWA electrodes can generate larger ablation zones than RFA electrodes, MWA can be also used for larger tumors (>4 cm in diameter) [9]. However, all the planning methods mentioned above are not suitable for treatment planning of larger tumors, as these methods do not address the optimization of multiple overlapping ablations. Planning of MWA for large tumors should achieve the following goals: (1) satisfy multiple clinical constraints including insertion length limit, liver capsule insertion angle limit, no crossing of critical structures and no collision between MWA electrodes; (2) minimize the number of electrodes and ablations to completely ablate the tumor; and (3) minimize damage to normal tissues. Typically, the number of required MWA electrodes can be reduced by increasing the size of the ablation zone, but a larger ablation zone may cause more damage to normal tissues. Therefore, it cannot be guaranteed that the above planning goals are optimized simultaneously. Several methods have been developed to optimize the multiple overlapping ablations for better tumor coverage [10–12]. These methods mainly focused on goals (2) and (3) mentioned above but did not consider the multiple clinical constraints during the optimization, which may generate plans that are not clinically acceptable. Moreover, the tradeoff between different objectives was not considered.

In this paper, we propose a novel multi-objective optimized planning method for MWA, which can be used for liver tumors of various sizes. Key features of our work are: (1) a 2-stages set cover-based method is proposed, which can integrate multiple clinical constraints; and (2) the concept of Pareto optimality is used. With different sizes of ablation zones, the set-cover based planning method can generate multiple plans, from which the Pareto optimal plans can be found with the suitable tradeoff between the number of electrodes and damage to normal tissues.

2   Methods

The method's framework is shown in Fig. 1. Since the ablation plan requires that the ablation zone should extend beyond the tumor to ensure complete tumor ablation, we define the tumor plus 5 mm safety margin as the *treatment zone*. We also define sets I and J as electrode's potential target and entry positions respectively and set K as points in the treatment zone.

2.1   Preprocessing

Our method requires 3D CT images with the liver, tumor, and critical structures (ribs, vessels, and lungs) segmented and resampled on a 1 mm × 1 mm × 1 mm voxel grid. The segmented structures are used by our method to find the optimal plan. To obtain set I (potential target positions), we calculated a convex hull encompassing the treatment

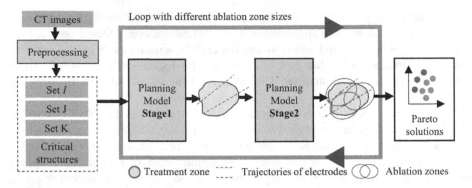

Fig. 1. The proposed method framework. Sets *I* and *J* are the potential target and entry positions of the electrodes respectively, and set *K* refers to points in the treatment zone.

zone, which was voxelized to generate a convex voxel-based volume. This was followed by 5 mm–10 mm morphological erosion, which was applied to the convex volume to obtain the treatment zone interior. Set *I* was then generated by down-sampling the treatment zone interior with 2 mm–6 mm voxel grid (depending on tumor size).

To obtain set J (potential entry positions), the anterior and lateral part of the abdominal skin, which covers the liver, were segmented. Then, the skin points were down-sampled to ensure that the distances between adjacent points ranged from 4 mm to 6 mm (approximately two to three times the diameter of a MWA electrode). Each skin point was then connected to all the positions in set *I* to generate all possible trajectories. To examine the clinical feasibility of these trajectories, a fast voxel traversal method [13] was used to check if trajectories cross any critical structures and to find the intersections between trajectories and the liver capsule. For each skin point, the number of feasible trajectories (defined as NF) was determined, and only the 500 skin points with highest NF were used to compose set *J*.

Set *K* (points in the treatment zone) was composed of two subsets: (i) Union of points down-sampled from the boundary of the treatment zone (with 2 mm–4 mm voxel grid) and vertices of the treatment zone's convex hull, and (ii) Points down-sampled from the treatment zone with coarser voxel grid (5 mm–7 mm depending on tumor size).

2.2   2-Stages Set Cover-Based Planning Method

First Stage. Given the ablation zone, the MWA planning method is similar to the minimum set cover problem. The treatment zone is considered as a universal set. An ablation zone determined by an entry and a target positions covers part of the treatment zone, which can be considered as a subset of the universal set, as shown in Fig. 1. The main goal of the planning method is to find the minimum number of ablation zones (subsets) to cover the treatment zone (the universal set). Typically, the ablation zone can be modeled as an ellipsoid or a sphere for each electrode. In clinical practice, multiple ablations can be performed along one electrode trajectory using the pullback technique. In this case, the ablation zone can be modeled as a cylinder. Based on the description above, the first stage of our model is formulated as follows:

$$\min\left(\sum_{ij}(N_K+M)W_{ij}+\sum_{ij\in\Omega}W_{ij}\cdot L_i-\sum_{ijk}W_{ij}\cdot \text{sgn}(C^{ca}_{ijk}+C^{ce}_{ijk})\right) \qquad (1)$$

$$\Omega=\left((i,j)|\sum_k W_{ij}\cdot sgn(C^{ca}_{ijk}+C^{ez}_{ijk})=N_K\right)$$

Subject to

$$\sum_i W_{ij}\leq 1 \quad \forall j \qquad (2)$$

$$\sum_{i,j}W_{ij}\times C^{ca}_{ijk}+\sum_{i,j}W_{ij}\times C^{ez}_{ijk}\geq 1 \quad \forall k \qquad (3)$$

$$\sum_{i,j}W_{ij}\times C^{ce}_{ijk}\leq 1\,\forall k \qquad (4)$$

$$W_{ij}\times P_{ij}\geq 1\,\forall i,j \qquad (5)$$

Where:

i, j, k: Indices for sets I, J and K, respectively.

N_K : The cardinality of set K;

M: A large constant number;

W_{ij}: A binary decision variable, equal to 1 if the trajectory determined by $I(i)$ and $J(j)$ is chosen;

C^{ca}_{ijk}, C^{ce}_{ijk}:Binary parameters, equal to 1 if $K(k)$ is within a cylindrical zone with an axis along the trajectory determined by $I(i)$ and $J(j)$. Cylinder ca has a radius smaller than the radius (perpendicular to the circular symmetry axis) of the given ellipsoidal ablation zone. Cylinder ce has a 4 mm–6 mm radius (approximately two to three times the electrode's diameter).

C^{ez}_{ijk}: A binary parameter, equal to 1 if $K(k)$ is within an ellipsoidal zone. The center of the ellipsoid is on position $I(i)$ and the circular symmetry axis is along the trajectory determined by positions $I(i)$ and $J(j)$.

P_{ij}: A binary parameter, equal to 1 if the trajectory determined by $I(i)$ and $J(j)$ satisfies the clinical constraints. P_{ij} can be obtained using a fast voxel traversal algorithm [13] from $J(j)$ to $I(i)$ in the segmented volume.

L_i: Distance between $I(i)$ and set K's center of gravity.

$sgn(\cdot)$: Sign function.

The objective function (1) minimizes the number of electrode trajectories and ablated healthy tissue. The first term in (1) preserves the main goal of minimizing the number of trajectories. The large constant M is used to keep the value of the objective function positive. The second term is valid only when the ablation zones along one single trajectory can cover the treatment zone and is used to keep the target position close to the treatment zone's center. The third term penalizes trajectories that result in increasing ablation of healthy tissues. Constraint (2) ensures that there can be at most one trajectory at each entry point. Constraint (3) ensures that each point in the treatment zone is covered by at least one cylindrical or ellipsoidal ablation zone. Constraint (4) ensures that only one trajectory is within l_c mm (4 mm–6 mm) from a point in the treatment zone, which is used to avoid collision between trajectories. Constraint (5) ensures that the trajectories satisfy the multiple clinical constraints.

Solving the above model can generate a minimum number of trajectories along which the electrodes can deliver ablation zones to cover the treatment zone (Fig. 1).

Second Stage. The second stage is quite similar with the first one, but sets I, J, and K are updated. Assuming that t optimized trajectories $T = \{(I(i_1), J(j_1)), (I(i_2), J(j_2)), \ldots (I(i_t), J(j_t))\}$ are generated in the first stage, the optimal target positions of the electrodes must be on the trajectories. Thus, the potential target positions are generated along the trajectories equidistant within the treatment zone, which compose the new set I. All the entry points found in the first step are the new set of entry positions J, and all points in the treatment zone are the new set K. Since the trajectories have been fixed, constraints (2) (3) (4) and (5) are no longer used and two new constraints are added.

$$\sum_{ij} W_{ij} \times C_{ijk}^{ez} \geq 1 \quad \forall k \tag{6}$$

$$W_{ij} = 0, \forall (I(i), J(j)) \, not \, parallel \, with \, any \, trajectories \, in \, T \tag{7}$$

Constraint (6) ensures that the whole treatment zone is covered, and constraint (7) guarantees that the ablation zones are along the generated trajectories.

Optimization. The above model can be solved using the branch-and-cut algorithm, which was implemented using the GAMS CPLEX solver [14]. During the optimization, a "relative gap" serves as a measure of the progress towards finding and proving optimality. When the "relative gap" equals to 0, the solution is optimal [14]. A time limit of 20 min was set during the optimization to generate one plan with a given ablation zone size. If the optimal solution was not found within the time limit, the optimization process was terminated, and a sub-optimal solution with a "relative gap" greater than 0 was generated.

2.3   Experiments and Evaluation

To evaluate the performance of our method, we used CT images from the "3D-IRCADb" database that had segmented boundaries of the liver, tumors, vessels and ribs [15]. To demonstrate the utility of the MWA planning method, six tumors from three patients were selected by the interventionalists as suitable for MWA using Cool-tip MWA electrodes. According to the manufacturer, the ablation zone of the Cool-tip electrode is spherical, and the maximum diameter is 42 mm. In our experiment, we used different ablation zones with diameters ranging from 28 mm to 42 mm (2 mm step). The maximum electrode's length is 150 mm, the minimum liver capsule insertion angle is 20°. The automatic MWA planning was implemented using PYTHON on a workstation (Intel(R) Xeon(R) E5-2620, 2.00 GHz, 64G RAM, Windows 10).

After the planning results were generated, the following evaluation metrics were calculated: (1) Number of electrode (NE); (2) Number of ablations (NA); (3) Coverage percentage (CP) = ablated volume within the treatment zone/volume of treatment zone; (4) Ablation efficiency (AE) = ablated volume within the treatment zone/total ablated volume. (5) The plan 1 with minimum number of electrodes and the plan 2 with maximum ablation efficiency were found. Also, visualization of the plans was provided to the interventionalists using the Visualization Toolkit (VTK).

3 Results and Discussion

Figure 2 shows MWA planning results for two tumors. For both tumors, eight plans were generated automatically. Figures 2(a)–(c) show the two Pareto optimal plans generated for a treatment zone with a corresponding minimum bounding box (55.9 mm × 49.3 mm × 37.8 mm) of a 13.2 cm^3 tumor. Plan 1, with minimum number of electrodes, used a 38 mm diameter ablation zone and required only 2 electrodes and 5 ablations. Its ablation efficiency was 46.7%. Plan 2, with maximum ablation efficiency, used a 32 mm diameter ablation zone and requires 3 MWA electrodes and 7 ablations. Its ablation efficiency was 60.6%. Figures 2(d) and (e) show one Pareto optimal plan for a treatment zone with a corresponding minimum bounding box (67.4 mm × 44.8 mm × 38.15 mm) of a 25.8 cm^3 tumor. Both plans 1 and 2 are optimized simultaneously. This plan used an ablation zone with 42 mm diameter and required 2 MWA electrodes and 5 ablations, resulting in an ablation efficiency of 65.9%.

Figure 3 shows the electrode trajectories' information for the three Pareto optimal plans shown in Fig. 2. All liver capsule insertion angles are larger than 20°, all insertions lengths are smaller than 150 mm, and all distances to critical structures are larger than 3 mm, which indicate that the plans satisfy the multiple clinical constraints. The running time (generating 8 plans) for the tumors in Figs. 2(a) and (d) was 47 min and 53 min respectively.

MWA planning was performed for all the tumors and the results are summarized in Table 1. Since the proposed method took into account the clinical constraints during the optimization, all the generated plans satisfied the clinical constraints. For each tumor, the proposed method can provide two plans with suitable tradeoff between the objectives: the plan with minimum number of MWA electrodes (called plan 1), and the plan with least damage to normal tissues (called plan 2). In some cases, it is possible to achieve the two goals with the same plan, such as cases 1 and 3 in Table 1. For plans with the minimum number of electrodes (plans 1) required at most 3 electrodes. The average ablation efficiency of all plans 2 is 58.9%, which is slightly less than Chen's results (60%–70%) [12], most likely due to our use of multiple constraints (not considered in Chen's method). Although this method was designed for MWA planning, it could be applied on RFA and cryoablation, which are very similar with MWA.

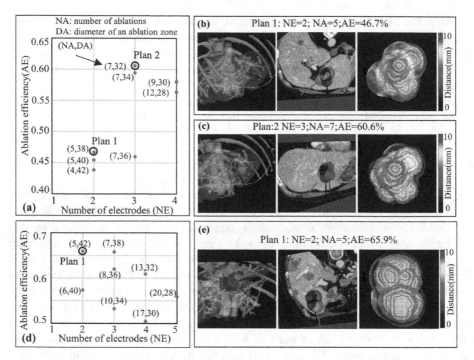

Fig. 2. (a) and (d) show the MWA planning results using electrodes with different ablation zone sizes for a 13.2 cm³ and 25.8 cm³ tumor volumes respectively. The red circles indicate the Pareto optimal plans. (b) and (c) are visualizations of the Pareto optimal plans in (a). (e) is the visualization of the Pareto optimal plan in (d). The right column of (b), (c) and (e) shows the ablation zones with color-coded distances from the ablation zone's boundary to the treatment zone boundary. The white solid indicates the treatment zone. (Color figure online)

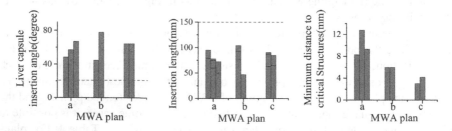

Fig. 3. Evaluation of the Pareto optimal plans in Fig. 2 to check if the clinical constraints are satisfied. Each column bar refers to one trajectory. Plan a, b refer to Plan 2, 1 in Fig. 2(a) respectively. Plan c refers to Plan 1 in Fig. 2(d).

Table 1. Pareto optimal plans for different size tumors. MBB = minimum bounding box of treatment zone; NE = number of electrodes; NA = number of ablations; AE = ablation efficiency; CP = coverage percentage.

Case#	Tumor size (cm^3)	MBB (mm)	Plan	NE	NA	AE	CP
1	25.8	67.4 × 44.8 × 38.1	1(2)	2	5	65.9%	100%
2	4.1	33.8 × 31.1 × 27.9	1	1	1	50.1%	100%
			2	2	4	58.5%	100%
3	16.6	48.2 × 49.2 × 39.1	1(2)	2	4	64.6%	100%
4	28.4	72.6 × 50.3 × 43.0	1	3	7	47.8%	100%
			2	6	25	48.3%	100%
5	13.2	55.9 × 49.3 × 37.8	1	2	4	43.9%	100%
			2	3	7	60.6%	100%
6	5.7	36.1 × 32.8 × 25.9	1	1	1	47.9%	100%
			2	2	4	55.7%	100%

4 Conclusions

We have shown that automated focal MWA planning for liver tumors can generate clinically useful plans. The potential of our method lies in: (1) the capability to integrate multiple clinical constraints, which ensures that the generated plans are feasible, and (2) the Pareto optimal solutions provide interventionalists with more options and allows them to choose the most suitable plan for the patient. Further work includes developing a fast model solver and testing our method in more liver tumor cases.

References

1. Simon, S.J., et al.: Microwave ablation: principles and applications. Radiographics **25**, 69–83 (2005)
2. Baegert, C., Villard, C., Schreck, P., Soler, L., Gangi, A.: Trajectory optimization for the planning of percutaneous radiofrequency ablation of hepatic tumors. Comput. Aided Surg. **12**, 82–90 (2007)
3. Altrogge, I., et al.: Towards optimization of probe placement for radio-frequency ablation. In: Larsen, R., Nielsen, M., Sporring, J. (eds.) MICCAI 2006. LNCS, vol. 4190, pp. 486–493. Springer, Heidelberg (2006). https://doi.org/10.1007/11866565_60
4. Schumann, C., et al.: Fast automatic path proposal computation for hepatic needle placement. In: Medical Imaging 2010: Visualization, Image-Guided Procedures, and Modeling, pp. 76251J. International Society for Optics and Photonics (2010)
5. Seitel, A., et al.: Computer-assisted trajectory planning for percutaneous needle insertions. Med. Phys. **38**, 3246–3259 (2011)
6. Schumann, C., et al.: Interactive multi-criteria planning for radiofrequency ablation. Int. J. Comput. Assist. Radiol. Surg. **10**, 879–889 (2015)
7. Zhai, W., Xu, J., Zhao, Y., Song, Y., Sheng, L., Jia, P.: Preoperative surgery planning for percutaneous hepatic microwave ablation. In: Metaxas, D., Axel, L., Fichtinger, G., Székely, G. (eds.) MICCAI 2008. LNCS, vol. 5242, pp. 569–577. Springer, Heidelberg (2008). https://doi.org/10.1007/978-3-540-85990-1_68

8. Liu, F., et al.: A three-dimensional visualisation preoperative treatment planning system in microwave ablation for liver cancer: a preliminary clinical application. Int. J. Hyperth. **29**, 671–677 (2013)
9. Poggi, G., Tosoratti, N., Montagna, B., Picchi, C.: Microwave ablation of hepatocellular carcinoma. World J. Hepatol. **7**, 2578 (2015)
10. Dodd III, G.D., Frank, M.S., Aribandi, M., Chopra, S., Chintapalli, K.N.: Radiofrequency thermal ablation: computer analysis of the size of the thermal injury created by overlapping ablations. Am. J. Roentgenol. **177**, 777–782 (2001)
11. Ren, H., Guo, W., Ge, S.S., Lim, W.: Coverage planning in computer-assisted ablation based on genetic algorithm. Comput. Biol. Med. **49**, 36–45 (2014)
12. Chen, R., Lu, F., Wang, K., Kong, D.: Semiautomatic radiofrequency ablation planning based on constrained clustering process for hepatic tumors. IEEE Trans. Biomed. Eng. **65**, 645–657 (2018)
13. Amanatides, J., Woo, A.: A fast voxel traversal algorithm for ray tracing. In: Eurographics, pp. 3–10 (1987)
14. GAMS - The Solver Manuals, GAMS Release 25.1.3 (2018)
15. D-IRCADb (3D Image Reconstruction for Comparison of Algorithms Database). http://www.ircad.fr/research/3dircadb/. Accessed 16 Feb 2019

Generating Large Labeled Data Sets for Laparoscopic Image Processing Tasks Using Unpaired Image-to-Image Translation

Micha Pfeiffer[1][✉], Isabel Funke[1], Maria R. Robu[2,3], Sebastian Bodenstedt[1], Leon Strenger[1], Sandy Engelhardt[4], Tobias Roß[5], Matthew J. Clarkson[2,3], Kurinchi Gurusamy[6], Brian R. Davidson[6], Lena Maier-Hein[5], Carina Riediger[7], Thilo Welsch[7], Jürgen Weitz[7,8], and Stefanie Speidel[1,8]

[1] Division of Translational Surgical Oncology, National Center for Tumor Diseases, Dresden, Germany
micha.pfeiffer@nct-dresden.de
[2] Wellcome/EPSRC Centre for Interventional and Surgical Sciences, University College London, London, UK
[3] Centre for Medical Image Computing, University College London, London, UK
[4] Faculty of Computer Science, Mannheim University of Applied Sciences, Mannheim, Germany
[5] Division of Computer Assisted Medical Interventions (CAMI), German Cancer Research Center (DKFZ), Heidelberg, Germany
[6] Division of Surgery and Interventional Science, University College London, London, UK
[7] Department for Visceral, Thoracic and Vascular Surgery, University Hospital Dresden, Dresden, Germany
[8] Centre for Tactile Internet with Human-in-the-Loop (CeTI), TU Dresden, Dresden, Germany

Abstract. In the medical domain, the lack of large training data sets and benchmarks is often a limiting factor for training deep neural networks. In contrast to expensive manual labeling, computer simulations can generate large and fully labeled data sets with a minimum of manual effort. However, models that are trained on simulated data usually do not translate well to real scenarios. To bridge the domain gap between simulated and real laparoscopic images, we exploit recent advances in unpaired image-to-image translation. We extend an image-to-image translation method to generate a diverse multitude of realistically looking synthetic images based on images from a simple laparoscopy simulation. By incorporating means to ensure that the image content is preserved during the translation process, we ensure that the labels given for the simulated images remain valid for their realistically looking translations. This lets us generate a large, fully labeled synthetic data set. We

Electronic supplementary material The online version of this chapter (https://doi.org/10.1007/978-3-030-32254-0_14) contains supplementary material, which is available to authorized users.

show that this data set can be used to train models for the task of liver segmentation in laparoscopic images. We achieve median dice scores of up to 0.89 in some patients without manually labeling a single laparoscopic image and show that using our synthetic data to pre-train models can greatly improve their performance. The synthetic data set is made publicly available, fully labeled with segmentation maps, depth maps, normal maps, and positions of tools and camera (http://opencas.dkfz.de/image2image).

Keywords: Unsupervised · GAN · Image translation · Segmentation

1   Introduction

With the increase in computing power, there is an obvious trend towards training larger and deeper networks. However, in the medical domain, the lack of large data sets is a strong limiting factor [10]. The difficulty of recording real patient data in an operating room, legal restrictions on sharing and the great expense of manual labeling by experts make it near impossible to generate large training benchmarks. An example application is the segmentation of laparoscopic images, where deep networks can achieve high accuracies, but can fail to generalize to new patients due to the lack of more labeled data [4]. A solution to this problem could be the usage of synthetic training data, which can be created automatically in computer simulations. The main issue here is that models trained on synthetic data usually do not generalize well to real data, due to the *domain gap* between the two.

We propose to use *image-to-image translation* techniques to translate images from the domain of simulated images in which labels are known (domain A), to the domain of real images in which we want to train our model (domain B).

The CycleGAN [13] has made it possible to translate images between two unpaired domains (i.e. no one-to-one mapping between the domains is known). It is based on the usage of two *Generative Adversarial Networks (GANs)* and a cycle consistency loss. A generator network G_B translates images from A to B which a discriminator network D_B tries to differentiate from real images in B. Generator G_A and discriminator D_A use the same method to translate images from B to A. The cycle consistency states that an image a translated to B and back to A must match the original image, i.e. $a = G_A(G_B(a))$ (and symmetrically for an image b). This cycle-loss can prevent mode collapse (where many diverse images are translated to a few very similar images), as it requires the original image to be reconstructed from the translation. However, architectures based on the CycleGAN have also been shown to be very effective at *steganography* (one generator hides information in the output images so that the other can use this information to reconstruct the original image) [2].

While the CycleGAN can only learn a one-to-one mapping (uni-modal), recent *multi-modal* image translation methods can learn to use different styles to generate multiple images from a single input image [6,8]. Here, the key idea is the separation of an image's *content* from its *style*. The assumption is that the content between domains remains the same, while the style is domain-specific (texture, lighting). An encoder E_A first extracts a *style-code* s_a and a *content-code* c_a from the source image and a generator G_B then uses this content-code together with a style-code s_b *from the target domain* to create the image b' in the target domain. The opposite direction works analogously. A cycle loss and various reconstruction losses bind the networks together. For more details, we refer the reader to the supplementary material and related literature [6,8].

In the present work, domain A consists of images from very simple laparoscopic 3D computer simulations while domain B is the domain of images from real laparoscopy video feeds. In order to use the translated data for training, care must be taken that (1) the translated images look realistic enough to bridge the domain gap and (2) the labels remain valid. Unpaired multi-modal image-to-image translations can output convincingly realistic results, but have mostly been tested on scenarios where the content stays similar in all images across both domains (such as faces to faces). In cases where the image content can change drastically between different viewpoints and between patients, we have found that the difference in domain distributions can lead to many wrongly added details, such as a gallbladder where there should only be liver or fat tissue replacing liver tissue, which compromises the validity of the synthetic labels. To avoid this, there have been a number of approaches to translate synthetic data to look like real data while preserving labels.

Related Work. SPIGAN [9] proposes to train an additional network which tries to predict the depth map from the translated image, arguing that this preserves image structure. In our experience, this bears the risk of co-adaptation between the networks. AugGAN [5] and GANTruth [1] bind the generators to the image structure via weight-sharing with segmentation networks. However, AugGAN requires segmentation labels to be known for both domains and GANTruth requires a pre-trained segmentation network in the target domain. Our goal is to not use labels during the translation process, simplifying the training procedure.

Contribution. In this work, we show how both realism as well as the preservation of label accuracy during translation can be achieved. First, we build an extension to the *Multimodal Unsupervised Image-to-Image Translation (MUNIT)* framework [6]. While the original MUNIT implementation treats both image domains the same, our modification of the framework does not require the simulated domain to have multiple styles, speeding up the process of creating the simulated data. Next, we incorporate an additional *multi-scale structural similarity loss* [12] and show empirically that it helps to preserve image content and structure despite large changes in camera viewpoint. We also show how the addition of noise in the encoders can inhibit steganography effects and thus help the cycle consistency in avoiding mode collapse. To validate the approach, we show that pre-training a segmentation model on the synthetic data can increase segmentation accuracy. As part of this work, we translate 100 000 images to domain B (see Fig. 1). This data set, fully labeled with segmentation maps, depth maps and further labels as well as the code is publicly available[1], with possible applications ranking from pre-training to benchmarking.

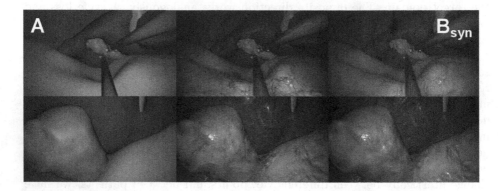

Fig. 1. Images from our simple laparoscopic computer simulation (domain A, first column) are translated to look like real laparoscopic video frames (synthetic B_{syn}, second and third column) using various styles. During the unpaired training process, a multi-scale structural similarity loss ensures that structures remain similar. This enables us to use the generated images along with labels from domain A as training data for various tasks.

2   Methods

2.1   Architecture

Our architecture is an adaptation of the MUNIT framework and can be seen in Fig. 2. The following outlines the differences to the original framework.

Asymmetrical Style: One of our aims is to reduce the amount of manual work required to generate data. In this spirit, we want to translate from a simple and easy to set up domain A to a very complex domain B and let the computer do the bulk of the work automatically. We remove the part of encoder E_A which extracts the style and the style-injection from G_A. As a result, our setup becomes asymmetrical and we do not need to worry about creating multiple textures or lighting styles in the simulated domain A, simplifying the simulation process. During training, both the style extracted by E_B as well as randomly drawn style vectors are used when translating from A to B. In this way, the network can later translate images either using a random style or the style taken from a real image.

Multi-scale Structural Similarity (MS-SSIM) Loss: Unpaired translation networks often modify the image structure, for example by inventing additional

---

[1] Data set and code available at: http://opencas.dkfz.de/image2image/.

details. This is likely due to two reasons: (1) Some structures and some view-points occur more in one of the two domains than in the other. For example, our domain B consists of images from cholecystectomies and contains more close-ups of the gallbladder than domain A, where random placement of the camera results in many close-ups of liver texture instead. The discriminator D_B will thus encourage close-ups of the gallbladder, resulting in the generator G_B often inventing an additional gallbladder in the close-ups of the liver. (2) Generative models are susceptible to *mode collapse*, where many diverse input images are mapped to a few similar output images. We add a multi-scale structural simi-larity [12] loss between an image a and its translation $b' = G_B(E_A(a), s_b)$ (and likewise in the other direction). The loss works on the image brightness (average over the channels) which ensures that brighter regions (such as the gallblad-der) remain brighter and darker regions remain dark while at the same time not penalizing style-dependent changes in hue.

Noise Against Steganography: Since the generators G_A and G_B are trained jointly to fulfill the cycle consistency, one generator learns to hide details of its input image in the translation which the other generator can use to reconstruct the input (an effect called steganography). Once the generators become adapt at steganography, they can start generating outputs which look very similar to the human eye (mode collapse) while satisfying the cycle-loss using the hidden information. To circumvent this effect, we add Gaussian noise to the input of each translation network. This removes hidden information from the images and, in our experience, also prevents mode collapse.

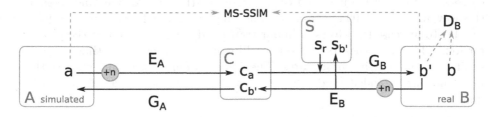

Fig. 2. Architecture of the final translation framework. Image a randomly drawn from A is translated to B and back to A, where a cycle loss ensures that a is reconstructed correctly. A discriminator D_B attempts to distinguish between the translation b' and real images b. The same steps are executed in the opposite direction for images drawn from B (not shown). During the translation process, images from A are encoded to a latent code c_a, while images from B are split into two latent codes: content c_b and style s_b. Unlike MUNIT, we do not have a style in A, which simplifies the creation of the rendered images. Furthermore, we add noise to all encoders to prevent the hiding of information and add the MS-SSIM loss between source images and their transla-tions. Various reconstruction losses ensure that the generators and encoders work as expected (please see the supplementary material for more details and a comparison with MUNIT).

2.2   Translation Data

To train our translation framework, we use two unpaired data sets, which both contain images with livers, gallbladders, tools, fat and abdominal wall (see examples in Fig. 3).

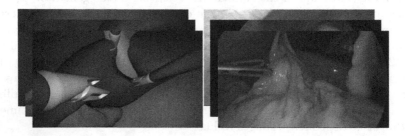

Fig. 3. Sample images from the two domains. Both contain similar objects, but no pairing information is known, and the distribution of content does not necessarily match.

Rendered Data Set - Domain A: We create six synthetic laparoscopic 3D-scenes using the liver and gallbladder surface meshes extracted from CT scans of six patients (3D-IRCADb 01 data set, IRCAD, France). We add meshes which represent fat tissue, ligament and the inflated abdominal wall. Each tissue type is assigned a distinctive texture with small random details. We randomly place the camera together with a light source (representing the laparoscope) and tools. In this way, we render 2000 images from random perspectives for each patient (data set A). To increase the diversity in our translated results, we repeat the process for four additional patients where no gallbladder is present, resulting in scenes similar to liver staging procedures. The images from all ten patients together make up our extended rendered data set A^+, consisting of 20 000 synthetic images.

Real Data Set - Domain B: The real images are taken from 80 videos of the Cholec80 data set (videos of 80 laparoscopic cholecystectomies) [11]. We first identify parts of the videos in which the gallbladder is still intact and then extract frames at five frames per second. We separate the resulting images into a training data set B_{tr} (75 patients, roughly 74 000 images) and a segmentation data set B_v (5 patients). We manually segment the liver in 196 images of B_v (at a rate of one frame every five seconds).

2.3   Experiments

We train the translation networks for 375 000 iterations on the data sets $A+$ and B_{tr}. Afterwards, we translate all images from A^+, using five randomly drawn style vectors for each image, resulting in 100 000 images which we call the synthetic data set B_{syn}.

Evaluating the image quality quantitatively is difficult. Instead, we test the usefulness of the synthetic data set as training data for a liver segmentation task in laparoscopic images. We train a TernausNet-11 [7] to segment the liver using various combinations of training data and then compare the median dice scores over the images. As a baseline, we first train on the real Cholec80 validation data set B_v in a leave-one-patient-out cross-validation (five models trained, each time one patient is left out of the training data to be used for testing). We then train the same network only on the synthetic data B_{syn} and validate it on all five patients in B_v. Furthermore, we test how the performance changes if the network which is already trained on B_{syn} is fine-tuned on the real data in the same cross-validation as before. These experiments are then repeated for a TernausNet which has previously been pre-trained on the ImageNet data set [3].

To see how our synthetic data helps in the adaptation to a wider diversity of images, we also evaluate the same networks on images from 13 liver staging sequences, in which a total of roughly 2000 images are segmented [4]. These images differ substantially from the Cholec80 data in that they don't show gallbladders, focus on the cranial side of the liver and have different lighting conditions.

3 Results

Using the MS-SSIM loss improves the preservation of image structure (example shown in Fig. 4, more translation results in the supplementary materials). In many images, correct assignment of texture to the various organs can be clearly seen and close-up shots of the liver surface result in highly detailed liver texture translations.

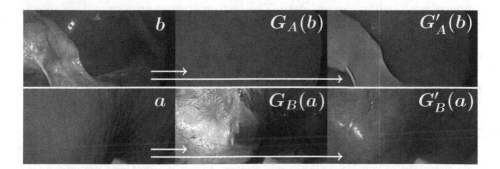

Fig. 4. Qualitative results for the MS-SSIM loss. During translation of images b and a, the networks tend to remove ($G_A(b)$) or add ($G_B(a)$) details. In contrast, networks G'_A and G'_B, which are trained with an MS-SSIM loss, preserve structures in both directions.

Results of training the TernausNet on the different data sets are shown in Table 1. Training on the ImageNet data I and our synthetic data B_{syn} yields

Table 1. Median dice scores on B_v (Patients 76 to 80 from Cholec80 data) and for the 13 staging procedures for networks trained on combinations of the real data B_v, synthetic data B_{syn} and ImageNet data I. In cases where B_v is part of the training *and* testing data, the reported results are from a leave-one-patient-out cross-validation.

Training data	P76	P77	P78	P79	P80	Staging procedures
B_v	0.50	0.68	0.42	0.52	0.56	
B_{syn}	0.73	0.70	0.13	0.74	0.76	
$B_{syn} + B_v$	0.74	0.72	0.40	0.64	0.61	
$I + B_v$	0.80	0.81	0.48	0.86	0.83	0.25
$I + B_{syn}$	0.89	0.80	0.12	0.80	0.85	0.61
$I + B_{syn} + B_v$	0.92	0.83	0.64	0.89	0.91	0.77

median dice scores of up to 0.89 without manually labeling a single laparoscopic image. Pre-training on our synthetic data improves the median dice score by an average of 8.4%. When the network was tested on the 13 staging procedures [4], the mean dice score using only real training data I and B_v was 0.25, and improved to 0.77 when the network was pre-trained with our synthetic data.

4   Discussion

In this work, we have shown that consistent translation results can be achieved despite having a large change in content and viewpoints. We find that the usage of this synthetic data can be beneficial for training segmentation networks. When using it to pre-train a network, we can demonstrate an increase in performance, compared with only using real data. The test on staging procedure data shows that the synthetic data can help a network in generalizing.

The translation results can vary in quality. While some images can be classified as synthetic even by untrained novices, other images look so realistic that expert surgeons had difficulties distinguishing them from real images. We note that to some extent, the goals we set for our networks contradict each other: Creating more realistic results would require the translation networks to modify the structure of the simulated images, which would destroy the correctness of the labels. In our experience, the realism can be greatly influenced by how well the synthetic images in A follow the structure of the images in B and by how the weight of the MS-SSIM loss is chosen. Investigating these dependencies systematically should be subject of future research.

Unpaired image-to-image translation is proving to be a very powerful tool in the generation of training data. Since the domain of surgical data science still mostly lacks large benchmarks and open data sets, it could greatly benefit from further development in this field.

References

1. Bujwid, S., Martí, M., Azizpour, H., Pieropan, A.: GANtruth - an unpaired image-to-image translation method for driving scenarios (2018)
2. Chu, C., Zhmoginov, A., Sandler, M.: CycleGAN, a Master of Steganography. ArXiv abs/1712.02950 (2017)
3. Deng, J., Dong, W., Socher, R., Li, L.J., Li, K., Fei-Fei, L.: ImageNet: a large-scale hierarchical image database. In: CVPR 2009 (2009)
4. Gibson, E., et al.: Deep residual networks for automatic segmentation of laparoscopic videos of the liver (2017)
5. Huang, S.-W., Lin, C.-T., Chen, S.-P., Wu, Y.-Y., Hsu, P.-H., Lai, S.-H.: Aug-GAN: cross domain adaptation with GAN-based data augmentation. In: Ferrari, V., Hebert, M., Sminchisescu, C., Weiss, Y. (eds.) ECCV 2018. LNCS, vol. 11213, pp. 731–744. Springer, Cham (2018). https://doi.org/10.1007/978-3-030-01240-3_44
6. Huang, X., Liu, M.Y., Belongie, S., Kautz, J.: Multimodal unsupervised image-to-image translation. In: The European Conference on Computer Vision (ECCV) (2018)
7. Iglovikov, V.I., Shvets, A.A.: TernausNet: U-Net with VGG11 Encoder Pre-Trained on ImageNet for Image Segmentation. CoRR abs/1801.05746 (2018)
8. Lee, H.Y., Tseng, H.Y., Huang, J.B., Singh, M., Yang, M.H.: Diverse image-to-image translation via disentangled representations. In: The European Conference on Computer Vision (ECCV) (2018)
9. Lee, K.H., Ros, G., Li, J., Gaidon, A.: SPIGAN: privileged adversarial learning from simulation. In: International Conference on Learning Representations (2019)
10. Maier-Hein, L., et al.: Surgical data science for next-generation interventions. Nat. Biomed. Eng. 1(9), 691 (2017)
11. Twinanda, A., Shehata, S., Mutter, D., Marescaux, J., De Mathelin, M., Padoy, N.: EndoNet: a deep architecture for recognition tasks on laparoscopic videos. IEEE Trans. Med. Imaging 36, 86–97 (2016)
12. Wang, Z., Simoncelli, E.P., Bovik, A.C.: Multiscale structural similarity for image quality assessment. In: The Thrity-Seventh Asilomar Conference on Signals, Systems Computers, vol. 2, pp. 1398–1402 (2003)
13. Zhu, J.Y., Park, T., Isola, P., Efros, A.A.: Unpaired image-to-image translation using cycle-consistent adversarial networks. In: 2017 IEEE International Conference on Computer Vision (ICCV) (2017)

Mask-MCNet: Instance Segmentation in 3D Point Cloud of Intra-oral Scans

Farhad Ghazvinian Zanjani[1,2](✉), David Anssari Moin[2], Frank Claessen[2],
Teo Cherici[2], Sarah Parinussa[2], Arash Pourtaherian[1], Svitlana Zinger[1],
and Peter H. N. de With[1]

[1] Eindhoven University of Technology, 5612 AJ Eindhoven, The Netherlands
f.ghazvinian.zanjani@tue.nl
[2] Promaton Co., Ltd., 1076 GR Amsterdam, The Netherlands

Abstract. Accurate segmentation of teeth in dental imaging is a principal element in computer-aided design (CAD) in modern dentistry. In this paper, we present a new framework based on deep learning models for segmenting tooth instances in 3D point cloud data of an intra-oral scan (IOS). At high level, the proposed framework, called *Mask-MCNet*, has analogy to the *Mask R-CNN*, which gives high performance on 2D images. However, the proposed framework is designed for the challenging task of instance segmentation of point cloud data from surface meshes. By employing the Monte Carlo Convolutional Network (MCCNet), the Mask-MCNet distributes the information from the processed 3D surface points into the entire void space (e.g. inside the objects). Consequently, the model is able to localize each object instance by predicting its 3D bounding box and simultaneously segmenting all the points inside each box. The experiments show that our Mask-MCNet outperforms state-of-the-art for IOS segmentation by achieving 98% IoU score.

Keywords: Deep learning · 3D point cloud · Instance segmentation ·
Intra-oral scan

1 Introduction

Modern dentistry, using digital equipment for both intra-oral and extra-oral imaging, demands for computer-aided design (CAD) systems to facilitate data analysis, e.g. for accurate treatment planning and diagnostic aid. In this study, we explore a segmentation methodology for intra-oral scans (IOS) based on recent deep learning advances, to support automated clinical workflow in implantology and orthodontic fields. Such CAD-based workflows require accurate segmentation of each individual tooth and gingiva (gums) in the imaging data. IOS imaging involves capturing the 3D geometrical profile of tooth crowns and

Electronic supplementary material The online version of this chapter (https://doi.org/10.1007/978-3-030-32254-0_15) contains supplementary material, which is available to authorized users.

gingiva in a high-spatial resolution. Processing of such high-detail information from the anatomic structures of tooth crowns is highly desirable for many clinical applications. An IOS consists of a large (e.g. hundreds of thousands) set of points in a 3D Cartesian coordinate system. These data can be represented either by a point cloud or a mesh (i.e. after applying a triangulation algorithm on the points). Each point is represented by its 3D coordinates and, depending on the type of scanner, other attributes such as color. In this paper, the semantic instance segmentation of an IOS refers to the assignment of a unique label to all the points belonging to each instance (i.e. an individual tooth) using a computational model. After the segmentation of the tooth instances, a post-processing stage follows for the standardization of the labels, where the model assigns to each detected tooth one label prescribed by the *Federation Dentaire Internationale* (FDI) dental notation for adult dentition.

In the sequel, we briefly introduce the related work on IOS segmentation, recent advances of deep learning in instance segmentation on point cloud data, and our contributions to both. Afterwards, we explain our proposed method and the obtained results in detail. Lastly, we provide discussions and conclusions.

2   Related Work

IOS Segmentation efforts are mostly based on conventional computer vision techniques, which are limited by finding the best handcrafted features, manual tuning of several parameters and lack of generalization and robustness [1]. Recently, Zanjani *et al.* [1] proposed an end-to-end learning model for IOS segmentation using a deep *PointCNN* [6] model. In their work, the label of each tooth is treated as a semantic label, which aims to be predicted directly at the output of the network. However, formulating the IOS segmentation using a point-based classification loss is ill-posed. This is mainly due to the low inter-class variability between neighbouring teeth, especially among the molar and premolar teeth. Hence, an accurate prediction of the labels requires not only the local geometrical information (i.e. crown shapes), but also the global context of e.g. the relative position, teeth arrangement and possible absence of other teeth.

Thus, to address this ill-posed statement, the segmentation problem is defined in the context of an instance segmentation task, which recognizes each tooth as an instance in the 3D point cloud. The learning model then localizes all instances with their 3D bounding boxes and simultaneously assigns a unique label to all points belonging to each instance. This approach has at least two advantages: (1) inference on the labeling of each tooth instance is not dependent on its relative position with respect to other teeth; (2) a patch-based training and subsequent processing of point cloud data at its original spatial resolution (without downsampling) is facilitated. This is possible since the network does not require the global context to assign a specific FDI label to all points in the tooth instance.

Deep Learning Instance Segmentation in 3D Point Cloud: Among the proposed deep learning models for point cloud analysis, only a few researchers have addressed the challenging issue of 3D instance segmentation. To better compare and position our proposed framework, we briefly survey the most related recent works. *FrustumNet* [8] proposes a hybrid framework involving two stages. The first stage detects the objects bounding boxes in a 2D image. The second stage processes the 3D point cloud in a 3D search space, partially bound by the initially set 2D bounding boxes. The *3D-SIS* model [4] also first processes the 2D images rendered from the point cloud through a 2D convolutional network (ConvNet). Afterwards, the learned features are back-projected on the voxelized point cloud data, where the extracted 2D features and the geometric information are combined to obtain the object proposal and per-voxel mask prediction. The dependency on 2D image(s) of both preceding models limits the application of them for 3D point cloud analysis. In another approach, the *GSPN* [12] follows an analysis-by-synthesis strategy and instead of directly finding the object bounding boxes in a point cloud, it utilizes a conditional variational auto-encoder (CVAE). However, GSPN training requires a separate two-stage training of the CVAE part and the region-based networks (which perform the classification, regression and mask generation on the proposals). In an alternative approach to detect object proposals, *SGPN* [11] and *MASC* [7] methods perform a clustering on the processed points for segmenting the instances. *SGPN* [11] uses a similarity matrix between the features of each pair of points in the embedded feature space, to indicate whether the given pair of points belong to the same object instance or not. However, computing such a pair-wise distance is impractical for large point clouds and especially for IOS data, where down-sampling would significantly affect the detection/segmentation performance. *MASC* [7] voxelizes the point cloud for processing the volumetric data by a 3D U-Net model. Similar to SGPN, MASC uses a clustering mechanism to find similarities between each pair of points by comparing their extracted features in several hidden layers of a trained U-Net. Unfortunately, as mentioned before, voxelization of a large fine-detailed point cloud greatly limits the performance of such approaches.

In this paper, we propose an end-to-end deep learning model for instance segmentation in 3D point cloud data. Our contribution is threefold.

1. We present a new instance segmentation model, called Mask-MCNet. Our proposed model is applied directly to an irregular 3D point cloud on its original spatial resolution and predicts the 3D bounding boxes of instances along with their masks, indicating the segmented points of each instance.
2. To the best of our knowledge, this is the first study which both detects and segments tooth instances in IOS data by a deep learning model.
3. We conduct an extensive experimental evaluation and show that the proposed model significantly outperforms state-of-the-art in IOS segmentation.

3   Method

At high level, the Mask-MCNet is similar to the Mask R-CNN [2] as it includes three main parts: the backbone network, Region Proposal Network (RPN), and three branches of predictor networks for classification, regression, and mask generation (see Fig. 1). Each part is explained in detail below.

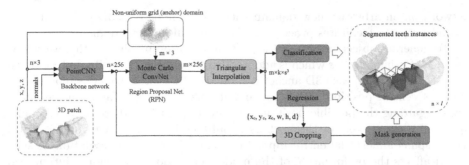

Fig. 1. Block diagram of the Mask-MCNet (see supplementary material for details).

The backbone network acts as a feature extractor and consists of a deep MLP-based network, which is applied on the entire or cropped 3D patches (depending on hardware limitations) of an input 3D point cloud. Every input patch includes n points (varying across patches), where each point is represented by its (x, y, z) 3D coordinates along with its normal vector (which can be computed by averaging over all normal vectors of faces which are connecting to that point). Hence, the input to the backbone model is an $n \times 6$ matrix. In this study, we choose to employ a PointCNN [6] for its fine-detail processing capacity and its small model size [1,6]. The backbone outputs an $n \times 256$ matrix of features (where n denotes the number of input points) which contain rich geometrical information around each point.

Monte Carlo ConvNet as Region Proposal Network (RPN). Since the points in the point cloud cover solely the surface of objects, the computed features from the backbone network only contain local geometrical representations on a manifold in 3D space. However, for a regression problem such as accurate localization of a 3D bounding box encompassing an object, the model requires awareness of several parts (or sides) of each object. Hence, voxelization of the data and employing a 3D ConvNet on the obtained volumetric data is a common approach. However, the shortcomings of it have been mentioned already. Therefore, in an alternative approach, for aggregating the computed feature vectors of the 3D points, we employ a Monte Carlo ConvNet (MCCNet) [3] for distributing and transferring the information from the surface of objects into the entire 3D space (e.g. into void space inside of the objects). The MCCNet consists of several modular MLP sub-networks of two hidden layers whose function resembles a set of convolution kernels. For more information regarding the mechanism of MCCNet, we refer to the original paper [3].

We employ the MCCNet as our region proposal network (RPN) because of two important properties: (1) its capability of computing the convolution on an arbitrary output point-set within the kernel's field of view (FOV), regardless of its presence within the set of input points; (2) its capability of handling the non-uniform distribution of points when computing the convolution. The first property makes it possible to transfer the computed features by the backbone network on an arbitrary new domain such as the node of a 3D grid, while the second property facilitates processing of a non-uniform grid domain.

To generate object proposals (i.e. 3D cubes encompassing teeth), we follow the idea of using *anchors* which is adopted from *Faster-RCNN* [10], but modified to a 3D space. Here, each 3D anchor is indicated by a cube, which is represented with its central position $[x_a, y_a, z_a]$ and its size $[w, d, h]$. Making no assumptions regarding the possible positions of objects (which leads to a more generic approach), the centers of the anchors should be located on a regular 3D grid which spans almost the entire input 3D space. The spatial resolution of such a grid affects the performance of the model, i.e. choosing a low-resolution grid leads to positioning too few anchors inside the small objects (e.g. incisor teeth), whereas a high-resolution grid causes the computation to be inefficient. Instead of imposing a naive uniform grid, we design a non-uniform grid that has dense nodes close to the object surface(s) and sparse nodes far from the surface. A non-uniform grid can be easily obtained by filtering out the nodes of an initial dense grid in the 3D space, according to the distance of each node from a closest point in the point cloud and a predefined lower bound for the grid resolution.

With the two above-mentioned properties, the MCCNet is able to transfer the received features from the backbone network into a new non-uniform grid domain with m nodes, through its first convolutional layer. By further processing of data through the hidden layers of MCCNet and based on the FOV of each convolutional kernel, the geometrical information of surface points becomes distributed on the entire grid domain. Reminding that each node on the non-uniform grid indicates the center of one ($k = 1$) or multiple-size ($k > 1$) anchor(s), the total amount of anchors is $k \times m$. As a classification task, the model predicts from the feature set inside each anchor whether the anchor contains an object or not. If so, a further regression task is performed on the prediction of the object's center-point and its size. As a fully-connected MLP with fixed-length input would be employed for performing such a classification and regression task, the feature set inside each anchor would require to have a fixed length. To do so, a fixed set of $s \times s \times s$ nodes (e.g. $s = 5$) is interpolated inside each anchor in 3D space by applying a triangular interpolation using the three nearest neighbour nodes of the grid and weighting their feature vectors based on their distance to the new node in 3D space. At this stage, for $k \times m$ positioned anchors in 3D input space, an output matrix of $k \times m \times s^3$ is obtained.

Predictor networks consist of three parallel branches for classification, regression, and mask generation. The classification and regression branches both consist of a fully-connected MLP network and receive the $k \times m \times s^3$ feature matrix from the RPN. The classification branch aims to make a binary classification, to indicate if each $k \times m$ anchors contain an object instance or not. In case of a positively detected anchor, its central position and size offset (i.e. residual vectors) are predicted at the output of the regression branch. In the training phase an anchor is labeled positive if it has an overlap with any tooth instances above a threshold (e.g. 0.4 IoU) and it is labeled negative if it is lower than a certain threshold (e.g. 0.2 IoU). Since the number of positive and negative anchors are highly imbalanced, about 50% of each training batch is selected from the positive and 25% from the negative anchors. The rest of the 25% sampled anchors in the training batch are selected from the marginal anchors ($0.2 < IoU < 0.4$), which are considered also as negative samples.

The mask-generation branch directly receives features from the backbone network. The architecture of the mask branch is similar to a PointCNN, which has been used as the backbone network, though it consists of only three $X-Conv$ layers [6]. The estimated 3D bounding boxes by the regression branch are used and the point cloud is cropped accordingly. The cropped point set along with their feature vectors at the output of the backbone network are passed on to the mask branch, which performs a binary classification of the points inside each anchor into two classes: (1) foreground points which belong to a tooth instance and (2) background points which belong to other teeth or gingiva.

The loss function of Mask-MCNet is similar to Mask R-CNN with an equal contribution of three terms. The first term is a cross-entropy loss value for the classification branch on its softmax output layer. The second term is a mean squared error at the linear output layer of the regression branch. Finally, the third term is a binary cross-entropy loss for classification of all points in each positive anchor at the output softmax layer of the mask branch. The regression loss and mask loss are involved only if the examined anchor is labeled positive.

Tooth Label Assignment as Constraint Satisfaction Problem: As mentioned earlier, for clinical purposes and consistency of the tooth labeling assignments, we use a post-processing stage for translating (via a look-up table) the instance labels predicted by the Mask-MCNet into the FDI standard labels. By measuring the average central positions and sizes of the FDI labels within the training data, a combinatorial search algorithm searches the most likely label assignment, which satisfies the predefined constraint (prior measurements on training data) in the context of a constraint satisfaction problem (CSP).

3.1 Implementation Details

Training of the entire Mask-MCNet model is done end-to-end by using a gradient descent and the Adam learning adaptation technique for 1000 epochs with a batch size of 32 (equally balanced between positive and negative anchors). The pre-processing of the input IOS only consists of normalizing the whole point cloud to obtain zero mean and unit variance. The input to the Mask-MCNet is a randomly cropped patch of the point cloud, which usually contains 2–4 tooth instances. As explained, the non-uniform grid domain is constructed by filtering out the nodes of a dense regular grid with 0.04 (lower bound) spatial resolution in each dimension. The upper bound for the grid resolution is set to be equal to 0.12. For creating sufficient overlap between anchors and both small and large objects (e.g. incisor and molar teeth, respectively), two types ($k = 2$) of anchors are employed (with size of [0.3, 0.3, 0.2] and [0.15, 0.2, 0.2]).

Inference on a new IOS is performed by applying the Mask-MCNet on several cropped overlapped patches. Giving the 3D patches and applying a regular grid with the highest defined resolution (e.g. 0.04), the anchors positioned on the grid are classified into object/no-object by the classification branch. The sizes and central positions of positively detected anchors are updated according to the estimated values by the regression branch. Since for each object multiple anchors might be detected, similar to Faster-RCNN, a non-maximum suppression algorithm is employed according to the highest objectiveness scores (from classification probabilities). It is worth mentioning that the non-maximum suppression also handles the repeated points by overlapping the input patches. After bounding box prediction, retrieving a mask for all points inside each bounding box from the mask prediction branch is straightforward. Network architecture of the Mask-MCNet is given in the supplementary material.

4 Experiments and Results

Data: Our dataset consists of 120 optical scans of dentitions from 60 adult subjects, each containing one upper and one lower jaw scan. The optical scan data was recorded by a 3Shape d500 optical scanner (3Shape AS, Copenhagen, Denmark), which obtains 180k points on the average (varying in a range interval of [100k, 310k]). The first dataset includes scans from healthy dentition with a variety of abnormalities among subjects.

All optical scans were manually segmented and their respective points were categorized according to the FDI standard into one of the 32 classes by a dental professional and reviewed and adjusted by one dental expert. Segmentation of each optical scan took 45 min on average, which shows that it forms an intensive laborious task for a human.

Experimental Setup: The performance of the Mask-MCNet in comparison with the state-of-the-art is evaluated by fivefold cross-validation. The average Jaccard Index (also known as mIoU) is used as a segmentation metric. On top of the mIoU, by treating each class individually as a binary (one-versus-all) segmentation problem and then by averaging on all measured precision and recall scores, we report the mean average precision (mAP) and mean average recall (mAR) for evaluating the multi-class teeth segmentation problem. In contrast to teeth semantic segmentation approach that preserving the global context information (e.g. relative tooth positions on the dental arch) is required for accurate label assignment, Mask-MCNet can be applied on the cropped scans (e.g. partitioned into five patches). This is because an instance segmentation approach first localizes the objects (teeth) and then performs segmentation by assigning a unique label to each instance. As earlier explained, in the post-processing stage, the assigned unique labels are converted into semantic tooth labels by applying the constraint satisfaction solver. Employing a patch processing technique allows Mask-MCNet to process an IOS in a higher resolution at the cost of longer execution time. Using 5 patches per scan, Mask-MCNet segments an IOS in a longer execution time as has been reported in Table 1.

The obtained results are shown in Table 1 and a number of segmented IOS are visualized in the supplementary material. As can be observed, the proposed

Mask-MCNet significantly outperforms the state-of-the-art networks in IOS segmentation.

Table 1. Instance segmentation performance of the Mask-MCNet, compared with state-of-the-art semantic segmentation models on multi-class tooth label assignment. The mean IoU (mIoU), mean average precision (mAP), mean average recall (mAR), and the execution time are reported.

Method	Metric			Exec.time *
	mIoU	mAP	mAR	(sec.)
PointNet [9]	0.76	0.73	0.65	**0.19**
PointGrid [5]	0.80	0.75	0.70	0.88
MCCNet [3]	0.89	0.88	0.84	1.01
PointCNN [6]	0.88	0.87	0.83	0.66
PointCNN++ [1]	0.94	0.93	0.90	6.86
Mask-MCNet (ours)	**0.98**	**0.98**	**0.97**	14.6

* NVIDIA Titan-X GPU

5   Discussion and Conclusion

In this study, we have presented a new instance segmentation framework, called Mask-MCNet, for tooth instance segmentation in a 3D point cloud of IOS data. In contrast to alternative deep learning models, our proposed end-to-end learning model does not follow a voxelization step for processing a point cloud. Consequently, the data can be processed by preserving its fine-detail geometrical information, which is important for a successful IOS segmentation. Furthermore, by employing the Monte Carlo ConvNet, the Mask-MCNet can handle the processing of the non-uniformly distributed information in a 3D space. This property leads to an efficient search of object proposals that is important for scalability of the method to be applicable for processing the IOS data with large point clouds (more than 100k points). The experiments have shown that the proposed framework achieves a 98% IoU score on the test data, thereby outperforming the state-of-the-art networks in the IOS segmentation task. This performance is close to the human level and obtained in only a few seconds of processing time, while it forms a lengthy and intensive laborious task for a human.

References

1. Zanjani, F.G., et al.: Deep learning approach to semantic segmentation in 3D point cloud intra-oral scans of teeth. In: Proceedings of the 2nd International Conference on Medical Imaging with Deep Learning (MIDL), vol. 102, pp. 557–571. PMLR (2019)

2. He, K., Gkioxari, G., Dollár, P., Girshick, R.: Mask R-CNN. In: Proceedings of the IEEE International Conference on Computer Vision, pp. 2961–2969 (2017)
3. Hermosilla, P., Ritschel, T., Vázquez, P.P., Vinacua, À., Ropinski, T.: Monte Carlo convolution for learning on non-uniformly sampled point clouds. In: SIGGRAPH Asia 2018 Technical Papers, p. 235. ACM (2018)
4. Hou, J., Dai, A., Nießner, M.: 3D-SIS: 3D semantic instance segmentation of RGB-D scans. In: Proceedings of IEEE Conference on Computer Vision and Pattern Recognition, pp. 4421–4430 (2019)
5. Le, T., Duan, Y.: PointGrid: a deep network for 3D shape understanding. In: Proceedings of IEEE Conference on Computer Vision and Pattern Recognition, pp. 9204–9214 (2018)
6. Li, Y., Bu, R., Sun, M., Wu, W., Di, X., Chen, B.: PointCNN: convolution on X-transformed points. In: Advances in Neural Information Processing Systems, pp. 820–830 (2018)
7. Liu, C., Furukawa, Y.: MASC: multi-scale affinity with sparse convolution for 3D instance segmentation. arXiv preprint arXiv:1902.04478 (2019)
8. Qi, C.R., Liu, W., Wu, C., Su, H., Guibas, L.J.: Frustum pointnets for 3D object detection from RGB-D data. In: Proceedings of IEEE Conference on Computer Vision and Pattern Recognition, pp. 918–927 (2018)
9. Qi, C.R., Su, H., Mo, K., Guibas, L.J.: PointNet: deep learning on point sets for 3D classification and segmentation. In: Proceedings of IEEE Computer Vision and Pattern Recognition, vol. 1, no. 2, p. 4 (2017)
10. Ren, S., He, K., Girshick, R., Sun, J.: Faster R-CNN: towards real-time object detection with region proposal networks. In: Advances in Neural Information Processing Systems, pp. 91–99 (2015)
11. Wang, W., Yu, R., Huang, Q., Neumann, U.: SGPN: similarity group proposal network for 3D point cloud instance segmentation. In: Proceedings of the IEEE Conference on Computer Vision and Pattern Recognition, pp. 2569–2578 (2018)
12. Yi, L., Zhao, W., Wang, H., Sung, M., Guibas, L.: GSPN: generative shape proposal network for 3D instance segmentation in point cloud. arXiv preprint arXiv:1812.03320 (2018)

Physics-Based Deep Neural Network for Augmented Reality During Liver Surgery

Jean-Nicolas Brunet[1], Andrea Mendizabal[1,2], Antoine Petit[1], Nicolas Golse[3], Eric Vibert[3], and Stéphane Cotin[1(✉)]

[1] INRIA, Strasbourg, France
stephane.cotin@inria.fr
[2] University of Strasbourg, ICube, Strasbourg, France
[3] Hôpital Paul-Brousse, Paris, France

Abstract. In this paper we present an approach combining a finite element method and a deep neural network to learn complex elastic deformations with the objective of providing augmented reality during hepatic surgery. Derived from the U-Net architecture, our network is built entirely from physically-based simulations of a preoperative segmentation of the organ. These simulations are performed using an immersed-boundary method, which offers several numerical and practical benefits, such as not requiring boundary-conforming volume elements. We perform a quantitative assessment of the method using synthetic and *ex vivo* patient data. Results show that the network is capable of solving the deformed state of the organ using only a sparse partial surface displacement data and achieve similar accuracy as a FEM solution, while being about 100× faster. When applied to an *ex vivo* liver example, we achieve the registration in only 3 ms with a mean target registration error (TRE) of 2.9 mm.

Keywords: Deep learning · Real-time simulation · Augmented reality

1 Introduction

In computer-assisted interventions, correctly aligning preoperative data to real-time acquired intraoperative images remains a challenging topic, especially when large deformations are involved and only sparse input data is available. This is typically the case when trying to provide an augmented view of an organ during surgery. In this context, just about 30% of the surface of the organ is visible due

---

J.-N. Brunet and A. Mendizabal—Contributed equally to the paper.

Electronic supplementary material The online version of this chapter (https://doi.org/10.1007/978-3-030-32254-0_16) contains supplementary material, which is available to authorized users.

D. Shen et al. (Eds.): MICCAI 2019, LNCS 11768, pp. 137–145, 2019.
https://doi.org/10.1007/978-3-030-32254-0_16

to the limited field of view of the laparoscopic camera or size of the incision [2]. Several works have demonstrated the benefits of physics-based models, particularly patient-specific biomechanical models, for accurate registration between different preoperative 3D anatomical model and intraoperative data [3–6]. These models are usually derived from continuum mechanics theory, where finite element (FE) methods are preferred due to their ability to numerically solve the complex partial differential equations associated with the constitutive models.

When considering augmented reality or, more generally, real-time tracking of the organ's deformation to provide up-to-date guidance, the computational efficiency of the FE method is essential. To this end, various solutions have been proposed, with different trade-offs regarding the ratio between computation time and model accuracy [5,7,8]. The choice of the model, and its parameterization, are obviously key to an accurate registration. It is usually acknowledged that a registration of internal structures below 5 mm is needed for best clinical impact, such as targeting relatively small tumors.

Without lack of generality, let us consider the scenario where an augmented view of the liver has to be provided during hepatic surgery. The intraoperative data is provided as a point cloud, reconstructed from the laparoscopic images [13,14] or direct camera view [9] of the operative field. Images are usually acquired at 20 Hz or more, and latency between data acquisition and display of the augmented image needs to be minimized. This leads to update times of less than 50 ms, during which image acquisition, image processing and model update need to take place. As a result, FE computation times should require less than 30 ms. This is usually achieved using efficient implementation of specific elastic models.

In surgery where only small deformations take place, achieving such computation times is feasible, as illustrated in [10]. However, when considering large, non-linear deformations, involving typical soft tissue hyper-elastic behavior, computation times become incompatible with augmented reality constraints. A solution towards this objective has been to use a co-rotational technique, allowing to cope with large displacements (but small strain) behavior [4,9]. Yet, if more advanced laws from biomechanics are to be used, these optimizations (and simplifications) no longer hold. Alternative solutions have been proposed to avoid these restrictions. For instance, Marchesseau et al. [11] introduced the Multiplicative Jacobian Energy Decomposition (MJED) which is an alternative to the Galerkin FEM formulation. This method for discretizing non-linear hyperelastic materials on linear tetrahedral meshes can lead to fast and realistic liver deformations including hyperelasticity, porosity and viscosity. Also, Miller et al. [12] introduced TLED, an efficient numerical algorithm for computing deformations of very soft tissues. By using a total Lagrangian formulation, most spatial derivatives can be pre-computed, leading to fast simulations of non-linear material.

In this paper, we propose a method allowing for extremely fast and accurate simulations by using an artificial neural network that partially encodes the stress-strain relation in a low-dimensional space. Such a network can learn the desired constitutive model, and predict deformations under new, complex, conditions. As a result it can be used for augmented reality applications, where both complex

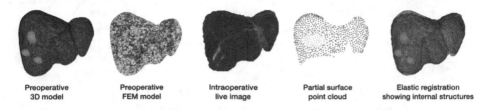

Preoperative   Preoperative   Intraoperative   Partial surface   Elastic registration
3D model   FEM model   live image   point cloud   showing internal structures

Fig. 1. Augmented reality pipeline: preoperative internal structures are mapped in real-time onto the live image of the organ using a FEM model.

tissue deformation and boundary conditions are involved. Our method consists in two main components: a deep network architecture, described in Sect. 2.1, which is derived from model order reduction techniques, and an immersed boundary method, used for generating patient-specific simulations, using hexahedral finite elements Sect. 2.2. Results presented in Sect. 3 show the efficiency of the method when applied to both synthetic and *ex vivo* scenarios.

2   Method

A typical pipeline for providing an augmented view of an organ during surgery is described by Fig. 1. The only assumption here is that we have a method for extracting a partial point cloud of the organ during surgery, either from a laparoscopic image or other system, such as RGB-D camera.

In such a pipeline we propose to accelerate the FE computation step by replacing it with a non-linear dimensionality reduction technique based on a U-Net architecture. Dimensionality reduction techniques have shown real benefits in speeding-up FE simulations. Among them, POD is a very popular one since it leads to very realistic real-time simulations. Although authors in [17] have shown good results using this method for large deformation, POD is better suited for linear or weakly non-linear processes. Our method uses a deep neural network to learn the relationship between sparse surface data and volumetric deformation of a given mesh.

2.1   U-Net Architecture

The 3D point cloud provided by the RGB-D sensor is a sparse and partial view of the surface deformation of the organ. Our problem consists of finding the function f that produces the best estimation of the internal deformation of the organ from such point cloud. The function f is found by minimizing the expected error over a training set $\{(\mathbf{u_s}^n, \mathbf{u_v}^n)\}_{n=1}^{N}$ of N samples:

$$\min_{\theta} \frac{1}{N} \sum_{n=1}^{N} \|f(\mathbf{u_s}^n) - \mathbf{u_v}^n\|_2^2. \tag{1}$$

where θ is the set of parameters of the network f, and $\mathbf{u_s}$ and $\mathbf{u_v}$ are the surface input and the volumetric output displacement fields of each sample.

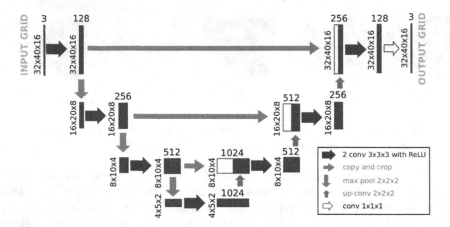

Fig. 2. U-Net architecture with 3 steps and 128 channels in the first layer for a padded input grid of size $32 \times 40 \times 16 \times 3$.

In order to characterize f, we propose to use the U-Net [1], a modified fully convolutional network initially built for precise medical image segmentations. As depicted in Fig. 2, the network is similar to an auto-encoder, with an encoding path to transform the input space into a low-dimensional representation, and a decoding path to expand it back to the original size. Additional skip connections transfer detailed information along matching levels from the encoding path to the decoding path. The encoding path consists of k sequences of two padded $3 \times 3 \times 3$ convolutions ($k = 4$ in [1]) and a $2 \times 2 \times 2$ max pooling operation (see Fig. 2). At each step, each feature map doubles the number of channels and halves the spatial dimensions. In the bottom part there are two extra $3 \times 3 \times 3$ convolutional layers leading to a 1024-dimensional array. In a symmetric manner, the decoding path consists of k sequences of an up-sampling $2 \times 2 \times 2$ transposed convolution followed by two padded $3 \times 3 \times 3$ convolutions. The features from the encoding path at the same stage are cropped and concatenated to the up-sampled feature maps. At each step of the decoding path, each feature map halves the number of channels and doubles the spatial dimensions. There is a final $1 \times 1 \times 1$ convolutional layer to transform the last feature map to the desired number of channels of the output (3 channels in our case). The up- and down-sampling process implies to use a grid-like structure for storing displacement information. Although this could be interpolated from a non-structured FEM mesh, we prefer here to rely on hexahedral mesh, as explained below.

2.2   Soft Tissue Deformation on Hexahedral Grids

To train our network, we need to generate many samples consisting of a volumetric output displacement field $\mathbf{u_v}$, given a nearly random input displacement $\mathbf{u_s}$. The simulation that generates this data needs to be as accurate as possible, yet computationally efficient to make it possible to generate data and train the

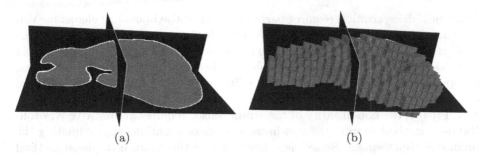

Fig. 3. Example of sparse grid discretization generated from a preoperative CT. Combined with an immersed boundary method, it allows the use of regular hexahedral meshes to simulate the deformation of the organ, and can be used with our CNN.

network in less than a day (i.e. in the shortest amount of time available between preoperative data acquisition and surgery). While several choices of constitutive models can be made to describe soft tissue biomechanics, we want here to emphasize the choice of elements used in our FE implementation. Instead of using 4-node tetrahedral elements, as it is very often the case in the literature, we choose here to rely on 8-node hexahedral elements. This choice is governed by their better convergence, and lock-free behavior, especially with close to imcompressible materials (such as the liver) and strong shear stresses [19]. In addition, we combine this choice of elements with an immersed-boundary method, which allows us to create a hexahedral mesh directly from the segmented image and produces a sparse, regular grid of elements which matches the structure of the first layer of our U-net. Since most soft tissue exhibit an hyperelastic behavior, we chose to implement a Saint Venant-Kirchhoff model, for its relative simplicity and computational efficiency. This hyperelastic material model is just an extension of the linear elastic material model to the nonlinear regime. It is derived from Cauchy's first law of motion, which states the conservation of linear momentum in a continuum. The second Piola-Kirchhoff stress tensor $S = 2\mu\epsilon + \lambda tr(\epsilon)I$ conveys the amount of stress (N/m^2) sustained by the material undergoing a certain deformation, described by the strain tensor $\epsilon(u) = \frac{1}{2}(\nabla u^T + \nabla u + \nabla u^T \cdot \nabla u)$. Here, λ and μ are the Lamé elasticity parameters and $u = [u\,v\,w]^T$ is a displacement vector from position x^0 in the undeformed state of the body to its deformed position $x = x^0 + u$. Cauchy's first law of motion can finally be translated into the system of partial differential equations $-\nabla \cdot \sigma = f_{ext}$ which pose our set of rules for the simulation process. The weak form of those rules, obtained from the principle of virtual work, brings forward the boundary terms and allows to solve the nonlinear system of equations of the Saint Venant-Kirchhoff model through a discretization of the domain into a finite set of hexahedral elements (Fig. 3).

The choice of discretizing the initial domain with a sparse and regular grid brings several benefits. The usual tri-linear interpolation functions of an 8-nodes hexahedral element are reduced to a linear mapping, and, similar to 4-nodes tetrahedral elements, its jacobian remains constant inside the element. However, using such discretization requires particular care of the boundary elements. Volume integration of the displacement field inside these partially filled cells is carried on by recursively subdividing the cell into 8 sub-cells. The stiffness matrix inside a boundary cell is then accumulated from its sub-cells using the linear mapping, as in [16]. Since we are using a fine mesh of the domain, only one level of subdivision is enough to obtain an accurate approximation of the volume integral. Finally, the non-linearity of the strain tensor requires an iterative Newton-Raphson method to solve the non-linear system of equations approximating the unknown displacement. Since the convergence of the Newton-Raphson method is only valid for a displacement near the solution, large external loads must be applied by small increments, which can in turn require a large number of iterations to converge. This is an important characteristic, as one would need to restrict those iterations during a simulation if such nonlinear model were to be used directly in the registration process. In our case, these computations are done in the training stage and do not need to meet real-time constraints.

2.3   Data Generation for U-Net Training

To train the U-Net, a data set of pairs $(\mathbf{u_s}, \mathbf{u_v})$ is generated, where the surface displacement corresponds to the mapped point cloud. We assume that, at most, half of the organ surface is visible from the camera. Hence, we uniformly sample 100 points on the visible surface mesh. Hundred simultaneous forces are then applied to this virtual point cloud with random amplitudes and directions. In order to generate a series of surface deformations (see Fig. 4(b)), these random forces are applied to their enclosing grid nodes using their barycentric coordinates. Patient-specific parameterization of the biomechanical model is not required since for homogeneous materials, the relation between the surface and the volumetric displacements is independent of the stiffness of the object [21], and only depends on the Poisson's ratio. As a result, we set the Poisson's ratio to 0.49 (soft tissues are generally incompressible).

3   Results

Results below are obtained using an *ex vivo* human liver data set, for which surface data was obtained with an RGB-D camera and ground truth data acquired at different stages of deformation using a CT scan. Markers were embedded in the liver to compute Target Registration Errors (TRE).

Predictions on Controlled Synthetic Deformations. To validate the performance of our network, we compare the predictions of the displacement field with the corresponding FE simulation, using the model described in Sect. 2.2. We generated 1,000 samples and used $N = 800$ samples to train the network by minimizing Eq. (1). The minimization is performed using the Adam optimizer: a stochastic gradient descent procedure with parameter-wise adjusted learning rates. The remaining 200 samples are then used for validation. For each sample, the average target registration error (TRE) is computed over 10 virtual markers. The obtained average TRE over the validation set is $\overline{\text{TRE}} = 1.96 \pm 3.46\,\text{mm}$.

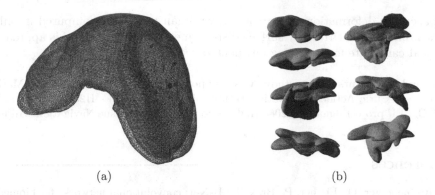

(a)   (b)

Fig. 4. (a) U-Mesh prediction in green, co-rotational FEM based registration in blue and ground truth in red. A mean TRE of 2.92 mm is achieved over the 10 markers in about 3ms. (b) Samples of the generated deformations using our FE method. The rest shape is shown in gray. (Color figure online)

Application to Augmented Reality. With a PyTorch implementation of the U-Net running on a GeForce 1080 Ti, the network can predict the volumetric deformation of the liver in only 3 ms. We can then apply this prediction each time the RGB-D camera generates a point cloud. Before computing the displacement field, the point cloud needs to be cropped to the portion of the surgical image that contains the liver. This is done by segmenting the associated color image, similarly as in [15]. The RGB-D point cloud is then interpolated onto the grid to obtain per-node displacements on the surface (i.e. u_s). Given this input, the network predicts the volumetric deformation, and the next point cloud can be processed. When compared to our *ex vivo* ground truth, the average TRE at the 10 markers is of only 2.92 *mm* with a maximal value of 5.3 mm. The same scenario, but this time using a co-rotational FE method, leads to an average TRE of 3.79 mm and is computed in about 25 ms. The solution of the Saint Venant-Kirchhoff model, used to train our model, gives nearly the same error (which was expected) but for a computation time of 1550 ms, even when using a very efficient linear solver (Pardiso[1]).

4   Conclusion

We have presented a deep neural network approach that can learn complex elastic deformations of a liver and generate its deformed state about 500× faster than a reference FE solution. Since the network takes as input a regular sparse grid where displacements are imposed, we have shown an efficient FE immersed-boundary method based on the same hexahedral discretization from which thousands of deformed configurations are generated to train the network. Based on a U-net architecture, which emulates a model order reduction technique, complex

---

[1] https://pardiso-project.org.

and accurate deformation of a preoperative organ model are computed in only a few milliseconds. Driven by surface displacement data, it makes this approach an ideal candidate for providing augmented reality during surgery.

Acknowledgements. This study was supported by H2020-MSCA-ITN Marie Skłodowska-Curie Actions, Innovative Training Networks (ITN) - H2020 MSCA ITN 2016 GA EU project number 722068 High Performance Soft Tissue Navigation (HiPer-Nav).

References

1. Ronneberger, O., Fischer, P., Brox, T.: U-Net: convolutional networks for biomedical image segmentation. In: Navab, N., Hornegger, J., Wells, W.M., Frangi, A.F. (eds.) MICCAI 2015. LNCS, vol. 9351, pp. 234–241. Springer, Cham (2015). https://doi.org/10.1007/978-3-319-24574-4_28
2. Plantefeve, R., et al.: Patient-specific biomechanical modeling for guidance during minimally-invasive hepatic surgery. Ann. Biomed. Eng. **44**(1), 139–153 (2016)
3. Clements, L.W., Chapman, W.C., Dawant, B.M., Galloway, R.L., Miga, M.I.: Robust surface registration using salient anatomical features for image-guided liver surgery: algorithm and validation. Med. Phys. **35**(6Part1), 2528–2540 (2008)
4. Haouchine, N., Dequidt, J., et al.: Image-guided simulation of heterogeneous tissue deformation for augmented reality during hepatic surgery. In: ISMAR, pp. 199–208 (2013)
5. Suwelack, S., Röhl, S., Bodenstedt, S., Reichard, D., et al.: Physics-based shape matching for intraoperative image guidance. Med. Phys. **41**(11), 111901 (2014)
6. Alvarez, P., et al.: Lung deformation between preoperative CT and intraoperative CBCT for thoracoscopic surgery: a case study. In: Medical Imaging, vol. 10576D (2018)
7. Modrzejewski, R., Collins, T., Bartoli, A., Hostettler, A., Marescaux, J.: Soft-body registration of pre-operative 3D models to intra-operative RGBD partial body scans. In: Frangi, A.F., Schnabel, J.A., Davatzikos, C., Alberola-López, C., Fichtinger, G. (eds.) MICCAI 2018. LNCS, vol. 11073, pp. 39–46. Springer, Cham (2018). https://doi.org/10.1007/978-3-030-00937-3_5
8. Peterlík, I., Duriez, C., Cotin, S.: Modeling and real-time simulation of a vascularized liver tissue. In: Ayache, N., Delingette, H., Golland, P., Mori, K. (eds.) MICCAI 2012. LNCS, vol. 7510, pp. 50–57. Springer, Heidelberg (2012). https://doi.org/10.1007/978-3-642-33415-3_7
9. Petit, A., Cotin, S.: Environment-aware non-rigid registration in surgery using physics-based simulation. In: ACCV - 14th Asian Conference on Computer Vision (2018)
10. Meier, U., López, O., Monserrat, C., et al.: Real-time deformable models for surgery simulation: a survey. Comput. Methods Programs Biomed. **77**(3), 183–197 (2005)
11. Marchesseau, S., Heimann, T., Chatelin, S., Willinger, R., Delingette, H.: Multiplicative Jacobian energy decomposition method for fast porous visco-hyperelastic soft tissue model. In: Jiang, T., Navab, N., Pluim, J.P.W., Viergever, M.A. (eds.) MICCAI 2010. LNCS, vol. 6361, pp. 235–242. Springer, Heidelberg (2010). https://doi.org/10.1007/978-3-642-15705-9_29
12. Miller, K., Joldes, G., Lance, D., Wittek, A.: Total Lagrangian explicit dynamics finite element algorithm for computing soft tissue deformation. Commun. Numer. Methods Eng. **23**(2), 121–134 (2007)

13. Collins, T., Pizarro, D., Bartoli, A., Canis, M., Bourdel, N.: Real-time wide-baseline registration of the uterus in monocular laparoscopic videos. In: MICCAI (2013)
14. Heiselman, J.S., et al.: Characterization and correction of intraoperative soft tissue deformation in image-guided laparoscopic liver surgery. J. Med. Imag. **5**(2), 021203 (2017)
15. Petit, A., Lippiello, V., Siciliano, B.: Real-time tracking of 3D elastic objects with an RGB-D sensor. In: IROS, pp. 3914–3921 (2015)
16. Düster, A., et al.: The finite cell method for three-dimensional problems of solid mechanics. Comput. Methods Appl. Mech. Eng. **197**(45–48), 3768–3782 (2008)
17. Niroomandi, S., et al.: Real-time deformable models of non-linear tissues by model reduction techniques. Comput. Methods Programs Biomed. **91**(3), 223–231 (2008)
18. Cifuentes, A., et al.: A performance study of tetrahedral and hexahedral elements in 3-D finite element structural analysis. Finite Elem. Anal. Des. **12**, 313–318 (1992)
19. Benzley, S.E., et al.: A comparison of all hexagonal and all tetrahedral finite element meshes for elastic and elasto-plastic analysis. In: 4th IMR, vol. 17, pp. 179–191 (1995)
20. Wang, E., Nelson, T., Rauch, R.: Back to elements-tetrahedra vs. hexahedra. In: Proceedings of the 2004 International ANSYS Conference (2004)
21. Miller, K., Lu, J.: On the prospect of patient-specific biomechanics without patient-specific properties of tissues. J. Mech. Behav. Biomed. Mater. **27**, 154–166 (2013)

Detecting Cannabis-Associated Cognitive Impairment Using Resting-State fNIRS

Yingying Zhu[1]([⊠]), Jodi Gilman[2], Anne Eden Evins[2], and Mert Sabuncu[1,3]

[1] School of Electrical and Computer Engineering, Cornell University, Ithaca, USA
zhuyingying2@gmail.com
[2] Center for Addiction Medicine, Massachusetts General Hospital, Boston, USA
[3] Meinig School of Biomedical Engineering, Cornell University, Ithaca, USA

Abstract. Functional near infrared spectroscopy (fNIRS), an emerging, versatile, and non-invasive functional neuroimaging technique, promises to yield new neuroscientific insights, and tools for brain-computer-interface applications and diagnostics. In this work, we consider the novel problem of detecting cannabis intoxication based on resting-state fNIRS data. We examine several machine learning approaches and present an innovative data augmentation technique suitable for resting-state functional data. Our experiments suggest that a recurrent neural network model trained on dynamic functional connectivity matrices, computed on sliding windows, coupled with the proposed data augmentation strategy yields the best accuracy for our application. We achieve up to 90% area under the ROC on cross-validation for detecting cannabis associated intoxication at the individual-level. We also report an independent validation of the best performing model on data not used in cross-validation.

1 Introduction

Cognitive impairment caused by intoxication is a factor in approximately 25% of motor vehicle accidents. After alcohol, $\delta 9$-tetrahydrocannabinol (THC) is the most frequently detected drug in drivers in car accidents [1]. THC is the primary psychoactive compound in cannabis. The prevalence of detectable THC in body fluids of those detained for DUI has steeply increased from 19% to 27% of drivers, between 2007 and 2014.

Recent studies have found that brain activity patterns at rest, particularly in the prefrontal cortex, exhibit a robust signal that can be used to discriminate individuals impaired by an intoxicant from those with normal cognitive ability [2,3]. Although functional magnetic resonance imaging (fMRI) and positron emission tomography (PET) are most commonly used to study resting-state activity, these modalities are not practical for widespread use in real-world settings. In this work, we employ the more portable functional near-infrared spectorsocpy (fNIRS) method to capture resting-state functional connectivity. fNIRS is a safe, non-invasive and inexpensive technique that uses light absorption properties of hemoglobin to measure oxygenated hemoglobin (HbO) concentrations

© Springer Nature Switzerland AG 2019
D. Shen et al. (Eds.): MICCAI 2019, LNCS 11768, pp. 146–154, 2019.
https://doi.org/10.1007/978-3-030-32254-0_17

that arise from cerebral blood flow associated with brain activity [4]. fNIRS detects a local hemodynamic response signal analogous to the blood oxygen level dependent (BOLD) response detected by fMRI. In this work, we collected resting-state fNIRS data using an array of 20 channels over the forehead designed to detect activity in the prefrontal cortex. These resting-state data are capturing spontaneous brain activity patterns in the absence of any external stimuli or experimental tasks.

Following the common strategy to exploit and characterize resting-state functional scans [5–7], one can compute the correlation between the time series of channel pairs in fNIRS data. This correlation metric, commonly called functional connectivity, can be interpreted as the strength of the functional coupling between the brain regions captured by the channels. The vast majority of resting state functional connectivity approaches, particularly those based on machine learning methods, employ so-called "static" metrics, which quantify the *average* strength of coupling between pairs of regions. Static measures do not take full advantage of the temporal dynamics in the signal, yet they have been very useful in offering neuroscientific insights or deriving clinical tools, e.g., for diagnosis [8]. Recently, there has been an increasing number of studies demonstrating the utility of examining the temporal dynamics in resting-state data beyond what static measures capture [6,9–12]. Motivated by this, an important goal in the present paper was to empirically assess the boost in prediction performance when going from static functional connectivity to a model that exploits dynamic connectivity metrics.

We also present a novel data augmentation strategy suitable for resting-state functional scans. Our results suggest that the proposed data augmentation can provide a significant increase in prediction performance.

This paper's main contribution is to consider different machine learning approaches for the novel problem of detecting THC-induced cognitive impairment from resting-state fNIRS data. We conduct a thorough set of experiments that offer following conclusions. A model that exploits dynamic connectivity can achieve substantially better prediction performance than a model trained with static connectivity measures. The best performing model was an RNN trained on dynamic connectivity matrices, computed with sliding temporal windows, coupled with the proposed augmentation technique. This model achieved up to 90% area under the ROC curve (AUC) on 11-fold cross-validation. We also provide an independent validation of the best-performing model, on data not used for cross-validation.

2 Methods

2.1 Individual-Level Prediction Based on Static Functional Connectivity

Let $\mathbf{s}_i \in \mathbb{R}^{M \times 1}$ denote the signal captured by the i'th channel ($i = 1, \cdots, N$), where M is the length of the time course and N is the total number of channels under consideration ($N = 20$ in our data-set). Note that each fNIRS channel is

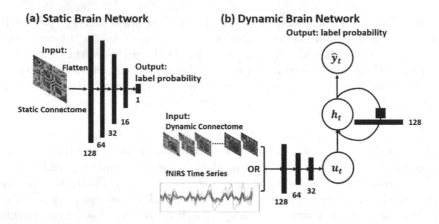

Fig. 1. Illustration of machine learning methods. (a) Fully connected neural network on static connectivity matrix. (b) RNN model on dynamic connectivity matrices or input fNIRS timeseries.

sensitive to a specific region in the brain. In this paper, an $N \times N$ static functional connectivity matrix $\mathbf{S}$ consists of pairwise correlations (Pearson's correlation coefficients) between the time series $\{\mathbf{s}_i\}$. To date, virtually all of the machine learning-based techniques used with resting state functional neuroimaging data have relied on such a static connectivity matrix, which is often vectorized and fed as input features $\mathbf{x}$ to some classifier that computes an individual-level prediction [13].

For this study, we experimented with multiple machine learning approaches on the static connectivity features (including SVMs and neural networks). We achieved best results with a fully connected neural network with 4 hidden layers (see Fig. 1a). The input to this model is a 190 dimensional feature vector, which is the lower triangle of the static connectivity matrix. The hidden layers have 128, 64, 32, and 16 nodes, all fully connected with tanh nonlinearities. The output is a single tanh node that computes the probability of cognitive impairment. Note we did not perform a thorough optimization of this architecture as we had access to a limited sample size and wanted to minimize the risk of over-fitting in our experiments. The model was trained with cross-entropy loss.

2.2   Dynamic Functional Connectivity

The most popular technique to study dynamic functional connectivity relies on connectivity matrices computed with sliding windows [14]. Each window corresponds to a small segment of the resting state scan and thus the correlation metrics are computed within this local clip. Let $\mathbf{s}_{it}$ denote the time course in sliding window t for channel i and the total number of sliding windows is T. In our experiments, we used a window length of 200 time points, and a skip of 50 time points. For each window t, we then can compute the instantaneous functional connectivity matrix based on correlating the $\mathbf{s}_{it}$'s.

In this work, we use a recurrent neural network (RNN) model to exploit the temporal dynamics in the data. We implement two versions of the RNN model. In one version, the input is the 20-channel fNIRS time courses. In the second version, the input is the instantaneous functional connectivity matrix. Thus the only architectural difference between these two models is the input layer. All other layers are the same between the two versions, and illustrated in Fig. 1b.

In the RNN architecture, we have a core component that is the same as the static connectivity network. This core consists of fully connected layers that map the input to a latent representation $\mathbf{u}_t$, which in turn feeds to a hidden state $\mathbf{h}_t$ with recurrent connections. A probabilistic prediction $\hat{y}_t$ is computed at every time point by applying a fully connected layer to the hidden state $\mathbf{u}_t$. As above, we used tanh for all nonlinearities. To sum, the RNN model implements following relationships:

$$\mathbf{u}_t = f(\mathbf{x}_t)$$
$$\hat{y}_t = g(\mathbf{h}_t)$$
$$\mathbf{h}_t = \phi(\mathbf{u}_t, \mathbf{h}_{t-1}),$$

where f is the core component that maps input $\mathbf{x}_t$ to a 32-dimensional latent representation $\mathbf{u}_t$; ϕ is another fully connected neural net with a single hidden layer of 128 dimensions and consists of recurrent connections that capture the temporal dynamics; and g is the output layer that maps the hidden state $\mathbf{h}_t$ to a probabilistic prediction $\hat{y}_t$. The output is the *current* estimation of the probability of the subject's cognitive impairment status. We used a weighted averaged cross-entropy loss to train the RNNs:

$$\sum_t -w_t y \log(\hat{y}_t) - w_t(1-y) \log(1 - \hat{y}_t),$$

where $\hat{y}_t$ is the model's probabilistic prediction, y is the ground truth label for that subject, and w_t is weight for the prediction at time-point t. We want to emphasize the predictions at later time-points, so in our experiments we used a weighting strategy that linearly changed from 0 to 1 between the first and last time points of an input sequence.

2.3   Data Augmentation

Data augmentation techniques have played a significant role in the recent success of deep learning, particularly in the context of limited sample sizes, which is the case in our application. Data augmentation is based on explicitly identifying the in-variance in the prediction problem and exploiting it via applying random transformations within the in-variance class. For example, in image-based classification a common in-variance is rotation or zoom. In resting-state functional imaging, the participant is scanned in the absence of any external conditioning.

Therefore, it is safe to assume that the exact start and end points of a resting state scan should not influence the prediction. This will be true if the target variable, e.g. cognitive impairment, is relatively stable throughout the scanning session. In our setting, the time required for cognitive recovery is much longer than the fNIRS scan time. To exploit this, we propose the following augmentation strategy. We randomly choose a start and end point. In our experiments, the start time was chosen between $t = 1$ and 300. The augmented scan length was fixed to 2500. At test time, we computed probabilistic predictions by averaging the outputs corresponding to the augmented copies of the test scan.

2.4   Implementation Details

We implemented the neural networks in Keras, with a TensorFlow back-end. We used grid search with hyper-parameters and Alternating Direction Method of Multipliers (ADMM) for optimization. Learning was terminated when validation loss stopped improving.

3   Experiment Results

3.1   Study Design

Our dataset includes 41 healthy adults, who were frequent cannabis users and aged 18–55. Frequent users were recruited because they are the population that is most likely to drive while intoxicated. For study inclusion, subjects were required to test positive for cannabis, and negative for all other illicit drugs at the screening visit.

Participants were asked to be abstinent overnight and received a single, physician determined dose of 5 to 50 mg MARINOL (dronabinol), an FDA-approved synthetic form of THC, or identical appearing placebo at each of two study visits, randomized for order, conducted at least 7 days apart. During each study visit, there were three fNIRS scans; one before the THC/placebo administration (called "Pre Scan"), another scan approximately 100 min after the dose was administered ("Post Scan"), which is when peak THC-associated effects are reported to occur, and finally 200 min after the study drug was administered ("Second Post Scan"). Heart rate and subjective intoxication measures were collected and used together with clinical impression and field sobriety test results to determine cognitive impairment status. The study physician aimed to give a dose of THC that would produce intoxication and also be well tolerated; dose determination was based on factors such as height, weight, age, sex, general health, and quantity and frequency of regular cannabis use to estimate tolerance to the effects of THC. We note not all participants became intoxicated after THC administration, likely because of greater than expected THC tolerance. Further, some participants were deemed by the field sobriety test to be cognitively impaired during a placebo visit, possibly due to drug use prior to the visit.

Data from such incongruent visits, where there was a disagreement between cognitive status and drug/placebo assignment were excluded from further analysis.

3.2   fNIRS Data

Functional data was collected using a continuous-wave NIRSport device (NIRx Medical Technology, New York), at a sampling frequency of 7.8 Hz, using two wavelengths of light (760 nm and 850 nm), from 8 sources, using 8 detectors (3 cm long source-detector separation) located on the forehead, following the international 10–20 system to cover prefrontal brain regions. This source-detector geometry resulted in 20 channels. Each fNIRS scan included a 6 min resting state segment. These data were pre-processed using standard steps, which included band-pass filtering between 0.009 and 0.08 Hz, removing possible physiological noise (e.g., hearth beat (0.8 Hz), cardiac cycles (1 Hz), and motion detection and frame removal followed by a spline interpolation.

3.3   Subject-Wise Cross-Validation

After excluding incongruent visits, there were 23 sessions where participants exhibited cognitive impairment after receiving THC, and 26 sessions where participants showed no cognitive impairment after receiving placebo. We used all "post scans" from the drug and placebo congruent visits , in addition to the available "second post" scans from the congruent placebo visits. This yielded a total of 23 fNIRS with a cognitively impaired label and 67 scans with an unimpaired label.

We implemented a 11-fold cross-validation strategy, where we ensured that two sessions from a single subject fell within the same set and thus treated the same as either training, validation or test data. All data were first partitioned into 11 non-overlapping sets, each with at least 2 impaired scans and 4 unimpaired scans. In each fold, one set was reserved as a test set, one set was treated as validation data and the remaining sets were used to train the model.

3.4   Machine Learning Approaches

In our experiments, we consider following machine learning strategies:

- A fully connected neural (FCN) network model trained on the static functional connectivity matrix
- A linear SVM trained on the static connectivity matrices
- An RNN trained on dynamic connectivity (DC) matrices
- An RNN trained directly on the 20-channel fNIRS data

We implemented these both with and without the proposed data augmentation.

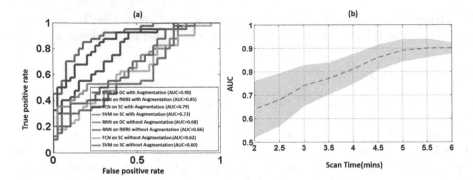

Fig. 2. (a) The ROC curves for the different machine learning models, on cross-validation (DC: dynamic connectivity and SC: static connectivity). (b) The AUC value of best-performed method for different fNIRS scan times. (Better viewed in color) (Color figure online)

3.5   Cross-Validation Results

Figure 2a shows the ROC curves for the aforementioned machine learning methods obtained via cross-validation. We observe that the proposed data augmentation strategy significantly improves the prediction performance for all three models. For the linear SVM model, data augmentation improves the AUC from 60% to 73% on the static connectivity matrices. For the static FCN model, augmentation boosts the AUC from 62% to 79%, whereas for the best-performing RNN, this increase is from 68% to 90%. On the other hand, we notice that the RNN models that capture the temporal dynamics in the data outperform the static model, demonstrating the value in going beyond static functional connectivity in individual-level predictions.

In a secondary analysis, we were interested in examining the effects of shortening the fNIRS scans, as this might help with more wide-spread adoption of this technology. We used the best-performing method, namely the RNN trained on dynamic connectivity matrices with augmentations, on fNIRS data that were artificially clipped at the end. We conducted the same 11-fold cross-validation on these shorter clips. Figure 2b shows how the AUC varies as a function of scan time. The confidence interval is computed as the standard deviation of the AUC metric across the folds. We observe that with as little as 4.5 min of data, we can achieve a promising performance level of about 85% AUC.

3.6   Independent Validation Results

In cross-validation, the models were trained on a subset of the scans from congruent visits: all post scans, and the second post scans from the placebo sessions. Thus, none of the "pre" scans from both sessions, and "second post" scans from the drug sessions were included in cross-validation. Here, we use these for independent validation.

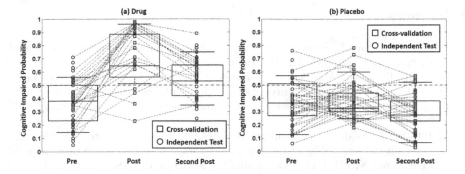

Fig. 3. Predicted probability of cognitive impairment across Pre, Post and Second Post scans of drug (THC) and Placebo sessions. Each datapoint is a single scan, and scans from the same participants are connected by lines. The circles show independent test scans and squares show scans used during cross-validation. Note, for the cross-validation datapoints, the predictions are unbiased and correspond to the fold where that participant was treated as a test case.

For the drug visits, Fig. 3(a) shows the predicted cognitive impairment probability on each of the fNIRS scans. We observe that the majority of these predictions are less than 50% for the pre-scans, and greater than 50% for the post and second post scans. Note that each dot corresponds to a scan and scans from same subject are connected with a line. We observe that for a vast majority of cases (all but 2), the post scans are predicted to be more impaired than the pre-scans. Furthermore, in all but three cases, the second post scans are predicted to be less impaired than the post scans. These are very consistent with our expectations of subjects achieving a peak high around the time of the post scan.

For the placebo visits, Fig. 3(b) shows the predicted cognitive impairment probability values. We observe that most of these predictions, particularly for the second post scans are less than 50% and the up-down pattern we observe in the drug sessions is not apparent. Again, these results are very consistent with our expectations for a placebo session, where some participants might have some residual cognitive impairment due to drug use before the visit.

4   Conclusion

In this work, we studied resting-state fNIRS data and its application to detecting cannabis-associated cognitive impairment. We evaluated several machine learning approaches on static brain connectivity, dynamic brain connectivity and pre-processed fNIRS data to solve this problem. Our results demonstrated that modeling the temporal dynamics in functional connectivity data can yield a significant boost in prediction performance. We also presented a novel data augmentation strategy suitable for resting state functional scans that can improve accuracy.

References

1. Sewell, R., Poling, J., Sofuoglu, M.: The effect of cannabis compared with alcohol on driving. Am. J. Addict. **18**, 185–193 (2009)
2. Keles, H., Radoman, M., Pachas, G., Evins, A., Gilman, J.: Using functional near-infrared spectroscopy to measure effects of delta 9-tetrahydrocannabinol on prefrontal activity and working memory in cannabis users. Front. Hum. Neurosci. **11**, 488–498 (2017)
3. McIntosh, M., Shahani, U., Boulton, R., McCulloch, D.: Absolute quantification of oxygenated hemoglobin within the visual cortex with functional near infrared spectroscopy (fNIRS). Invest. Ophthalmol. Vis. Sci. **51**(9), 4856–4860 (2010)
4. Quaresima, V., Ferrari, M.: Functional near-infrared spectroscopy (fNIRS) for assessing cerebral cortex function during human behavior in natural/social situations: a concise review. Organ. Res. Methods **22**(1), 46–68 (2019)
5. Wee, C., Yap, P., Shen, D.: Diagnosis of autism spectrum disorders using temporally distinct resting-state functional connectivity networks. CNS Neurosci. Ther. **22**, 212–219 (2016)
6. Eavani, H., Satterthwaite, T.D., Gur, R.E., Gur, R.C., Davatzikos, C.: Unsupervised learning of functional network dynamics in resting state fMRI. In: Gee, J.C., Joshi, S., Pohl, K.M., Wells, W.M., Zöllei, L. (eds.) IPMI 2013. LNCS, vol. 7917, pp. 426–437. Springer, Heidelberg (2013). https://doi.org/10.1007/978-3-642-38868-2_36
7. Wee, C., Yap, P., Zhang, D., Wang, L., Shen, D.: Group-constrained sparse fMRI connectivity modeling for mild cognitive impairment identification. Brain Struct. Funct. **219**, 641–656 (2014)
8. Lv, J., Jiang, X., Li, X., Zhu, D., Chen, H., Zhang, T.: Sparse representation of whole-brain fMRI signals for identification of functional networks. Med. Image Anal. **20**, 112–134 (2015)
9. Kiviniemi, V., et al.: A sliding time-window ICA reveals spatial variability of the default mode network in time. Brain connectivity **1**(4), 339–347 (2011)
10. Chang, C., Glover, G.H.: Time-frequency dynamics of resting-state brain connectivity measured with fMRI. NeuroImage **50**, 81–98 (2010)
11. Di, X., Biswal, B.: Dynamic brain functional connectivity modulated by resting-state networks. Brain Struct. Funct. **220**, 37–46 (2015)
12. Leonardi, N.: Principal components of functional connectivity: a new approach to study dynamic brain connectivity during rest. NeuroImage **83**, 937–950 (2013)
13. Khosla, M., Jamison, K., Ngo, G.H., Kuceyeski, A., Sabuncu, M.R.: Machine learning in resting-state fMRI analysis. Magn. Reson. Imaging (2019)
14. Leonardi, N., Ville, D.V.D.: On spurious and real fluctuations of dynamic functional connectivity during rest. Neuroimage **104**, 430–436 (2015)

Cross-Domain Conditional Generative Adversarial Networks for Stereoscopic Hyperrealism in Surgical Training

Sandy Engelhardt[1,3]([✉]) [ID], Lalith Sharan[1,3], Matthias Karck[2],
Raffaele De Simone[2], and Ivo Wolf[1]

[1] Faculty of Computer Science, Mannheim University of Applied Sciences,
Mannheim, Germany
s.engelhardt@hs-mannheim.de
[2] Department of Cardiac Surgery, Heidelberg University Hospital,
Heidelberg, Germany
[3] Department of Simulation and Graphics and Research Campus STIMULATE,
Magdeburg University, Magdeburg, Germany

Abstract. Phantoms for surgical training are able to mimic cutting
and suturing properties and patient-individual shape of organs, but lack
a realistic visual appearance that captures the heterogeneity of surgical
scenes. In order to overcome this in endoscopic approaches, hyperrealistic concepts have been proposed to be used in an augmented reality-
setting, which are based on deep image-to-image transformation methods. Such concepts are able to generate realistic representations of phantoms learned from real intraoperative endoscopic sequences. Conditioned
on frames from the surgical training process, the learned models are able
to generate impressive results by transforming unrealistic parts of the
image (e.g. the uniform phantom texture is replaced by the more heterogeneous texture of the tissue). Image-to-image synthesis usually learns a
mapping $G : X \rightarrow Y$ such that the distribution of images from $G(X)$ is
indistinguishable from the distribution Y. However, it does not necessarily force the generated images to be consistent and without artifacts. In
the endoscopic image domain this can affect depth cues and stereo consistency of a stereo image pair, which ultimately impairs surgical vision. We
propose a cross-domain conditional generative adversarial network approach (GAN) that aims to generate more consistent stereo pairs. The
results show substantial improvements in depth perception and realism
evaluated by 3 domain experts and 3 medical students on a 3D monitor
over the baseline method. In 84 of 90 instances our proposed method was
preferred or rated equal to the baseline.

Keywords: Generative adversarial networks · Minimally-invasive
surgical training · Augmented reality · Mitral valve simulator ·
Laparoscopy

D. Shen et al. (Eds.): MICCAI 2019, LNCS 11768, pp. 155–163, 2019.
https://doi.org/10.1007/978-3-030-32254-0_18

1   Introduction

Minimally invasive surgery is characterized by a restricted view of the surgical target. In many such procedures, the only way to observe the surgical field is with endoscopic vision on an external display, which is commonly associated with an impaired depth perception. This situation requires an excellent hand-eye coordination, exceptional skills and dexterity with instruments, which should be trained with surgical simulators before performing it on patients. On such simulators, the photo-realistic fidelity and depth perception is a key feature that can improve the transfer ratio of trainees to real surgeries. However, most virtual or physical simulators lack such properties, due to limited capabilities of modelling realistic textures or by current material that is used for phantoms.

In our previous work [1], a deep learning-based concept to tackle the issue of photo-realism of surgical simulations was presented. The approach was coined *hyperrealism*, which is able to map patterns learned from intraoperative video sequences onto the video stream captured during simulated surgery on anatomical replica. Used within an augmented reality setting, *hyperrealism* is defined as a new augmented reality paradigm on the Reality-Virtuality continuum [2], which is closer to 'full reality' in comparison to other concepts where artificial overlays are superimposed on a video frame. In a hyperrealistic surgical training environment, the parts of the simulated environment that look unnatural are replaced by realistic appearances. Parts that already look natural ideally stay the same. It is shown that such an approach greatly improves reproduction of the intraoperative appearance during training and therefore makes minimally-invasive surgical training more realistic. The approach is in principle also employable for enhancing photo-realism of virtual training simulators, as shown by Luengo et al. [3] who used a deep learning approach that relies on style transfer.

Methodologically, our proposed approach is based on so-called unpaired deep image-to-image transformation methods [4]. The underlying concept is to use adversarial training of a generator and a discriminator network, and to employ a cycle between the two input domains to generate realistic looking images. The key to the success of such generative adversarial networks (GANs) is the idea of an adversarial loss that forces the generated images to be, in principle, indistinguishable from real images. Such concepts are able to generate realistic representations of phantoms learned from real intraoperative endoscopic sequences [1]. Conditioned on frames from the surgical training process, the learned models are able to generate impressive results by transforming unrealistic parts of the image (e.g. the uniform phantom texture is replaced by the more heterogeneous texture of the tissue). However, the traditional CycleGAN approach [4] neither enforces temporal coherence, which was incorporated in our previous contribution [1], nor enforces a stereo pair to be consistent.

A recent work published at CVPR 2018 [5] was the first to address stereoscopic neural style transfer. Approaches beforehand only dealt with monocular style transfer. The authors showed that independent application of stylization approaches to left and right views of stereoscopic images does not preserve the original disparity consistency in the final stylization results, which causes 3D

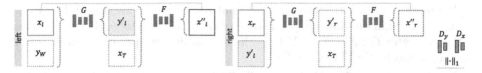

Fig. 1. Proposed architecture that shows the $X \to Y \to X$-cycle for a stereo pair (x_l, x_r). In contrast to classical generators, each generator G and F takes two inputs and generates one output. The second input image, e.g. y_W, x_T, is taken from the other domain and can be chosen randomly. To enable a better consistency, the output of G, which is y'_l, is chosen as a second input in the generation cycle of the right image. Discriminators D_y and D_x evaluate real and fake images marked in orange and green. (Color figure online)

fatigue to the viewers on a 3D display [5]. Chen et al. [5] incorporated a disparity loss into the style loss function that is employable in virtual scenes with known disparity information. In this contribution, we want to tackle the same issue for physical surgical simulators, i.e. generation of more consistent stereo-images without relying on ground truth disparity, which is more complicated to obtain in the medical domain. In order to achieve this, a novel cross-domain conditional GAN is introduced in the following.

2   Methods

Given unpaired training samples in two image domains X and Y, the Cycle-GAN model proposed by Zhu et al. [4] learns a mapping (generator) $G : X \to Y$ and the reverse mapping $F : Y \to X$. These generators are trained to produce outputs that are indistinguishable from real images in the respective target domains for discriminator networks D_Y and D_X. Additionally, the consistency of the cyclic mappings $F(G(x))$ and $G(F(y))$ with the respective inputs $x \in X$ and $y \in Y$ is enforced by using the L_1-norm. The proposed method builds upon this idea to learn a style transfer between an image stream from the source domain X of *surgical simulation* to a target domain Y of *intraoperative surgeries* and vice versa in the absence of paired endoscopic image samples.

2.1   Cross Domain Conditional GAN

For our task, the forward generator $G : X \to Y$ of the standard CycleGAN tended to create unrealistic colors and artifacts in the generated intraoperative scenes. To overcome this, we introduce *cross domain conditional GANs*.

Traditional *conditional GANs* [6] learn a mapping from an observed input domain X and random noise Z to the output domain Y, $G : X \times Z \to Y$. Isola et al. [7] found the additional random noise vector to be ineffective and dropped it from the paired image translation predecessor of the unpaired CycleGAN as well as from the CycleGAN itself (in contrast to the concurrent DualGAN [8]).

We propose to re-introduce an additional input, but to use a sample y from the target domain distribution p_Y instead of random noise to guide the training of the generator $G : X \times Y \rightarrow Y$ to realistic coloring and preservation of detail (and analogously $F : Y \times X \rightarrow X$).

For our stereo image translation task, we use a random sample $y_W \sim p_Y$ for the translation of the left image x_l of the stereo pair and the generated output of the generator $y'_l := G(x_l, y_W)$ for generating the right image $y'_r := G(x_r, y'_l)$ to additionally support the generation of consistently colored stereo pairs, see Fig. 1.

2.2 Network Architectures

The used network architectures of the generators and discriminators are largely the same as in the original CycleGAN approach [4]. A TensorFlow implementation provided on GitHub[1] was used as the basis and extended. All discriminators take the complete input images, which is different from the 70×70 PatchGAN approach [4]. For the generators, 7 instead of 9 residual blocks are used, because experiments on our data showed better results for this configuration. Moreover, the generators were changed to handle a 6-channel input.

3   Evaluation

A minimally invasive mitral valve repair simulator (MICS MVR surgical simulator, Fehling Instruments GmbH & Co. KG, Karlstein, Germany) was extended with patient-specific silicone mitral valves. In comparison to other simulators, the valve replica consist of all anatomical parts, i.e. the annulus, the leaflets, the chordae tendineae and the papillary muscles. Details on the valve model production are elaborated on in a previous work [9].

An expert segmented pathological mitral valves on the end-systolic time step from echocardiographic data, which are represented as virtual models. From these models, 3D printable molds and suitable prosthetic rings were automatically generated and 3D-printed. Subsequently, 15 silicone valves were manufactured that could be anchored in the simulator onto a custom valve holder. We asked different experts and trainees to perform mitral valve repair techniques (annuloplasty, triangular leaflet resection, neo-chordae implantation) on these valves and recorded the endoscopic video stream [10].

3.1   Data and Training of Network

In total, approx. 240,000 stereo pair frames from the surgical training procedures were captured in full HD resolution or larger, which sums up to 9 h of video material. Most of the videos were captured at 25 fps. Due to change in recording equipment, a subset of approx. 20,000 stereo frames was acquired at 1 fps. The

---

[1] https://github.com/LynnHo/CycleGAN-Tensorflow-PyTorch-Simple.

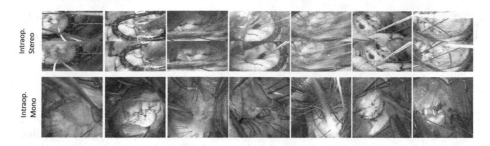

Fig. 2. Mono- and stereoscopic examples from mitral valve repair. The scenes are diverse: with or without prosthetic ring, sutures, instruments and needles, blood etc.

training data for the network was sampled every 240th frame or every 40th frame, respectively. In total, the network training set consists of 1400 stereo pair frames from the training with the surgical phantom. To avoid overfitting of the model, valve replica shown in videos for network training were not used for network testing.

Intraoperatively, more than 620,000 stereo pairs were captured during three minimally invasive mitral valve repair surgeries. The frame rate varied between 60 fps and 25 fps. Scenes where the valve itself was not visible were neglected. For network training, a stereo pair after each 120th or 240th frame was sampled retrospectively from these videos, which sums up to approx. 1200 stero pairs for network training. The scenes are highly diverse, as the valve's appearance drastically changes over time (e.g. due to cutting of tissue, implanting sutures and prostheses, fluids such as blood and saline solution), see Fig. 2. Furthermore, occlusions or lens fogging often disturbed the recording.

Besides the just described stereo data collection, we pre-trained our network on a monoscopic data base. The strength of our proposed method is that, it does not solely rely on a stereo pair as input, but can be also trained un-stereo-paired. The monoscopic data was put together from recordings during four open mitral valve surgeries with a monocular endoscope, in which case fewer lens occlusions and less fogging occurred. For the phantom recordings, half of the frames used for the monoscopic pre-training are also represented in the stereo data set. In total, the source and target domain consisted of approx. 1500 single frames each.

All monoscopic frames or each left and right image of the pair were randomly cropped and re-scaled to 256×512. Further data augmentation was performed by random horizontal flipping and intensity re-scaling. For all the experiments, the consistency loss was weighted with $\lambda = 20$. The Adam solver with a batch size of 1 and a learning rate of 0.0001 without linear decay to zero was used. Similar to Zhu et al. [4], the objective was divided by 2 while optimizing D, which slows down the rate at which D learns relative to G. Discriminators are updated using a history of 50 generated images rather than the ones produced by the latest generative networks [4]. The CycleGAN network was pre-trained for 40 epochs on the monoscopic data and then trained on the left image of the stereo pair for another 40 epochs. Similarly, our proposed network was trained on $40 + 40$

epochs. For using the proposed network in the monoscopic case, y_W is randomly chosen from the other domain in the $X{\to}Y{\to}X$ cycle and x_W accordingly in the reverse cycle.

3.2 Evaluation

The most important factors for the proposed application are related to perception. Therefore, we first evaluated whether three domain experts (cardiac surgeons who each at least assisted mitral valve repair surgeries) and three non-experts (medical students) are able to perceive depth on a 3D monitor on interlaced stereo pairs. Secondly, we asked the surgeons how real the generated intraoperative stereo frames appear from their experiences. All answers had to be given on a 5-point Likert Scale, with 5 being the answer with the highest agreement. Related to this, we found it crucial to ask clinical questions to the domain experts in order to show the reliability of the transformation, which is associated with a change in appearance of the scene. Reliability of the transformation requires the scene to not change too drastically, meaning that neither the shape of objects should be altered, nor additional parts should be added or taken away. The surgeons were asked (1) to diagnose the pathology of the presented valve, (2) to name the surgical instrument visible in the scene, and (3) to state which phase of the surgery is presented. We evaluated these questions by extracting 15 random samples from our test set; each sample was shown in interlaced format on a 3D monitor. For each frame, the corresponding result from the original CycleGAN was shown directly afterwards, therefore enabling a direct comparison between our results and the baseline. At the start of the experiments we asked the participants of the study to rate the depth for two realistic stereo frames from the surgical phantom, in the following referred to as *Test1* and *Test2* example.

4 Results

Example results of our method in comparison to the baseline CycleGAN are provided in Fig. 3. A rough visual analysis shows that the structure of the valves and of the instruments are better preserved in our method. Furthermore, the left and right image of the stereo pair appeared to be very consistent. The same was confirmed by the user study.

Figure 4 illustrates the ratings by the non-experts for depth perception for each of the presented scenes. The median for each participant on our results in comparison to the baseline are 3 to 2, 4 to 3 and 3 to 3, which means that our method was clearly favored over the baseline and that the participants had a three-dimensional impression from the synthesized stereo images. Figure 4 also shows that depth perception even on real images of the silicone phantom is not assessed as completely perfect (*Test1* and *Test2*). These ratings help to relate the assessment of the generated stereo images to samples taken from the real world. In 39 instances, our method was preferred over the baseline by the participants

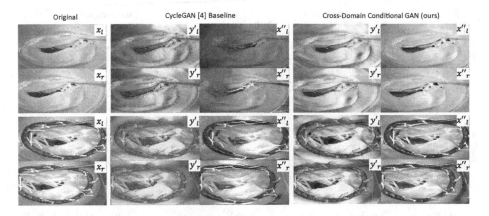

Fig. 3. Examples from CycleGAN baseline [4] and our proposed method.

(10 instances are better by $\Delta 2$ and 29 are better by $\Delta 1$). In three instances, both methods were assessed as equally good and in three other instances, our method was rated worse in stereo consistency.

Considering the evaluation by the expert, a similar picture can be drawn. The respective diagram on assessment of depth perception is provided in Fig. 4. In 35 instances, our method was preferred over the baseline by the experts (1 instance better by $\Delta 3$, 8 instances better by $\Delta 2$ and 26 instances better by $\Delta 1$). In seven cases, both methods were assessed as equal and in three other instances, our method was assessed as worse in comparison to the baseline. When referring to the realism, our method is also superior, and was conceived as less artifact-prone and more related to an intraoperative scene. Figure 4 illustrates the ratings by the experts. In 37 cases, our method was preferred over the baseline by the experts (5 instances better by $\Delta 3$, 10 instances better by $\Delta 2$ and 22 instances better by $\Delta 1$). Pathology assessment on the synthesized stereo frames yielded a good result. 37 of 45 correct decisions were made solely by watching the generated stereo pair. Furthermore, in 42 of 45 cases, the correct instrument that is shown in the scene, was named. Please note that in some instances, the instruments are only visible by a small margin on the actual clipped image. Moreover, motion artifacts complicated the assessment in 2 cases (example 13, 14). In 43 of 45 assessments, the right surgical phase has been identified by the participants.

5 Discussion

To the best of our knowledge, the presented approach is the first to address stereo-endoscopic scene transformation for minimally-invasive surgical training. In this paper, we propose a novel cross domain conditioning GAN, which is superior in synthesizing consistent and more realistic stereo data in comparison to the unpaired CycleGAN approach [4]. Due to conditioning on a second image, which is drawn from the target domain (real or generated content), the network

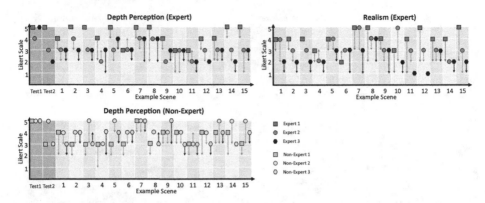

Fig. 4. Expert and non-expert ratings for depth perception and realism. Symbols indicate the rating per participant of the generated samples by cross-domain conditional GAN. Arrows show the difference to CycleGAN [4].

is also able to generate images with less artifacts and with more realistic color, heterogeneous textures, specularities and blood. The reliability of the generated samples was indirectly assessed by asking clinically relevant end points considering visible pathology, surgical instrument and surgical phase. We want to especially emphasize that almost all of the questions could be correctly answered with high confidence. In general, we decided against the conduction of a Visual Turing Test, as some shape-related features in the scene (e.g. a personalized ring shape instead of a standard commercial ring) would have been easily identified by an expert surgeon.

Future work includes usage of the presented approach together with depth sensing technologies which are currently not applicable during surgery due to sterilization restrictions. The acquired depth information can be leveraged as ground truth data for training disparity estimation models from transformed mono- or stereo-endoscopic images.

Acknowlegments. The research was supported by the German Research Foundation DFG project 398787259, DE 2131/2-1 and EN 1197/2-1. The GPU was donated by Nvidia small scale grant.

References

1. Engelhardt, S., De Simone, R., Full, P.M., Karck, M., Wolf, I.: Improving surgical training phantoms by hyperrealism: deep unpaired image-to-image translation from real surgeries. In: Frangi, A.F., Schnabel, J.A., Davatzikos, C., Alberola-López, C., Fichtinger, G. (eds.) MICCAI 2018. LNCS, vol. 11070, pp. 747–755. Springer, Cham (2018). https://doi.org/10.1007/978-3-030-00928-1_84
2. Milgram, P., Kishino, F.: A taxonomy of mixed reality visual displays. IEICE Trans. Inf. Syst. **77**(12), 1321–1329 (1994)

3. Luengo, I., Flouty, E., Giataganas, P., Wisanuvej, P., Nehme, J., Stoyanov, D.: Surreal: enhancing surgical simulation realism using style transfer. In: British Machine Vision Conference 2018, BMVC 2018, Northumbria University, Newcastle, UK, 3–6 September 2018, p. 116 (2018)
4. Zhu, J.Y., Park, T., Isola, P., Efros, A.A.: Unpaired image-to-image translation using cycle-consistent adversarial networks. In: IEEE International Conference on Computer Vision (ICCV) 2017, pp. 2242–2251 (2017)
5. Chen, D., Yuan, L., Liao, J., Yu, N., Hua, G.: Stereoscopic neural style transfer. In: The IEEE Conference on Computer Vision and Pattern Recognition (CVPR), pp. 6654–6663, June 2018
6. Mirza, M., Osindero, S.: Conditional Generative Adversarial Nets. arXiv:1411.1784, November 2014
7. Isola, P., Zhu, J.-Y., Zhou, T., Efros, A.A.: Image-to-image translation with conditional adversarial networks. arXiv:1611.07004, November 2016
8. Yi, Z., Zhang, H., Tan, P., Gong, M.: DualGAN: unsupervised dual learning for image-to-image translation. In: The IEEE International Conference on Computer Vision (ICCV), pp. 2868–2876, October 2017
9. Engelhardt, S., Sauerzapf, S., Preim, B., Karck, M., Wolf, I., De Simone, R.: Flexible and comprehensive patient-specific mitral valve silicone models with chordae tendinae made from 3D-printable molds. Int. J. Comput. Assist. Radiol. Surg. (IPCAI Spec. Issue) 14(7), 1177–1186 (2019)
10. Engelhardt, S., Sauerzapf, S., Brčić, A., Karck, M., Wolf, I., De Simone, R.: Replicated mitral valve models from real patients offer training opportunities for minimally invasive mitral valve repair. Interact. Cardiovasc. Thorac. Surg. 29, 43–50 (2019)

Free-View, 3D Gaze-Guided Robotic Scrub Nurse

Alexandros Kogkas[1]([✉])(iD), Ahmed Ezzat[1](iD), Rudrik Thakkar[2], Ara Darzi[3](iD), and George Mylonas[1](iD)

[1] HARMS Lab, Department of Surgery and Cancer, Imperial College London, St Mary's Hospital, London, UK
a.kogkas15@imperial.ac.uk
[2] St George's, University of London, London, UK
[3] Department of Surgery and Cancer, Imperial College London, St Mary's Hospital, London, UK

Abstract. We introduce a novel 3D gaze-guided robotic scrub nurse (RN) and test the platform in simulated surgery to determine usability and acceptability with clinical teams. Surgeons and trained scrub nurses performed an ex vivo task on pig colon. Surgeons used gaze via wearable eye-tracking glasses to select surgical instruments on a screen, in turn initiating RN to deliver the instrument. Comparison was done between human- and robot-assisted tasks (HT vs RT). Real-time gaze-screen interaction was based on a framework developed with synergy of conventional wearable eye-tracking, motion capture system and RGB-D cameras. NASA-TLX and Van der Laan's technology acceptance questionnaires were collected and analyzed. 10 teams of surgical trainees (ST) and scrub nurses (HN) participated. Overall, NASA-TLX feedback was positive. ST and HN revealed no statistically significant difference in overall task load. Task performance feedback was unaffected. Frustration was reported by ST. Overall, Van der Laan's scores showed positive usefulness and satisfaction scores following RN use. There was no significant difference in task interruptions across HT vs RT. Similarly, no statistical difference was found in duration to task completion in both groups. Quantitative and qualitative feedback was positive. The source of frustration has been understood. Importantly, there was no significant difference in task workflow or operative time, with overall perceptions towards task performance remaining unchanged in HT vs RT.

Keywords: Smart operating room · Gaze interactions · Robotic scrub nurse.

1 Introduction

Technology advances within surgery have seen operating habits transform over the past years. Certain surgeries have seen traditional techniques replaced by robotic assistance, now accepted by the surgical community as mainstream practice [7].

Electronic supplementary material The online version of this chapter (https://doi.org/10.1007/978-3-030-32254-0_19) contains supplementary material, which is available to authorized users.

ⓒ Springer Nature Switzerland AG 2019
D. Shen et al. (Eds.): MICCAI 2019, LNCS 11768, pp. 164–172, 2019.
https://doi.org/10.1007/978-3-030-32254-0_19

Thus, more research has targeted the development of further assistive robotic systems to improve operating practice. Healthcare associated human error has been reported as a leading cause of preventable patient harm and has at times resulted in avoidable patient death [8].

Systems such as *Gestix* has relied on predetermined hand gestures and 2D cameras to enable a particular action such as magnifying or changing the image [13]. *HERMES VRI* is a voice-command system which was trialed in laparoscopic surgery and shown faster operating times [2]. More recently, there has been an expansion of research directed at gaze-controlled navigation due to perceived advantage in practicality and limitations of the interruptions of hand gesture control, as well as difficulty of voice recognition when scrubbed within the noisy operating environment [1].

Surgical robotic assistance that can augment human teams is an area attracting a lot of research with much promise. Such devices include the da Vinci^{TM} (Intuitive Surgical, Inc.); an established robotic system controlled by the surgeon via a computer-based console. Other examples include automated laparoscopic devices relying on the surgeon's head position to move the instrument and show up to 15% reduction in task completion time [4]. *Gestonurse* is a magnetic based robotic scrub nurse which uses hand gesture to select and deliver surgical instruments [5]. *Penelope* has been described as the first robotic scrub nurse successfully used in surgery, reported as a semi-autonomous system relying on verbal commands to predict, pick up and deliver the desired instrument [11].

More recently, we have introduced the perceptually-enabled smart operating room concept, based on a novel real-time framework for theater-wide and patient-wise 3D gaze localization in a simultaneous and unrestricted/mobile fashion [6]. The framework facilitates seamless and meaningful integration of human and technology in the theater, aiming at improved safety, collaboration and clinical outcome. An extension of this framework is presented here, that allows hands-free gaze-driven interactions with a screen and a robotic arm, which acts as a robotic scrub nurse (RN) assistant by transferring surgical instruments to the surgeon. The introduction of a RN as an integral component may address nursing shortages and empower the team by enabling the usability and acceptability by the operating team, during realistic surgical procedures.

2   Methods

The core functionality of the real-time framework is to provide the user's 3D point of regard (PoR) in a world coordinate system (WCS), defined by multiple co-registered RGB-D sensors fixed in the theater. It relies on (a) estimating the pose of the scene camera integrated with the eye-tracking glasses (ETG) in the WSC and (b) tracing the gaze ray provided by the ETG on the head frame of reference onto the 3D reconstructed space. The ETG scene camera pose is estimated with the employment of a motion capture system (MCS) and spherical markers mounted on the ETG. The provided camera pose, 2D fixation and parameters provided by an offline calibration process, enable gaze control of a screen in space. A graphical user interface (GUI) designed allows gaze selection of surgical instruments to be delivered by a robot arm.

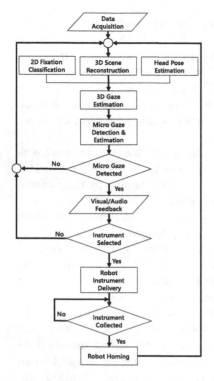

Fig. 1. Flow chart of the RN system.

Equipment. For eye-tracking, the wireless SMI (SensoMotoric Instruments GmbH) glasses are used; for RGB-D sensing the Microsoft Kinect v2; for head pose tracking the OptiTrack MCS, with 4 Prime 13 cameras. The robot is a UR5 (Universal Robots), with the Robotiq FT-300 F/T sensor attached. The instrument selection GUI is shown on a 42" LG screen with 1920×1080 px resolution. A Windows 10 PC is used for acquiring and streaming ETG and MCS data and a Linux PC with Ubuntu 14.04 for all other modules.

Offline Calibration. In an offline calibration routine, the following are defined: (a) rigid transformation between the MCS coordinate system (MCS CS) and the WCS, (b) screen position in the WCS. (c) surgical instruments positions in the robot coordinate system (RCS). The rigid transformations between the ETG rigid body–ETG scene camera (Y) and MCS CS – WCS (X) is estimated by solving the hand-eye calibration problem $AX = YB$ [10]. This involves simultaneously capturing 6 DOF poses of the ETG rigid body in the MCS CS and the ETG scene camera in the WCS. The *screen corners'* 3D coordinates in the WCS are manually selected on the Kinect RGB image and the 3D points are generated. The *surgical instruments* are positioned in fixed positions on a tray. The robot is manually moved over each instrument and the target pose is calibrated. 9-point *eye-tracking calibration* is performed before every task.

Application Workflow. The system is developed in *ROS* with C++, to facilitate the hardware agnostic aspect of the framework. User head-pose (equivalent to the ETG's scene camera pose) provided by the MCS and transformed to the WCS, can be used to map 2D gaze to a unique 3D fixation in the WCS. The 3D gaze ray is used to detect fixations on the screen fixed in space (microfixation). The GUI consists of two parts: instrument selection (left) and image navigation (right). The image navigation part shows task workflow steps. The user can navigate through it by fixating on the right top and bottom of the

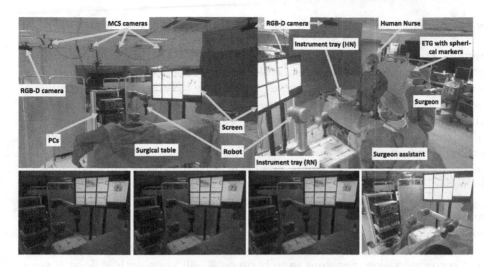

Fig. 2. Top: The experimental setup. Bottom: Egocentric view. From left to right, the surgeon looks at an instrument (red), the instrument is preselected (orange), then selected (green) and the robot delivers it to the ST. (Color figure online)

screen. Micro-fixation on any of the instrument blocks initiates a traffic light sequence (red-amber-green) followed by relevant audio feedback. After a certain dwell time the robot routine is triggered. The robot moves towards a surgical instrument selected by the user, grasps it with a magnetic gripper and transfers it to the user. When the F/T sensor mounted on the robot senses the instrument is picked up, it returns to its homing pose (Fig. 1).

3   Experiments

Surgeons (surgical trainees – ST) were recruited to perform ex vivo resection of a pig colon and hand sewn end-to-end anastomosis. Each surgeon performed two experiments in randomized order:

- A *human nurse only task (HT)* with the assistance of a human scrub nurse (HN).
- A *robot and human nurse task (RT)* with the assistance of both robotic (RN) and human (HN) scrub nurses.

In both experiments, a surgeon assistant aids the surgeon and a scrub nurse assistant the HN. The instrument tray inventory consists of the 6 most frequently utilized instruments during this particular task: a suture scissors, a Mcindoe (curved) scissors, a non-toothed forceps, two artery clips and a hand suture attached to an artery clip. The main stages of the task are presented on the right part of the screen (Fig. 2).

For the RT, the surgeon uses the ETG and is asked to fixate on 9 predefined points to perform eye-tracking calibration. Familiarization with the system setup is offered for 1 min. During the task, the surgeon looks at the screen to select an instrument and once it is delivered and collected, the surgeon assistant responds to verbal command or prior experience to return the instrument to its predefined position on the instrument tray (See supplementary material). The surgeon uses verbal command directed towards the HN when further instruments are required. In case the wrong instrument is delivered, the surgeon expresses the error verbally. If eye-tracking recalibration is necessary, the task continues after recalibration. During the HT the setup is identical. The screen and RN are switched off and the surgeon relies entirely on the HN to deliver instruments based on verbal commands. ETG is utilized to capture and analyze visual behavior.

During both experiments, distractions are introduced to the HN. The scrub nurse assistant asks the HN to stop and perform an instrument count twice and solve a puzzle at specific task stages.

10 surgical trainee specialists (ST) participated (7 male and 3 female). Two had corrected vision. Surgeons were between 30–40 years with at least 6 years surgical experience. 5 trained theater scrub nurses (HN) were recruited. One surgical trainee, with 2 years surgical experience, acted as surgeon assistant and one medical student acted as scrub nurse assistant for all experiments.

4   Results

Performance, Usability and Workflow Metrics. Overall *task completion time* was 22:35 ± 6:30 min vs 26:04 ± 4:50 min (HT vs RT, respectively). The RT mean duration includes system recalibration intervals (Table 1).

Workflow interruptions were measured for both tasks. During the HT, interruptions are defined as the events of a wrong instrument delivery by the HN and the interruption of the task by the ST for >3 s waiting for instrument delivery. During the RT, the same interruptions are measured (HN-derived) in addition to the RN-derived events, namely incorrect instrument delivery and eye-tracking recalibrations (Fig. 3).

After each task, the ST and HN were asked to complete a *NASA-TLX* questionnaire and the results are depicted in (Fig. 3).

Technology usability and satisfaction feedback was collected immediately following the RT (*Van der Laan*). ST reported usefulness score of 0.5 ± 0.73 and

Table 1. ANOVA of number of interruptions and task completion time (*mm : ss*) between the HT and RT.

Task	Interruptions				Task completion time			
	Lower	Upper	Mean	SD	Lower	Upper	Mean	SD
HT	1	5	2.4	1.26	16:02	37:17	22:35	6:30
RT	1	4	2.3	0.95	20:18	34:35	26:04	4:50
ANOVA	$F(1, 18) = 0.040$, p $= 0.844$				$F(1, 18) = 1.849$, p $= 0.191$			

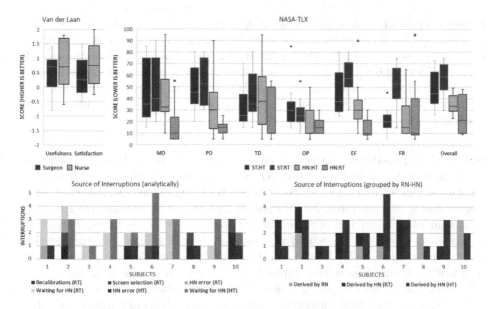

Fig. 3. Top left: Technology acceptance results. Top right: NASA-TLX results, consisting of mental demand *(MD)*, physical demand *(PD)*, temporal demand *(TD)*, performance *(OP)*, effort *(EF)* and frustration *(FR)*. *ST:HT* refers to ST feedback on human nurse only task (HT). Bottom: Source of interruptions analytically (left) and grouped by RN- and HN- derived

satisfying score of 0.43 ± 0.74. ST reported that the RN was likable 0.4 ± 0.84, useful 0.5 ± 1.08 and pleasant 0.8 ± 0.79. ST feedback was neutral about RN desirability 0.1 ± 0.99. HN feedback reported usefulness score of 0.76 ± 0.92 and satisfying score of 0.78 ± 0.79. HN reported RN was likable 0.6 ± 1.26, useful 0.7 ± 1.42 and pleasant 0.9 ± 0.99. RN was perceived as desirable 0.7 ± 0.82.

Comparative Analysis. No significant difference was found in overall *task completion time* (p $= 0.19$) in RT vs HT with $26{:}04 \pm 4{:}50$ vs $22{:}35 \pm 6{:}30$ min, respectively (Table 1).

The comparative analysis of the total number of *interruptions* per task is shown in Table 1. No significant difference incurred (p $= 0.844$) between RT and HT (2.3 ± 0.95 vs 2.4 ± 1.26, respectively).

Upon comparison of ST vs HN using RN there was no statistically significant difference in *technology acceptance* domains. Overall responses were positive in ST and HN groups (usefulness score of 0.5 ± 0.73/satisfying score of 0.43 ± 0.74 vs usefulness score of 0.76 ± 0.92 and satisfying score of 0.78 ± 0.79, respectively).

ST subjective feedback (*NASA-TLX*) reported no significant difference overall. ST did not report any significant change on task performance mean 33.5 ± 20 vs 27.5 ± 12.3 (HT vs RT), p $= 0.779$. ST did report significant frustration using RN 22 ± 10.6 vs 51.5 ± 19.3, p $= 0.013$. HN feedback reported no significant difference overall. There was no significant difference in task performance; 18 ± 14.2 vs 16 ± 7, p=0.989. Frustration remained unchanged; 24.5 ± 18.3 vs 25.5 ± 29.1, $p = 1.0$. Comparison of ST vs HN using RN showed significant difference overall $(57.5 \pm 15.8$ vs 24.6 ± 15.9, $p < .001)$ and specifically in mental, physical demand and effort, in so demonstrating reduced HN demands. Perception on task performance was non-significant $(p = 0.282)$. There was a significant difference in frustration $(p = 0.035)$.

Subjective Feedback. Overall feedback was positive with all participants expressing that RN had potential. All STs expressed looking away from surgical field can affect task flow whilst seven STs highlighted verbal commands may augment the platform. All STs highlighted that a more intuitive RN platform that can predict the next instrument would improve usability. Three STs expressed a view that RN would not respond as well as HN in unpredictable events or emergency. All HN reported positively about the RN platform and dismissed any concerns it may replace their role entirely. All HNs agreed the RN would allow them to perform other tasks more efficiently, especially in big operations where multiple instrument sets and assemblies are required. All HNs reported RN would have a role in surgery.

5 Discussion and Conclusion

A novel robotic scrub nurse has been proposed, enabling surgeons to visually select an instrument, using an ETG device, to retrieve and then deliver it to the surgeon to complete a surgical task.

Subjectively, RN was received positively. NASA-TLX data demonstrated no statistically significant difference between HT vs RT across perceptions by ST and HN on overall task load. This affirms a perception of safety towards the platform. ST reported no significant difference across mental, physical or temporal demands in delivering the task. Furthermore, Van der Laan technology acceptance scores were positive across ST vs HN participants.

Objectively, RT incurred no significant difference in number of task interruptions, compared with HT. RN related interruptions were attributed to recalibration where the surgeon visual gaze was not accurately represented on the instrument monitor. The RN selected the correct instrument in 100% of tasks. In comparison, HT interruptions included incorrect instrument transfers or delays in instrument delivery. HT interruptions and resulting errors occurred during HN disruptions during an ongoing task (instrument count/puzzle). These findings are supported by literature into healthcare interruptions [9], with reported error rates of nearly 3.5% in drug administration when nurses were interrupted, impacting directly on patient safety and related outcomes. In tandem, patient mortality has been shown to increase due to scrub nurses shortage [12]. This has big implications in longer and more complicated surgical tasks where more disruptions exist and more personnel is required. This is partly accounted for by the person shifting cognitive load towards the "new" disruption (the puzzle for instance), in so taking longer in performing the primary task or not all [3].

We demonstrated no significant difference in overall experiment duration. Whilst, mean duration is longer in RN group, this is in part accounted for by recalibration which will be improved in the hardware-agnostic platform modifications through the use of techniques for online ETG displacement compensation.

ST frustration was significant using RN, although all experiments were completed. Qualitative feedback revealed frustration related to looking away from the operative field to select an instrument. ST proposed verbal commands may enhance the platform. Verbal commands alone may not be reliable due to surrounding noise [1]. In one study surgeons needed to repeat their verbal commands up to three times 30% of the time, using verbally based *Penelope* platform [11].

Our aim is to further develop our visually aided RN by enabling real-time recognition and tracking of the surgical instruments and screen position in space. We aim for the RN to deliver and return the instruments. Finally, we aim to introduce an intuitive RN, to automatically respond to surgeon instrument selection behaviors, through work flow segmentation and task phase recognition, imitating the HN's greatest advantage of instrument anticipation [12], as was emphasized in our subjective feedback.

We introduce a robotic scrub nurse system, visually controlled in a mobile and unrestricted fashion. This is the first platform of its kind. Subjective feedback was positive. Task duration was similar across RT vs HT. Surgeon frustration was highlighted and can be improved by future sophisticated versions. Perception over performance was unchanged.

Acknowledgements. This research project is supported by the NIHR Imperial Biomedical Research Centre (BRC).

References

1. Ebert, L.C., Hatch, G., Ampanozi, G., Thali, M.J., Ross, S.: You can't touch this: touch-free navigation through radiological images. Surg. Innov. **19**(3), 301–307 (2012). https://doi.org/10.1177/1553350611425508
2. El-Shallaly, G.E.H., Mohammed, B., Muhtaseb, M.S., Hamouda, A.H., Nassar, A.H.M.: Voice recognition interfaces (VRI) optimize the utilization of theatre staff and time during laparoscopic cholecystectomy. Minim. Invasive Ther. Allied Technol. (2005). https://doi.org/10.1080/13645700500381685
3. Gillie, T., Broadbent, D.: What makes interruptions disruptive? A study of length, similarity, and complexity. Psychol. Res. (1989). https://doi.org/10.1007/BF00309260
4. Hong, N., Kim, M., Lee, C., Kim, S.: Head-mounted interface for intuitive vision control and continuous surgical operation in a surgical robot system (2018). https://doi.org/10.1007/s11517-018-1902-4
5. Jacob, M.G., Li, Y.T., Wachs, J.P.: Gestonurse: a multimodal robotic scrub nurse. In: 2012 7th ACM/IEEE International Conference on Human-Robot Interaction (HRI), vol. 1, pp. 153–154 (2012). https://doi.org/10.1109/ICSMC.2011.6083972

6. Kogkas, A.A., Darzi, A., Mylonas, G.P.: Gaze-contingent perceptually enabled interactions in the operating theatre. Int. J. Comput. Assist. Radiol. Surg. 1–10 (2017). https://doi.org/10.1007/s11548-017-1580-y
7. Laviana, A.A., Williams, S.B., King, E.D., Chuang, R.J., Hu, J.C.: Robot assisted radical prostatectomy: the new standard? Minerva urologica e nefrologica = Ital. J. Urol. Nephrol. **67**(1), 47–53 (2015)
8. Makary, M.A., Daniel, M.: Medical error-the third leading cause of death in the US. BMJ (Online) (2016). https://doi.org/10.1136/bmj.i2139
9. Rivera-Rodriguez, A.J., Karsh, B.T.: Interruptions and distractions in healthcare: review and reappraisal (2010). https://doi.org/10.1136/qshc.2009.033282
10. Shah, M.: Solving the robot-world/hand-eye calibration problem using the kronecker product. J. Mech. Robot. **5**(3), 31007 (2013). https://doi.org/10.1115/1.4024473
11. Treat, M.R., Amory, S.E., Downey, P.E., Taliaferro, D.A.: Initial clinical experience with a partly autonomous robotic surgical instrument server. Surg. Endosc. Other Intervent. Tech. (2006). https://doi.org/10.1007/s00464-005-0511-0
12. Velasquez, C.A., Mazhar, R., Chaikhouni, A., Zhou, T., Wachs, J.P.: Taxonomy of communications in the operating room. In: Duffy, V., Lightner, N. (eds.) AHFE 2017. AISC, vol. 590, pp. 251–262. Springer, Cham (2018). https://doi.org/10.1007/978-3-319-60483-1_25
13. Wachs, J.P., et al.: A gesture-based tool for sterile browsing of radiology images. J. Am. Med. Inf. Assoc. (2008). https://doi.org/10.1197/jamia.M2410

Haptic Modes for Multiparameter Control in Robotic Surgery

Philipp Schleer[✉][ⓘ], Sergey Drobinsky, Tahany Hmaid,
and Klaus Radermacher

Chair of Medical Engineering, Helmholtz Institute for Biomedical Engineering,
Pauwelsstraße 20, 52074 Aachen, Germany
schleer@hia.rwth-aachen.de

Abstract. Accurate manual execution of a pre- or intraoperatively generated plan is an essential ability of surgeons and can be related to a successful outcome of a surgery. Therefore, surgeons regularly need to control multiple parameters simultaneously which increases control complexity, particularly if the information has to be derived and fused from multiple reference frames (e.g. displays). In master-slave or cooperative robotic settings haptic assistances can be provided to facilitate manual control of e.g. milling tasks. Haptic assistances present the information in the human hand reference frame and therefore can make mental transformation obsolete. Additionally, in contrast to autonomous robotic milling, the surgeon remains in the control loop and is able to customize the plan according to his expertise and intraoperative requirements. This paper experimentally investigates effects on usability of different haptic assistances in separate degrees of freedom during a multiple parameter control task. Subjects had to apply a force and follow a path with a constant velocity, while different levels of haptic assistance were provided. Results indicate that each assistance provides a statistically significant improvement with respect to the associated measure (i.e. force, position, velocity) and the task-associated perceived workload is reduced. Consequently, haptically assisted milling allows for an efficient control of milling parameters during surgery whose performance lies in between completely manual and autonomous robotic execution while keeping the surgeon in the control loop.

Keywords: Robotic surgery · Haptics · Virtual fixtures

1 Introduction

Manual guidance of surgical instruments is a multidimensional sensomotoric control task, which varies in complexity and often involves the control of multiple parameters simultaneously. Dynamic control parameters include forces, to avoid damage of sensitive tissues, position and orientation along trajectories of motion, which vary in their geometric complexity, as well as velocity (e.g. to comply with optimal milling parameters of bone) [1, 2].

However, complexity of control increases with every additional parameter that needs to be controlled. Therefore, while tasks with two degrees of freedom (DOF) are

© Springer Nature Switzerland AG 2019
D. Shen et al. (Eds.): MICCAI 2019, LNCS 11768, pp. 173–181, 2019.
https://doi.org/10.1007/978-3-030-32254-0_20

still relatively easy to perform, tasks with three DOFs are already challenging (e.g. riding a bike) and five DOFs tasks (e.g. riding a unicycle) already need a comparably high amount of practice and induce higher workloads [3]. Workload associated with sensomotoric tasks also depends on the complexity of mental transformations necessary to process the perceived input information (e.g. from different reference frames) to generate an appropriate manual response, e.g. in case of eye-hand-coordination of visually controlled surgical navigation tasks [2, 4]. One way to reduce task complexity is to provide haptic guidance or virtual fixtures respectively. Haptic devices (in contrast to visual guidance) present guidance information in the human hand reference frame and therefore can make mental transformation obsolete. A study [5] showed that usability (efficiency, effectiveness, user satisfaction) in typical surgical instrument motion control tasks can be affected by incorporation of different haptic assistance modes. Thereby, improvements also depend on the number of tasks that are superimposed. If there is solely one task, tracking a trajectory, improvements can be seen with respect to efficiency (mean velocity of movement) or the task associated perceived workload. If participants have to control two parameters simultaneously, tracking a trajectory and applying a constant force, improvements with respect to efficiency cannot be seen, however, effectiveness improvements (mean deviation from trajectory) are observed.

For accurate and efficient milling of bone e.g. in orthopedics or craniofacial surgery [6] apart from tool pose, velocity control of the movement is crucial. Milling velocity influences the efficiency of the milling process as well as (in combination with the tool revolution speed and geometry) milling forces or temperature rise respectively which can lead to bone damage [7]. Reported feed rates in literature vary between 2–82.5 mm/s [7, 8]. Whereas dynamic control of all relevant milling parameters (e.g. position, force, feed rate, …) for efficient bone milling can be a major benefit of autonomous robotic milling, manual motion control requires additional guidance cues.

There have already been efforts to give haptic guidance information on movement velocities without a specific trajectory that needs to be followed [9, 10]. Another work investigates tracking of a trajectory with a specific velocity profile [11] which showed promising results, however, lacked a comprehensive user study. So far no user study including multiple subjects has been performed to statistically evaluate benefits of haptic assistance to track a trajectory with a defined velocity. With regard to robotic surgery sometimes not only position and velocity along a trajectory is important but also the applied force. One example is the control of the milling depth along the inner cortical layer of skull bone on basis of force sensor information in a master-slave robot setting to preserve underlying sensitive structures in craniofacial surgery [6]. Therefore, we investigated if haptic assistance can improve usability of a control task with three parameters position, velocity and force, in the context of robotic surgery.

2 Materials and Methods

A Phantom OMNI (SensAble Technologies Inc., Wilmington, MA, USA) haptic device was used in association with Matlab Simulink (The MathWorks Inc., Natick, MA, USA) and the real-time control software QUARC (Quanser, Markham, ON, Canada).

An experiment was designed such that subjects had to control three parameters in separate degrees of freedom simultaneously, which are:

- Applying a constant force of 1.5 N in the depth direction orthogonal to the main visual plain,
- tracking a 2D trajectory in the main visual plane, and
- maintaining a constant velocity of 15 mm/s along the trajectory.

Furthermore, four haptic modes were designed for the experiments which consecutively introduce assistance in additional degrees of freedom to reduce the complexity of the task. The different haptic modes and their assisted DOFs are listed in Table 1.

Table 1. Haptic assistance modes.

Mode	DOF	Haptic assistance
No	0	No haptic feedback (reference mode)
F	1	Haptic feedback for force application in the depth direction
F+P	2	In addition to mode F haptic assistance for position guidance on the path in the main visual plane
F+P+V	3	In addition to mode F+P assistance for velocity guidance along the path

Thereby, haptic feedback concerning the force application (Mode F) was implemented using a unidirectional PD controller. Haptic assistance based on the deviation from the path (Mode P) was implemented using a proxy method to avoid skipping of the reference point along the trajectory in association with a PD controller [12]. Velocity assistance (Mode V) was implemented using a PD controller on the current velocity whose force output was limited to 1 N to avoid an uncomfortable strong pull along the trajectory. All PD gains were tuned experimentally to suit the different assistances.

During experiments users received a graphical representation of the scene which can be seen in Fig. 1, which displayed the experimental path (inspired by a milling path) and the currently active assistance mode. Additionally, several visual elements (Table 2) were implemented such that all control parameters could also be perceived visually.

The experimental workflow consisted of a tutorial which all participants underwent first to accustom to the different assistance modes until they were confident. During experiments participants were first haptically guided to the start point of the trajectory. Afterwards, they were asked to apply the target force of 1.5 N supported by a randomly

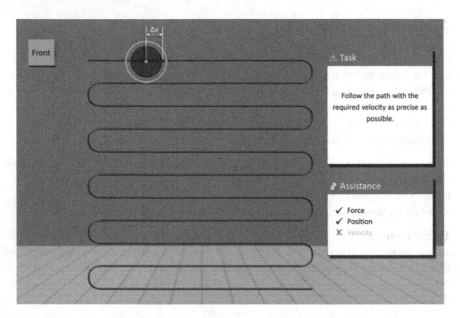

Fig. 1. Graphical user interface (GUI) during the experiments (labeling of Δv is not part of the GUI and only inserted here to support understanding). (Color figure online)

Table 2. Elements used for visualization of control parameters.

Visual element	Explanation
Yellow dot	Current user input position
Yellow ring	Target force that needs to be applied
Circle	Currently applied force scaled with reference to the target force (1.5 N, yellow ring), additionally the color of the circle changes to red in case a deviation of 0.5 N is exceeded
Green dot	Current reference point on the trajectory shifted forward depending on the current velocity deviation Δv, scaling factor is set such that for the expected maximum forward shift equals the radius of the yellow ring (Δv = 15 mm/s if v = 0 mm/s)

selected assistance mode. As soon as they were ready to start recording they pressed the space bar of the computer keyboard and started the task. Each participant performed the task with every haptic mode resulting in four test runs for each participant.

Dependent variables for the experiments were chosen based on usability evaluation criteria for medical electrical equipment defined in DIN EN 60601-1-6 and constituted of:

- Effectiveness
  - Mean absolute deviation from path
  - Mean absolute force deviation
  - Mean absolute velocity deviation
- User satisfaction
  - Perceived Workload obtained by the NASA-TLX questionnaire

Thereby, participants completed the NASA-TLX rating scales after each run and the NASA-TLX source of workload questionnaire after all runs were completed. Efficiency variables were not evaluated as a fixed tracking velocity was specified.

10 right-handed subjects took part in the experiments consisting of 6 males and 4 females. Subjects were aged between 22 and 43 and had a high technical affinity demonstrated by high ATI scores (Mean = 5.14, STD = 0.54) [13]. Furthermore, introductory questionnaires showed that on average subjects perfom tasks requiring high manual dexterity (e.g. playing computer games/an instrument, sewing) once a week.

3 Results

Statistical evaluation was done using analysis of variance (ANOVA) with a post-hoc test using the Tukey-Kramer method. In Figs. 2 and 3 statistically significant differences ($\alpha = 0.05$) are marked with (*), while higher significance levels of $p < 0.01$ and $p < 0.001$ are marked with (**) and (***) respectively. Boxplots are used for representation of the results, thereby the central line indicates the median, bottom and top edges of the box represent the 25th and 75th percentiles, the whiskers display the most extreme data points and outliers are marked with the "+" symbol.

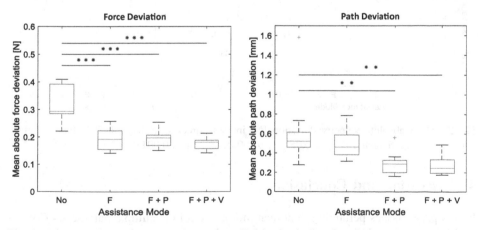

Fig. 2. Mean absolute force deviation [N] applied in depth direction (left) and mean absolute deviation [mm] from the path (right) in directions of the graphical representation (*: $p < 0.05$; **: $p < 0.01$; ***: $p < 0.001$).

Figure 2 (left) illustrates the mean absolute force deviation depending on the different assistance modes. A statistically significant difference is observed ($F(3, 36) = 24.62$, $p < 0.001$). Furthermore, the post-hoc test reveals a difference between "No" and all other modes ($p < 0.001$).

The mean absolute path deviation can be seen in Fig. 2 (right) and statistically significant differences are observed ($F(3, 36) = 6.53$, $p = 0.0012$). Additionally, the post-hoc test indicates a difference between modes "No" and "F + P" ($p = 0.0063$) and modes "No" and "F + P + V" ($p = 0.0032$). The p-values for comparison of modes "F" and "F + P" or "F + P + V" are $p = 0.1433$ and $p = 0.0861$ respectively.

Figure 3 (left) shows the mean absolute velocity deviation for different assistance modes for which a statistically significant difference is also proven ($F(3, 36) = 5.66$, $p = 0.0028$). Moreover, the post-hoc test reveals a difference between modes "No" and "F + P + V" ($p = 0.0013$). The p-values for comparison of modes "F + P + V" and "F" or "F + P" are $p = 0.077$ and $p = 0.093$ respectively.

Results of the TLX ratings are illustrated in Fig. 3 (right) and a statistically significant difference is proven ($F(3, 36) = 4.91$, $p = 0.0058$). The post-hoc test reveals additionally that there is a difference between modes "No" and "F + P" ($p = 0.042$) and modes "No" and "F + P + V" ($p = 0.004$). The P-value for comparison of modes "No" and "F" is $p = 0.1662$.

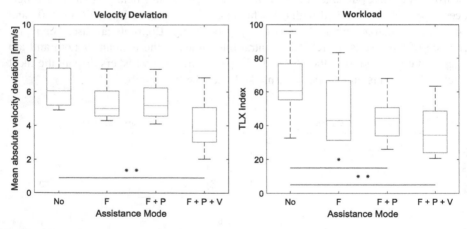

Fig. 3. Mean absolute velocity deviation [N] in path direction (left) and TLX Index (right) obtained by questionnaire (*: $p < 0.05$; **: $p < 0.01$; ***: $p < 0.001$).

4   Discussion and Conclusion

In this paper, issues pertaining to human motor control of multiple parameters (force, position, velocity) during robotic surgery have been outlined. A potential solution to the associated problems is to utilize haptic assistance to reduce the complexity of the task and consequently improve human-machine system performance. Several haptic assistances have already proven effective [14]; however, so far no comprehensive user study regarding a haptic velocity assistance has been performed. An experiment has been described to evaluate the influence of different haptic assistance modes on human-machine-system performance during a multiple parameter control task.

Results show that each assistance, force, position and velocity, significantly improves human-machine-system performance of the respective measure compared to the reference mode. Furthermore, significant decreases in perceived workload can be achieved as soon as force and position are assisted.

Considering the results of the force application in detail it can be seen that the absolute force deviation improves from between 0.3 N and 0.4 N (**No**) to around 0.2 N (**F**). Thereby, the latter force is only slightly higher than the just noticeable difference found by Allin et al. [15] of approximately 10% of the base force which would be 0.15 N for our experiments. The slight difference of 0.05 N could be due to inherent delays in the perception-cognition-action chain, which are prevalent in human manual control [16].

Absolute positional deviations of the reference mode (**No**) between 0.5 mm and 0.6 mm are only slightly lower than literature average values for manual bone milling of eleven neurosurgeons (mean deviation 0.7 mm) [17]. As soon as haptic assistance is provided the positional deviation reduces to about 0.3 mm. Compared to an automatic robotic milling process (mean deviation 0.2 mm [8]) deviations are still slightly increased. However, keeping surgeons in the control loop reduces negative side effects such as low situational awareness, overreliance, dependency on the system and retention of skills [18]. Additionally, interactive robotic systems enable surgeons to adapt surgical plans based on their expert appraisal of the intraoperative situation, thereby increasing the versatility and robustness of robot assisted surgery. Tendencies also indicate a slight positional improvement as soon as the feedback on the force application is activated, but sample sizes were too small for statistical approval.

Average deviations with respect to velocity are around 6 mm/s in the reference mode (**No**) and are reduced to 4 mm/s with haptic assistance (**F+P+V**). This finding is in coherence with literature, however, the performed study has a low level of evidence as trials were only performed with one user [11]. Tendencies also indicate a slight improvement as soon as haptic feedback concerning the force application (**F**) is activated, however, sample sizes were too small for statistical approval.

For the NASA TLX perceived workload there seems to be an improvement with each additional assistance which could also be observed in [5]. Statistical approval is observed for all assistance modes that provide haptic assistance for both force and position (**F+P, F+P+V**). Tendencies indicate an improvement if feedback on the force application (**F**) is provided, but sample sizes were too small for statistical approval.

Limitations of the study include that the investigated user group did not consist of surgeons. The study was based on a computer simulation scenario, whereas the real surgical context of use could potentially induce additional constraints or boundary conditions. Knowledge of the subjects concerning the active haptic mode could have influenced their subjective workload ratings. Learning effects could have influenced results, however, due to randomization they constitute a random and not a systematic error.

All things considered, results of the presented experiment indicate that for multi-parameter control tasks the execution accuracy with haptic assistance lies between the completely manual and the completely automated execution. In case of telerobotic surgery, accuracy could be further improved by motion scaling. Thereby, accuracy would largely depend on the executing slave robot. The task associated perceived workload is decreased with haptic assistance enabling the surgeon to shift his attention to higher level decisions. Consequently, haptic assistance seems to be a potential solution to improve accuracy as well as decrease complexity for the human operator while keeping him in the control loop in robotic surgery.

References

1. Troccaz, J., Peshkin, M., Davies, B.: Guiding systems for computer-assisted surgery: introducing synergistic devices and discussing the different approaches. Med. Image Anal. **2**, 101–119 (1998)
2. Radermacher, K.: Computerunterstützte Operationsplanung und-ausführung mittels individueller Bearbeitungsschablonen in der Orthopädie. Shaker (1999)
3. Luczak, H.: Prinzipien menschlicher Informationsverarbeitung-Analytik und Gestaltung informatorisch-mentaler Arbeit. In: Luczak, H. (ed.) Arbeitswissenschaft, pp. 126–213. Springer, Heidelberg (1993). https://doi.org/10.1007/978-3-662-21634-7_7
4. Wickens, C.D., Hollands, J.G., Banbury, S., Parasuraman, R.: Engineering Psychology and Human Performance. Pearson, London (2013)
5. Schleer, P., Drobinsky, S., Radermacher, K.: Evaluation of different modes of haptic guidance for robotic surgery. IFAC-PapersOnLine **51**, 97–103 (2019). https://doi.org/10.1016/j.ifacol.2019.01.035
6. Cunha-Cruz, V., et al.: Robot-and computer-assisted craniotomy (CRANIO): from active systems to synergistic man—machine interaction. Proc. Inst. Mech. Eng. Part H: J. Eng. Med. **224**, 441–452 (2010)
7. Denis, K., et al.: Influence of bone milling parameters on the temperature rise, milling forces and surface flatness in view of robot-assisted total knee arthroplasty. In: International Congress Series, pp. 300–306. Elsevier (2001)
8. Engelhardt, M., Bast, P., Lauer, W., Rohde, V., Schmieder, K., Radermacher, K.: Manual vs. robotic milling parameters for development of a new robotic system in cranial surgery. In: International Congress Series, pp. 533–538. Elsevier (2004)
9. Fu, Y., Yin, H., Pan, B.: Fuzzy based velocity constraints of virtual fixtures in tele-robotic surgery. In: 2014 IEEE International Conference on Robotics and Biomimetics (ROBIO), pp. 2625–2630. IEEE (2014)
10. Kouskoulas, Y., Renshaw, D., Platzer, A., Kazanzides, P.: Certifying the safe design of a virtual fixture control algorithm for a surgical robot. In: Proceedings of the 16th International Conference on Hybrid Systems: Computation and Control, pp. 263–272. ACM (2013)
11. Pezzementi, Z.A., Okamura, A.M., Hager, G.D.: Dynamic guidance with pseudoadmittance virtual fixtures. In: ICRA, pp. 1761–1767 (2007)
12. Bowyer, S.A., Davies, B.L., Rodriguez, Y., Baena, F.: Active constraints/virtual fixtures: a survey. IEEE Trans. Robot. **30**, 138–157 (2014). https://doi.org/10.1109/tro.2013.2283410
13. Franke, T., Attig, C., Wessel, D.: A personal resource for technology interaction: development and validation of the Affinity for Technology Interaction (ATI) scale. Int. J. Hum.–Comput. Interact. **35**(6), 456–467 (2018)
14. Enayati, N., De Momi, E., Ferrigno, G.: Haptics in robot-assisted surgery: challenges and benefits. IEEE Rev. Biomed. Eng. **9**, 49–65 (2016)

15. Allin, S., Matsuoka, Y., Klatzky, R.: Measuring just noticeable differences for haptic force feedback: implications for rehabilitation. In: Proceedings of the 10th Symposium on Haptic Interfaces for Virtual Environment and Teleoperator Systems, HAPTICS 2002, pp. 299–302. IEEE (2002)
16. Peon, A.R., Prattichizzo, D.: Reaction times to constraint violation in haptics: comparing vibration, visual and audio stimuli. In: World Haptics Conference (WHC), pp. 657–661. IEEE (2013)
17. Bast, P., Engelhardt, M., Lauer, W., Schmieder, K., Rohde, V., Radermacher, K.: Identification of milling parameters for manual cutting of bicortical bone structures. Comput. Aided Surg. **8**, 257–263 (2003)
18. Abbink, D.A., Mulder, M., Boer, E.R.: Haptic shared control: smoothly shifting control authority? Cogn. Technol. Work **14**, 19–28 (2012)

Learning to Detect Collisions
for Continuum Manipulators
Without a Prior Model

Shahriar Sefati[1(✉)], Shahin Sefati[2], Iulian Iordachita[1], Russell H. Taylor[1],
and Mehran Armand[1,3]

[1] Laboratory for Computational Sensing and Robotics, Johns Hopkins University,
Baltimore, MD 21218, USA
{sefati,iordachita,rht}@jhu.edu
[2] Comcast Applied AI Research, Comcast, Washington D.C. 20005, USA
shahin_sefati@comcast.com
[3] Johns Hopkins University Applied Physics Laboratory, Laurel 20723, USA
mehran.armand@jhuapl.edu

Abstract. Due to their flexibility, dexterity, and compact size, Continuum Manipulators (CMs) can enhance minimally invasive interventions. In these procedures, the CM may be operated in proximity of sensitive organs; therefore, requiring accurate and appropriate feedback when colliding with their surroundings. Conventional CM collision detection algorithms rely on a combination of exact CM constrained kinematics model, geometrical assumptions such as constant curvature behavior, *a priori* knowledge of the environmental constraint geometry, and/or additional sensors to scan the environment or sense contacts. In this paper, we propose a data-driven machine learning approach using only the available sensory information, without requiring any prior geometrical assumptions, model of the CM or the surrounding environment. The proposed algorithm is implemented and evaluated on a non-constant curvature CM, equipped with Fiber Bragg Grating (FBG) optical sensors for shape sensing purposes. Results demonstrate successful detection of collisions in constrained environments with soft and hard obstacles with unknown stiffness and location.

Keywords: Collision detection · Continuum Manipulator · Minimal invasive surgery · Machine learning

1 Introduction

Compared to conventional rigid-link robots, CMs exhibit higher dexterity, flexibility, compliance, and conformity to confined spaces, making them suitable for

Electronic supplementary material The online version of this chapter (https://doi.org/10.1007/978-3-030-32254-0_21) contains supplementary material, which is available to authorized users.

D. Shen et al. (Eds.): MICCAI 2019, LNCS 11768, pp. 182–190, 2019.
https://doi.org/10.1007/978-3-030-32254-0_21

minimally invasive interventions. Examples of the use of CMs in medical applications include, but not limited to neurosurgery, otolaryngology, cardiac, vascular, and abdominal interventions [3]. In these medical interventions, the CM may be used for steering in curvilinear pathways, manipulating tissue, or merely as a flexible pathway for navigation of flexible instruments to a desired surgical site, all of which accentuating the necessity of detecting CM collision or contact with bone, tissue, or organs.

Detecting CM collisions with the environment is of great importance and has been studied in the literature. In [2], CM collisions were detected by monitoring the distance between expected and the actual instantaneous screw axis of motion, measured from the unconstrained CM kinematics model and electromagnetic sensory information, respectively. In [10], collisions were detected by obtaining the exact model of a continuum manipulator featuring multiple constant-curvature sections and a modeled object using polygonal mesh. In [1], two model-dependent approaches were presented: (1) using the deviation of joint forces from the nominal CM model, and (2) using a modified CM kinematics model to detect contacts. These studies, in addition to sensory information, required exact modeling of the CM or objects, relying on geometrical assumptions and properties specific to the choice of continuum manipulator.

This study aims at enhancing safety during teleoperation or autonomous control of CMs in proximity of sensitive organs in confined spaces. We propose a data-driven machine learning algorithm that solely relies on data from any already-available sensor, independent of the CM kinematics model, without any prior assumption or knowledge regarding the geometry of the CM or its surrounding environment. The key idea behind our proposed method is to define the problem of collision detection as a classification problem, with sensory information as the input, and occurrence/no-occurrence of CM collision with the environment as the output classes. A machine learning model is trained preoperatively on the sensory data from the CM, and is then used intraoperatively to detect collisions with the unknown environment. This information can then be conveyed to the surgeon as audio or haptic feedback to safeguard against potential trauma and damage to sensitive organs.

Different sensing methods such as electromagnetic tracking and intraoperative imaging have been used for sensing in CMs [18]. In recent years, FBG optical sensors have offered advantages over other sensing methods such as not requiring a direct line of sight, high streaming rate (up to 1 KHz), and minimal effects on compliance and compactness. FBG sensors have been used for shape, force, and torsion sensing in applications with CMs, biopsy needles, catheters, and other flexible medical instruments [7–9, 12–14, 19]. To this end, we implement our proposed method on a CM previously developed for MIS applications, equipped with FBG sensors for shape estimation [15–17]. Using the proposed method, the FBG sensor will serve as a dual-purpose simultaneous shape sensor and collision detector, preserving CM small size from additional sensors.

The contributions of this work include (1) the development of a supervised machine learning algorithm for data-driven CM collision detection with audio feedback, without requiring additional sensors, a prior model of the CM, obstacle location, or environment properties, (2) training and tuning of the hyper-parameters for the machine learning algorithm, and (3) verification of the algorithm by performing a series of experiments involving CM collision with hard and soft objects with unknown properties and locations.

2   Method

We define the problem of collision detection as a supervised classification problem with two classes: collision, and no collision. The input to this method is the sensory data obtained from the CM and the output is the corresponding class of collision. Similar to other supervised learning algorithms, the proposed method consists of an offline dataset creation step during which, the sensory data is labeled with correct collision class. A supervised machine learning model is trained on the collected dataset to learn the nonlinear mapping from sensory data to the appropriate class of collision. The trained model is optimized by tuning the hyper-parameters via a K-fold cross validation by splitting the data to training and validation sets. Performance of the tuned model is then evaluated on unseen test data from CM collisions with obstacles with different stiffness and properties (hard and soft), placed at random unknown locations relative to the CM.

2.1   Dataset Creation

To create an appropriate dataset, a vision-based algorithm based on a connected components labeling algorithm [6] is used to segment preoperative images captured via an overhead camera looking at the CM and the surrounding obstacles. The images are first converted to binary format by applying appropriate thresholds. An erosion morphological operation [4], followed up with a dilation, both with small kernel sizes are applied to the binary image to remove potential background noise and ensure robust connected region detection. The connected

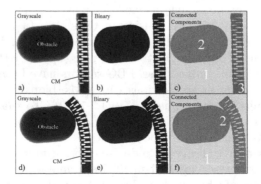

Fig. 1. Image collision labeling based on number of connected components. Top and bottom rows demonstrate no collision and collision labels, respectively.

components labeling algorithm then segments the binary image to distinguish between the background, the CM, and obstacles present in the scene. A particular sensor sample is labeled with the collision class, if the CM and the obstacle form a connected region in the corresponding image frame. Figure 1 indicates the segmented regions in collision and no collision instances during the training phase.

To follow a simple and easy-to-repeat dataset creation procedure, a random-sized oval-shaped obstacle was 3D-printed and placed in five random locations in the CM surrounding volume. The CM was then actuated to collide with the obstacles, while capturing synchronized sensory data and overhead camera images. The captured images were then segmented using the vision-based algorithm to generate the corresponding collision labels.

2.2 Data-Driven Collision Detection Framework

Most conventional CM collision detection algorithms are physics- and geometric-based models. These approaches may lead to very complex models that do not accurately detect collisions. This might be in part due to the lack of knowledge of reliable physical models of the components, and/or due to lack of knowledge of the topology of interacting components. To this end, we propose a data-driven approach to directly identify a collision detection model for CMs based on empirical data. We formulate the collision detection problem as a machine learning classification problem. In particular, we use a gradient boosting classifier to learn and build a collision detection model for CMs. Gradient boosting trees, similar to most other ensemble models, are less likely to overfit to training data which are suitable for generalization of the model to different obstacles placed at unseen locations. Figure 2 demonstrates the proposed framework.

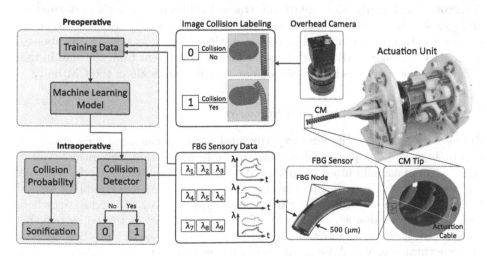

Fig. 2. Experimental setup and the proposed framework: preoperative phase involving model training using sensory data and camera images, and intraoperative phase for collision detection and sonification using only sensory data.

Gradient Boosting Classifier. Gradient boosting is a powerful machine learning technique for classification and regression problems. Gradient Boosting builds a model in a sequential way and combines an ensemble of relatively weak simple models (base learners) [5]. Let $\{x_k\}_{k=1}^{N}$ be a sequence of observations, where $x_k \in \mathbb{R}^n$ (n is the number of FBG sensory data at frame k) represents the observation at frame k. Let y_k be their corresponding labels (1 collision, 0 no collision). Given the training data, we train a Gradient Boosting Classifier to detect collision. The classifier scores can be used as probability of predicting collection.

2.3   Real-Time Sonification

Visual feedback is one of the most common means of conveying information to the surgeon during surgery. However, augmentation of this feedback method with many sources of information is prone to the risk of missing crucial information. As a workaround to these challenges, we convey the information associated with the collision detection via sonification of the probability of predicting collision (classifier score).

3   Experiments

3.1   Experiment Design

To create the dataset explained in Sect. 2.1, we 3D printed an oval-shaped obstacle from plastic ABS material, placed it at five random locations around the CM body, and collected the sensory data and overhead images, which we refer to as *offline* dataset. This dataset was the baseline for training and tuning the collision detector. Additionally, to evaluate the trained collision detector's performance and robustness on unseen data, we designed experiments that involved CM collisions with objects with different shapes and stiffness, such as soft gelatin, sponge foam, and also plastic ABS, but placed at locations different from the ones in the *offline* dataset, and also hand collisions at various points along the CM body.

3.2   Experimental Setup and Software

Figure 2 demonstrates the used experimental setup. It consisted a cable-driven CM previously developed for MIS, constructed from a 35 mm-long nitinol (NiTi) tube with outside and inner diameters of 6 mm and 4 mm, respectively, suitable for passing flexible instruments through the CM. The CM was equipped with a fiber optic sensor consisted of 3 FBG fibers (each with 3 FBG nodes) attached to 0.5 mm outside diameter NiTi wire. The CM cables were actuated by two DC motors (RE16, Maxon Motor Inc. Switzerland) with velocity or position control of the actuation cables. A Flea2 1394b (FLIR Integrated Imaging Solutions Inc.) camera was used to capture the overhead images for dataset creation. Model training and testing were programmed in Python using Scikit-learn open source library [11], and UDP communication transferred the trained model's output data to Max/MSP (Cycling '74, San Francisco, USA) for sonification. FBG data and camera images are streamed and recorded at 100 Hz and 30 Hz, respectively.

4   Results

To establish a baseline for optimal collision detection performance, the boosting tree hyper-parameters such as learning rate, number of max features, max depth, and boosting iterations (number of estimators) were tuned by running a randomized k-fold cross-validation on the *offline* dataset. To avoid overfitting to the particular *offline* dataset, and to enhance generalization to future unseen observations, we explored different regularization techniques such as shrinkage (learning rate < 1), stochastic gradient boosting (subsample < 1), and variation on maximum number of features (using all or $log2$ of the features). An initial a k-fold ($k = 4$) validation on different number of estimators ($\{100, 250, 500\}$) and max depths ($\{3, 5, 7\}$) yielded optimal performance with these parameters set to 500 and 3, respectively. Figure 3 demonstrates the performance results on the *offline* dataset with 57000 samples for five experiments, over 500 boosting iterations, with max depth of 3, and with different combinations of learning rates ($\{1, 0.8, 0.6, 0.4, 0.2\}$) and subsampling values ($\{1, 0.2\}$). It is observed that shrinkage yields improvements in model's generalization ability over gradient boosting without shrinking (left figure). Additionally, subsampling can increase performance when combined with shrinkage (right figure and Table 1). Table 1 summarizes boosting tree performance results for various combinations of learning rates, subsampling values, number of maximum features, and training times. Comparing the results, the optimal hyper-parameters (shown in bold font in Table 1) are chosen to maximize the k-fold mean accuracy and minimize the standard deviation of performance among all combinations of training and testing sets in a k-fold split. The performance of this optimized model is then evaluated on unseen data in real-time collisions with hard and soft objects different from the ones in the *offline* dataset, placed at new locations around the CM. Figure 4 indicates successful CM collision detection with hand, gelatin, and foam. The collision probabilities from the gradient boosting collision detector with 9 FBG sensory data as input are shown and compared to ground truth

Table 1. K-fold ($k = 4$) cross validation results for hyper-parameter tuning.

Learning rate	0.2				**0.6**				1			
Max features	all		log2		all		**log2**		all		log2	
Sub-sample	1.0	0.2	1.0	0.2	1.0	0.2	**1.0**	0.2	1.0	0.2	1.0	0.2
Mean accuracy (%)	97.8	97.8	97.7	97.5	97.7	98.2	**98.6**	98.0	97.0	93.5	82.1	97.9
Std. deviation (%)	0.05	0.07	0.07	0.03	1.48	0.14	**0.04**	0.20	2.06	6.95	18.0	0.23
Training time (s)	108.0	65.3	47.5	40.4	94.7	64.2	**46.1**	40.0	77.9	64.5	41.9	37.9

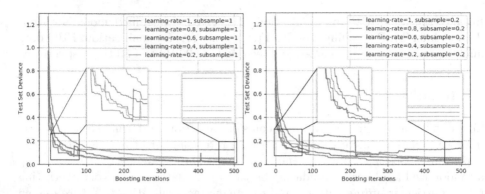

Fig. 3. Regularization via shrinkage and subsampling to avoid overfitting and enhance generalization. X and Y axis correspond to boosting iterations and loss on test data, respectively.

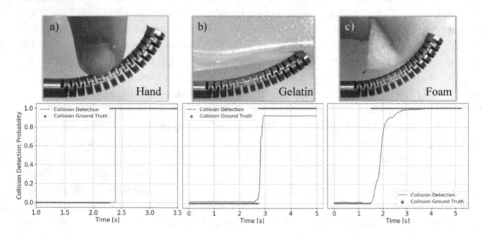

Fig. 4. Real-time collision detection on unseen data (unknown obstacle stiffness and location). CM collides with (a) hand (b) soft gelatin phantom, and (c) soft sponge foam.

collisions from the overhead camera. Please refer to the supplementary material for additional scenarios of CM collision with other materials at unknown locations with different properties. Of note, the time needed for *offline* dataset collection is within a few minutes, depending on the number of locations for obstacle placement during the training phase.

5   Discussion and Conclusion

We proposed a data-driven machine learning approach to collision detection in CMs without prior models, using only the available sensory data such as FBG. The proposed framework consisted of a preoperative offline training and tuning step via k-fold cross validation on a dataset created with a 3D-printed object placed at five locations around the CM, and an intraoperative online collision detection step, as well as sonification, during which only the FBG data was fed to the trained model. Results demonstrated successful detection of collisions on unseen data in constrained environments with soft and hard obstacles of different properties and unknown location. It should be noted that other types of sensors (e.g. Electromagnetic tracking) could be substituted for FBGs, since the algorithm only relies on the raw sensory data. Additionally, even though the CM used in the experiments is restricted to planar bending, the FBG sensor is capable of detecting 3D motions (since using 3 fibers), therefore, the method could potentially be extended to 3D manipulators. Such collision detection algorithm could enhance safety in minimally invasive interventions where the CM is operating in confined cluttered spaces near sensitive organs. Future work includes extension of this work to localizing contact point, exploring other machine learning algorithms, as well as the analysis and study of the generalization capability of the proposed method to other CMs and sensors.

References

1. Bajo, A., Simaan, N.: Finding lost wrenches: using continuum robots for contact detection and estimation of contact location. In: 2010 IEEE International Conference on Robotics and Automation, pp. 3666–3673. IEEE (2010)
2. Bajo, A., Simaan, N.: Kinematics-based detection and localization of contacts along multisegment continuum robots. IEEE Trans. Robot. **28**(2), 291–302 (2012)
3. Burgner-Kahrs, J., Rucker, D.C., Choset, H.: Continuum robots for medical applications: a survey. IEEE Trans. Robot. **31**(6), 1261–1280 (2015)
4. Comer, M.L., Delp, E.J.: Morphological operations for color image processing. J. Electron. Imaging **8**(3), 279–290 (1999)
5. Friedman, J.H.: Greedy function approximation: a gradient boosting machine. Ann. Stat. **29**(5), 1189–1232 (2001)
6. He, L., Chao, Y., Suzuki, K., Wu, K.: Fast connected-component labeling. Pattern Recogn. **42**(9), 1977–1987 (2009)
7. Jäckle, S., Strehlow, J., Heldmann, S.: Shape sensing with fiber Bragg grating sensors. Bildverarbeitung für die Medizin 2019. I, pp. 258–263. Springer, Wiesbaden (2019). https://doi.org/10.1007/978-3-658-25326-4_58
8. Khan, F., Denasi, A., Barrera, D., Madrigal, J., Sales, S., Misra, S.: Multi-core optical fibers with Bragg gratings as shape sensor for flexible medical instruments. IEEE Sens. J. (2019)
9. Lai, W., Cao, L., Xu, Z., Phan, P.T., Shum, P., Phee, S.J.: Distal end force sensing with optical fiber Bragg gratings for tendon-sheath mechanisms in flexible endoscopic robots. In: 2018 IEEE International Conference on Robotics and Automation (ICRA), pp. 1–5. IEEE (2018)
10. Li, J., Xiao, J.: Exact and efficient collision detection for a multi-section continuum manipulator. In: 2012 IEEE International Conference on Robotics and Automation, pp. 4340–4346. IEEE (2012)
11. Pedregosa, F., et al.: Scikit-learn: machine learning in Python. J. Mach. Learn. Res. **12**, 2825–2830 (2011)

12. Rahman, N., Deaton, N.J., Sheng, J., Cheng, S.S., Desai, J.P.: Modular FBG bending sensor for continuum neurosurgical robot. IEEE Robot. Autom. Lett. **4**(2), 1424–1430 (2019)
13. Sefati, S., Alambeigi, F., Iordachita, I., Armand, M., Murphy, R.J.: FBG-based large deflection shape sensing of a continuum manipulator: manufacturing optimization. In: 2016 IEEE SENSORS, pp. 1–3. IEEE (2016)
14. Sefati, S., Alambeigi, F., Iordachita, I., Taylor, R.H., Armand, M.: On the effect of vibration on shape sensing of continuum manipulators using fiber Bragg gratings. In: 2018 International Symposium on Medical Robotics (ISMR), pp. 1–6. IEEE (2018)
15. Sefati, S., Hegeman, R., Alambeigi, F., Iordachita, I., Armand, M.: FBG-based position estimation of highly deformable continuum manipulators: Model-dependent vs. data-driven approaches. In: 2019 International Symposium on Medical Robotics (ISMR), pp. 1–6. IEEE (2019)
16. Sefati, S., et al.: FBG-based control of a continuum manipulator interacting with obstacles. In: 2018 IEEE/RSJ International Conference on Intelligent Robots and Systems (IROS), pp. 6477–6483. IEEE (2018)
17. Sefati, S., Pozin, M., Alambeigi, F., Iordachita, I., Taylor, R.H., Armand, M.: A highly sensitive fiber Bragg grating shape sensor for continuum manipulators with large deflections. In: 2017 IEEE SENSORS, pp. 1–3. IEEE (2017)
18. Shi, C., et al.: Shape sensing techniques for continuum robots in minimally invasive surgery: a survey. IEEE Trans. Biomed. Eng. **64**(8), 1665–1678 (2017)
19. Xu, R., Yurkewich, A., Patel, R.V.: Curvature, torsion, and force sensing in continuum robots using helically wrapped FBG sensors. IEEE Robot. Autom. Lett. **1**(2), 1052–1059 (2016)

Simulation of Balloon-Expandable Coronary Stent Apposition with Plastic Beam Elements

Camille Krewcun[1]($\boxtimes$), Émilie Péry[1], Nicolas Combaret[2], Pascal Motreff[2], and Laurent Sarry[1]

[1] Université Clermont Auvergne, CNRS, SIGMA Clermont,
Institut Pascal, 63000 Clermont-Ferrand, France
`camille.krewcun@uca.fr`
[2] Université Clermont Auvergne, CHU Clermont-Ferrand,
CNRS, SIGMA Clermont, Institut Pascal, 63000 Clermont-Ferrand, France

Abstract. The treatment of the coronary artery disease by balloon-expandable stent apposition is a fully endovascular procedure. As a consequence, limited imaging data is available to cardiologists, who could benefit from additional per-operative information. This study aims at providing a relevant prediction tool for stent apposition, in the form of a mechanically precise simulation, fast enough to be compatible with clinical routine. Our method consists in a finite element discretisation of the stent using 1D connected beam elements, with nonlinear plastic behaviour. The artery wall is modelled as a surface mesh interacting with the stent. As a proof of concept, the simulation is compared to micro-CT scans, which were acquired during the apposition of a stent in a silicone coronary phantom. Our results show that the simulation is able to accurately reproduce the stent final geometry, in a computational time greatly lower than for classic 3D finite element codes. Although this first validation step is preliminary, our work is to be extended towards more realistic scenarios, notably with the introduction of a personalised artery model and the corresponding *in vivo* validation.

Keywords: Simulation · Stent deployment · Finite Element Method · Beam element · Plasticity

1 Introduction

The coronary artery disease results from a physiological ageing process causing a progressive narrowing (*stenosis*) of the artery lumen. In this study, we focus on the treatment of the disease by balloon inflation (i.e. angioplasty) and stent deployment. The procedure outcomes highly depend on the stent final geometry and on the accuracy of the deployment. Consequently, numerical simulation, if reliable, can be a valuable asset to minimise complications.

© Springer Nature Switzerland AG 2019
D. Shen et al. (Eds.): MICCAI 2019, LNCS 11768, pp. 191–199, 2019.
https://doi.org/10.1007/978-3-030-32254-0_22

We find in literature an important number of studies using the Finite Element Method (FEM) to simulate the deployment of coronary stents. Several studies aim at the stent design optimisation: see for instance [8] (stent alone), [3] (stent and balloon) or [12] (stent, balloon, and artery). As design optimisation gives priority to precision over computational time (e.g. 48 h in [3]), the corresponding models can not be used directly in a clinical environment.

In this paper, we propose a faster simulation routine to model accurately the deployment of a balloon-expandable stent. Our objective is to reach an execution time compatible with clinical routine, so that our simulation method could be used in practice as a relevant prediction tool (typically in patient-specific applications). We decide to base our model on the discretisation of the stent geometry by 1D serially linked beam elements. Similar work was proposed by Čanić and Tambača in [11], where the stent structure is modelled by an assembly of 1D rod elements. Although limited to a linear elastic behaviour (auto-expandable stents), the simulation is much faster than for design optimisation.

We decide to use beam elements in a similar way, in order to model the more complex (nonlinear) deformation undergone by a balloon-expandable stent. The use of connected beam elements has already been proved efficient in medical simulation to model slender structures, such as endovascular coils for brain aneurysm in [4] or flexible needles in [1]. The use of beam elements in these studies allows to achieve low computational times (up to interactive simulations), but once again is limited to elastic deformations.

2 Method

2.1 Stent Discretisation

In order to benefit from the slender shape of the stent struts, we use serially linked 1D beam elements to discretise the entire stent structure.

Each beam element is represented by two nodes, each of them described by 6 Degrees of Freedom (DoF), 3 for position, and 3 for orientation. The approximation of the continuous medium between the nodes can be written in matrix form as:

$$\mathbf{u}(x,y,z) = \mathbf{N}(x,y,z)\tilde{\mathbf{u}}, \tag{1}$$

where $\mathbf{u}$ is the continuous displacement field inside the element, (x,y,z) are the material coordinates, and $\tilde{\mathbf{u}}$ is the 12×1 vector of nodal displacement. $\mathbf{N}$ is a 3×12 matrix containing Timoshenko interpolation shape functions, which expression is given in [2]. The Timoshenko beam model notably allows to take into account shear deformations and describe 'thick' beams more accurately. We encounter this type of beams in highly curved parts of the stent.

The mesh conception is made with Computer Aided Design. The dimensions of the stent are retrieved from the micro-CT acquisition of a crimped metallic stent. From these measures, we can reproduce a flat version of the stent mesh, composed of 2D edges. The mesh is then wrapped up into a cylindrical shape, each edge corresponding to a beam element.

2.2   Finite Element Workflow

Our Finite Element (FE) implementation entirely relies on the open simulation framework SOFA[1]. A thorough description of most of the mechanisms involved in the SOFA simulation workflow can be found in [5].

Very briefly, we base our simulation on the (implicit) Backward Euler numerical scheme. This leads to solving at each time step the following mechanical system:

$$\underbrace{(\mathbf{M} - h\mathbf{B} - h^2\mathbf{K})}_{A} \Delta\mathbf{v}_{t+h} = \underbrace{h\mathbf{f}_t(\mathbf{x}, \mathbf{v}) + h^2\mathbf{K}\mathbf{v}_t}_{b}, \tag{2}$$

in which $\mathbf{M}$ is the mass matrix of the discretised mechanical system (i.e. if the system is described by n DOFs, then $\mathbf{M}$ is a $n \times n$ matrix), $\mathbf{x}$ is the global position vector, and $\mathbf{v}$ the velocity. Subscript $_t$ indicates that the variable is considered at time t, and h is the time step. $\mathbf{f}$ stands for the forces, $\mathbf{K} = \frac{\partial \mathbf{f}}{\partial \mathbf{x}}$ for the stiffness matrix and $\mathbf{B} = \frac{\partial \mathbf{f}}{\partial \mathbf{v}}$ the damping matrix.

The system in (2) is solved in $\Delta\mathbf{v}_{t+h}$ at each time step. From this, the simulation can be progressed forward in time.

2.3   Mechanical Model

Elasticity. In elasticity, the relation between the stress tensor σ and the strain tensor ϵ is given by Hooke's law, and can be written in matrix form as:

$$\sigma = \mathbf{C}\epsilon. \tag{3}$$

The explicit expression of $\mathbf{C}$ as a matrix can be found in [9]. We stress out that ϵ and σ are actually second order tensors, which can be written as 6×1 vectors without loss of information thanks to symmetry.

From (3) and the virtual work principal, the 12×12 element stiffness matrix $\mathbf{K_e}$ can be expressed as:

$$\mathbf{K_e} = \int_\Omega \mathbf{B_e}^T \mathbf{C} \mathbf{B_e} \, \mathrm{d}\Omega, \tag{4}$$

where Ω is the 3D domain on which the element is defined, and $\mathbf{B_e}$ is a 6×12 matrix obtained by spatial derivation of $\mathbf{N}$. Expression of $\mathbf{B_e}$ results from the small strain hypothesis, which is expressed in [9]. For details of the computation of $\mathbf{K_e}$ from the principle of virtual work, we also refer the reader to [9].

Plasticity. In plasticity theory, the constitutive law (3) varies during the deformation, following two phases:

- an elastic phase, during which the internal stress depends linearly on the strain, as in (3),

---

[1] www.sofa-framework.org.

– a plastic phase, during which part of the strain can be distinguished as resulting from plastic energy dissipation, and the stress-strain relation becomes
nonlinear.

The transition from the elastic to the plastic phase is described by a yield criterion $f : \mathbb{R}^6 \to \mathbb{R}$, defined on the stress space. In this study, we use the Von
Mises yield function, which expression is given in [6].

The computation of an acceptable plastic stress state relies on the decompo-
sition of the strain into a plastic and an elastic component: $\epsilon = \epsilon^{el} + \epsilon^{pl}$. In the
following, we adopt a model of *perfect plasticity*, as described in [6]. The term
'perfect' indicates that the yield surface, described by $f(\boldsymbol{\sigma}) = 0$ in the stress
space, also remains unchanged.

The evolution of the plastic strain is described by an *associative flow rule*,
expressed as:

$$d\epsilon^{pl} = d\lambda \frac{\partial f}{\partial \boldsymbol{\sigma}}, \tag{5}$$

where $d\lambda$ is called the plastic multiplier and defines the norm of $d\epsilon^{pl}$. We use
the *radial return algorithm* as described in [6], to compute a new plastic stress
state $\boldsymbol{\sigma}_{t+h}$ at each time step. Details of the computation can be found in [6].

Once $\boldsymbol{\sigma}_{t+h}$ is known, we may finally compute the resulting internal forces,
and linearised stiffness matrix, so that they are taken into account in the global
mechanical system (2).

The new internal forces are simply computed by integration:

$$\mathbf{f}_{int}(\boldsymbol{\sigma}_{t+h}) = \int_\Omega \mathbf{B_e}^T \boldsymbol{\sigma}_{t+h} \, d\Omega. \tag{6}$$

The linearised version of the stiffness matrix (or tangent stiffness matrix) $\mathbf{K}_t$
can be expressed in a similar analysis way as for (4), leading to:

$$\mathbf{K}_t = \int_\Omega \mathbf{B_e}^T \left(\frac{d\boldsymbol{\sigma}}{d\epsilon} \right) \mathbf{B_e} \, d\Omega. \tag{7}$$

Starting from Hooke's law, we have:

$$d\boldsymbol{\sigma} = \mathbf{C} d\epsilon^{el} = \mathbf{C}(d\epsilon - d\epsilon^{pl}) = \mathbf{C}(d\epsilon - d\lambda \frac{\partial g}{\partial \boldsymbol{\sigma}}).$$

Using the consistency condition ($df = 0$), we can express $d\lambda$ in terms of $\frac{\partial f}{\partial \sigma}$ and
$d\epsilon$, and replace it in the expression of $d\boldsymbol{\sigma}$, to obtain:

$$d\boldsymbol{\sigma} = \left(\mathbf{C} - \frac{\mathbf{C} \frac{\partial f}{\partial \sigma} \frac{\partial f}{\partial \sigma}^T \mathbf{C}}{\frac{\partial f}{\partial \sigma}^T \mathbf{C} \frac{\partial f}{\partial \sigma}} \right) d\epsilon = \mathbf{C}^{ep} d\epsilon. \tag{8}$$

This allows to explicitly express the tangent stiffness as:

$$\mathbf{K}_t = \int_\Omega \mathbf{B_e}^T \mathbf{C}^{ep} \mathbf{B_e} \, d\Omega. \tag{9}$$

In practice, we use Gaussian reduced integration to compute the stress and the element internal forces with (6), at each time step during the simulation. We update the tangent stiffness matrix with (9). Once $\mathbf{K_e}$ is computed for each element, all the matrices are assembled into the global stiffness matrix $\mathbf{K}$ in (2).

2.4 Balloon and Contact Constraints

We simulate the balloon indirectly by attaching a spring to each of the stent nodes. The other end of each spring is attached to a particle on a virtual surface, representing the balloon membrane. At time $t = 0$, the springs rest lengths are defined to maintain the system in equilibrium.

During the simulation, the surface particles are moved in the radial direction so that the diameter of the virtual membrane corresponds to the one given in the balloon *compliance table*. This table, provided by the stent manufacturer, gives the expected stent and balloon diameters for given pressures (typically every 1 atm from $P = 8$ to $P = 20$ atm). During the simulation, we gradually increment a virtual pressure to reproduce the actual increase in pressure carried out by the physician. The characteristics of the springs (stiffness and damping) are fixed so that the stent diameter in the simulation is coherent with the compliance table. As the table does not provide information for low pressures (<8 atm), we complete it with two entries, corresponding to 0 atm, and to the first pressure measured experimentally for which the stent becomes fully cylindrical (p_{cyl}). We then use a linear-by-parts model for pressure increasing in the simulation: the first part is a linear interpolation between 0 atm and p_{cyl}, while the second part is fitted on the p_{cyl} value and the constructor compliance table.

We handle contacts between the topological primitives composing the stent (edges) and the artery (triangles) with a collision pipeline available in SOFA. At each time step, if a collision between two primitives is detected, a response is computed accordingly in the form of a Lagrangian constraint.

Briefly, the addition of constraints involves an additional step in the numerical solution:

- At first, (2) is solved without constraints, giving a new position (free motion).
- Then, a modified constrained system is solved from the free motion:

$$\mathbf{A}\Delta\mathbf{v}_{t+h} = \mathbf{b} + h\mathbf{H}^T\boldsymbol{\lambda}, \tag{10}$$

where $\mathbf{H}$ is the Jacobian of the constraint expressions, and $\boldsymbol{\lambda}$ contains the Lagrange multipliers associated to each constraint. In SOFA, this system is typically solved iteratively using a Gauss-Seidel algorithm. A more detailed description of the process is available in [5].

2.5 Experimental Validation

To propose a first assessment of the simulation, we conducted an experiment involving the apposition of a stent in a perfectly straight coronary artery phantom. We chose silicone (Sylgard 184, Dow Corning, Midland, Michigan, U.S.A.)

to reproduce the artery, as the material has already been successfully used to create phantom vessels. In order to exactly control the vessel geometry, we used additive manufacturing to create a plastic mould and a water-soluble stick made in PolyVinyl Alcohol (PVA). The mould gives the external shape of the phantom, while the lumen geometry is entirely define by the stick (once dissolved).

Following the phantom creation, we actually expand a stent inside the mock artery, under micro-CT supervision. We proceed by gradually incrementing the inflation pressure of the balloon, and realising a CT acquisition at each incremental step. The resulting 3D reconstructions contain the geometry of the stent in transient states, from a pressure of 0 atm (crimped stent) to the nominal pressure (fully expanded stent). The deformation can be compared to the output of the simulation.

As the artery phantom was obtained from 3D-printed elements, the 3D artery geometry to be included in the simulation is known. In this case, we use a surface mesh, on which we add an elastic behaviour [10], already implemented in SOFA.

3   Results

As a first validation, we simulated the expansion of a Synergy II coronary stent (Boston Scientific, Marlborough, Massachusetts, U.S.A) in a perfectly cylindrical artery model, which we reproduced experimentally. For Hooke's Law, we use $E = 203\,\mathrm{GPa}$ (Young's modulus) and $\nu = 0.285$ (Poisson ratio), corresponding to the Pt-Cr alloy [7] used for the Synergy II. The artery diameter is chosen to match the stent nominal diameter (3 mm). Pressure in the experiment is increased from 0 atm to 11 atm, while carrying out micro-CT acquisition at 5, 6, 7, 9 and 11 atm. We increment the pressure in the simulation by following the linear-by-parts model mentioned above. We export the stent geometry at regular pressure increments (every 200 iterations, i.e. every 0.44 atm) between 0 and 11 atm.

Comparison is made between a pointset extracted from the micro-CT 3D reconstruction, and the stent nodes. We register the two pointsets in two steps: first by superimposing the principal axes of inertia and centres of gravity (rigid transform), and then by minimising the Euclidean distance between simulated points and their closest neighbours in the CT pointset (rigid rotation around the common axis).

We compare the poinset of each acquisition to all the exported stent geometries. We choose as best correspondence the one minimising the mean radial distance $\bar{d}_r$ and Euclidean distance $\bar{d}_E$ between the pairs of points. Table 1 gives the best matching simulated stent state for each micro-CT acquisition, with the number of iterations (it), the corresponding simulated pressure and diameter, and the minimised metrics values. 3D rendering of the registration output is given in Fig. 1 for a crimped and a deployed configurations.

Table 1. Comparison between experimental and simulated stent expansions.

Experimental		Theoretical (compliance)	Simulation best correspondence				
P (atm)	∅ (mm)	∅ (mm)	it	P (atm)	∅ (mm)	$\bar{d}_r$ (μm)	$\bar{d}_E$ (μm)
5	2.496	–	2000	4.4	2.540	40	150
6	2.580	–	2000	4.4	2.540	30	150
7	2.710	–	2200	4.84	2.714	30	80
9	2.876	2.96	3200	7.04	2.884	30	90
11	3.004	3.08	4400	9.68	2.992	27	90

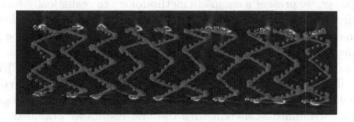

Fig. 1. 3D rendering of the rigid registration between the last micro-CT acquisition (deflated balloon) and the simulation best correspondence. The CT reconstruction is displayed in grey, while the simulation mesh nodes are superimposed as red points (Color figure online).

4   Discussion and Conclusion

The first remark which has to be made regarding our results is the significant difference between the experimental pressure and the simulated pressure in the best corresponding configuration. This discrepancy can be explained both by the fact that we export geometries only every 200 iterations (thus limiting the number of candidates for best correspondence), and by the complete lack of data in the compliance table, for $P < 8$ atm. Consequently, the first part ($P \leq 5$ atm) of the model that simulates the pressure increase is too approximative. This is evidenced by the almost identical diameters measured in the acquisitions for $P = 5$ atm and $P = 6$ atm, which can't correspond to a linear model.

An issue with developing a more accurate pressure/diameter model for low pressure values is that the stent experience asymmetrical deformation for $P \leq 5$ atm. As presented by De Beule *et al.* in [3], this phenomenon, called *dog boning* can only be reproduced if a realistically folded balloon is simulated.

If we don't consider early transient states, Zahedmanesh *et al.* showed in [12] that an approximated balloon model is able to accurately retrieve the final configuration of the stent. In this study, it is indeed the case for the nominal pressure of 11 atm, for which the acquisition and the simulation are in accordance. In addition to that, considering only the diameter independently of the pressure, we can see that the simulation is also able to reproduce transient states as long as the stent is fully cylindrical. On the correspondences we obtain, the distance errors are thus in the same order of magnitude as the stent strut thickness ($50\,\mu$m for the Synergy II). We consider this error reasonable regarding stent apposition.

Regarding the computational time, the plastic mechanical model we implemented can be handled at 4 Frames Per Second (FPS), allowing a stent mesh composed of 1622 beam elements to reach the artery diameter in about 15 min, without any form of optimisation (single thread CPU execution on an Intel Xeon E3-1270 v5 (8CPUs) 3.6 GHz, 16 GB RAM, Windows10 64 bits). As soon as contact occurs, the number of FPS decreases, but the computational time stays significantly lower than for fully volumetric meshes.

In this paper, we present a complete methodology to realistically simulate the plastic deformation of a balloon-expandable stent with 1D serially linked beam elements, in a reasonable time. The long-term goal of this work is to be included in a workflow where we could retrieve a patient's artery geometry and mechanical properties using endovascular Optical Coherence Tomography (OCT) imaging, run the simulation, and provide the physicians with a personalised prediction of stent apposition, before deployment. For this, we aim at a computational time lower than a few minutes, coherent with the first results we obtained.

Presently, clinical assessment of stent apposition almost exclusively relies on the evaluation by the physicians of the artery diameter, before and after the procedure. In this context, we believe that a stent apposition simulation could provide additional (mechanical) information to the physician. In order to progress towards this clinical use, we started to develop simulations and experiments with more realistic artery geometries. In parallel, the use of OCT to complete the clinical workflow is currently under investigation. Finally, we also intend to improve the present simulation by optimising our code (addressing the issue of computational time), and compare the results with equivalent 3D codes from the literature.

Acknowledgements. The authors would like to thank Arnaud Briat from the multimodal imaging facility IVIA (In Vivo Imaging Auvergne), Clermont-Ferrand, France, for their assistance in the acquisition of the micro-CT images. We also thank François Wastable for helping with the phantom manufacturing.

References

1. Adagolodjo, Y., Goffin, L., Mathelin, M.D., Courtecuisse, H.: Inverse real-time finite element simulation for robotic control of flexible needle insertion in deformable tissues. In: IEEE/RSJ International Conference on Intelligent Robots and Systems (IROS) (2016)
2. Bazoune, A., Khulief, Y.A., Stephen, N.G.: Shape functions of three dimensional timoshenko beam element. J. Sound Vib. **259**, 473–480 (2003)
3. Beule, M.D., Mortier, P., Carlier, S.G., Verhegghe, B., Impe, R.V., Verdonck, P.: Realistic finite element-based stent design: the impact of balloon folding. J. Biomech. **41**, 383–389 (2008)

4. Dequidt, J., Marchal, M., Duriez, C., Kerien, E., Cotin, S.: Interactive simulation of embolization coils: modeling and experimental validation. In: Metaxas, D., Axel, L., Fichtinger, G., Székely, G. (eds.) MICCAI 2008. LNCS, vol. 5241, pp. 695–702. Springer, Heidelberg (2008). https://doi.org/10.1007/978-3-540-85988-8_83
5. Faure, F., et al.: SOFA: a multi-model framework for interactive physical simulation, pp. 283–321. Springer, Berlin (2012). https://doi.org/10.1007/8415_2012_125
6. Hughes, T.J.R.: Theoretical Foundation for Large-Scale Computations of Nonlinear Material Behavior, Chap. II. Springer, Berlin (1984). https://doi.org/10.1007/978-94-009-6213-2
7. Idziak-Jabłońska, A., Karczewska, K., Kuberska, O.: Modeling of mechanical phenomena in the platinum-chromium coronary stents. J. Appl. Math. Comput. Mech. **16**, 29–36 (2017)
8. Migliavacca, F., Petrini, L., Colombo, M., Auricchio, F., Pietrabissa, R.: Mechanical behavior of coronary stents investigated through the finite element method. J. Biomech. **35**, 803–811 (2002)
9. Przemieniecki, J.S.: Theory of Matrix Structural Analysis, 1st edn. McGraw-Hill, New York (1968)
10. Tournier, M., Nesme, M., Gilles, B., Faure, F.: Stable constrained dynamics. ACM Trans. Graph. **34**, 132:1–132:10 (2015)
11. Čanić, S., Tambača, J.: Cardiovascular stents as PDE nets: 1D vs. 3D. IMA J. Appl. Math. **77**, 748–770 (2012)
12. Zahedmanesh, H., Kelly, D.J., Lally, C.: Simulation of a balloon expandable stent in a realistic coronary artery-determination of the optimum modelling strategy. J. Biomech. **43**, 2126–2132 (2010)

Virtual Cardiac Surgical Planning Through Hemodynamics Simulation and Design Optimization of Fontan Grafts

Byeol Kim[1]([✉]), Yue-Hin Loke[2], Florence Stevenson[1], Dominik Siallagan[1], Paige Mass[2], Justin D. Opfermann[1,2], Narutoshi Hibino[3], Laura Olivieri[2], and Axel Krieger[1]

[1] University of Maryland, College Park, MD 20742, USA
{star,axel}@umd.edu
[2] Sheikh Zayed Institute for Pediatric Surgical Innovation, Children's National, Washington DC 20010, USA
[3] Division of Cardiac Surgery, The Johns Hopkins Hospital, Baltimore, MD 21287, USA

Abstract. For complex congenital heart disease (CHD) involving a single functioning ventricle, the Fontan operation is performed which results in a circulation where deoxygenated venous blood passively flows into the pulmonary arteries without a ventricular pump. However, conventional Fontan graft designs may result in suboptimal cardiovascular hemodynamics leading to post-surgical complications. Patient-specific designs are thus promising in the Fontan operation. This paper reports the virtual simulation and designs of patient-specific Fontan grafts with the aid of computational fluid dynamics (CFD). CFD parameters including meshing, wall layers, and solver choices were studied to bolster accuracy while minimizing computational time. CFD simulations of original Fontan design were performed to evaluate three hemodynamic parameters: indexed power loss (iPL), hepatic flow distribution (HFD), and percentage of the non-physiological wall shear stress (%WSS, a novel surrogate marker for clot risk). New designs were then created to target these parameters with iterative optimization technique. This overall approach was utilized to redesign the Fontan grafts of patients (n = 2). The re-designed Fontan grafts showed significant improvements in all three hemodynamic parameters when compared to the original designs. Our unique integration of surgical design and flow simulation has the potential to enable cardiac surgeons to effectively simulate patient specific designs for the Fontan operation, potentially improving the surgical outcomes of patients with complex CHD.

This work is supported by the National Institutes of Health under award numbers R01HL143468 and R21HD090671. The content is solely the responsibility of the authors and does not represent the official views of the National Institutes of Health.
The authors acknowledge the University of Maryland supercomputing resources (http://hpcc.umd.edu) made available for conducting the research reported in this paper.

D. Shen et al. (Eds.): MICCAI 2019, LNCS 11768, pp. 200–208, 2019.
https://doi.org/10.1007/978-3-030-32254-0_23

Keywords: Virtual surgical planning · Computational fluid dynamics · Patient specific model

1   Introduction

Congenital heart disease (CHD) affects 0.8% of the population, with $\frac{1}{4}$ of infants requiring life-saving intervention as a neonate [9]. For patients with complex CHD involving a single functioning ventricle, surgeons perform a series of open-heart surgeries to modify the venous circulation. The third surgery, the Fontan operation, connects the inferior vena cava into the superior cavopulmonary anastomosis via intracardiac patch (lateral tunnel Fontan) or a conduit (extracardiac Fontan) [6]. The Fontan graft's geometry influences hemodynamics of blood flow into the pulmonary arteries, and novel designs such as a y-shaped (bifurcated) graft have been previously proposed [11]. Despite significant development in the Fontan operation, graft designs are still constrained by material type and availability, potentially resulting in suboptimal cardiovascular hemodynamics and post-surgical complications including cardiac performance impairment [1], pulmonary arteriovenous malformation [14], and thrombosis [8]. Many studies approached this problem via simulating the blood flow inside Fontan and predicting hemodynamics using the computational fluid dynamics (CFD) [7,13], none have addressed the risk of thrombosis in a Fontan graft.

The simulation approach can be combined with a manufacturing process using computer-aided design (CAD), CFD and electrospinning of tissue-engineered vascular grafts (TEVGs) to create patient-specific designs as part of virtual surgical planning [13]. With the use of these, patient-specific Fontan graft designs may be the key to improving the quality of surgery and patient outcomes. As patient-specific Fontan grafts become closer to reality, we continue to refine the workflow of virtual surgical planning by identifying an accurate, time-efficient and clinically relevant CFD approach to virtual surgical planning of Fontan grafts. The objective of this study is to investigate and propose the best set of CFD parameters (i.e. meshing strategy, wall layering, and CFD solver choice) for the Fontan circulation simulation. Additionally, along with CFD simulation of conventional hemodynamic parameters such indexed power loss and hepatic flow distribution (CFD), we introduce a novel hemodynamic parameter, non-physiological wall shear stress, that acts as a surrogate for risk of thrombosis.

2   Methods

This section summarizes the sequential steps for simulating and optimizing the Fontan designs. Our approach consists of seven steps (see Fig. 1) including two previously reported steps on manufacturing and implanting patient specific 3D printed grafts [5], which we will combine in the future for improving Fontan surgeries. Sections 2.1 and 2.2 entails the methods for MRI data acquisition (i.e. anatomy and boundary flow data), image segmentation, and geometry preparation. Section 2.3 lays out the details of the CFD simulation (i.e. meshing, number

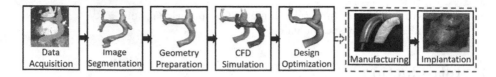

Fig. 1. Schematic workflow diagram of the virtual Fontan design optimization.

of wall layers, and solver settings). Based on the calculated hemodynamics, various Fontan design parameters are optimized in three iterations to correct the flow and pressure in the graft, which is explained in Sect. 2.4.

2.1 Data Acquisition and Image Segmentation

The magnetic resonance angiogram (MRA) data, consisting of a late-phase, non-gated, breath-held acquisition with pixel size ~1.4 × 1.4 mm, served as a road-map to build a 3-dimensional (3D) Fontan model, including the proximal cavae and branch pulmonary arteries, using a commercially available image segmentation software (Mimics; Materialise, Leuven, Belgium). Both automatic thresholding and manual methods were used to identify the blood pool of the Fontan in each slice of the angiogram, allowing for the creation of a 3D Fontan model them exported using the stereolithography (STL) file format. This STL file was hollowed and smoothed. Following, retrospectively-gated, through plane phase-encoded velocity maps were acquired across the IVC, SVC, LPA, and RPA using standard sequences, reconstructing 30 phases per cardiac cycle with a velocity encoding threshold of $150 \frac{cm}{second}$. The time-averaged IVC and SVC flow rates were derived from the phase velocity data and prescribed as inlet boundary conditions to the CFD simulations. The time-averaged RPA and LPA flow rates were prescribed as outlet flow splits (the ratio of LPA to RPA). All patient data was collected with the Institutional Review Board approval.

2.2 Geometry Preparation

All models were modified by a "Deform" function which globally smooth out the models' surfaces, reducing irregular surfaces, using Meshmixer (Autodesk Inc., San Rafael, CA). Deformation of the original model from smoothing was minimized by applying "Shape Preserving" method. Since the smoothed models were extremely fine meshed and caused some software to crash, the mesh size was reduced by 50%, leaving us with around 30,000 triangles per model. Then, 50 mm long extensions were added at the each end of the boundaries for two important purposes. The inlet extensions enabled the velocity profiles to fully develop before the blood enters the computationally interesting areas. The outlet extensions allowed the numerical flow data to stabilize and provide more accurate results [13,15]. The boundary cuts were adjusted in CAD (SolidWorks, Dasault, France) to ensure smooth extensions of the boundaries. The final model was converted

Table 1. Impact of smoothing and cutting on cell quality.

Designed model		Aspect ratio	Max skewness	Min orthogonal
P1	Non-edited	30.303	0.975	2.548e−2
	Smoothed	17.355	0.917	8.310e−2
	Smoothed & cut	16.927	0.802	0.198
P2	Non-edited	32.315	0.927	7.309e−2
	Smoothed	17.602	0.817	0.183
	Smoothed & cut	17.005	0.797	0.203

into the text-based Parasolid file and showed improved cell qualities including aspect ratio, maximum skewness, and minimum orthogonal values (Table 1), the deterministic features for the numerical computation accuracy and stability [4].

2.3   CFD Simulation

Performance Metric. The blood flow inside the Fontan graft was virtually simulated through CFD (ANSYS, Pennsylvania, USA) to determine its performance by the indexed power loss (iPL), hepatic flow distribution (HFD), and the non-physiological wall shear stress percentage (%WSS). iPL, a deterministic factor of the abrupt blood flow changes causing cardiac performance impairment [1], was calculated using the Eq. 1, derived from power loss (Eq. 2):

$$iPL = \frac{PL}{\rho Q_s^3 / BSA^2} \tag{1}$$

$$PL = \sum_{inlets} \int_A (p + \frac{1}{2}\rho v^2)v \times dA - \sum_{outlets} \int_A (p + \frac{1}{2}\rho v^2)v \times dA \tag{2}$$

where p being the static pressure, ρ the density, A the boundary area, v the velocity, Q_s the systemic venous flow, and the BSA the body surface area [7]. Unbalanced HFD overstresses the heart and progresses malformation of pulmonary arteriovenous [14]. HFD was estimated by computing the ratio of the number of particles passed through each outlets from the IVC. The particles at the IVC was evenly spaced with a 0.1 mm marker size and 1 mm spacing factor setting. The percentage of Fontan and outlet areas falling below 1 $\frac{dynes}{cm^2}$ in WSS were estimated since the low WSS represents the low-flow in venous stasis causing deposition of procoagulant [8]. In summary, Fontan models with iPL lower than 0.03, HFD between 40:60 or 60:40, and %WSS below 10% were considered to have healthy hemodynamic performance.

Meshing. Mesh size was tested to bolster the computation accuracy and time efficiency. The meshing could either be uniform where the elements are roughly the same size or non-uniform with a max element size defined. Our test runs

Table 2. Hemodynamics results between non-uniform and uniform meshing.

Simple, 0.7 mm, 5 layers		iPL	HFD (LPA%)	%WSS	Computing time (hr:min)
P1	Non-uniform	0.036	57.68	1.035	15:12
	Uniform	0.036	58.08	1.128	39:21
P2	Non-uniform	0.008	33.25	13.628	14:52
	Uniform	0.008	31.80	13.323	18:02

Table 3. Impact of max element size on cell quality.

Original model		Aspect ratio	Max skewness	Min orthogonal
P1	0.70 mm	15.004	0.887	0.114
	1.00 mm	23.259	0.953	4.697e−2
	1.25 mm	19.017	0.944	5.571e−2
	1.50 mm	16.492	0.912	8.844e−2
P2	0.70 mm	18.069	0.883	0.117
	1.00 mm	20.615	0.906	9.384e−2
	1.25 mm	19.197	0.931	6.928e−2
	1.50 mm	19.451	0.937	6.318e−2

confirmed that the CFD results between uniform and non-uniform were similar, but non-uniform meshing performed much faster (see Table 2). Following, the max element sizes, between 0.7 mm to 1.5 mm, were tested to identify the best size for creating mesh around the sharp corners and minimize numerical errors (Table 3). The recommended minimum orthogonal quality is 0.01, and only the 0.7 mm max mesh size was able to get sufficing values. Also considering that the lowest aspect ratio and lowest max skewness was with 0.7 mm, a max element size of 0.7 mm was selected for non-uniform meshing.

Wall Layer. The number of wall layers was explored to obtain accurate WSS measurements. Considering previously reported wall layer values, [3,12], the range of three to six was tested. These variations had minimal impact on the Fontan hemodynamics and the computing time (Table 4). Thus, the study concluded to use five layers, which is the default setting in ANSYS.

Solver. We compared the pressure-based segregated algorithms including simple, coupled, and PISO. Despite the PISO and coupled algorithms known to be computationally heavy but more accurate, results were close to that of simple algorithm (Table 5). Hence, simple solver was applied to solve the laminar flow, which was confirmed by the Reynolds number. The simulated blood was assumed to be a Newtonian fluid with $1060 \frac{kg}{m3}$ density and $3.71\,mPas$ viscosity [13]. Our CFD simulation used the 3D unsteady Navier-Stokes equations with 40 iterations with each iteration timestep lasting 0.001 s. The x, y, z-velocity and mass conservation residual convergence values were set to 10^{-5} [13].

Table 4. Hemodynamics results under the varying number of wall layers.

PISO, 1.25 mm		iPL	HFD (LPA%)	%WSS	Computing time (hr:min)
P1	3	0.0355	57.69	0.90	13:04
	4	0.0357	57.62	0.92	14:11
	5	0.0360	57.90	1.03	15:12
	6	0.0362	58.45	1.06	15:15
P2	3	0.0083	32.74	13.32	14:42
	4	0.0082	32.94	13.51	14:41
	5	0.0082	32.97	13.56	14:51
	6	0.0083	33.08	13.29	14:17

Table 5. Hemodynamics results under various solver algorithms.

0.7 mm, 5 layers, non-uniform		iPL	HFD (LPA%)	%WSS	Computing time (hr:min)
P1	Simple	0.036	57.68	1.035	13:65
	Coupled	0.036	58.02	0.998	18:51
	PISO	0.035	57.89	1.075	15:12
P2	Simple	0.008	33.25	13.628	08:23
	Coupled	0.008	33.28	13.863	23:54
	PISO	0.008	33.23	13.647	14:52

2.4   Design Optimization

Fontan grafts were optimized by three consecutive iterations of design modifications based on the patient's anatomy and the performance metric results (Fig. 2). The first iteration included identifying possible paths and anastomoses regions with the assistance of experienced cardiologists. The possible paths avoided colliding with the surrounding anatomy, including heart, major vessels, and spine. Then, the surgically adequate tube-shaped and the y-shaped (bifurcated) Fontan grafts were designed. For a tube-shaped graft, a 3D spline was drawn between 2 points. The starting point was placed at the center of the IVC and the end point was chosen at the center of an ellipse drawn on the identified anatomoses region at the SVC. The IVC's outline and the ellipse on the SVC with the 3D spline as the centerline were selected for 3D lofting. For easier spline control, 1 or 2 extra points along the intended spline path were added. The bifurcated graft was made with two ellipses on the SVC and connecting it with the IVC using the 2D surface loft function in CAD. Manipulating the curvature of the graft was accomplished by adding an ellipse in between the SVC and IVC, similar to adding 1 or 2 spline points for a tube-shaped graft. The bifurcated Fontan grafts were not always feasible if the identified path was too narrow for two ellipses to be connected. The second iteration involved changing the geometrical parame-

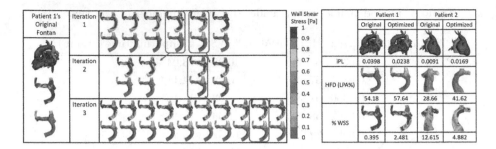

Fig. 2. Left: Iterative design for optimizing the first patient's Fontan graft, Right: Comparison of performance for original and optimized Fontan grafts.

ters of the prior designs considering the hemodynamic performance. The entry angle and the center curve of the Fontans were adjusted when the iPL was higher than 0.03. The location, dimensions, and angles of the ellipse on the anastomoses region acted as the manipulator tool of the direction and the amount of the inlet flow heading to Glenn, adjusting the HFD. High %WSS was controlled by reducing the girth of the Fontans. The significance of each geometrical parameter on the hemodynamic performance was summarized and applied for making slight adjustments to further improve Fontan performance during the third iteration. The Fontan grafts were optimized to achieve the lowest iPL, while maintaining below 10% for %WSS and between 40:60 and 60:40 HFD.

3   Result

The Fontan grafts were optimized hemodynamically for each patient (Fig. 2) using our approach. The optimized Fontan designs had significant improvements on hemodynamics with 40% decrease in iPL for patient one (P1) with a y-shaped graft and 45% increase in flow distribution to the LPA and 61% reduction in %WSS for the second patient (P2) with a tube-like graft.

4   Discussion and Conclusion

We developed 3 benchmark parameters that were based off Haggerty et al.'s larger CFD cohort simulation of 100 patients [7]. This ensured providing patient-specific designs in the hemodynamic optimal when compared to other Fontan patients. %WSS is completely a novel parameter, but is based on relevant clinical data [8] and should be incorporated in all Fontan simulations moving forward. Of note, our method creates a tradeoff between iPL and risk of thrombosis, as larger Fontan grafts will have less power loss but increased risk of thrombosis. This is clinically appropriate given the risk of thrombosis in patients with Fontans [2].

Reducing computational time whilst maintaining accuracy allows more time for feedback from the surgeon and the design team before the Fontan operation.

Inevitable, some adjustments are needed in the initial proposed designs, and shorter computational time allows for more design iterations. Our decisions on CFD simulations were made to balance the accuracy and computational time. Rigid wall was assumed in the current CFD simulations. However, fluid-structure interaction is known to provide higher accuracy in WSS calculation [10] and should be implemented in future studies.

This study introduces the unique virtual simulation workflow and computational fluid dynamics for optimizing the Fontan graft design. The re-designed Fontan grafts of two patients using this approach showed significant improvements in hemodynamic parameters (i.e. iPL, HFD, and %WSS). We believe that our unique integration of surgical design and flow simulation has the potential to enable cardiac surgeons to effectively simulate patient specific designs for the Fontan operation, potentially improving the surgical outcomes of patients with complex CHD. Future studies will entail applying this approach on more patient models and manufacturing the designs for implantation.

References

1. Ascuitto, R.J., Kydon, D.W., Ross-Ascuitto, N.T.: Pressure loss from flow energy dissipation: relevance to Fontan-type modifications. Pediatr. Cardiol. **22**(2), 110–115 (2001)
2. Atz, A.M., et al.: Longitudinal outcomes of patients with single ventricle after the Fontan procedure. J. Am. Coll. Cardiol. **69**(22), 2735–2744 (2017)
3. Biglino, G., et al.: Using 4D cardiovascular magnetic resonance imaging to validate computational fluid dynamics: a case study. Front. Pediatr. **3**, 107 (2015)
4. Diskin, B., Thomas, J.: Effects of mesh regularity on accuracy of finite-volume schemes. In: 50th AIAA Aerospace Sciences Meeting including the New Horizons Forum and Aerospace Exposition. Aerospace Sciences Meetings (2012)
5. Fukunishi, T., et al.: Preclinical study of patient-specific cell-free nanofiber tissue-engineered vascular grafts using 3-dimensional printing in a sheep model. J. Thorac. Cardiovasc. Surg. **153**(4), 924–932 (2017)
6. Gewillig, M.: The fontan circulation. Heart **91**(6), 839–846 (2005)
7. Haggerty, C.M., et al.: Fontan hemodynamics from 100 patient-specific cardiac magnetic resonance studies: a computational fluid dynamics analysis. J Thorac. Cardiovasc. Surg. **148**(4), 1481–1489 (2014)
8. Hathcock, J.J.: Flow effects on coagulation and thrombosis. Arterioscler. Thromb. Vasc. Biol. **26**(8), 1729–1737 (2006)
9. Hoffman, J.I.E., Kaplan, S.: The incidence of congenital heart disease. J. Am. Coll. Cardiol. **39**(12), 1890–1900 (2002)
10. Long, C.C., Hsu, M.C., Bazilevs, Y., Feinstein, J.A., Marsden, A.L.: Fluid-structure interaction simulations of the fontan procedure using variable wall properties. Int. J. Numer. Methods Biomed. Eng. **28**(5), 513–527 (2012)
11. Marsden, A.L., et al.: Evaluation of a novel Y-shaped extracardiac Fontan baffle using computational fluid dynamics. J. Thorac. Cardiovasc. Surg. **137**(2), 394–403.e2 (2009)
12. Ni, M.W., et al.: Computational investigation of a self-powered Fontan circulation. Cardiovasc. Eng. Technol. **9**(2), 202–216 (2018)

13. Siallagan, D., et al.: Virtual surgical planning, flow simulation, and 3-dimensional electrospinning of patient-specific grafts to optimize Fontan hemodynamics. J. Thorac. Cardiovasc. Surg. **155**(4), 1734–1742 (2018)
14. Trusty, P.M., et al.: The first cohort of prospective Fontan surgical planning patients with follow-up data: how accurate is surgical planning? J. Thorac. Cardiovasc. Surg. **157**(3), 1146–1155 (2019)
15. Wei, Z.A., et al.: Can time-averaged flow boundary conditions be used to meet the clinical timeline for Fontan surgical planning? J. Biomech. **50**, 172–179 (2017)

3D Modelling of the Residual Freezing for Renal Cryoablation Simulation and Prediction

Caroline Essert[1]($\boxtimes$), Pramod P. Rao[1,2], Afshin Gangi[1,2], and Leo Joskowicz[3]

[1] ICube, Université de Strasbourg, Strasbourg, France
essert@unistra.fr
[2] Department of Radiology, University Hospital of Strasbourg, Strasbourg, France
[3] CASMIP, The Hebrew University of Jerusalem, Jerusalem, Israel

Abstract. Percutaneous cryoablation has become a popular alternative to open surgery for the treatment of abdominal tumors. The preoperative planning of such interventions is an essential but complicated task. It consists in predicting the best placement for several cryoprobes to optimize the resulting iceball shape, that has to cover the whole tumor, while preserving healthy tissue and surrounding sensitive structures. In the past few years, methods have been proposed to simulate the propagation of cold within the tissue, in order to anticipate the final coverage. However, all the proposed models considered the source of cold as limited to the active tip of the cryoprobe, thus omitting a residual freezing along the probe's body. The lack of precision of the resulting models can cause an underestimation of the predicted iceball leading to potential damages to healthy tissue or pain. In this paper, we describe the extension of an existing freezing simulation model to account for this effect. We detail the experimentation of our model on 5 retrospective cases, and demonstrate the improvement of the accuracy and realism of our simulation.

1 Introduction

Cryoablation is an alternative to open surgery in the treatment of abdominal tumors. It consists in destroying the malignant cells using an extreme cold propagated from the tip of multiple cryoprobes inserted in the abdomen of the patient. This kind of interventions being lighter than open surgery and providing a faster recovery, it has become popular in the past decades to treat tumors of a reasonable size. However, a strong expertise is necessary to perform it, due to the difficulty to find a safe and optimal position for the cryoprobes, and to predict accurately the final shape of the iceball produced by the combination of the multiple freezing sources. This paper focuses on the second issue, with the aim of assisting the surgeon in predicting the final iceball using computer simulation.

Early approaches for computer assistance to cryoablation planning were mostly using ellipsoids to represent the shape of the iceball, with the idea of mimicking the theoretical measurements provided by the cryoprobes manufacturers [1]. However, in reality the combined effect of the multiple probes produces

© Springer Nature Switzerland AG 2019
D. Shen et al. (Eds.): MICCAI 2019, LNCS 11768, pp. 209–217, 2019.
https://doi.org/10.1007/978-3-030-32254-0_24

a final iceball which is very different from the union of all theoretical shapes. This approach also misses the effects of the surrounding warming structures that deform the iceball, such as large vessels. In the past years, simulations of the thermal propagation inside soft tissue for cryoablation have been investigated by a few groups. Most of the approaches implement an iterative algorithm to model the thermal propagation with a cube surrounding the tumor. The implementation is usually based on Pennes' bioheat equation [10], which is a complex but accurate representation of the phenomenon.

Magalov *et al.* [9] and Ge *et al.* [2] both proposed simplified models to simulate iceball growth in gels. More recently, Ge *et al.* [3,4] applied their model to human properties, including a simulation of the influence of vascular systems during freezing. Similar models were presented with application to various organs, e.g., the prostate [6] or the lungs [7,8]. In most of these models, the accuracy and realism of the model come at the cost of high computation times. In 2011, Rieder *et al.* [11] described a GPU-based implementation of heat propagation for radio frequency ablation procedures, which is another popular type of thermal ablation using extreme heat. Their model, designed for a single probe, is based on weighted distance fields, and has been simplified to allow real-time computation. More recently, we proposed a formulation of the propagation of cold in the tissue, and an efficient implementation on GPU within a cube of interest [5].

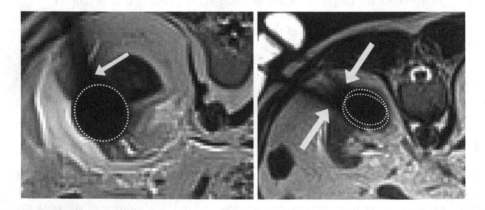

Fig. 1. Examples of residual freezing along the cryoprobe's body on two patients images, with respectively one (left) and two (right) visible cryoprobes. The dotted white lines represent the theoretical ellipsoidal shapes of the iceballs, while the red arrows highlight the residual freezing (Color figure online).

All of the above cited approaches consider that the localization of the production of cold is limited to the freezing shaft, and that the body of the needle, supposed to be insulated, is completely passive. For all those models, the source of cold is then limited to the tips of the cryobrobes. However the well-known phenomenon, sometimes called "comet-tail effect" by radiologists, and that is very well visible on the intra-operative images, contradicts this theory. The actual dark shape of the iceball, as illustrated on Fig. 1, is not perfectly ellipsoidal but rather drop-shaped, elongated along the cryoprobe's body. This effect is mostly due to a residual freezing along the body of the cryoprobe that is imperfectly insulated. An omission of this effect can lead to an underestimation of the predicted iceball during the planning and potential damages to healthy tissue.

In this paper, we present a method improving our previous approach to account for the residual freezing. In Sect. 2, we present our method to model the decreasing freezing along the cryoprobe, and how it is included in the simulation. In Sect. 3, we explain the experiment we conducted to validate our approach and detail the results before discussing and concluding.

2 Materials and Methods

In our previous work [5], we proposed an approach to simulate the thermal propagation within a cubic grid of voxels of 10 cm centered on the tumor, where some voxels were labeled as freezing or cooling structures with a fixed and constant temperature assigned to each label. The sources of cold were limited to the active tips of the cryoprobes.

2.1 Modelling of the Cryoprobe's Body Temperature

To model the residual freezing along the probes, we propose an enhanced variant. We label voxels as being part of one of the three categories: (1) freezing elements (including cryoprobe's body), (2) cooling structures and (3) normal tissue. But instead of associating a temperature to a whole set of voxels sharing the same label, we associate to each individual voxel of categories 1 or 2 its own operating temperature. This approach allows to have different temperatures, constant over time, within the same structure.

The voxels of the freezing shaft are labeled "1" and homogeneously associated with the freezing temperature T_f of the corresponding cryoprobe model given by the manufacturer. The voxels located inside the vessels are labeled "2" and homogeneously associated with the body temperature T_b.

The voxels located in the body of the cryoprobe are labeled "1", and assigned an increasing temperature along its shape towards the entry point, as shown on Fig. 2.

Let us denote L the length of the part of the cryoprobe's body that is emitting residual freezing, p_f, δ_f, and T_f are respectively the center, the length, and the temperature of the freezing shaft, p_b the point along the cryoprobe's body where the residual freezing stops and the cryoprobe's body starts being at body temperature T_b, and $\overrightarrow{v}$ is the outwards direction vector of the cryoprobe. The notations are illustrated on Fig. 3. Temperature T at an intermediary point p along the cryoprobe is given by Eq. 1:

$$T = \lambda.T_f + (1 - \lambda).T_b \tag{1}$$

where $\lambda = l/L$, with $l = \|p_b - p\|$, and $p_b = p_f + (L + \frac{\delta_f}{2}).\overrightarrow{v}$.

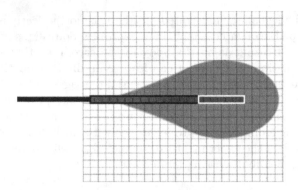

Fig. 2. Part of the cubic grid in which the simulations are computed. The voxels are labeled "1" if they are located along the cryoprobe. The blue color represent the freezing temperature T_f, red represents the body temperature T_b, and the color gradient represents the residual temperature gradient along the cryoprobe's body. Voxels of the freezing shaft are represented with a yellow border. (Color figure online)

The voxels labeled "0" as part of normal tissue are assigned T_b as an initial temperature, and considered as variable. The temperature of all other voxels is considered as constant.

Once built, the tridimensional matrix of labels and temperatures is passed to the thermal propagation simulation algorithm to compute the variation of temperatures over time. The advantage of assigning the constant temperatures as an initial step in a grid is that increasing the sources of cold does not have any significant influence over the computation time.

After this initial step, we use an iterative simulation algorithm that can be found in the literature, based on a discrete approximation of Pennes heat equation used in a finite space:

$$T^{new}_{i,j,k} = T_{i,j,k} + \frac{\Delta t.\beta}{C_{i,j,k}(\Delta x)^3}.H_{i,j,k} + C_b.\omega_b(T_{i,j,k}).(T_b - T_{i,j,k}) + Q_m \quad (2)$$

where $T^{new}_{i,j,k}$ denotes the new temperature to be computed at voxel (i,j,k) after a time step of Δt, $T_{i,j,k}$ and $C_{i,j,k}$ are respectively the current temperature and the volumetric heat capacity at the same voxel, β is a relaxation factor set to 1.95, $H_{i,j,k}$ is the heat flow computed from the six neighbouring cells spaced of Δx from the current voxel, C_b denotes the heat capacity of blood, ω_b is the blood perfusion rate, and Q_m is the metabolic heat rate of tissue. We refer the reader to [5] for a detailed description of the algorithm and the parameters used.

2.2   Placement of the Cube of Interest

It is important to ensure that the simulated residual freezing is fully included within the cube in which the simulation is performed. If the cube of interest is centered on the center of gravity of the cryoprobe's tips, the shape of the residual

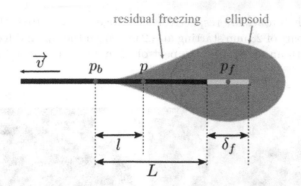

Fig. 3. The drop-shaped iceball (gray) is elongated along the cryoprobe's body. Point p_f is the center of the active freezing shaft (yellow). A residual freezing is observed over a length l of the body of the cryoprobe, up to point p_b. Intermediary point p_i produces residual freezing at a temperature T_i. (Color figure online)

freezing might be too close to the borders of the cube where boundary conditions apply, which would alter the simulation, then reducing and deforming the final shape.

One possibility is simply to enlarge the cube enough to ensure a good coverage of the whole final iceball. However, this approach is very time consuming as an increase of 10% of the size of the cube implies an increase of 33% of the computation time. If the computation time, and thus the reduction of the size of the cube, is an important issue, then a good centering of the final iceball including the residual freezing will be essential to ensure a fast and accurate computation and avoid simulations in irrelevant parts of the volume.

In order to avoid this effect, it is recommended to shift the center of the cube along the vector $\vec{V}$ averaging the direction vectors of all cryoprobes. For N cryoprobes, if $\vec{v_n}$ is the direction vector of the nth cryoprobe, $\vec{V} = \frac{\sum_{n=1}^{N} \vec{v_n}}{N}$.

The amount of the shift will depend on several factors, among which the size of the cube of interest, the chosen value of L, the cryoprobe model (on which depends the size of the iceball), and the global orientation of the cryoprobes (towards a corner or a side of the cube). In this work, we considered a cube of 8 cm to be in most cases a good compromise.

3   Experiment and Results

We experimented our simulation on 5 datasets of patients who underwent renal cryoablation interventions. For all interventions, intraoperative T1 MR images were acquired during the maximal freezing session, showing quite clearly the hypodense signal corresponding to the iceball generated from the cryoprobes. The interventions were performed using 3 to 5 cryoprobes of two models: IceRod and IceEdge from Galil Medical, interacting to produce a large iceball covering the whole tumor. Each patient case had only one single model of probes. The dimensions of the probes are respectively: IceEdge 2.4 mm (10G) thick, with an active freezing part of 28 mm starting at 5.2 mm from the tip, and IceRod 1.5 mm (17G) thick, with an active freezing part of 31 mm starting at 4.2 mm from the tip.

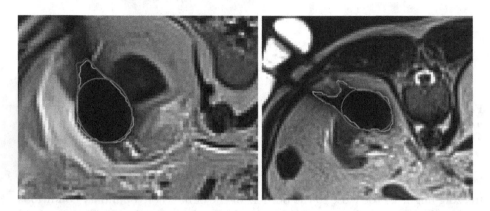

Fig. 4. Result of the simulation on cases 3 (left) and 4 (right): simulated iceball shapes with residual freezing $\mathcal{I}_{RF}$ (blue) and without $\mathcal{I}_{ELL}$ (green), and segmented shape $\mathcal{I}_{SEG}$ (red). (Color figure online)

For each dataset, the iceball including the residual freezing ($\mathcal{I}_{SEG}$) was interactively segmented and the entry and tip points of each cryoprobe were manually selected under the supervision of an expert radiologist. The simulation was computed twice: once using our approach considering the residual freezing (RF), and once using the approach from the literature [5] without residual freezing (ELL), producing the respective resulting shapes $\mathcal{I}_{RF}$ and $\mathcal{I}_{ELL}$ corresponding to the 0°C isotherm surfaces. Simulation with no residual freezing was achieved by labelling "0" the cryoprobes bodies. All the simulations were run on a desktop computer equipped with a core-i5 3.20 GHz CPU with 32 Gb RAM and a GeForce GTX-760 GPU.

In all cases a cube of 8 cm was used to allow space around the iceball and avoid the direct influence of the boundary condition. Length L has been chosen empirically according to the cryoprobes types and their respective size: 45 mm for IceRod, and 60 mm for IceEdge. A shift of 15% of L has been used in all cases.

Each experiment simulated a full standard procedure with alternating freezing/thawing cycles: 10 min of active freezing, followed by 9 min of passive thawing and 1 min of active thawing, and again 10 min of active freezing. We used the parameters provided by the manufacturer: the freezing temperature at the cryoprobe's tip was set to −138.0°C for IceEdge, and to −119.40°C for IceRod. Results are illustrated on Fig. 4.

To evaluate the accuracy of our simulation, $\mathcal{I}_{RF}$ and $\mathcal{I}_{ELL}$ were compared to $\mathcal{I}_{SEG}$ by computing the Hausdorff distance and the Dice coefficient. The results, along with computation times, are presented on Table 1.

Table 1. Dice coefficient and Hausdorff distance (HD, in mm) measurements between the computed and the ground truth iceball segmentation shapes, and computation times, for simulations with and without residual freezing.

Patient case	Nb of probes	With (RF)			Without (ELL)		
		Dice	HD	Time (s.)	Dice	HD	Time (s.)
1	5	0.789	9.333	16.05	0.536	21.601	15.82
2	4	0.792	9.654	18.15	0.536	22.965	18.22
3	4	0.912	8.101	16.21	0.520	21.562	16.10
4	3	0.813	9.020	16.08	0.369	31.105	15.82
5	2	0.799	10.590	15.87	0.598	17.189	15.70
Average		0.821	9.340	16.47	0.512	22.884	16.33
STD		0.052	0.908	0.95	0.085	5.085	1.07

It can be observed that the simulated shape $\mathcal{I}_{RF}$ fits the segmented shape $\mathcal{I}_{SEG}$ better than $\mathcal{I}_{ELL}$. The average Dice coefficient is 0.821, and the average Hausdorff distance is 9.340 mm, improving the results of the simulation without residual freezing. As expected, the computation time is not significantly different when considering a simulation with or without residual freezing. The computation time mostly depends on the size of the cube, *i.e.* the number of voxels to explore during the simulation.

This first attempt of simulating the residual freezing has been designed assuming that the increase of temperature along the cryoprobe's body was linear. It would be interesting to perform experimental measurements to validate this theory, and get more accurate parameters to refine our model. Non linearity of the temperature distribution could be achieved by replacing Eq. 1 by a more complex model.

In our experiments, we chose to use a cube size of 8 cm, as a trade-off between a full inclusion of the simulated iceball within the cube with enough distance to the boundaries, and a reduced computation time. For case 5, a smaller cube of 6 cm could have been used, as the number and model of cryoprobes are smaller. However, it could be interesting to investigate the automatic suggestion of an optimal cube size, based on the number of cryoprobes, their orientation in the image, and their model.

Previous works in the literature obtained simulation results that were usually compared against theoretical shapes of iceballs (pure ellipsoids) or segmented iceballs in which the residual freezing part was usually not included. Yet, modelling the residual freezing is clinically relevant and important, as an underestimation of the predicted iceball shape may result in potential damage to healthy cells, causing pathologies or pain. With the objective in mind to include such a simulation within a preoperative treatment planning framework, with an automatic computation of optimal placements for the cryoprobes, an accurate and complete prediction of the iceball is essential.

4   Conclusion

In this paper we presented a first approach to model the residual freezing along the cryoprobes bodies during renal cryoablation. This phenomenon was usually ignored in previously published works, although it may result in an underestimation of the predicted frozen area and to potential damage to healthy tissue, or cause pain. Our approach consists in modelling a temperature linearly increasing along the cryoprobe's body but constant over time, and use it as a source of cold during the simulation. We experimented our model on 5 retrospective patient datasets, and showed that our model fits the segmented iceball with a reasonable accuracy. We determined that a size of 8 cm for the simulation cube, with an appropriate shift, is enough to simulate the whole 30 mn process and produce the shape of the resulting iceball in less than 20 s. Further experiments should be performed in future works to confirm these first results.

Acknowledgments. This work was partially supported by a grant from the Maimonide France-Israel Research in Biomedical Robotics, funded jointly by the French Ministry of Higher Education, Research and Innovation, the French Ministry for the Economy and Finance, and Israel Ministry of Science, Technology and Space, 2016–18, and by Grant 53681 (METASEG) from the Israel Ministry of Science, Technology and Space, 2016–2019.

References

1. Butz, T., et al.: Pre-and intra-operative planning and simulation of percutaneous tumor ablation. In: Delp, S.L., DiGoia, A.M., Jaramaz, B. (eds.) MICCAI 2000. LNCS, vol. 1935, pp. 317–326. Springer, Heidelberg (2000). https://doi.org/10.1007/978-3-540-40899-4_32
2. Ge, M., Chua, K., Shu, C., Yang, W.: Analytical and numerical study of tissue cryofreezing via the immersed boundary method. Int. J. Heat Mass Transfer **83**, 1–10 (2015)
3. Ge, M., Shu, C., Chua, K., Yang, W.: Numerical analysis of a clinically-extracted vascular tissue during cryo-freezing using immersed boundary method. Int. J. Therm. Sci. **110**, 109–118 (2016)
4. Ge, M., Shu, C., Yang, W., Chua, K.: Incorporating an immersed boundary method to study thermal effects of vascular systems during tissue cryo-freezing. J. Therm. Biol. **64**, 92–99 (2017)
5. Golkar, E., Rao, P.P., Joskowicz, L., Gangi, A., Essert, C.: Fast GPU computation of 3D isothermal volumes in the vicinity of major blood vessels for multiprobe cryoablation simulation. In: Frangi, A.F., Schnabel, J.A., Davatzikos, C., Alberola-López, C., Fichtinger, G. (eds.) MICCAI 2018. LNCS, vol. 11073, pp. 230–237. Springer, Cham (2018). https://doi.org/10.1007/978-3-030-00937-3_27

6. Hossain, S.C., Zhang, X., Haider, Z., Hu, P., Zhao, G.: Optimization of prostatic cryosurgery with multi-cryoprobe based on refrigerant flow. J. Therm. Biol. **76**, 58–67 (2018)
7. Kumar, A., Kumar, S., Katiyar, V., Telles, S.: Phase change heat transfer during cryosurgery of lung cancer using hyperbolic heat conduction model. Comput. Biol. Med. **84**, 20–29 (2017)
8. Kumar, M., Upadhyay, S., Rai, K.: A study of cryosurgery of lung cancer using modified legendre wavelet galerkin method. J. Therm. Biol. **78**, 356–366 (2018)
9. Magalov, Z., Shitzer, A., Degani, D.: Isothermal volume contours generated in a freezing gel by embedded cryo-needles with applications to cryo-surgery. Cryobiology **55**(2), 127–137 (2007)
10. Pennes, H.H.: Analysis of tissue and arterial blood temperatures in the resting human forearm. J. Appl. Physiol. **1**(2), 93–122 (1948)
11. Rieder, C., Kroeger, T., Schumann, C., Hahn, H.K.: GPU-based real-time approximation of the ablation zone for radiofrequency ablation. IEEE Trans. Visual. Comput. Graph. **17**(12), 1812–1821 (2011)

A Generative Model of Hyperelastic Strain Energy Density Functions for Real-Time Simulation of Brain Tissue Deformation

Alejandro Granados[1]([✉]), Martin Schweiger[1], Vejay Vakharia[2],
Andrew W. McEvoy[2], Anna Miserocchi[2], John S. Duncan[2,3],
Rachel Sparks[1], and Sébastien Ourselin[1]

[1] School of Biomedical Engineering and Imaging Sciences,
King's College London, London, UK
alejandro.granados@kcl.ac.uk
[2] National Hospital of Neurology and Neurosurgery, London, UK
[3] Department of Clinical and Experimental Epilepsy,
UCL Queen Square Institute of Neurology, London, UK

Abstract. *Purpose.* The goal of this paper is to build a simulation environment that allows for the prediction of patient-specific tissue response by drawing samples from a generative model with a probability distribution. We propose a Gaussian Process (GP) regression approach to learn distributions over strain energy density functions including elastography, linear and hyperelastic models reported in the literature. *Methods.* We gather a total of 73 models characterising elastic properties of brain white matter, grey matter and abnormalities and express them as strain energy density functions. A multi-output GP is used to quantify means and confidence intervals across each anatomical region and model. We sample the GP distribution and use nonlinear optimisation to fit a Neo-Hookean meta-model to guarantee stable strain energy functions. We validate the Neo-Hookean meta-model by fitting known strain energy density functions from the literature and report optimisation cost. We also validate the ability of the GP to approximate elastic properties of tissue given a reference deformed state using simulation. *Results.* The GP was able to capture confidence intervals of varying strain ranges; the GP parameters and optimisation costs indicated a higher variability of hyperelastic models compared to elastography and linear models. Although one term is insufficient to fully capture hyperelastic models with higher number of terms, the resulting meta model is stable for real-time simulation within a wider range of stretches captured during mechanical characterisation of soft tissue. We demonstrated that our approach was able to approximate known elastic properties of tissue with a root-mean-squared error of 0.6 mm of node displacements when drawing six samples from a distribution of hyperelastic white matter. *Conclusion.* In this initial proof-of-concept, we demonstrated a GP-based approach to estimate the elastic behaviour of brain tissue through simulation by sampling a generative model comprising elastic models found in the literature.

© Springer Nature Switzerland AG 2019
D. Shen et al. (Eds.): MICCAI 2019, LNCS 11768, pp. 218–226, 2019.
https://doi.org/10.1007/978-3-030-32254-0_25

Keywords: Biomechanics · Brain deformation · Gaussian Processes

1 Introduction

The motivation of this paper is to build a simulation environment to predict patient-specific tissue response caused by mechanical stimuli. This is particularly important in scenarios where an estimate of such behaviour is available from the population but is not patient-specific. For instance, given the deformed state of a human organ or even the effect of tools interacting with it, the main goal is to sample elastic behaviour from a probability distribution that best characterises the observations.

Soft tissue characterisation is typically performed either *in-vivo* using Magnetic Resonance Elastography (MRE) via shear wave propagation within a small window of strain (e.g. 500 μm) [6] or *ex-vivo* by mechanical loading of small blocks of resected tissue. For human tissue, linear models are only appropriate for small strains (where tissue behaves roughly linearly) and nonlinear hyperelastic models are more appropriate for larger strains. Brain tissue has been widely investigated [11] and recent studies report Ogden hyperelastic models best fit the observations [3,8,9]. However, whilst computer-assisted interventions mostly take into account patient-specific anatomy, elastic behaviour is typically modelled with average values reported from the literature. Although it is relevantly easy to compare linear models (*Lamé coefficients*), it is more difficult to compare hyperelastic models due to differences in model order and coefficient heterogeneity. Furthermore, reported parameters fit observations over a smaller range of strains than necessary for real-time simulation of deformable bodies.

Few generative models have been proposed for sampling mechanical behaviour. In animation, *Martin et al.* [7] proposed the simulation of complex material behaviour via interpolation in strain space of an *example manifold* and then compute a force based on elastic potentials to attract a solid to that configuration. This approach later became the foundation of projective dynamics [4]. In multi-scale modelling, *Bhattacharjee et al.* [2] proposed a model reduction using manifold learning (isomap) and neural networks for hyperelastic heterogeneous materials. Stochastic processes have also been used to model phenomena as random functions including the mechanical characterisation of soft tissue [10].

In this paper, we propose a Gaussian Process for regression to learn a distribution over strain energy density functions that allows for sampling elastic properties of human brain tissue (brain in general, white matter, grey matter and abnormalities) from MRE, linear and hyperelastic models reported in the literature. A Neo-Hookean hyperelastic meta-model is then used to fit samples drawn from the distribution whilst guaranteeing a valid strain energy density function that can be used for real-time simulation.

2 Methods

Elasticity of Brain Tissue. From the literature we collected a total of 73 elastic models with reported coefficients corresponding to MRE, linear and hyperelastic models as *strain energy density functions* [3,8,9,11]. A strain energy density function Ψ, or *elastic potential*, relates strain (represented by the deformation tensor $\boldsymbol{F}$) to stress (obtained using the gradient of Ψ with respect to F). We can define a nonlinear hyperelastic model $\Psi(\lambda_1, \lambda_2, \lambda_3)$ in terms of its principal stretches λ_i, where $\hat{\boldsymbol{F}}$ is calculated using a rotation variant SVD [14,16] from F with rotations $\boldsymbol{U}$ and $\boldsymbol{V}$ (Eq. 1). For instance, Eq. 1 defines a Neo-Hookean hyperelastic model in terms of λ_i and shear modulus μ. Although Ψ can also be defined in terms of the invariants of the right Cauchy-Green deformation tensor $\boldsymbol{C} = \boldsymbol{F}^T \boldsymbol{F}$ [15], it becomes difficult to express all materials, e.g. Ogden [16].

MRE and linear models were also defined in terms of their strain energy density function $\Psi_{linear}(\boldsymbol{F}) = \mu_L \boldsymbol{\epsilon} : \boldsymbol{\epsilon} + \frac{\lambda_L}{2} tr^2(\boldsymbol{\epsilon})$, where $\boldsymbol{\epsilon} = \frac{1}{2}(\boldsymbol{F} + \boldsymbol{F}^T) - I$ is the small strain tensor, and μ_L, λ_L are the *Lamé coefficients* which are related to the material properties (i.e. *Young's modulus* and *Poisson's ratio*) [13]. We use compression and tension strain ranges when reported in the literature, which was only for hyperelastic models (20, 30, 40, and 45%), otherwise we assume strain ranges of $\pm 5\%$ for MRE studies and $\pm 10\%$ for linear models (Fig. 1 top). Recent studies report fitted parameters of a hyperelastic model independently for compression and tension [3] and these are treated accordingly.

$$F = U\hat{F}V^T$$

$$\hat{F} = \begin{bmatrix} \lambda_1 & 0 & 0 \\ 0 & \lambda_2 & 0 \\ 0 & 0 & \lambda_3 \end{bmatrix} \tag{1}$$

$$\Psi_{N-H} = \frac{\mu}{2}(\lambda_1^2 + \lambda_2^2 + \lambda_3^2 - 3)$$

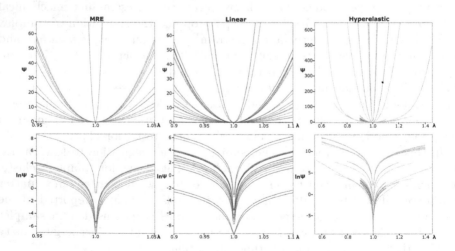

Fig. 1. Brain tissue models from the literature expressed in terms of their strain energy density function Ψ. Horizontal axis represents stretch λ during rest (=1), compression (<1) and tension (>1). Different ranges of compression/tension tests are shown for MRE (5%), linear (10%) and hyperelastic (<45%) studies. *Top:* Ψ in Pascals. *Bottom:* natural log transform of Ψ.

Generative Model. Gaussian Process (GP) regression is a non-parametric Bayesian approach to learn distributions over functions [12]. We define a multi-task GP following an Intrinsic Coregionalization Model (ICM) [1] where we assume correlation among the tasks with heterotopic data D_t ($N = 73$) sampled from different patients/brain regions and under different experimental conditions (Eq. 2). We define a total of $T = 12$ tasks ($f_{\mathcal{GP}_t}(\boldsymbol{\lambda}_t)$, $t = 1, \ldots, T$) related to the combination of brain tissue types (brain in general, white matter, grey matter and abnormalities) and elastic model types (MRE, linear, hyperelastic). Each curve is discretised in $I = 100$ points and the number of curves in each task may vary ($n \in t$). Ψ varies significantly across stretches finding their log space ($ln\Psi$) easier to optimise. Each task $f_{\mathcal{GP}_t}(\boldsymbol{\lambda}_t)$ is a multiple output vector-valued function that takes as inputs stretches $\boldsymbol{\lambda}_t \in \Re^{1xI}$ (x-axis of Fig. 1) and as outputs strain energy density functions in log space ($ln\Psi$, y-axis in Fig. 1 bottom) with Gaussian noise $\epsilon_t \sim \mathcal{N}(0, \sigma_t^2)$ (Eq. 3). The proposed kernel structure is a *Matérn 3/2* covariance kernel $k(\boldsymbol{\lambda}_t, \boldsymbol{\lambda}_t') = k_{M3/2}$ that captures the covariance within tasks. The covariance across tasks is mapped with the coregionalization matrix $\boldsymbol{B}$, which is positive-definite and defined by $\boldsymbol{B} = \boldsymbol{W}\boldsymbol{W}^T + \kappa_t \boldsymbol{I}$, where $\boldsymbol{W}$ is of rank 1 and relates to coefficients used for the linear interpolation of $f_{\mathcal{GP}_t}(\boldsymbol{\lambda}_t)$ and κ reflects the variance across tasks (Eq. 4). The GP regression optimisation has 38 parameters (*Matérn* length scale and variance, as well as 12-valued vectors $\boldsymbol{W}$, κ_t and σ_t^2). $k_{M3/2}$ is initialised with a unit variance (fixed), and length scale of 0.01. After GP optimisation, we draw samples from the distribution $f_{\mathcal{GP}_t}(\boldsymbol{\lambda}_t)$ for a task t and a range of stretches $\boldsymbol{\lambda}_t$. We sample over a range of $\mu_s \pm 1.96\sigma_s$, where μ_s and σ_s are the mean and standard deviation of the distribution, respectively.

$$D_t = \{(\lambda_{i,n}, ln\ \Psi_n(\lambda_{i,n})) \mid i \in I, n \in N, t \in T, n \in t\} \tag{2}$$

$$ln\ \Psi_{\mathcal{GP}_t}(\boldsymbol{\lambda}_t) \sim \mathcal{GP}(0, k(\boldsymbol{\lambda}_t, \boldsymbol{\lambda}_t'))$$
$$f_{\mathcal{GP}_t}(\boldsymbol{\lambda}_t) = ln\ \Psi_{\mathcal{GP}_t}(\boldsymbol{\lambda}_t) + \epsilon_t \tag{3}$$

$$\begin{bmatrix} f_{\mathcal{GP}_1}(\boldsymbol{\lambda}_t) \\ \vdots \\ f_{\mathcal{GP}_T}(\boldsymbol{\lambda}_T) \end{bmatrix} \sim \mathcal{N}\left(\begin{bmatrix} 0 \\ \vdots \\ 0 \end{bmatrix}, \boldsymbol{B} \otimes \boldsymbol{K} + \sigma_t^2 \boldsymbol{I} \right) \tag{4}$$

Hyperelastic Meta-model. We define a compressible Neo-Hookean hyperelastic meta-model Ψ_{meta} (Eq. 5a) using *Lamé* coefficients μ_m, λ_m, principal stretches $\lambda_{i=1,2,3}$ (Eq. 1) and $J = \lambda_1 \lambda_2 \lambda_3$ to fit the samples described above. For a uniaxial tension/compression mechanical test, Ψ_{meta} can be reduced to $\Psi_{opt}(\lambda_1, \lambda_1^{-\frac{1}{2}}, \lambda_1^{-\frac{1}{2}}) = \frac{\mu_m}{2}(\lambda_1^2 + 2\lambda_1^{-1} - 3)$. $ln\Psi_{opt}$ is then used to fit the sample via non-linear least squares optimisation with a bound on weight μ_m to be positive. For real-time simulation, we define Ψ_{meta} in terms of its principal stretches λ_i and express it using the Valanis-Landel hypothesis (Eq. 5b) similar to [16], where $f(\lambda_i)$, $g(\lambda_i \lambda_j)$ and $h(\lambda_1 \lambda_2 \lambda_3)$ are one-dimensional strain energy density functions for uniaxial, biaxial and triaxial strain, respectively.

$$\Psi_{meta} = \frac{\mu_m}{2}(\lambda_1^2 + \lambda_2^2 + \lambda_3^2 - 3) - \mu_m lnJ + \frac{\lambda_m}{2}(lnJ)^2 \tag{5a}$$

$$f(\lambda_i) = \frac{\mu_m}{2}(\lambda_i^2 - 1), \qquad g(\lambda_i\lambda_j) = 0, \qquad h(J) = -\mu_m lnJ + \frac{\lambda_m}{2}(lnJ)^2 \tag{5b}$$

Implementation. The presented generative model is implemented in Python (3.6). For each elastic model from the literature, we describe Ψ in terms of their principal stretches λ_i using symbolic mathematics with SymPy (1.3) and evaluate it for a uniaxial tensile/compressible mechanical test. The GP is implemented in GPy (1.9.6) [5] and its parameters are optimised using the default bound constrained optimisation L-BFGS-B algorithm in SciPy (1.2.1). Least square minimisation of Ψ_{opt} was performed with the Trust Region Reflective (trf) method in SciPy. For real-time simulation, we implemented a hyperelastic Finite Element Model partly based on VegaFEM (http://run.usc.edu/vega/) and following [14,16] as a native C++ plugin executed using the Unity3D game engine.

Validation. We evaluate the performance of the GP by reporting learnt parameters and inference across the confidence interval given a brain tissue and elastic model type. We report the performance of Ψ_{meta} and validate our approach by running real-time nonlinear hyperelastic FEM simulation (see above) for each inferred strain energy density functions when applying external forces (10 N) to a subset of nodes of a volumetric tetrahedral mesh obtained from a human brain segmented using a T1-w MRI and Geodesic Information Flow (GIF) parcellation (Fig. 2). The volumetric deformable model (in yellow) consists of 437 tetrahedra and 163 nodes, whereas the surface model (in pink) consists of 50,000 triangles and 24580 vertices. Dirichlet fixed boundary conditions (in green) where defined on 10 vertices at the base of the brain and falx cerebri (as in [11]) based on two primitive boxes (in green).

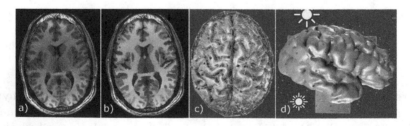

Fig. 2. From a T1-weighted MRI (a) we determine a brain parcellation using GIF (b). The parcellation is used to create a fine surface and coarse volumetric mesh of the human brain. (c) Volumetric elements are shown in yellow with red spheres indicating nodes where external forces (10 N) are applied to in the direction towards the screen. (d) Boundary conditions are defined by fixing nodes inside green boxes located at the base of the brain and falx cerebri. (Color figure online)

3   Results

Table 1 reports the variance (κ_t) and noise (σ_t^2) for the best fit GP, using a *Matérn* 3/2 kernel, $T = 12$ tasks and rank $W = 1$. As shown in the table, the hyperelastic models had the highest variance and noise for the task considered. We found the GP converged and better fit means and confidence intervals (including extended ranges of stretches than those reported in the literature) compared to other kernels tested including squared exponential, linear, bias and simple combinations of these.

Table 1. Number of samples (n), GP parameters (κ_t, σ_t^2) and nonlinear least squares optimisation cost of Ψ_{opt} for a total of $T = 12$ tasks (elastic model and tissue types).

Model	Tissue	n	κ_t	σ_t^2	Ψ_{opt} *lsq* cost
MRE	Grey matter	5	0.184	0.24	0.001 (6.5e−7)
	White matter	5	0.467	0.57	0.001 (1.07e−6)
	Brain	1	0.319	0.0	0.001
	Abnormal	1	4.986	0.0	0.001
Linear	Grey matter	1	0.0	0.0	0.008
	White matter	1	0.063	0.0	0.008
	Brain	16	0.409	1.33	0.008 (0.008)
	Abnormal	7	1.034	9.66	0.043 (0.06)
Hyperelastic	Grey matter	10	8.929	0.13	7.097 (1.447)
	White matter	10	9.810	0.11	12.36 (4.325)
	Brain	15	28.006	8.67	11.444 (9.889)
	Abnormal	1	1.096	7.52	1.039

Validation of Meta-model. We evaluated the performance of Ψ_{opt} to represent Ψ models from the literature using nonlinear least squares optimisation. We observe higher optimisation costs of hyperelastic models compared to linear models (Table 1). The highest errors are observed in cases where multiple terms are used and tension/compression tests are modelled independently (Fig. 3).

Validation of Generative Model. We examine three learnt GP functions (Fig. 4). The proposed GP is able to fit well the mean and variance of strain energy density functions in log space ($ln\Psi$) for linear models in general. Small variations in log space are translated into significant changes in Ψ, where differences are noticeable between grey matter and white matter tissue. When generating samples for linear models and fitting the proposed Neo-Hookean meta-model, smooth and uniform samples (lines in grey colour) are obtained within the confidence interval. Related to hyperelastic models, we were also able to capture a function spanning different

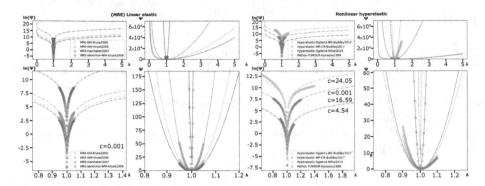

Fig. 3. Full (top) and close-up view (bottom) of meta-model (dash/solid) fitted to four linear elastic (left) and four hyperelastic (right) models (circles) in $ln\Psi$ and Ψ space. Although the meta-model adequately fits linear data, it underperforms fitting hyperelastic models with n-terms (pink) or are defined as mixed models (grey/orange). (Color figure online)

ranges of stretches. However, the fluctuations observed in Ψ space of healthy brain tissue are the result of the variability reported in the literature. The data used for white matter (Fig. 4 centre) describes Ψ in two different parts (one for tension and one for compression) that one Neo-Hookean meta-model with a single term is unable to capture, resulting in regions of the meta-model falling outside of the confidence interval. Despite this limitation, the meta-model is able to cope with fluctuations and therefore avoids negative slopes in the gradient that cause instabilities during real-time simulation.

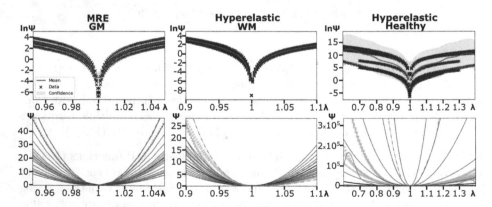

Fig. 4. *Top:* GP of three tasks (MRE-GM, hyperelastic-WM and -healthy brain tissue) learnt in $ln\Psi$ showing data (+), mean (blue), and confidence interval CI (light blue). *Bottom:* CI is transformed to Ψ space (dashed lines) with 10 samples drawn from the distribution (circles) and fitted to a Neo-Hookean meta-model (black lines). (Color figure online)

Validation of Generative Model and Meta-model. We demonstrate our approach by estimating the elastic parameters of brain tissue given a reference deformed state, a hyperelastic model of white matter (corpus callosum) consisting of two models (compression and tension) [3], which is loaded into our simulation platform and where external forces are applied as in Fig. 2. To validate our approach six samples are drawn from the hyperelastic white matter distribution (Fig. 4 centre) within $-2\sigma_s$ and $+2\sigma_s$ from the mean μ_s, i.e. from soft to hard, respectively (Fig. 5 blue series). Each sample is then fitted to the proposed meta-model (Fig. 5 orange series) and the optimised shear modulus μ_m is used to initialise the nonlinear hyperelastic FEM before applying an external force of 10 N to a subset of nodes (Fig. 2). After 3 s, we compute node displacements with respect to the reference nodes and quantify similarity by means of root-mean-squared error (RMSE) of node displacements (Fig. 5 bottom). Given the RMSE, we confirmed that the reference elastic behaviour is between $+1.2\sigma$ and $+2\sigma$ from the mean. Although external forces are difficult to measure during a real scenario, recent approaches attempt to estimate these using machine learning algorithms. With better boundary conditions and accounting for different types of regions in the brain, we envisage that the presented generative model could be used similarly as the validation described above to estimate elastic properties that characterise nonlinear deformation.

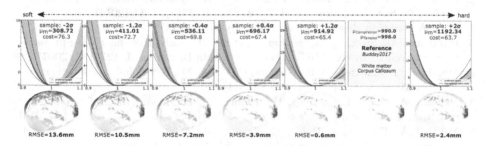

Fig. 5. Estimating elastic behaviour by drawing six samples $[\mu_s - 2\sigma_s, \mu_s + 2\sigma_s]$ from white matter hyperelastic distribution. *Top:* Mean and confidence interval (grey), sample from distribution (blue), and meta-model (orange) for each sample along a reference picked from the literature. *Bottom:* Colour map indicating (red) the Euclidean distance of each volumetric node to those nodes of a reference state with similarity quantified as root-mean-squared error in mm. (Color figure online)

4   Conclusion and Future Work

Our approach allows for sampling strain energy density functions from a GP regression method to approximate elastic behaviour of human brain tissue. There are numerous ways of extending this work in the future. Further studies could incorporate combined load and other factors such as age, fibre orientation or differentiate between different regions of similar type of tissue. Further work will investigate other strategies of GP kernel choice and extend our meta-model to models with more terms such as Ogden.

Acknowledgements. This research was funded/supported by the Health Innovation Challenge Fund (WT106882), the Wellcome/EPSRC Centre for Medical Engineering [WT203148/Z/16/Z], and the National Institute for Health Research (NIHR) Biomedical Research Centre based at Guy's and St Thomas' NHS Foundation Trust and King's College London and/or the NIHR Clinical Research Facility. We are grateful to the Wolfson Foundation and the Epilepsy Society for supporting the Epilepsy Society MRI scanner. The views expressed in this publication are those of the authors and not necessarily those of the Wellcome Trust, NHS, the NIHR or the Department of Health.

References

1. Álvarez, M.A., Rosasco, L., Lawrence, N.D.: Kernels for vector-valued functions: a review. J. Found. Trends Mach. Learn. **4**(3), 195–266 (2012)
2. Bhattacharjee, S., Matouš, K.: A nonlinear manifold-based reduced order model for multiscale analysis of heterogeneous hyperelastic materials. J. Comput. Phys. **313**, 635–653 (2016)
3. Budday, S., Sommer, G., Birkl, C., et al.: Mechanical characterization of human brain tissue. Acta Biomater. **48**, 319–340 (2017)
4. Bouaziz, S., Martin, S., Liu, T., et al.: Projective dynamics: fusing constraint projections for fast simulation. ACM Trans. Graph. **33**(4), 1–11 (2014)
5. GPy: A Gaussian Process Framework in Python (2014)
6. Hamhaber, U., Sack, I., Papazoglou, S., et al.: 3D analysis of shear wave propagation observed by in vivo MRE of the brain. Acta Biomater. **3**, 127–137 (2007)
7. Martin, S., Thomaszewski, B., Grispun, E., Gross, M.: Example-based elastic materials. ACM Trans. Graph. **30**(4), 1–8 (2011)
8. Mihai, L.A., Chin, L., Janmey, P.A., Goriely, A.: A comparison of hyperelastic constitutive models applicable to brain and fat tissues. Royal Soc. **12**, 1–12 (2015)
9. Mihai, L.A., Budday, S., Holzapfel, G.A., et al.: A family of hyperelastic models for human brain tissue. J. Mech. Phys. Solids **106**, 60–79 (2017)
10. Mihai, L.A., Wooley, T.E., Goriely, A.: Stochastic isotropic hyperelastic materials: constitutive calibration and model selection. Proc. Royal Soc. A **474**, 1–20 (2018)
11. Morin, F., Chabanas, M., Courtecuisse, H., Payan, Y.: Biomechanical modelling of brain soft tissues for medical applications. In: Biomechanics Living Organs, pp. 127–146 (2017)
12. Schulz, E., Speekenbrink, M., Krause, A.: A tutorial on GP regression: modelling, exploring, and exploiting functions. J. Math. Psychol. **85**, 1–16 (2018)
13. Sifakis, E.D.: FEM Simulation of 3D Deformable Solids: a practitioner's guide to theory, discretization and model reduction. SIGGRAPH Course, pp. 1–32 (2012)
14. Stomakhin, A., Hower, R., Schroeder, C., Teran, J.M.: Energetically consistent invertible elasticity. In: Eurographics, pp. 1–8 (2012)
15. Teran, J., Sifakis, E., Irving, G., Fedkiw, R.: Robust quasistatic finite elements and flesh simulation. In: EG/SIGGRAPH Symposium on Computer animation, pp. 1–11 (2005)
16. Xu, H., Sin, F., Zhu, Y., Barbic, J.: Nonlinear material design using principal stretches. ACM Trans. Graph. **34**(4), 1–11 (2015)

Variational Shape Completion for Virtual Planning of Jaw Reconstructive Surgery

Amir H. Abdi$^{(\boxtimes)}$, Mehran Pesteie, Eitan Prisman, Purang Abolmaesumi,
and Sidney Fels

University of British Columbia, Vancouver, Canada
{amirabdi,mehranp,purang,ssfels}@ece.ubc.ca, eitan.prisman@ubc.ca

Abstract. The premorbid geometry of the mandible is of significant relevance in jaw reconstructive surgeries and occasionally unknown to the surgical team. In this paper, an optimization framework is introduced to train deep models for completion (reconstruction) of the missing segments of the bone based on the remaining healthy structure. To leverage the contextual information of the surroundings of the dissected region, the voxel-weighted Dice loss is introduced. To address the non-deterministic nature of the shape completion problem, we leverage a weighted multi-target probabilistic solution which is an extension to the conditional variational autoencoder (CVAE). This approach considers multiple targets as acceptable reconstructions, each weighted according to their conformity with the original shape. We quantify the performance gain of the proposed method against similar algorithms, including CVAE, where we report statistically significant improvements in both deterministic and probabilistic paradigms. The probabilistic model is also evaluated on its ability to generate anatomically relevant variations for the missing bone. As a unique aspect of this work, the model is tested on real surgical cases where the clinical relevancy of its reconstructions and their compliance with surgeon's virtual plan are demonstrated as necessary steps towards clinical adoption.

Keywords: Conditional variational autoencoder · 3D shape completion · V-Net · Mandible reconstruction

1 Introduction

Head and neck cancer comprises of a set of malignant tumors in the upper respiratory tract which constitutes 3–4% of cancer cases in North America [8]. Surgery is the first line of treatment for the majority of these cases. Despite the advances in tools and techniques, mandibular reconstruction after segmental mandibulectomy is still a challenging procedure. Moreover, due to the mandible's

Electronic supplementary material The online version of this chapter (https://doi.org/10.1007/978-3-030-32254-0_26) contains supplementary material, which is available to authorized users.

© Springer Nature Switzerland AG 2019
D. Shen et al. (Eds.): MICCAI 2019, LNCS 11768, pp. 227–235, 2019.
https://doi.org/10.1007/978-3-030-32254-0_26

vital role in mastication, speech, and swallowing, the functional and aesthetic requirements of mandibular reconstructions are quite high.

The vascularized free fibula flap is the most utilized technique for mandibular reconstruction [4] where the linear shape of the fibula bone is dissected, contoured, and modelled to complete the curved geometry of the ablated bone. In the past decade, three-dimensional (3D) virtual surgical planning (VSP) has gained traction. In the VSP-enhanced free fibula flap, the modelling and shaping of the fibula are virtually planned based on the pre-operative records.

One of the challenges in mandibular reconstruction is the unknown pre-incident shape of the missing (distorted) bony elements. In cases where the shape of the target bony element is unknown, three strategies are taken to anticipate the original anatomy [10]. In rare cases where previous medical records of the craniofacial skeleton is available, patient's own bone morphology serves as the reference. For unilateral defects, the uninvolved contralateral side is mirrored and manually positioned to create an estimated reconstruction reference. However, this approach becomes less reliable for defects with anteromedial extensions and is inapplicable in midline crossing lesions. Standard anatomic templates are seldom utilized to fill the missing bony elements after subjet-specific adjustments.

Related Work. Shape completion is an ill-posed inverse problem in computer vision and graphics. Data-driven models, including deep neural networks, are more intriguing as they directly learn the completion under supervision particularly because of the non-deterministic ground-truth and multiple acceptable solutions for the reconstruction problem. In the realm of 3D generative deep models, applicability of adversarial training (GAN) in 3D shape and point cloud syntheses are investigated [2, 11]. Varitional autoencoders (VAE) have also been able to learn semantically meaningful latent spaces for realistic completions [6]. The closest research to our work is a recent study where they empirically proved the feasibility of generating mandible shapes from a predefined set of landmarks [1].

Contributions. We introduce optimization approaches to train deep convolutional models to reconstruct the missing bone segment from the remaining healthy mandible. Our contributions are three-fold. First, we design a framework to randomly generate samples for training of shape completion models in deterministic and probabilistic paradigms. We introduce the Voxel-weighted Dice loss that prioritizes the target (removed) region over the rest of the geometry while ensuring consistency in reconstruction by leveraging the contextual information from the rest of the shape. Our main contribution is the Target-weighted variational objective function which addresses the one-to-many reality of shape reconstruction. We report the quantified gain in performance and demonstrate the model's ability to predict variations of the missing bone. Moreover, as a unique aspect of this work, qualitative results on real surgical cases are provided as a notion of clinical relevancy and compliance with surgeon's virtual plans.

2   Method

2.1   Network Architecture

The input (X) to the deep model is a 3D binary voxel-grid of size c^3 containing a mandible with a missing (dissected) contiguous segment. The output of the model is a 3D probability map $(\hat{Y})$ of size c^3 where the predicted volume is the union of all voxels with $Y_{ijk} > 0.5$. Architecture of the learning system is summarized in Fig. 1. We investigate two reconstruction approaches, deterministic and probabilistic. In heart of both lies a V-Net [5] consisting of four down-transition and four up-transitions with skip connections to forward feature maps from the encoding to the decoding stream. Each down-transition consists of strided 3D convolutions and batch-normalization. Similarly, the up-transitions contain transposed strided 3D convolution (deconvolution) and batch-normalization. ELU activation layers are used throughout the V-Net. Activations of the main stream of the last two down-transitions and the first two up-transitions are dropped out with a probability of 0.5. The final up-transition generates four 3D feature maps of size c^3, same size as the input and the target occupancy maps. More details of the architecture are available in the supplementary material.

In deterministic shape reconstruction, the final four feature maps are convolved with P_{gen} kernels of size 2 followed by a sigmoid function. In the probabilistic approach, the four feature maps of the V-Net are first concatenated with the tiled latent values (see Sect. 2.2) and convolved with 8 kernels in two consecutive layers of P_{comb} prior to P_{gen} (Fig. 1).

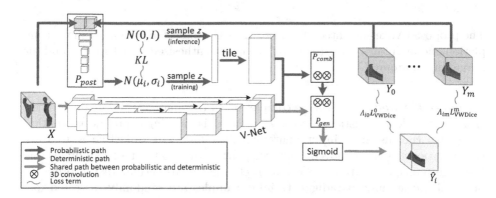

Fig. 1. Architecture of the deterministic and weighted multi-target probabilistic learning framework for anatomy completion with 3D convolutional models.

2.2   Loss Functions

During the mini-batch gradient decent optimization, each training sample is randomly dissected by a cuboid (B) with an arbitrary size and orientation, which forms a binary occupancy map inside a 3D grid of size c^3. The cuboid cuts the mandible to create input and target shapes as follows,

$$X = S \circ B' \quad \text{and} \quad Y = S \circ B, \tag{1}$$

where $P \circ Q$ denotes the Hadamard product of the tensors P and Q, and B' is the complement of the binary cuboid. X and Y are the input and target (Fig. 2).

Voxel-Weighted Dice. This objective function enables the model to leverage the contextual information from the surroundings of the dissected region. Hence, voxels of the predicted 3D probability map are weighted adversely by their distance from the removed bony segment. To do so, a 3D normal distribution, $\mathcal{N}_w(\bar{Y}, \sigma_w^2 I)$, with a diagonal covariance matrix is instantiated at the center of the target segment ($\bar{Y}$). The 3D weight matrix W of size c^3 is then defined as

$$W_{ijk} = \begin{cases} 1 & B_{ijk} = 1 \\ (2\pi\sigma_w)^{\frac{3}{2}}\mathcal{N}_w(i,j,k) & B_{ijk} = 0 \end{cases}. \tag{2}$$

Eq. 2 prioritizes the voxels inside the volume of the dissection cuboid (B) and ignores distant voxels. Here, σ_w is set to $c/3$ to encourage smoother contours. Based on the weight matrix, W, the proposed Voxel-weighted Dice loss is

$$\mathcal{L}_{\text{VWDice}}(X, Y, \hat{Y}, W) = 1 - \frac{2 * \sum\limits_{ijk}\left[\hat{Y} \circ (Y + X) \circ W\right]_{ijk}}{\sum\limits_{ijk}\left[(\hat{Y} + Y + X) \circ W\right]_{ijk}}. \tag{3}$$

The proposed Voxel-weighted Dice prioritizes the dissected region for shape completion and maintains consistency between the synthesized structure ($\hat{Y}$) and the remaining anatomy (X).

Target-Weighted Loss. Shape completion in the anatomical domain is inherently a non-deterministic process, *i.e.*, there is no single ground-truth that completes the dissected input anatomy. Therefore, our objective is to learn the variations of the removed bony segment from a dataset of mandibles and generate multiple solutions to reconstruct a given dissection. In the proposed probabilistic learning paradigm, training samples are randomly dissected, on-the-fly, and the removed segment is considered the best known reconstruction target, referred to as Y_0 hereafter. In the proposed multi-target approach, m random training samples are selected and dissected at the same location using the same cuboid and registered on Y_0 to create the set of possible reconstructions, $\mathcal{Y} = \{Y_0, Y_1, ..., Y_m\}$. Among $\mathcal{Y}$, only Y_0 perfectly completes X while others do not necessarily match the input. Therefore, the metric $\Lambda_{ij}(\mathcal{Y})$ is defined as the degree of geometrical conformity between members i and j of the set $\mathcal{Y}$.

All target nominees ($\mathcal{Y}$) are then independently concatenated with X and mapped to the latent position μ_i, with uncertainty σ_i, via the posterior encoder network (P_{post}). The resultant mappings are considered as parameters of an independent multivariate normal distribution $(\mathcal{N}(\mu_i, \sigma_i))$. A sample from this distribution is tiled and concatenated with the feature maps of the V-Net. The resultant 4D tensor is processed by P_{comb} and P_{gen} to predict the target:

$$\hat{Y}_i = P_{gen}(P_{comb}(V_{Net}(X), \mu_i)), \quad P_{post}(.|X, Y_i) = \mathcal{N}(\mu_i, \sigma_i). \qquad (4)$$

This process is repeated for all $m + 1$ nominee targets in the $\mathcal{Y}$ set of sample S.

Each predicted shape $(\hat{Y}_i)$ is compared with its corresponding target (Y_i) using the Voxel-weighted Dice. Since target nominees, other than Y_0, involve deviations from the input morphology (X), each target's conformity (Λ_{i0}) with the best known solution (Y_0) is taken into account in the proposed Target-weighted (TW) loss function. As a result, the final objective function is the weighted average of all loss functions with respect to the conformities of their targets. The proposed objective is formulated as follows:

$$\mathcal{L}_{\text{VWDice-TW}} = \alpha \sum_{i=0}^{m} \Lambda_{0i}(\mathcal{Y}) \, \mathcal{L}^i_{\text{VWDice}}(X, Y_i, \hat{Y}_i, W_i) + \gamma KL(P_{post} || \mathcal{N}(0, I)), \quad (5)$$

where, α is a normalizing parameter set as the sum of all m conformity values, and γ is a weighting constant. As shown in Eq. 5, during optimization, the Kullback– Leibler (KL) divergence of the posterior latent distribution with a fixed normal distribution, from which we sample during inference, is minimized.

The $\mathcal{L}_{\text{VWDice-TW}}$ loss function considers all targets as partially acceptable solutions for the probabilistic completion. In our experiments, $\Lambda(.)$ was set as the Dice coefficient between the shapes, where clearly $\Lambda_{00}(\mathcal{Y}) = Dice(Y_0, Y_0) = 1$.

3 Experiments

3.1 Data and Training

A total of 48 mandibles were collected from the archives of Vancouver General Hospital (VGH) through a data sharing agreement.

The 3D meshes were rigidly registered based on their point clouds using the group-wise student's-t mixture model algorithm with 50 mixture components [7]. Using ray testing, each surface mesh was voxelized into an isotropic binary occupancy voxel map with 1 mm increments to mimic mandibles segmented from CT scans with isotropic voxels. The occupancy maps of all mandibles were symmetrically zero padded to create voxel-grid cubes of size 141^3, *i.e.* size of the largest sample, which also matches the maximum facial width reported in the comprehensive dataset of the FaceBase project [3]. The dataset was randomly partitioned into test (15%), training (70%), and validation (15%) sets.

During the mini-batch gradient decent optimization, each sample was randomly rotated, translated (shifted), and mirrored across the sagittal plane. Adam optimizer was used with default momentum parameters along with ℓ_2 regularization of $1e - 5$. The learning rate was initialized at $1e - 2$ and exponentially

Table 1. Quantitative comparison of the proposed methods against other baselines.

	Method	DSC%	Comp	Acc	HD95
Determ.	$\mathcal{L}_{Dice}(X + Y, \hat{Y})$	0.4	N/A	N/A	N/A
	$\mathcal{L}_{Dice}(Y, \hat{Y})$	84.9 ± 0.2	0.85 ± 0.13	0.61 ± 0.13	2.95 ± 1.43
	$\mathcal{L}_{\text{VWDice}}(X, Y, \hat{Y})$ (ours)	$\mathbf{88.3 \pm 0.2}$	$\mathbf{0.65 \pm 0.10}$	$\mathbf{0.44 \pm 0.10}$	$\mathbf{2.64 \pm 1.83}$
Prob.	CVAE$_{\text{basic}}$ [9]	79.8 ± 0.6	1.20 ± 0.34	0.87 ± 0.18	3.98 ± 3.16
	CVAE$_{\text{VWDice-TW}}$ (ours)	$\mathbf{80.8 \pm 0.5}$	$\mathbf{1.11 \pm 0.31}$	$\mathbf{0.83 \pm 0.14}$	$\mathbf{3.74 \pm 2.44}$

decayed with a rate of 0.98 at each epoch until convergence. Size of the latent space was set to 8. Same random seeds were used for all the experiments.

The data processing pipeline and the models were implemented using the PyTorch deep learning platform and made publicly available: github.com/ amir-abdi/prob-shape-completion. For the experiments to be reproducable, the voxelized version of the data accompanies the code, according to each dataset's respective license and data sharing agreements.

3.2   Evaluation and Results

Shape completion is a non-deterministic process where no single answer is the ground-truth. However, to quantify the performance of the proposed learning methods, a dentist manually removed bone segments from the healthy mandibles of the test set and created nearly 100 test cases. The manually removed bone segments were considered as fair targets for evaluation and compared with the predicted reconstructions. We assessed the models based on Dice coefficient (DSC; $2 \times$ intersection/sum of volumes), completeness (Comp; average distance from target surface to predicted surface), accuracy (Acc; average distance from predicted surface to target surface), and Hausdorff distance at the 95th percentile (HD95). Except for the DSC, lower values of the metrics are preferred. For a fair comparison of non-deterministic CVAE models, and with only a single target reconstruction available, latent values during the quantitative analysis were set to the mean of the fixed distribution $\mathcal{N}(0, I)$.

The quantitative results are reported in Table 1 and a set of reconstructed samples from the test set are visualized in Fig. 3. As reported in the top row of Table 1, a vanilla Dice loss with the entire shape as its target (*i.e.* $L_{Dice}(X + Y, \hat{Y})$) equally treats all the voxels and ignores the dissected region. This model acts like an autoencoder which only regenerates the input (X). On the contrary, focusing only on the dissected target bone (*i.e.* $L_{Dice}(Y, \hat{Y})$) does not penalize the discrepancies in the margins of the reconstruction. Therefore, the predicted shape shows inconsistencies and discontinuities with respect to the surrounding anatomy. The performance gain achieved with the proposed objective function (Eq. 3) was assessed to be statistically highly significant ($p < 0.001$).

To demonstrate the effectiveness of the proposed contributions, two CVAE models were trained: one without any enhancements (CVAE$_{\text{basic}}$), and one with the objectives function described in Eqs. 3 and 5 (CVAE$_{\text{VWDice-TW}}$). Network

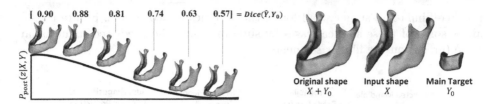

Fig. 2. Negative correlation between the deviation of the latent values from the mode $(\hat{P}_{post})$ and the conformity of the predicted shapes with the main target (Y_0).

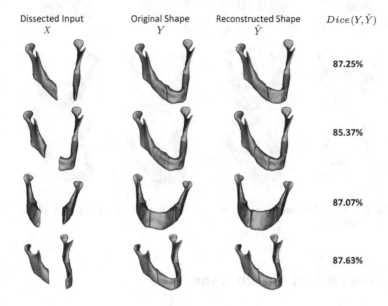

Fig. 3. Reconstructed samples of the test set along with their Dice metric when compared with the original anatomy.

architectures and hyper-parameters were kept the same across experiments for results to be comparable. The differences between the Dice metrics of the two models was observed to be statistically highly significant $(p < 0.001)$.

Thanks to the proposed Target-weighted variational objective, a strong negative correlation was observed between the deviation of a latent vector from its distribution's mode $(|z - \hat{P}_{post}|)$ and the similarity of its corresponding predicted shape with the main target (Y_0). This phenomenon is demonstrated in Fig. 2. The same was not true for the CVAE$_{basic}$ model.

Surgical Cases. We evaluated the performance of the variational model on real surgical cases who were treated with the virtually planned free fibula flap technique. Here, the affected mandibular bones were already removed by the clinicians. The dissected mandibles were reconstructed using the trained variational model. An expert assessed the reconstructions against surgeon's virtual plans of the free fibula flap surgery and found them clinically acceptable. Figure 4 visualizes some of these surgical cases by superimposing the predicted mandibular bone (green) on the fibular segments.

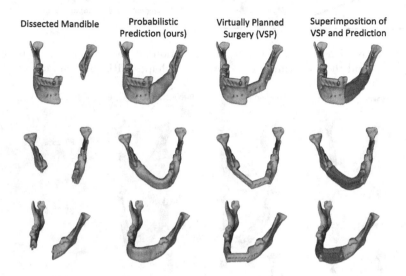

Fig. 4. Comparison of model predictions (green) with virtual surgical plans (VSPs). (Color figure online)

4   Discussion and Conclusions

In this paper, we introduced optimization approaches for training of deep variational models for anatomical 3D shape completion. The proposed Voxel-weighted objective improves the accuracy of reconstructions compared to similar approaches and guarantees smoothness between the predicted bony segment and the remaining contours of the mandible. The proposed variational method takes into account the many acceptable solutions for the shape completion problem and is able to generate realistic variations for the missing segment.

Among the limitations of our study is the inconsistency in the presence of teeth across the samples. While there were toothless mandibles in the dataset, the majority of samples had all or parts of their dentition. However, except for their correlation with the bone-loss, teeth have little to no role to play in determining the missing anatomy of mandible. Therefore, the presence of dentition in the target dissections adversely affected the performance. To mitigate this issue teeth should be excluded from the data, either manually or automatically.

The proposed probabilistic approach is among the first works in deep anatomical shape reconstruction. It can be applied to other anatomies as well as general computer graphics. Comparison with real surgical cases is demonstrated here as a step for clinical adoption. Our method requires no post processing, except in converting voxel-grids to and from surface meshes. Therefore, our next logical step is to switch from voxel-grids to graph representations to speedup the processing pipeline for better clinical acceptance.

References

1. Abdi, A.H., et al.: AnatomyGen: deep anatomy generation from dense representation with applications in mandible synthesis. Technical report (2019)
2. Achlioptas, P., et al.: Representation learning and adversarial generation of 3D point clouds. **2**(3), 4 arXiv preprint arXiv:1707.02392 (2017)
3. Brinkley, J.F., et al.: The FaceBase consortium: a comprehensive resource for craniofacial researchers. Development **143**(14), 2677–2688 (2016). www.facebase.org
4. Hidalgo, D.A.: Fibula free flap: a new method of mandible reconstruction. Plast. Reconstr. Surg. **84**(1), 71–79 (1989)
5. Milletari, F., et al.: V-Net: fully convolutional neural networks for volumetric medical image segmentation. In: 2016 Fourth International Conference on 3D Vision (3DV). IEEE (2016)
6. Nash, C., Williams, C.K.I.: The shape variational autoencoder: a deep generative model of part-segmented 3D objects. Comput. Graph. Forum **36**(5), 1–12 (2017)
7. Ravikumar, N., Gooya, A., Çimen, S., Frangi, A.F., Taylor, Z.A.: A multi-resolution T-mixture model approach to robust group-wise alignment of shapes. In: Ourselin, S., Joskowicz, L., Sabuncu, M.R., Unal, G., Wells, W. (eds.) MICCAI 2016. LNCS, vol. 9902, pp. 142–149. Springer, Cham (2016). https://doi.org/10.1007/978-3-319-46726-9_17
8. Siegel, R.L., et al.: Cancer statistics. CA Cancer J. Clin. **67**(1), 7–30 (2017)
9. Sohn, K., et al.: Learning structured output representation using deep conditional generative models. In: Cortes, C., et al. (ed.) Advances in Neural Information Processing Systems, vol. 28, pp. 3483–3491. Curran Associates, Inc. (2015)
10. Stranix, J.T., et al.: A virtual surgical planning algorithm for delayed maxillomandibular reconstruction. Plast. Reconstr. Surg. **143**(4), 1197–1206 (2019)
11. Wu, J., et al.: Learning a probabilistic latent space of object shapes via 3D generative-adversarial modeling. In: Advances in Neural Information Processing Systems, pp. 82–90 (2016)

Markerless Image-to-Face Registration for Untethered Augmented Reality in Head and Neck Surgery

Christina Gsaxner[1,2,3]($\boxtimes$) ⓘ, Antonio Pepe[1,3] ⓘ, Jürgen Wallner[2,3],
Dieter Schmalstieg[1] ⓘ, and Jan Egger[1,2,3] ⓘ

[1] Institute of Computer Graphics and Vision, Graz University of Technology,
Graz, Austria
gsaxner@tugraz.at
[2] Division of Oral-, Maxillofacial Surgery, Medical University of Graz, Graz, Austria
[3] Computer Algorithms for Medicine Laboratory, Graz, Austria

Abstract. In the treatment of head and neck cancer, physicians can benefit from augmented reality in preparing and executing treatment. We present a system allowing a physician wearing an untethered augmented reality headset to see medical visualizations precisely overlaid onto the patient. Our main contribution is a strategy for markerless registration of 3D imaging to the patient's face. We use a neural network to detect the face using the headset's depth sensor and register it to computed tomography data. The face registration is seamlessly combined with the headset's continuous self-localization. We report on registration error and compare our approach to an external, high-precision tracking system.

Keywords: Augmented reality · 3D registration · Head and neck cancer

1 Introduction

Medical applications can benefit from augmented reality (AR) interfaces, e.g., by providing a more intuitive mental mapping from 3D imaging data to the patient [1]. In particular, immersive AR systems combine natural 3D interaction with an increased spatial perception of 3D structures [2]. In this contribution, we present a method for immersive medical visualization in the head and neck area using a commercial AR headset with optical see-through display, the Microsoft HoloLens (Microsoft Corporation, Redmond, WA, USA). Our system works in an unprepared environment and achieves registration based on facial surface matching at real-time frame rates by registering 3D imaging data directly to the patient's face as observed by the headset's depth sensor. Moreover, we take

Supported by FWF KLI 678-B31 (enFaced), COMET K-Project 871132 (CAMed) and the TU Graz LEAD project "Mechanics, Modeling and Simulation of Aortic Dissection".

advantage of the built-in self-localization capabilities of the headset. The combination of facial detection and self-localization enables fully untethered, real-time markerless registration.

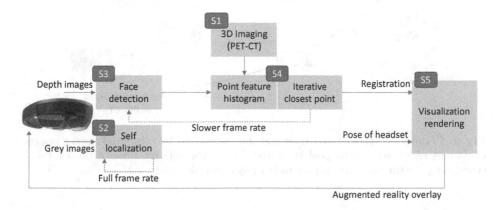

Fig. 1. Overview of the proposed five-step registration pipeline.

Related Work. Usually, image data is acquired offline, e.g., through magnetic resonance (MRI) or computed tomography (CT) imaging, and must be registered to the patient in the physician's view with high accuracy, thus establishing a relationship between physical and virtual space. Several studies for medical AR do not estimate this relationship at all, instead relying on the manual placement of medical content with respect to the virtual world [3,4]. Others establish this correspondence using outside-in tracking based on markers rigidly attached to the patient [5], or external devices, e.g., optical or depth sensors [6,7]. However, such outside-in approaches require complicated preparation and must be calibrated *in situ*, which disrupts clinical workflow and therefore hinders acceptance. As an alternative, inside-out methods utilizing self-localization techniques have recently been explored in the context of medical AR using intra-operative X-ray images or manually selected landmarks as a registration strategy [8,9].

Contribution. For applications involving the face, such as in surgery planning of head and neck cancer, the opportunity arises to use facial features for both registration and tracking. Thus, in our contribution, we present a strategy for markerless, inside-out image-to-face registration, which, in combination with the self-localization of the headset, enables untethered real-time AR to aid physicians in the treatment and management of head and neck cancer.

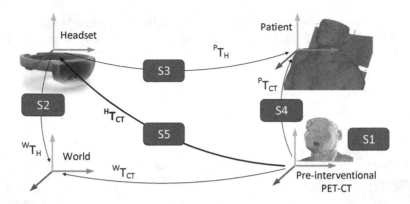

Fig. 2. Coordinate systems and their transformations to be computed during image-to-patient registration. The goal is to find $^{H}T_{CT}$, the relative pose of the PET-CT coordinate system CT with respect to the physician, denoted by H.

2   Methods

Our goal was to build a system for 3D image registration using only the headset hardware. Our solution combines two sensor pipelines, the headset's self-localization and facial localization using the headset's depth sensor. The self-localization runs an algorithm for simultaneous localization and mapping (SLAM) on a dedicated hardware accelerator, fed by multiple cameras on the headset, and delivers robust and accurate camera poses [10]. The depth sensor provides the ability to detect the patient's face as represented in the 3D image data. The depth sensor faces forward and is pre-registered with the user's field of view, conveniently allowing direct superposition of computer-generated visuals. We build a pipeline that performs competitive sensor fusion [11] between the self-localization component and a custom pipeline for face registration in five steps, labeled S1–S5, as shown in Fig. 1:

S1 Obtain and preprocess medical image data
S2 Obtain an update from the self-localization
S3 Apply a neural network for face detection on incoming depth images, followed by extraction of a point cloud
S4 Coarsely register the 3D image data to the depth image using point feature histograms; refine the registration using an iterative closest point method
S5 Render overlay using the registration obtained by combining S2 with S3/S4

Out of these five steps, only S1 is performed offline. All other steps are run online, but S3/S4 can be run at a lower than full frame without affecting overall system performance. To correctly overlay virtual content with the physical world, we need to estimate $^{H}T_{CT}(t)$, the rigid 3D transformation which correctly positions content in the coordinates of pre-interventional CT acquisitions CT with respect to the physician wearing the headset H at time t. Consequently, a series of transformations (Fig. 2) has to be estimated as follows:

$$^{H}T_{CT}(t) = {}^{W}T_{H}^{-1}(t) \cdot {}^{W}T_{H}(t_0) \cdot {}^{P}T_{H}^{-1}(t_0) \cdot {}^{P}T_{CT}(t_0), \tag{1}$$

with W and P representing the world and patient coordinate system, respectively. $^{H}T_{CT}(t)$ aligns the patients face and $\mathbf{P}_{CT}$, denoting the point cloud representation of the patients' skin surface recovered from CT, obtained in S1. We describe each of the steps S1–S5 in detail in the following sections.

2.1 Medical Imaging Data Processing

In the pre-interventional, offline step S1, we acquire ^{18}F-fluorodeoxy-D-glucose positron emission tomography-computed tomography (^{18}F-FDG PET-CT) data, which is essential in the diagnosis and evaluation of head and neck carcinomae due to its ability to combine functional information from PET with anatomical information from CT [12]. Volumetric CT image data of the patient is segmented into skin surface and anatomically relevant structures for visualization, and checked using Studierfenster (`studierfenster.at`). Polygonal meshes are extracted using Marching Cubes algorithm; then, a point cloud representation of the skin surface $\mathbf{P}_{CT}$ is created for usage in consecutive registration steps. Similarily, tumor sufaces are extracted from co-registered ^{18}F-FDG PET acquisitions, which exhibit high contrast for metabolically active tumors.

2.2 Self-localization

Step S2 obtains $^{W}T_{H}$, the poses of the surgeon's viewpoint with respect to world coordinates, using the headset's SLAM-based self-localization system [13]. We use the camera poses delivered by the headset and associate them with the face model created in S3 using the registration procedure of S4. We do not use the geometric model of the SLAM system, since it is too coarse for our purposes.

2.3 Face Detection and Extraction

Step S3 denotes the acquisition of a point cloud representation of the patient's face from the depth sensor. A region of interest (ROI) around the patient's head is found automatically and in real-time by using a neural network. It relies on a single-shot-multibox detector (SSD) [14] using a ResNet-10 architecture, pretrained for face detection. SSD performs object localization in a single forward pass by regressing a bounding box around objects. If detection is successful, the ROI is mapped to the depth image to create a point cloud using an inverse perspective transformation $(^{P}T_{H})^{-1}$. Given a position in the depth frame $\mathbf{m} = [u, v]$ in pixel units and the depth camera's intrinsic matrix K, the corresponding scene point in camera coordinates $\mathbf{p} = [x, y, z]^{T}$ can be calculated by

$$\mathbf{p} = \begin{bmatrix} x \\ y \\ z \end{bmatrix} = K^{-1} \begin{bmatrix} u \\ v \\ 1 \end{bmatrix} d(u,v) = \begin{bmatrix} f_x & 0 & c_x \\ 0 & f_y & c_y \\ 0 & 0 & 1 \end{bmatrix}^{-1} \begin{bmatrix} u \\ v \\ 1 \end{bmatrix} d(u,v), \tag{2}$$

where $d(u, v)$ denotes the depth at $[u, v]$. This inverse projection is applied to all pixels within the ROI around the patient's face, resulting in a point cloud $\mathbf{P}_P = \{\mathbf{p}_2, \mathbf{p}_2, ..., \mathbf{p}_N\}$ which represents the face in headset coordinates.

2.4   Aligning Pre-interventional Data with the Patient

For step S4, we take advantage of the distinctive nature of a human's facial features to enable a markerless, automatic, two-stage registration scheme inspired by the method proposed by Holz et al. [15]. Since the facial surface of humans is usually not subject to any major soft tissue deformations, a rigid transformation $^P T_{CT}$, which aligns the point cloud from pre-interventional imaging $\mathbf{P}_{CT}$ with the target point cloud representing the patient $\mathbf{P}_P$, is estimated. To compute an initial alignment, we adopt registration based on fast point feature histograms (FPFH) [16]. FPFH features are computed in both point clouds and reciprocally matched using 1-nearest-neighbor search, resulting in $\kappa_f = \{(\mathbf{f}_P, \mathbf{f}_{CT})\}$, a set of correspondence points found by matching FPFH features of $\mathbf{P}_P$ and $\mathbf{P}_{CT}$. The fast global registration algorithm by Zhou et al. [17] is applied to compute an initial transformation $^P \hat{T}_{CT}$ such that distances between corresponding points are minimized:

$$E(^P \hat{T}_{CT}) = \sum_{(\mathbf{f}_P, \mathbf{f}_{CT}) \in \kappa_f} \rho(||\mathbf{f}_P - ^P \hat{T}_{CT} \mathbf{f}_{CT}||), \qquad (3)$$

where $\rho(.)$ is a scaled German-McClure estimator, a robust penalty for optimization. The initial transformation $^P \hat{T}_{CT}$ is then refined using point-to-plane ICP [18], resulting in the final alignment $^P T_{CT}$. We define the correspondence set as the actual 1-nearest-neighboring points $\kappa = \{(\mathbf{p}_P, \mathbf{p}_{CT})\}$ and optimize

$$E(^P T_{CT}) = \sum_{(\mathbf{p}_P, \mathbf{p}_{CT}) \in \kappa} ((\mathbf{p}_P - ^P T_{CT} \mathbf{p}_{CT}) \cdot \mathbf{n}_{pp})^2, \qquad (4)$$

where $\mathbf{n}_{pp}$ is the normal of point $\mathbf{p}_P$. This combination of rapid feature matching and ICP refinement allows a robust, accurate and fast computation of $^P T_{CT}$.

2.5   Visualization Using Augmented Reality

In step S5, we use the transformation obtained in previous steps to render virtual content in a way that it is anchored to world coordinates using $^W T_{CT}$. As long as the patient remains stationary, $^W T_{CT}$ can be computed at a much lower framerate than $^W T_H$. This makes the system comfortable to use, allowing the surgeon to look away from the patent's face and preserve registration of virtual objects when returning to the patient, even without re-detection of the face, simply by receiving an update of $^W T_H(t)$. If the patient moves, re-detection of the face leads to instant re-registration of the overlaid virtual objects, by simply updating $^P T_{CT}$. Figure 3 shows an example of bones and tumoral masses registered with the patient.

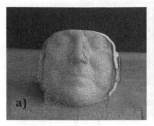 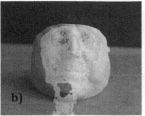 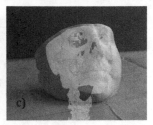

Fig. 3. Example AR visualization on a patient phantom. By registering a point cloud to the patient's face as in (a), bones and a tumoral mass can be overlaid as shown in (b). Registration persists if the physician changes his viewpoint, seen in (c).

3   Experiments and Results

We evaluted end-to-end registration using phantom heads by 3D-printing CT scans from step S1. We chose eight subjects with cancerous tumors in the head/neck area, for which PET-CT imaging was available. Furthermore, we show our application's feasability with a human subject. To avoid unjustifiable radiation exposure, a MRI scan was used to extract the isosurface of the skin.

3.1   Target Registration Error

The target registration error (TRE) is computed to evaluate the end-to-end registration accuracy of the proposed system. It is defined by

$$TRE = \frac{1}{N_k} \sum_{k=1}^{N_k} ||^H T_{CT} \mathbf{m}_k^{CT} - \mathbf{m}_k^H||, \tag{5}$$

where N_k is a number of reference points; $\mathbf{m}^{CT}$ and $\mathbf{m}^H$ are the reference points in the CT data and the headset's view, respectively. Since data obtained from the clinical routine is used in this study, there are no fiducial markers in pre-interventional data, which could be used as reference points for TRE computation. Therefore, $N_k = 5$ landmarks, namely, the left/right inner canthus, the tip of the nose and the left/right labial commissure of mouth, were labeled manually in CT data and later selected in the operator's view to obtain $\mathbf{m}^H$ and $\mathbf{m}^{CT}$. We repeated TRE measurement 10 times for each patient phantom as well as the human subject, at distances ranging from 50 cm to 90 cm between operator and patient, using slightly changing viewing angles. Table 1 summarizes the TRE for phantoms 1–8 as well as the human subject, averaged over all measurements.

3.2   Comparison with a High-Precision External Tracking Device

We compare $^H T_{CT}$ derived from our application with the transformation computed by an external infrared tracking system, consisting of 15 OptiTrack Flex

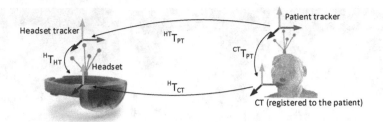

Fig. 4. Coordinate systems for comparing $^H T_{CT}$ to $^{HT} T_{PT}$ from an external infrared tracking system. $^{CT} T_{PT}$ and $^H T_{HT}$ are estimated using hand-eye calibration.

Table 1. Target registration error (TRE) of five reference points, as well as error in translation E_t and rotation E_r between the transformation $^S T_{CT}$ and the equivalent transformation $^S T_{CT}^{OT}$ obtained from an external infrared tracking system.

Subject		1	2	3	4	5	6	7	8	Human	Total
TRE (mm)	Mean	9.4	9.4	10.2	6.7	10.5	11.4	7.1	10.2	8.1	9.2
	Sd	2.3	0.8	1.7	1.3	2.2	2.2	0.7	1.4	1.0	1.5
E_t (mm)	Mean	5.4	2.0	3.1	6.7	3.1	2.3	7.0	3.0	4.3	3.9
	Sd	2.1	1.9	3.0	1.8	1.7	1.7	2.3	2.0	1.7	1.8
E_r (°)	Mean	4.9	5.7	5.4	11.0	2.9	2.4	4.4	5.6	9.8	4.9
	Sd	3.7	2.4	3.5	2.5	1.8	1.9	1.9	3.2	1.8	2.4

13 cameras (NaturalPoint, Inc., Corvallis, OR, USA). We rigidly attached a set of non-collinear retro-reflective markers to the headset and our patient phantoms or human subject for the computation of $^{HT} T_{PT}$, the relative pose of the patient tracker with respect to the HoloLens tracker from the OptiTrack. To correlate these transformations, $^H T_{HT}$, which calibrates the headset tracker and the virtual camera of the HoloLens, as well as $^{CT} T_{PT}$, the transformation from the patient tracker to the CT coordinate system (already registered to the patient), needed to be estimated by hand-eye calibration methods [19], as shown in Fig. 4.

This is performed in two steps. First, for estimating $^H T_{HT}$, we built a custom calibration object using ArUco markers [20] augmented with retro-reflective optical markers, which allows tracking of the object with both the headsets RGB camera and the OptiTrack system. Similarly, to compute $^{CT} T_{PT}$, we utilize face pose estimation to track faces in RGB frames together with the infrared tracking system. By observing those objects through different viewing angles, we estimate $^H T_{HT}$ and $^{CT} T_{PT}$. Thus, we can compute $^H T_{CT}^{OT}$, the reference transformation obtained by the OptiTrack system, as $^H T_{CT}^{OT} = {}^H T_{HT} \cdot {}^{HT} T_{PT} \cdot ({}^{CT} T_{PT})^{-1}$. To quantify the error between transformations, we evaluate the error in distance as well as the angular error separately. Again, measurements were taken at 10 different time points, under varying angles and distances, and averaged. The results obtained from all patient phantoms, as well as the results from our experiments with a human subject, are summarized in Table 1.

4   Discussion and Conclusion

We presented a novel end-to-end solution to the image-to-patient registration problem in AR using optical see-trough headsets. Our markerless registration scheme works fully automatically in an unprepared environment, by exploiting the distinct characteristics of human faces. It computates the transformation aligning pre-interventional 3D data with the patient in the surgeon's view. We evaluated accuracy with patient phantoms and a human test person, reporting a mean TRE of 9.2 ± 1.5 mm and an average error in comparison to a high-precision optical tracking system of 3.9 ± 1.8 mm in translation and $4.9 \pm 2.4°$ in rotation. The accuracy of $^{H}T_{CT}$ is subject to several error sources, partly due to hardware restrictions: A residual error remains due to the rather low quality of point cloud representation acquired from the headset's depth sensor. Moreover, inaccuracies and latency of the HoloLens self-localization may affect the overall precision, and hologram stability could be an issue [21]. Finally, optical see-through display calibration was not considered, as we expect that future hardware will support auto-calibration using eye tracking.

While our system does not yet achieve the sub-millimeter precision required for image-guided intervention, it represents a promising all-in-one tool for immersive treatment and intervention planning in the management of head and neck cancer. As others before us [2,8], we believe that the Microsoft HoloLens has great potential for clinical and educational applications in medicine, especially considering the imminent release of the HoloLens 2, which has much improved hardware and software capabilities.

As a next step, we plan a clinical evaluation of our system involving a patient study, for which ethics approval has recently been obtained. This study should demonstrate the benefits of AR to physicians in the treatment of head and neck cancer. Other future work includes a more refined visualization and 3D interaction to provide guidance to surgeons during intervention planning.

References

1. Sielhorst, T., Feuerstein, M., Navab, N.: Advanced medical displays: a literature review of augmented reality. J. Disp. Technol. 4(4), 451–467 (2008)
2. de Oliveira, M.E., Debarba, H.G., Lädermann, A., Chagué, S., Charbonnier, C.: A hand-eye calibration method for augmented reality applied to computer-assisted orthopedic surgery. Int. J. Med. Robot. 15(2), e1969 (2019)
3. Pratt, P., et al.: Through the HoloLens™ looking glass: augmented reality for extremity reconstruction surgery using 3D vascular models with perforating vessels. Eur. Radiol. Exp. 2(1), 2 (2018)
4. Incekara, F., Smits, M., Dirven, C., Vincent, A.: Clinical feasibility of a wearable mixed-reality device in neurosurgery. World Neurosurg. 118, e422–e427 (2018)
5. Ahn, J., Choi, H., Hong, J., Hong, J.: Tracking accuracy of a stereo-camera-based augmented reality navigation system for orthognathic surgery. J. Oral Maxillofac. Surg. 77(5), 1070-e1 (2019)

6. Chen, X., et al.: Development of a surgical navigation system based on augmented reality using an optical see-through head-mounted display. J. Biomed. Inform. **55**, 124–131 (2015)
7. Hsieh, C.H., Lee, J.D., Wu, C.T.: A Kinect-based medical augmented reality system for craniofacial applications using image-to-patient registration. Neuropsychiatry **07**(06), 927–939 (2017)
8. Hajek, J., et al.: Closing the calibration loop: an inside-out-tracking paradigm for augmented reality in orthopedic surgery. In: Frangi, A.F., Schnabel, J.A., Davatzikos, C., Alberola-López, C., Fichtinger, G. (eds.) MICCAI 2018. LNCS, vol. 11073, pp. 299–306. Springer, Cham (2018). https://doi.org/10.1007/978-3-030-00937-3_35
9. Mahmoud, N., et al.: On-patient see-through augmented reality based on visual SLAM. Int. J. Comput. Assist. Radiol. Surg. **12**(1), 1–11 (2017)
10. Klein, G.: Registration on HoloLens. Keynote talk at ISMAR (2017)
11. Durrant-Whyte, H.F.: Sensor models and multisensor integration. Int. J. Robot. Res. **7**(6), 97–113 (1988)
12. Castaldi, P., Leccisotti, L., Bussu, F., Miccichè, F., Rufini, V.: Role of (18)F-FDG PET-CT in head and neck squamous cell carcinoma. Acta Otorhinolaryngol. Ital. **33**(1), 1–8 (2013)
13. Klein, G., Murray, D.: Parallel tracking and mapping for small AR workspaces. In: ISMAR, pp. 1–10 (2007)
14. Liu, W., et al.: SSD: single shot multibox detector. In: Leibe, B., Matas, J., Sebe, N., Welling, M. (eds.) ECCV 2016. LNCS, vol. 9905, pp. 21–37. Springer, Cham (2016). https://doi.org/10.1007/978-3-319-46448-0_2
15. Holz, D., Ichim, A.E., Tombari, F., Rusu, R.B., Behnke, S.: Registration with the point cloud library: a modular framework for aligning in 3-D. IEEE Robot. Autom. Mag. **22**(4), 110–124 (2015)
16. Rusu, R.B., Blodow, N., Beetz, M.: Fast point feature histograms (FPFH) for 3D registration. In: ICRA, pp. 3212–3217 (2009)
17. Zhou, Q.-Y., Park, J., Koltun, V.: Fast global registration. In: Leibe, B., Matas, J., Sebe, N., Welling, M. (eds.) ECCV 2016. LNCS, vol. 9906, pp. 766–782. Springer, Cham (2016). https://doi.org/10.1007/978-3-319-46475-6_47
18. Chen, Y., Medioni, G.: Object modelling by registration of multiple range images. Image Vis. Comput. **10**(3), 145–155 (1992)
19. Tsai, R.Y., Lenz, R.K.: A new technique for fully autonomous and efficient 3D robotics hand/eye calibration. IEEE Trans. Robot. Autom. **5**(3), 345–358 (1989)
20. Garrido-Jurado, S., Muñoz-Salinas, R., Madrid-Cuevas, F.J., Marín-Jiménez, M.J.: Automatic generation and detection of highly reliable fiducial markers under occlusion. Pattern Recogn. **47**(6), 2280–2292 (2014)
21. Vassallo, R., Rankin, A., Chen, E.C., Peters, T.M.: Hologram stability evaluation for microsoft hololens. In: SPIE Medical Imaging, vol. 10136, p. 1013614 (2017)

Towards a Mixed-Reality First Person Point of View Needle Navigation System

Leah Groves[1]([✉])(iD), Natalie Li[2], Terry M. Peters[1,2,3](iD),
and Elvis C. S. Chen[1,2,3](iD)

[1] School of Biomedical Engineering, Western University, London, Canada
lgroves6@uwo.ca
[2] Medical Biophysics, Western University, London, Canada
[3] Robarts Research Institute, London, Canada

Abstract. Ultrasound-guidance has reduced complications, such as carotid artery punctures, during central venous catherization (CVC). The continued prevalence of these complications has promoted the use of mixed-reality systems for surgical needle navigation. We have developed a surgical navigation system that renders the calibrated ultrasound (US) image and tracked models of the probe, needle and needle-trajectory. We compared the effectiveness of this guidance system on a desktop monitor or within a head-mounted display (HMD) to the US-only approach in a phantom-based user study with 33 expert clinical practitioners. These users performed one needle insertion on each of the two vessel sets within the phantom, where the first insertion was used as training and the second was used for analysis. The guidance system rendered within the HMD significantly improved the safety margin, defined as number of successful needle insertions, where the final needle position was within the lumen of the vessel, as 31 users performed successful insertions with the HMD system compared to 21 successful insertions under US-only guidance. Furthermore, the HMD system significantly improved the distance from the final needle tip to the vessel wall, as clinicians more consistently position the needle such that it was within the vessel lumen but far from the vessel wall when using the HMD system. The clinicians' performance using the monitor system was comparable to the US-only guidance. Therefore, using a HMD to align the visual and motor fields of the clinician is imperative to successful needle guidance, promoting the continued pursuit of HMD guidance research.

Keywords: Surgical navigation · Mixed reality · Needle guidance ·
Tracking · Calibration · Perception · User performance

1 Introduction

In the United States, over five million central venous catheterizations (CVCs) are performed annually [6], with the internal jugular vein (IJV) being the most

© Springer Nature Switzerland AG 2019
D. Shen et al. (Eds.): MICCAI 2019, LNCS 11768, pp. 245–253, 2019.
https://doi.org/10.1007/978-3-030-32254-0_28

utilized insertion site [2]. The current gold standard is the blind technique, rely-ing on the clinician to palpate surrounding anatomical structures to identify the insertion site (Fig. 1a). Ultrasound-(US)-guided CVC is becoming the preferred technique as it has the potential to reduce complications including accidental punctures to structures such as the carotid artery (CA) [7,8]. The US-guided approach relies on real-time US video, depicting cross-sections of the anatomy on a 2D monitor, to guide the needle insertion (Fig. 1b). Despite US-guidance improving complication rates, clinical studies have found rates of CA puncture to be 7.8 % for US-guided trainees [5].

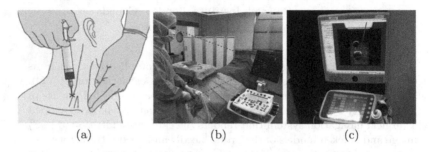

(a)   (b)   (c)

Fig. 1. Comparison of guidance techniques for CVC (a) Anatomical Guidance (b) US-only guidance and (c) AV guidance. Image (a, b) courtesy of Google

The common use of US-guided interventions has resulted in development of many US-guided computer-assisted surgical navigation systems. To address the aforementioned limitations of US-guided CVC, an augmented virtuality (AV) monitor-based surgical navigation system was developed for needle guidance [1]. Their system employed magnetic tracking to render tracked virtual models of the US probe, needle and needle trajectory, onto a front-facing US image (Fig. 1c). This system did not demonstrate significant improvement in the com-plications associated with the needle insertion compared to the US-only tech-nique for expert users [1]. Two potential factors that may have influenced the success of this system were the fixed face-on view provided to the user and the discrepancy between the visual and motor fields, as the user had to rely on a monitor exterior to the visual field of the phantom [1]. Despite the inconclu-sive results, their promising work has motivated our development of surgical navigation environments to reduce complications associated with CVC.

We investigated the efficacy of a first-person immersive mixed reality (MR) system for CVC needle navigation. Toward the long-term goal of clinical deploy-ment, we first aim to understand how the method to visualize the surgical infor-mation affects the rate of complication during US-guided CVC. Our surgical navigation system combines a spatially tracked head-mounted display (HMD) system with a surgical magnetic tracking system, allowing magnetically tracked surgical instruments to be visualized in 3D inside the HMD with submillimetre accuracy. For this work, we compare US-only guidance to a MR guidance system displayed on a 2D monitor or within a HMD. We hypothesize that the HMD will improve the success of needle insertions compared to the US-only and 2D monitor systems. This work aims to highlight the importance of coherent visual and motor fields for surgical applications. Aside from the technical advancement, our contribution is a comprehensive user study involving 33 clinical practitioners.

2   Materials and Methods

A patient-specific neck vasculature phantom was constructed, comprising of a hollow (wall-less) vascular structure embedded in an US compatible solid medium [9] (Fig. 2a). The positive models of both the CA and IJV were manufactured using 3D printer based on the manual segmentation of a patient computed tomography (CT). These 3D printed vessel models were embedded into, and later removed from, the US-compatible medium, leaving the exact negative imprint of vessel geometries. The phantom was housed in a plastic container with 8 hemi-spherical fiducial markers and scanned in CT (O-Arm, Medtronic, USA). The segmentation of the vessels and fiducial markers served as the basis for visualization and registration with the tracking system. This phantom serves as a surrogate for patient anatomy, producing anatomically realistic US images (Fig. 2b) compared to those obtained from healthy volunteers (Fig. 2c and d).

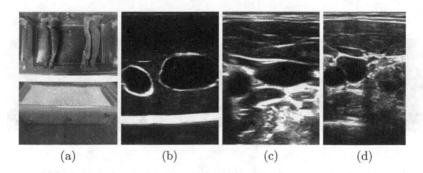

| (a) | (b) | (c) | (d) |

Fig. 2. (a) Phantom development, (b) Phantom under US, (c) and (d) health human neck vasculature under US. Image (c, d) courtesy of health volunteer.

The surgical guidance system comprises of a monitor or mixed-reality (MR) HMD (HTC VIVE Pro, HTC, Taiwan ROC), a magnetic tracking system (Aurora, NDI, Canada), a clinical US scanner (SonixTouch, BK Medical, USA), and a surgical hypodemic needle (7 cm metallic needle with 10 ml syringe, Fig. 3b). A linear transducer (L14-5,BK Medical, USA) was used to acquire real-time images of the phantom (depth of 6 cm with gain of 42 %). The US transducer, neck phantom, and surgical needle were magnetically tracked, spatially calibrated, and registered into a common coordinate system. As the HTC VIVE Pro has its own tracking system, it is co-registered with the magnetic tracking by means of a co-tracked apparatus that registers the magnetically tracked tools into the HMD (Fig. 3a) [4]. The co-calibration method was previously validated using a Computerized Numerical Control machine with reported accuracy of less than 1 mm and 1° (trueness plus precision) [4]. The magnetically tracked US transducer was calibrated using a Procrustean method [3], and the surgical needle was calibrated using a template-based approach (Fig. 3b). A visual assessment of the system accuracy, comprising of trackers co-calibration, tool calibration and patient registration is shown in Fig. 3c.

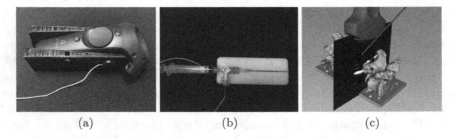

(a)   (b)   (c)

Fig. 3. (a) The co-calibration apparatus tracked by the VIVE controller and magnetic pose sensor (b) the calibration apparatus for the syringe, and (c) Visual representation of the total system accuracy

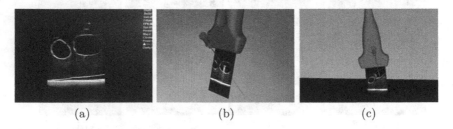

(a)   (b)   (c)

Fig. 4. Visual representation of each mode of visualization where (a) is the US-only system, (b) is the monitor system, and (c) is the HMD system. Images (b) and (c) comprise of models of the US probe, needle, needle trajectory and the calibrated US image.

Three modes of visualization were implemented and evaluated: (1) the traditional US-only, displayed on the US scanner, (2) an AV system displayed on a 2D monitor, (3) a MR system displaying the streaming US and tracked tools in their registered and tracked pose using the HMD, as depicted in Fig. 4. In both AV and MR visualizations, streaming US video, virtual representation of the tracked probe and needle, as well as a needle trajectory represented as a 10 cm blue extension from the needle tip were displayed for surgical guidance.

Thirty-three expert clinicians were recruited with consent according to the local REB regulation (Western University REB 107254). To accommodate hospital scheduling, the study was designed to take be 15-minutes in duration. Prior to the experiment, each participant was briefed on and introduced to the needle insertion required for CVC using the neck phantom. The vasculature on the left side of the neck phantom was used to train the users on all of the systems. The participants were given time to perform needle insertions using the US-only, MR on a monitor, and MR in the HMD system, until the user felt they were comfortable with all of the modes of visualization. The study was conducted using the vessels on the right hand side of the phantom. The order for each set of insertions was randomized for each participant. The participant was required to perform one insertion into the vessel on the right hand side of the phantom for each of the modes of visualization. Sufficient time was provided in between switching modes of visualization to allow the participant to rest and adapt to the new mode. The streaming US video, time, and tracked trajectories were recorded. After performing the experiment, the users filled out a questionnaire.

3   Results

The recorded data were processed to produce the following metrics: time, distance from the final needle tip position to the vessel wall, and path length. The recorded tracking information for all tracked apparatus were used to generate the needle path, visualized as heatmap-coded spheres in Fig. 5. Red spheres indicate the beginning of the needle insertion, transitioning into cold colour as time progresses. The needle path relative to vascular structure was analyzed to extract: the number of successful insertions define by insertions with the final needle tip within the IJV with no CA punctures (Fig. 5a); the number of insertions where the needle tip ended exterior to the IJV (Fig. 5b); and the number of CA punctures (Fig. 5c) . The questionnaire responses were in the form of a continuous scale where the centre and two ends were anchored with written descriptions. If the user agreed with one of the given responses they could mark that part of the scale or alternative anywhere along the scale. The questionnaire responses were converted into a numeric 10.0 scale and summarized in Table 1.

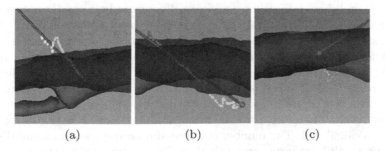

(a)   (b)   (c)

Fig. 5. (a) Successful insertion (b) Needle tip position exterior to the IJV (c) CA puncture (color figure online)

Table 1. User questionnaire results

Question	Average score
Do you think the HMD is a viable equipment to use in the OR?	4.35 ± 2.82
If the system was clinically available how often would you use it?	4.75 ± 2.70
Do you think the HMD system would be useful for training?	7.04 ± 2.25
How was the comfort associated with wearing the HMD?	7.64 ± 2.62

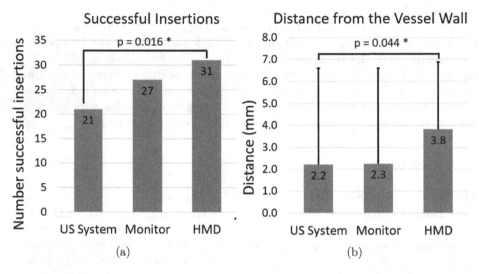

Fig. 6. (a) Graphical depiction of the number of successful insertions performed for each of the guidance systems, and (b) Graphical depiction of the average distance from the final needle tip position to the vessel wall for each of the guidance systems.

The continuous results, such as time, distance to vessel wall and path length, were individually compared across the three conditions US-only, monitor, and HMD using a repeated measures ANOVA. The ANOVA for the distance from the vessel wall returned a p-value less than 0.05 and therefore a least squared distance mutli-comparison post-test was conducted to compare between each pair of conditions. This post-test returned the p-value 0.044 for the US-only and HMD conditions indicating significant differences between these two conditions for the distance from the vessel wall. The mean and standard deviation of the distance from the vessel wall were calculated for each conditon, as the ANOVA for this metric returned a significant p-value. For the discrete results, including the number of successful insertions and CA punctures, the McNemar test was performed. Using this test to compare the number of successful insertions between the US-only and HMD returned a p-value of 0.0106 indicating a significant result. Therefore, the total number of successful insertions for all conditions was calculated. The number of successful needle insertions and distance to the vessel wall have been summarized in Fig. 6, with significant combinations ($p < 0.05$) denoted. All metrics that were not significant were not reported.

4   Discussion

The HMD system significantly improved the number of successful insertions and increased the distance from the final needle tip position to the vessel wall such that the needle tip was more centred within the lumen of the vessel compared to the US-only system. Thirty-one of the thirty-three clinicians performed successful insertions using the HMD system, whereas only twenty-one performed successful insertions using the US-only system. The HMD system had an average distance to the vessel wall of 3.8 ± 3.1 mm, whereas the US-only system had an average distance of 2.2 ± 4.4 mm. If the needle tip was within the vessel lumen the distance was denoted as positive, whereas if the needle tip was exterior to the vessel the distance was denoted as a negative. Therefore, a large positive number is desired as it is representative of the needle tip position within the vessel but far from the vessel wall. Clinicians using the HMD system produced a significantly larger distance on average with a smaller standard deviation compared to the US-only system. Thus, on average, clinicians more consistently targeted the centre of the vessel with the HMD system compared to the US-only system. However, other metrics that were calculated, such as path length and time, were not significantly different between any of these conditions. While these metrics did not show significant improvement, the HMD system allowed for improved guidance compared to the US-only and monitor systems without having a significant impact on the insertion time or path length.

There was no significant improvement in the clinicians' needle guidance when using the monitor based system compared to the US-only system. This result is consistent with the work done by Ameri et al.[1], where a similar monitor based system showed no significant improvements for expert users' needle guidance compared to an US-only system. The lack of improvement is likely due to disparities between the clinicians' motor and visual fields when using both the US-only and monitor based systems. Despite the fact that the monitor system had additional information intended to improve the needle guidance, clinicians' performance was comparable between the US-only systems. However, the HMD system did have significantly improved guidance compared to the US-only system. These results emphasize the importance of coherent visual and motor fields of needle guidance, which can be accomplished using a HMD. While monitor based systems would be more simple to integrate into a clinical workflow, the results presented here suggest that using HMD to bring needle guidance information directly into the line of sight of the clinician is important for successful needle guidance, promoting the continued pursuit of HMD research.

The rates of CA puncture are low and were not significant and therefore are not reported in this paper. The lack of CA punctures is likely due to the simplicity of the phantom as the IJV and CA had a simple orientation with limited overlap, as the CA was positioned laterally to the IJV. However, as depicted in Fig. 2(c and d), the appearance and configuration of the human neck vasculature is variable. The number of insertions that resulted in the final needle position external to the IJV could be representative of the potential puncture risk to important adjacent anatomical structures due to this variability of the anatomy.

Therefore, the reduction of the number of final needle placements outside of the IJV using the HMD could be a surrogate for a reduction in overall complications.

While this study supports the use of HMDs for needle guidance, it is important to consider the feasibility of clincial integration. Questionnaire responses showed that the current HMD system used for this study may be more useful for training rather than clinical use, as on average clinicians ranked the clinical viability of the system a 4.35 out of 10 compared to a 7.04 for usefulness for training. The centre of the scale (5/10) for the question on clinical viability represented the response "viable with proper assistance". Thus, on average, clinicians reported that with assistance this technology could be used in the operating room. However, on average, more clinicians see the potential of this system as a training tool. Furthermore, on average clinicians (4.75/10) indicated they would use this technology on a case by case basis, as more complicated cases would benefit from this high level of guidance. Future work will include continued development of the HMD system to include more real-world information to improve clinical feasbility. This study was performed entirely in VR to isolate the effects of the visual and motor fields. However, many of the clinicians did not think the current system was fully clinically viable due to the lack of real world information. Integrating feed from stereo camera would allow the clinician to visualize the guidance information and the real world simultaneously. Alternatively, the monitor based system is more clinically feasible due to the similarity to current US-only guidance platforms.

5   Conclusion

We developed an advanced needle guidance system that renders tracked tools such as the US probe, needle, and needle trajectory as well as the calibrated US image on a 2D monitor or within a HMD. The aim of this research was to compare needle insertion performance using US-only guidance, the advanced guidance system on a monitor, and the advanced guidance system in the HMD. Thirty-three expert users were trained on all three systems and then used each system to perform a needle insertion on the phantom. The HMD system significantly improved the number of successful needle insertions, as 31 out of 33 clinicians had a final needle tip position within the vessels lumen compared to 21 out of 33 clinicians using US-only guidance. The HMD system also significantly improved the distance from the final needle tip position to the vessel wall. Clinicians using the HMD system had an average distance of 3.8 ± 3.1 mm compared to 2.2 ± 4.4 mm using the US-only system, meaning they were consistently closer to the centre of the lumen of the vessel compared to the US-only approach. The monitor system did not show any siginficant improvements compared to the US-only system. Therefore, using a HMD to align the visual and motor fields is an important factor in promoting successful needle guidance, encouraging the continued pursuit of HMD surgical navigation research.

References

1. Ameri, G., Baxter, J.S.H., Bainbridge, D., Peters, T.M., Chen, E.C.S.: Mixed reality ultrasound guidance system: a case study in system development and a cautionary tale. Int. J. Comput. Assist. Radiol. Surg. **13**(4), 495–505 (2018)
2. Chao, A., et al.: Performance of central venous catheterization by medical students: a retrospective study of students' logbooks. BMC Med. Educ. **14**(1), 168 (2014)
3. Chen, E.C.S., Peters, T.M., Ma, B.: Which point-line registration? In: Webster, R.J., Fei, B. (eds.) Proceedings of the SPIE 10135, Medical Imaging 2017: Image-Guided Procedures, Robotic Interventions, and Modeling, p. 1013509 (2017)
4. Groves, L.A., et al.: Accuracy assessment for the co-registration between optical and VIVE head-mounted display tracking. Int. J. Comput. Assist. Radiol. Surg. **14**(7), 1207–1215 (2019)
5. Hameeteman, M., Bode, A.S., Peppelenbosch, A.G., der Sande, F.M.V., Tordoir, D.J.H.: Ultrasound-guided central venous catheter placement by surgical trainees: a safe procedure? J. Vasc. Access **11**(4), 288–292 (2010)
6. Raad, I.: Intravascular-catheter-related infections. Lancet (Lond. Engl.) **351**(9106), 893–898 (1998)
7. Saugel, B., Scheeren, T.W.L., Teboul, J.L.: Ultrasound-guided central venous catheter placement: a structured review and recommendations for clinical practice. Crit. Care **21**(1), 225 (2017)
8. Soni, N.J., et al.: Use of ultrasound guidance for central venous catheterization: a national survey of intensivists and hospitalists. J. Crit. Care **36**, 277–283 (2016)
9. Surry, K.J.M., Austin, H.J.B., Fenster, A., Peters, T.M.: Poly(vinyl alcohol) cryogel phantoms for use in ultrasound and MR imaging. Phys. Med. Biol. **49**(24), 5529–5546 (2004)

Concept-Centric Visual Turing Tests
for Method Validation

Tatiana Fountoukidou(✉) and Raphael Sznitman

ARTORG Center, University of Bern, Bern, Switzerland
{tatiana.fountoukidou,raphael.sznitman}@artorg.unibe.ch

Abstract. Recent advances in machine learning for medical imaging have led to impressive increases in model complexity and overall capabilities. However, the ability to discern the precise information a machine learning method is using to make decisions has lagged behind and it is often unclear how these performances are in fact achieved. Conventional evaluation metrics that reduce method performance to a single number or a curve only provide limited insights. Yet, systems used in clinical practice demand thorough validation that such crude characterizations miss. To this end, we present a framework to evaluate classification methods based on a number of interpretable concepts that are crucial for a clinical task. Our approach is inspired by the *Turing Test* concept and how to devise a test that adaptively questions a method for its ability to interpret medical images. To do this, we make use of a Twenty Questions paradigm whereby we use a probabilistic model to characterize the method's capacity to grasp task-specific concepts, and we introduce a strategy to sequentially query the method according to its previous answers. The results show that the probabilistic model is able to expose both the dataset's and the method's biases, and can be used to reduce the number of queries needed for confident performance evaluation.

1 Introduction

The field of medical image computing (MIC) has radically changed with the emergence of large neural networks, or Deep Learning (DL). For MIC tasks that were long considered extremely challenging, such as image-based pathology classification and segmentation, DL methods have now reached human-level performances on a variety of benchmarks.

Yet, as these methods have become increasingly powerful, the overall methodology to validate them has largely remained intact. For instance, challenge competitions compare different methods on a common dataset by using metrics most often borrowed from the computer vision literature. As recently noted in [9], challenge competition rankings and outcomes are very often highly skewed to the dataset or metrics used, and rarely relate to the clinical task. To tackle this, recent developments in visual question answering (VQA) [1,5,8,14] methods, which answer questions related to image content, show the ability to infer concepts beyond traditional classification. Here again, however, the metrics used to evaluate VQA's remain inadequate.

© Springer Nature Switzerland AG 2019
D. Shen et al. (Eds.): MICCAI 2019, LNCS 11768, pp. 254–262, 2019.
https://doi.org/10.1007/978-3-030-32254-0_29

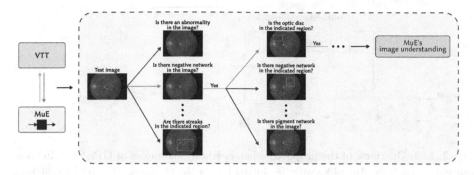

Fig. 1. Visual Turing Test (VTT) fundus image screening. Green arrows correspond to selected questions, and orange lines to the answers given by the MuE. (Color figure online)

Instead, we consider an alternative approach to validating MIC methods, one inspired by Alan Turing's *Turing Test* concept [13], where a human unknowingly communicates either with another human or an Artificial Intelligence system that produces answers. The aim of the test is to distinguish between the two based on a set of asked questions. Turing tests have been used in medical imaging to evaluate the quality of adversarial attacks, by seeing if an expert can distinguish between a real and an adversarial example [3,12]. Another approach, focusing on the interpretability of methods that infer semantic information from images (e.g. classification, segmentation etc.) is seen in the work of Geman et al. [4] on automated Visual Turing Tests (VTT). In their work, an algorithm adaptively selects images and questions to pose to a method under evaluation (MuE) such that the answers can not be predicted from the history of answers. While this approach has increased explanatory power, it is limited to manually fabricated story lines to guide questioning. This makes it ill suited for medical applications where such story lines are hard to formalize.

For this reason, we propose a novel VTT framework to evaluate MIC methods (see Fig. 1). In particular, our approach focuses on evaluating MIC classification methods and we present a framework that tests if the method has correctly *understood* the relevant medical concepts when inferring test data. We do this by formulating our problem as a Twenty Questions game [2,7] in which we model the likelihood of a given MuE to provide correct answers for different concepts present in test images. Our framework then sequentially picks test images and concepts such that the uncertainty of this model is reduced as quickly as possible. We demonstrate our framework in the context of three different multi-label classification problems where each concept is encoded by a given binary label.

2   Method

Our proposed VTT framework evaluates how a MuE, a MIC classification method in this case, performs with respect to core concepts relevant to the task

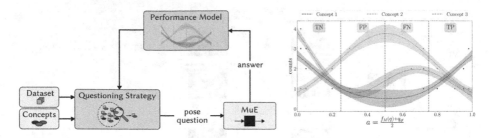

Fig. 2. Left: Overview of the proposed scheme. Right: Examples of GPs for 3 different concepts (points are the observations, dotted line is the mean of a GP and the shaded area corresponds to the 95% confidence region).

for which it was trained. To do this, we make use of a validation image dataset that the MuE has never had access to, $\mathcal{D} = \{\mathbf{s}_i\}_{i=1}^{N_S}$, where $\mathbf{s}_i$ is an available test sample, such as an image or an arbitrary region within an image. As such, N_S can be excessively large, as potentially millions of regions can be extracted from a single test image. For each $\mathbf{s}_i$, we denote the potential concepts that could be present in the sample as, $\mathcal{C} = \{c_j\}_{j=1}^{N_C}$. From this, we define a "question", $q = (\mathbf{s}_q, c_q) \in \mathcal{D} \times \mathcal{C} = \mathcal{Q}$, of the form "Is concept c_q present in sample $\mathbf{s}_q$?". We let $q_{gt} \in \{0, 1\}$ be the true answer to question q. In this work, we consider MuEs that perform multi-label classification tasks, $f : \mathcal{Q} \to [0, 1]$, taking as input the question q and producing the probability of the answer being "Yes" (see Fig. 1).

Given that evaluating all elements of $\mathcal{Q}$ may be computationally intractable, our VTT framework instead only evaluates a subset of $\mathcal{Q}$. We do this iteratively and adaptively, where we use the history of previously asked questions and their answers to build a *performance model* (Sect. 2.1). We then use a *questioning strategy* to determine which element of $\mathcal{Q}$ should be asked to the MuE. In particular, we propose a novel strategy that selects the element that maximally reduces the uncertainty in the performance model (Sect. 2.2). The process terminates after a fixed number of questions have been asked or when the uncertainty in the model has been reduced to an acceptable level. Figure 2 (Left) illustrates our framework and we detail our performance model and questioning strategy next.

2.1 Performance Model

From a set of questions and the corresponding MuE responses, we aim to model the MuE performance with respect to concepts $\mathcal{C}$. While the relation between concepts could in practice be complex, we model them as independent here.

By its definition, the MuE provides answers to binary questions, and for any concept, there are 4 possible outcomes to a question: a True Negative (TN), a False Positive (FP), a False Negative (FN) or a True Positive (TP). Our goal then is to model the relation between the frequency of these outcomes and the inputs to the MuE. To do this, we define a discrete random variable Y_c for every

---

Algorithm 1. Concept Centric VTT

Require: Dataset: $\mathcal{D}$, Concepts: $\mathcal{C}$, stopping criteria: τ and MuE: f

$\quad \mathcal{Q} \leftarrow \mathcal{D} \times \mathcal{C}$

$\quad$ Initialize $f_c^{\mathcal{GP}}, c \in \mathcal{C}$

$\quad$ **while** $\#$ questions asked $< \tau$ **do**

$$\mathcal{Q}_{candidates} \leftarrow \left\{ q \in \mathcal{Q} : c_q \in \arg\max_{c \in \mathcal{C}} \left(\max \left(u_c^-, u_c^+ \right) \right) \text{ and } q_{gt} = o_{c_q} \right\}$$

$\quad\quad$ **if** select based only on uncertainty **then**

$\quad\quad\quad q^* \leftarrow$ randomly select $q \in \mathcal{Q}_{candidates}$

$\quad\quad$ **else if** select based on uncertainty & unpredictability **then**

$\quad\quad\quad q^* \leftarrow$ random $q \in \{q \in \mathcal{Q}_{candidates} : |p(f(q) = \text{"Yes"}|\mathcal{H}) - 0.5| < \epsilon\}$

$\quad\quad$ **end if**

$\quad\quad$ Compute $f(q^*)$, a_c

$\quad\quad$ Update $f_c^{\mathcal{GP}}$

$\quad\quad \mathcal{H} \leftarrow \{\mathcal{H}, (q^*, f(q^*))\}$

$\quad\quad \mathcal{Q} \leftarrow \{\mathcal{Q} \setminus q^*\}$

$\quad$ **end while**

---

concept $c \in \mathcal{C}$ which encodes the counts[1] of outcomes given by f. We achieve this by means of a Gaussian Process (GP) [11] of the form,

$$f_c^{\mathcal{GP}}(a_c) \sim \mathcal{GP}\left(\mu_c(a_c), k_c(a_c, a_c')\right), \tag{1}$$

where $\mu_c(\cdot)$ and $k_c(\cdot, \cdot)$ are the mean and kernel functions of the GP, respectively, and

$$a_c = \frac{f(q) + q_{gt}}{2}, \tag{2}$$

describes the answer of f with respect to the question q. The mean function μ_c is initialized to 0, and the covariance function (kernel) k_c is a squared exponential $k_c(a_{c,m}, a_{c,n}) = \sigma_f \cdot e^{-\frac{1}{2l^2}(a_{c,m} - a_{c,n})^2} + \sigma_n \delta_{mn}$, with characteristic length-scale $l = 0.1$, initial signal variance $\sigma_f = 1$ and noise variance $\sigma_n = 0.025$.

To then infer the value of Y_c for any a_c, we store the pairs $\{(a_c^{(i)}, y_c^{(i)})\}$ where $y_c^{(i)}$ is the number of times f has given $a = a_c^{(i)}$, and use these as observations to infer the complete model $f_c^{\mathcal{GP}}$ using standard inference [11]. In practice, we discretized the range of a in bins of $\Delta a = 0.01$.

A consequence of this model is that we can now visualize the performance of f with respect to the concepts in $\mathcal{C}$, the selected q's and the dataset $\mathcal{D}$. In Fig. 2 (Right), we illustrate $f_c^{\mathcal{GP}}$ in terms of a for each c. Such a visualization depicts any bias that both f and the dataset $\mathcal{D}$ may have (e. g., $\mathcal{D}$ contains few samples regarding a specific concept). Note that by summing up the observations over concepts or integrating over the four different subregions of the support set, one retrieves the total TN, FP, FN and TP, and other subsequent metrics.

---

[1] The approach would be unchanged if the outcome frequency was used.

2.2   Questioning Strategy

With the performance model above and the fact that the validation dataset $\mathcal{D}$ may be intractably larger, we now describe how to select samples from $\mathcal{Q}$ to verify that the MuE has grasped relevant concepts.

To do this, we present a strategy that looks to select samples $\mathbf{s}$ and concepts c that are likely to reduce our model's uncertainty. We do this by computing the uncertainty of a concept as the integral of the 95% confidence region of the GP over its support set (i.e., 2 standard deviations). That is, for concept $c \in C$,

$$u_c = 4 \int_0^1 k_c(a, a) da, \tag{3}$$

which can be decomposed as $u_c^- = 4 \int_0^{0.5} k_c(a, a) da$ and $u_c^+ = 4 \int_{0.5}^1 k_c(a, a) da$, corresponding to the uncertainty associated with negative and positive samples in $\mathcal{D}$, respectively. Visually this corresponds to the area over the intervals $a = [0, 0.5]$ and $a = [0.5, 1]$ (see Fig. 2, Right).

Our strategy then chooses which concept to ask, and whether to ask a sample that has or does not have this concept in it. This is performed by selecting

$$q^* \in \left\{ q \in \mathcal{Q} : c_q \in \arg\max_{c \in C} (\max(u_c^-, u_c^+)) \text{ and } q_{gt} = o_{c_q} \right\}, \tag{4}$$

where $o_{c_q} = 0$ if $\max(u_c^-, u_c^+) = u_c^-$ or 1 if $\max(u_c^-, u_c^+) = u_c^+$.

From this, q^* is selected either randomly, or based on its unpredictability. As in [4], the latter is computed using the same dataset $\mathcal{D}$ and the history of already answered questions $\mathcal{H}$. An overview of the questioning strategy can be seen in Algorithm 1.

3   Experiments and Results

We choose to evaluate our framework on multi-label classification tasks where concepts are directly linked to groundtruth labels. In the following, we outline the different datasets and MuEs we use, and our experimental setup.

3.1   Datasets and MuE

Indian Diabetic Retinopathy image Dataset (IDRiD) [10]: 143 fundus images from both healthy and diabetic retinopathy subjects, with the task of identifying 4 different lesion types (hemorrhage, hard and soft exudates, microaneurysm). The multilabel MuE is a ResNet [6] with pre-trained weights, trained with 100 images. The remaining 43 images were used as samples in $\mathcal{D}$.

ISIC 2018 Skin Lesion Analysis[2]: 1,876 dermoscopic images of skin lesions. Here $N_C = 5$, consisting of different skin lesions types: pigment network, negative

---

[2] https://challenge2018.isic-archive.com/.

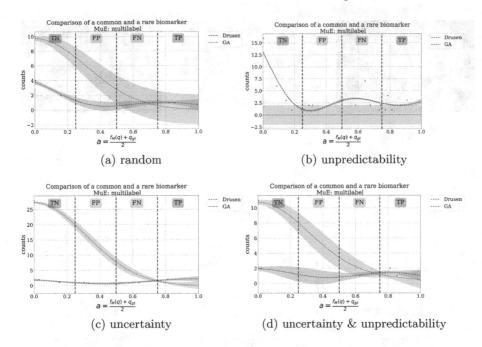

Fig. 3. Performance model for the 4 questioning strategies. The most common concept (Drusen) and a rare concept (Geographic Atrophy - GA) are shown after 100 questions are posed to the multilabel MuE.

network, globules, milia like cysts and streaks. The MuE is a pre-trained ResNet [6] trained with 70% of data. A hundred randomly chosen images from the 30% test images were used to populate $\mathcal{D}$.

OCT: 200 OCT cross-sectional slices from Age-Related Macular Degeneration and Diabetic Macular Edema patients. Eleven different biomarkers potentially can be present in any cross-section ($N_C = 11$). All 200 images are used for $\mathcal{D}$ and a seperate trained Dilated Residual Network [15] is used for the MuE.

Given that we are not focused on optimizing the performance of a specific MuE but rather on evaluating relative behavior with respect to concepts, we also provide a set of synthetically generated MuEs for which we understand their performance fully. That is, given that the distribution of concepts in $\mathcal{D}$ is not uniform for any of the datasets, we wish to compare each MuE to a "biased" MuE. To do this, we simulate a biased MuE that answers with 90% accuracy questions regarding the most common concept and 50% on all others. Similarly, we simulate a MuE with a 50% accuracy for the most common concept, and 90% on all others. Last, we also simulate an unbiased algorithm, with a 70% accuracy regardless of the concept or class imbalance.

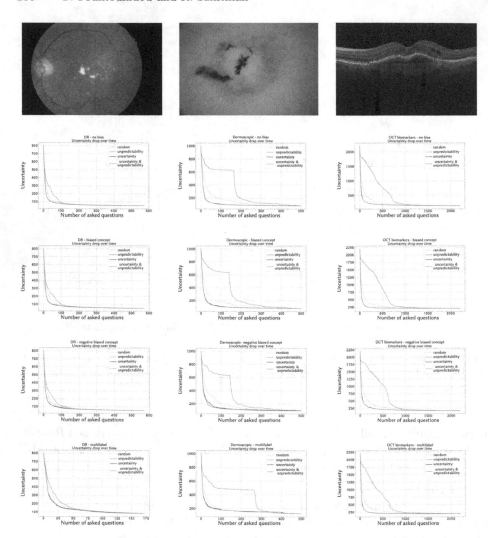

Fig. 4. Uncertainty of the performance model with respect to the number of questions asked for different MuEs. Each column corresponds to a dataset. **Rows, from top to bottom:** image example, uncertainty for unbiased MuE, uncertainty for biased to most common concept MuE, uncertainty for negatively biased to most common concept MuE and uncertainty for trained multilabel classifier.

3.2   Experiments

To evaluate our framework, we compare four questioning strategies: (a) random, (b) based on the predictability of the question given the previous questions and the dataset [4], (c) based on the uncertainty of the question as defined in Sect. 2.2, and (d) based on the combination of the above two, as described in Sect. 2.2.

Figure 3 depicts the state of the performance for two concepts (GA and Drusen) after a hundred questions have been asked on the **OCT** dataset using the trained MuE. In all plots the bias in concept occurrence can be observed and we see that both the random strategy, and the one relying solely on the unpredictability criteria, are prone to not ask many questions about rare concepts (GA concept), thus delaying the assessment of the MuE's on this concept. Both uncertainty based methods however manage to sample adequately and are more confident in the performance model.

In another experiment, we ask all possible questions following each one of the four described strategies. That is, the state of the performance model is the same after all questions have been asked. We repeat the experiments 10 times, and monitor the average uncertainty as questions are asked. The results are shown in Fig. 4. Here we observe that the proposed questioning strategies reach saturated levels of uncertainty quicker than the other strategies, and would require fewer questions for confident assessments.

4   Discussion

To summarize, we present a more informative and interpretable performance model for evaluating closed-end, "Yes/No" inference methods. To this, we propose a strategy to sample from the - possibly intractable - set of questions, in order to reach high certainty in the performance model characterizing the MuE and the validation data. We assess our method on three different medical imaging datasets and show that the performance model is able to capture the data distribution information and the MuE biases. Moreover, the questioning strategy allows for faster convergence of the performance model to a low uncertainty state. We will look to extend this concept to segmentation problems in future work.

References

1. Antol, S., et al.: VQA: visual question answering. In: The IEEE International Conference on Computer Vision (ICCV), December 2015
2. Bendig, A.: Twenty questions: an information analysis. J. Exp. Psychol. **5**, 345–348 (1953)
3. Chuquicusma, M.J., Hussein, S., Burt, J., Bagci, U.: How to fool radiologists with generative adversarial networks? a visual turing test for lung cancer diagnosis. In: 2018 IEEE 15th International Symposium on Biomedical Imaging (ISBI 2018), pp. 240–244. IEEE (2018)
4. Geman, D., Geman, S., Hallonquist, N., Younes, L.: Visual turing test for computer vision systems. Proc. Natl. Acad. Sci. **112**(12), 3618–3623 (2015)
5. Hasan, S.A., Ling, Y., Farri, O., Liu, J., Lungren, M., Müller, H.: Overview of the ImageCLEF 2018 medical domain visual question answering task. In: CLEF 2018 Working Notes (2018)
6. He, K., Zhang, X., Ren, S., Sun, J.: Deep residual learning for image recognition. In: Proceedings of the IEEE Conference on Computer Vision and Pattern Recognition, pp. 770–778 (2016)

7. Jedynak, B., Frazier, P., Sznitman, R.: Twenty questions with noise: Bayes optimal policies for entropy loss. J. Appl. Probab. **1**, 114–136 (2012)
8. Lau, J.J., Gayen, S., Abacha, A.B., Demner-Fushman, D.: A dataset of clinically generated visual questions and answers about radiology images. Sci. Data **5**, 180251 (2018)
9. Maier-Hein, L., et al.: Author correction: why rankings of biomedical image analysis competitions should be interpreted with care. Nat. Commun. **10**(1), 588 (2019)
10. Prasanna, P., et al.: Indian diabetic retinopathy image dataset (IDRiD) (2018)
11. Rasmussen, C.E.: Gaussian Processes for Machine Learning. MIT Press, Cambridge (2006)
12. Schlegl, T., Seeböck, P., Waldstein, S.M., Langs, G., Schmidt-Erfurth, U.: f-AnoGAN: fast unsupervised anomaly detection with generative adversarial networks. Med. Image Anal. **54**, 30–44 (2019)
13. Turing, A.: Computing machinery and intelligence. Mind **49**(236), 433–460 (1950)
14. Wu, Q., Teney, D., Wang, P., Shen, C., Dick, A., van den Hengel, A.: Visual question answering: a survey of methods and datasets. Comput. Vis. Image Underst. **163**, 21–40 (2017)
15. Yu, F., Koltun, V., Funkhouser, T.: Dilated residual networks, May 2017

Transferring from *ex-vivo* to *in-vivo*: Instrument Localization in 3D Cardiac Ultrasound Using Pyramid-UNet with Hybrid Loss

Hongxu Yang[1][✉], Caifeng Shan[2], Tao Tan[1], Alexander F. Kolen[2], and Peter H. N. de With[1]

[1] Eindhoven University of Technology, Eindhoven, The Netherlands
h.yang@tue.nl
[2] Philips Research, Eindhoven, The Netherlands

Abstract. Automated instrument localization during cardiac interventions is essential to accurately and efficiently interpret a 3D ultrasound (US) image. In this paper, we propose a method to automatically localize the cardiac intervention instrument (RF-ablation catheter or guidewire) in a 3D US volume. We propose a Pyramid-UNet, which exploits the multi-scale information for better segmentation performance. Furthermore, a hybrid loss function is introduced, which consists of contextual loss and class-balanced focal loss, to enhance the performance of the network in cardiac US images. We have collected a challenging *ex-vivo* dataset to validate our method, which achieves a Dice score of 69.6% being 18.8% higher than the state-of-the-art methods. Moreover, with the pre-trained model on the *ex-vivo* dataset, our method can be easily adapted to the *in-vivo* dataset with several iterations and then achieves a Dice score of 65.8% for a different instrument. With segmentation, instruments can be localized with an average error less than 3 voxels in both datasets. To the best of our knowledge, this is the first work to validate the image-based method on *in-vivo* cardiac datasets.

Keywords: Instrument localization · 3D US · Pyramid-UNet · Hybrid loss

1 Introduction

Cardiac intervention therapies, such as cardiac electrophysiology (EP) and transcatheter aortic valve implantation (TAVI), have been broadly applied to achieve lower risk and shorter recovery time for patients. To guide the instruments inside the heart during intervention, fluoroscopy imaging is typically considered using a contrast agent to visualize the vessel and tissue. However, radiation dose, harmful agents, invisible soft tissue and lack of 3D spatial information in X-ray imaging complicate the interpretation of the instrument during the interventions.

© Springer Nature Switzerland AG 2019
D. Shen et al. (Eds.): MICCAI 2019, LNCS 11768, pp. 263–271, 2019.
https://doi.org/10.1007/978-3-030-32254-0_30

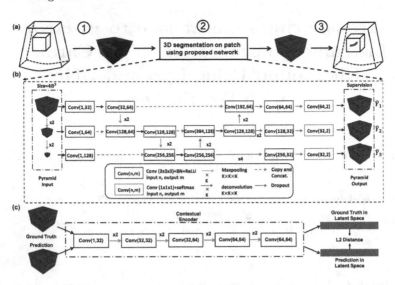

Fig. 1. (a) Block diagram of our method; (b) Pyramid-UNet structure for segmentation, the outputs are supervised by hybrid loss; (c) Encoding for contextual loss.

To address this, 3D ultrasound (US) is considered as an alternative solution for intervention guidance, which has a richer spatial information and no radiation exposure. Nevertheless, the low-resolution and low-contrast imaging of 3D US lead to difficulty for a sonographer to timely localize the instrument during the surgery. Therefore, automatic instrument segmentation and localization methods are highly demanded for clinical practice. As a promising approach, 3D US image-based instrument localization has been studied in recent years [1,5,6,8,9]. Conventional machine learning approaches with handcrafted features were applied to localize the catheter in a phantom heart or an *ex-vivo* dataset [5,9]. However, the limited discriminating capacity of handcrafted features cannot always handle the complex anatomical structures in 3D US images. More recently, deep learning methods, such as convolutional neural networks (CNNs), have achieved a significant performance improvement in medical applications. For instruments detection or localization in 3D US using deep learning, two main approaches have been studied: voxel-based classification by a CNN [6,8] and slice-based semantic segmentation [6]. Although they achieved better results than the approaches with handcrafted features, these deep learning methods still have limitations. Particularly for the slice-based semantic segmentation method, the authors [6] employ a 2D convolution method on the decomposed 2D slices. However, the 3D contextual information in 3D US cannot be fully exploited.

To better exploit 3D contextual information, we propose as the first contribution a 3D CNN for instrument localization in 3D US, which is shown in Fig. 1. More specifically, we propose a compact UNet with pyramid structure (Pyramid-UNet), which is able to keep both high-level and low-level features simultaneously at different image scales, while reducing the complexity of the standard

UNet [2,10]. From our experiments, our proposed Pyramid-UNet improves the segmentation performances when compared to a standard UNet structure. Moreover, as the second contribution, we design a hybrid loss function, which consists of contextual loss and class-balanced focal loss, to learn a better discriminating representation. The contextual loss controls the CNN towards high-level contextual information encoding for the prediction domain. The class-balanced focal loss enables the network to balance and focus more on challenging voxels of difficult structures. To validate our method, we first performed an experiment on the collected *ex-vivo* dataset for RF-ablation catheter localization (for EP operation), which successfully segmented the instrument with Dice score 69.6%. Furthermore, we conducted an experiment on an *in-vivo* dataset for guidewire localization (for TAVI operation). With limited images of the *in-vivo* dataset, we performed fine-tuning on this dataset by using the pre-trained model from the *ex-vivo* dataset, which achieved Dice score of 65.8%. Based on the successful segmentation result, the instrument's tip can be localized with an average error less than 3 voxels on both datasets. To the best of our knowledge and as the third contribution, this paper is the first one to validate the image-based cardiac instrument localization in an *in-vivo* dataset.

2 Methods

The block diagram of our proposed method is shown in Fig. 1, which is based on three stages: (1) the input 3D image is decomposed into smaller patches; (2) each patch is segmented by our proposed network and the output patches are combined back; (3) the instrument axis and its tip are extracted after the segmentation, which can then be visualized for clinical experts.

2.1 Pyramid-UNet

We adopt the popular segmentation net 3D UNet [2,10] as our backbone architecture, but we introduce the following modifications for our application, as shown in Fig. 1(b). Because of the limited amount of images in the dataset, we experimentally reduce the number of multi-scale levels of UNet and convolutional channels at each level, which leads to less trainable parameters and avoids overfitting. When compared to a standard UNet (19.4M parameters), our re-designed compact UNet is more compact and efficient (4.6M parameters). Typically as the network goes deeper, the discriminating information at low level can vanish or be omitted. Although UNet [2] employs skipping connections to preserve low-level information, it still cannot fully preserve the information at different levels. To address this, we design a Pyramid-UNet, which is shown in Fig. 1(b). We consider the multi-scale inputs at different UNet levels to preserve more low-level information within the encoding stage. The proposed image pyramid scaling at the input is attractive, since it potentially compensates the information loss during the feature pyramid of UNet [4]. Furthermore, to better supervise and synchronize the features at different scales, we employ deep supervision at the decoding stage [3], but introduce an extra convolutional block for a better stability. Specifically, we apply the deconvolution operation at each decoding level to generate the prediction with original patch size, which avoids further artifacts in the ground truth and preserves the accuracy. By combining the pyramid inputs and outputs, the proposed network potentially preserves more information at different feature scales than the standard UNet for US images.

2.2   Hybrid Loss Function

To better supervise the Pyramid-UNet and to enforce learning more contextual information rather than a conventional voxel-based loss function, such as cross-entropy and Dice loss, we propose a hybrid loss function. It consists of a contextual loss and a class-balanced focal loss. As shown in Fig. 1(b), the three outputs of the 3D Pyramid-UNet are denoted as $\hat{Y}_1$, $\hat{Y}_2$ and $\hat{Y}_3$. The hybrid loss function is defined as

$$Loss(\hat{Y}_1, \hat{Y}_2, \hat{Y}_3, Y) = \sum_{i=1}^{3} \alpha_i (Loss_{FL}(\hat{Y}_i, Y) + Loss_{CL}(\hat{Y}_i, Y)), \tag{1}$$

where Y is the ground truth of the input patch, $Loss_{FL}$ denotes the class-balanced focal loss and $Loss_{CL}$ is the contextual loss.

Typically, networks are learned by employing a voxel-wise loss function, such as cross-entropy or Dice loss, which are ignoring the high-level difference between prediction and ground truth. To enforce the network to learn a better contextual representation, we introduce a novel contextual loss, which formulates the contextual difference in a latent space. The prediction and ground truth are encoded by a contextual encoder, which is depicted in Fig. 1(c), to generate a high-level representation in latent space, denoted as $S_{\hat{Y}}$ and S_Y, respectively. As a consequence, the contextual loss $Loss_{CL}$ is characterized by

$$Loss_{CL}(\hat{Y}, Y) = ||CE(\hat{Y}) - CE(Y)||_2 = ||S_{\hat{Y}} - S_Y||_2, \tag{2}$$

where $|| \cdot ||_2$ is the norm-2 distance and $CE(\cdot)$ is the context encoder in Fig. 1(c).

The loss function, such as Dice or cross-entropy, is typically applied for segmentation tasks in medical imaging. However, it is not optimized when segmented objects have large size variations and imbalanced class distribution in the ground truth [7]. Moreover, when the instrument has a small size in 3D space and hard/challenging classified boundary voxels are more important than easy classified voxels at the center part of the instrument, the commonly used loss functions might not be optimized. Therefore, to focus more on challenging voxels and concerning the imbalanced classes of the previous focal loss [7], we adopt them into the class-balanced hybrid focal loss function, which is defined as

$$Loss_{FL}(\hat{Y}, Y) = \eta \left(1 - \frac{(1+\beta^2)\sum_{i=1}^{N} y_{ci}\hat{y}_{ci}}{(1+\beta^2)\sum_{i=1}^{N} y_{ci}\hat{y}_{ci} + \beta^2 \sum_{i=1}^{N} y_{ci}\hat{y}_{ni} + \sum_{i=1}^{N} y_{ni}\hat{y}_{ci}}\right)^{\gamma}$$

$$- (1 - \eta)\left(\sum_{i=1}^{N} \omega_{ci}(1 - \hat{y}_{ci})^{\sigma} \log(\hat{y}_{ci}) + \sum_{i=1}^{N} \omega_{ni}(1 - \hat{y}_{ni})^{\sigma} \log(\hat{y}_{ni})\right),$$

$$(3)$$

where y_{ci} denotes an instrument voxel from the ground truth, $\hat{y}_{ci}$ represents the voxel's prediction probability for the instrument class, while y_{ni} and $\hat{y}_{ni}$ are a non-instrument voxel and its corresponding prediction probability, respectively. Parameters β and ω are controlling the weight between different classes, which are calculated as the square root of the inverse of the classes ratio. Parameters γ and σ are controlling the slope of the loss curve, which are empirically selected as $\gamma = 0.3$ and $\sigma = 2$, respectively. Parameter η is the weight between two different focal losses, which is empirically chosen as $\eta = 0.8$.

2.3   Training Stage: Dense Sampling

The common training strategy for patch-wise segmentation is based on a random patch cropping from the full volumes [10]. However, this approach fails to train the network for instrument segmentation in 3D US, since the instrument occupies relatively small space in the volume and random cropping leads to an extremely imbalanced information distribution. To address this, we propose a dense sampling approach on catheter voxels: for each instrument voxel in the training volume, a 3D patch with size 48^3 voxels is generated that surrounds the voxel being at the center. As a result, the training patches are focusing on a subspace surrounding the instruments rather than sampling irrelevant information. The network is trained by minimizing the joint loss function of Eq. (1) using the Adam optimizer with initial learning rate equal to 0.001. Empirically, we empirically select loss weights in Eq. (1) as $\alpha_1 = 1$, $\alpha_2 = 0.6$ and $\alpha_3 = 0.4$, respectively. The learning is terminated after convergence. To generalize the network, data augmentations are applied on-the-fly, like random mirroring, flipping, contrast transformation, etc. The dropout rate is 0.5 during the training.

2.4   Instrument Localization

The full volume of 3D US is decomposed into patches to generate the segmentation results, which are combined back into a volume as the segmentation output, as shown in Fig. 1(a). A typical instrument localization method is using a predefined model to fit the instrument in 3D space [9], which could be complex and time-consuming. In our method, with the high segmentation performance of the proposed network, we directly extract the largest connected group as the instrument after the segmentation. As a result, our method avoids a complex post-processing stage. With the selected group, the instrument axis is extracted and the instrument's tip is localized as the point closest to the image center.

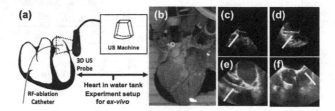

Fig. 2. (a) Our *ex-vivo* dataset collection setup with RF-ablation catheter; (b) Porcine heart placed in the water tank, the US probe is placed under the heart while the catheter is going through the vein; (c) (d) Example slices of ***ex-vivo*** image with **RF-ablation catheter**; (e) (f) Example slices of ***in-vivo*** image with **guidewire**.

Table 1. Segmentation performance for different methods in Dice Score (DSC) and Hausdorff Distance (HD), which are shown in mean ± std. All the methods are validated on our datasets. (−means failed to calculate the result due to memory overflow)

Method	*ex-vivo*		*in-vivo*	
	DSC (%)	HD (voxels)	DSC (%)	HD (voxels)
GF-SVM [5]	3.3 ± 8.5	-	1.0 ± 1.7	-
MF-AdaB [9]	36.5 ± 19.0	19.1 ± 8.5	37.6 ± 23.3	23.9 ± 18.2
ShareFCN [6]	52.8 ± 21.0	15.6 ± 16.7	55.9 ± 12.1	11.6 ± 7.8
LateCNN [8]	58.5 ± 10.7	11.5 ± 7.7	58.6 ± 7.9	11.0 ± 5.1
3D-UNet [10]	24.6 ± 24.9	38.3 ± 22.3	53.2 ± 14.7	18.8 ± 11.0
Compact-UNet	62.2 ± 20.0	13.3 ± 15.6	63.8 ± 9.2	9.8 ± 5.5
Pyramid-UNet	65.8 ± 18.9	11.3 ± 13.8	64.5 ± 8.3	8.8 ± 3.2
Proposed	**69.6 ± 10.9**	**9.0 ± 4.6**	**65.8 ± 9.2**	**8.4 ± 3.8**

3   Experiments

3.1   Experiment on *ex-vivo* dataset

Materials: We have first validated our method on an *ex-vivo* dataset, examples of data collection setup and corresponding US images are shown in Fig. 2. The *ex-vivo* dataset consists of 92 3D cardiac US images from porcine hearts. During the recording, the hearts were placed in water tanks with an RF-ablation catheter for EP (diameter range from 2.3 mm to 3.3 mm) inside the left ventricle or right atrium. The US probes were placed next to the heart to capture the images containing the catheter. The dataset includes the volumes of size range 120 × 69 × 92 to 294 × 283 × 202 voxels, in which the voxel size was isotropically resampled to the range of 0.4–0.7 mm. The datasets were manually annotated by clinical experts to generate the binary segmentation mask as the ground truth. The *ex-vivo* dataset was randomly divided into 62/30 volumes for training/testing. The evaluation metrics are Dice Score (DSC) and Hausdorff Distance (HD).

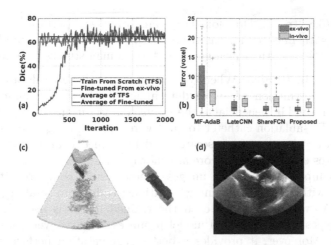

Fig. 3. (a) Learning curves for testing patches under two different scenarios at first 2k iterations in *ex-vivo*, with corresponding Dice score on testing volumes. (b) Box-plots of instrument tip error in different segmentation methods. (c) 3D volume with ground truth (green), segmentation (red), and enlarged visualization. (d) 2D slices of 3D volume, which is tuned to have the best view. (Color figure online)

Segmentation in *ex-vivo*: We have extensively compared our method with state-of-the-art medical instrument segmentation approaches on the *ex-vivo* data-set, including handcrafted feature methods using Gabor features (GF-SVM) [5], Multi-scale and multi-definition features (MF-AdaB) [9], LateCNN for voxel-based catheter classification (LateCNN) [8], and ShareFCN using a cross-section approach to decompose 3D information for needle segmentation (ShareFCN) [6]. Moreover, we also compared a standard 3D UNet for 3D US in another task (3D-UNet) [10]. The results are compared with our method and shown in Table 1. Ablation studies are also performed to validate our proposed compact UNet with standard Dice loss (Compact-UNet), Pyramid-UNet with standard Dice loss and our Pyramid-UNet with hybrid loss (denoted as Proposed in the Table). From the results in Table 1, the Compact-UNet has better performance than 3D-UNet because of using less parameters and avoiding of over-fitting. Moreover, it also has better performance than other medical instrument segmentation approaches. Our proposed Pyramid-UNet with hybrid loss is able to further boost the performance by exploiting more semantic information.

3.2 Experiment on *in-vivo* dataset

Materials: The collected *in-vivo* dataset includes 18 volumes from TAVI operations. During the recording, the sonographer recorded images from different locations of the chamber without any influence on the procedure. The volumes were recorded with a mean volume size of $201 \times 202 \times 302$, where the volume voxel size was resampled to 0.6 mm. The applied instrument in the *in-vivo* dataset is a guidewire (0.889 mm). Threefold cross-validation was performed on the *in-vivo* dataset with fine-tuning, based on the pre-trained *ex-vivo* model for the RF-ablation catheter. All ethical guidelines for human studies were followed.

Segmentation in *in-vivo*: When comparing our challenging datasets, *ex-vivo* possess more information of 3D cardiac images because of a larger training dataset, which could be beneficial to the *in-vivo* dataset using the concept of fine-tuning (from RF-ablation catheter to guidewire). As a consequence, we trained the model on *ex-vivo* data from scratch and fine-tuned it on the *in-vivo* data. Example curves of testing Dice score are shown in Fig. 3(a), which are obtained by random samples from testing images. These results come from two different scenarios with respect to training iterations: train from scratch (TFS) and fine-tuning. As we can observe, even the trained model is used for different instrument types, the pre-trained model promises a fast convergence less than 10 iterations. Moreover, it provides a better segmentation performance when compared to training from scratch. The fine-tuned model has 4% higher Dice score with 2,000 iterations than training from scratch with 20,000 iterations. Corresponding segmentation results are shown in Table 1.

3.3   Instrument Localization

With a robust segmentation performance, instruments are directly localized by selecting the largest connected component. The accuracy of instrument localization is evaluated in terms of instrument tip error, defined as the point-plane distance between the tip on the ground truth to the cross-section plane containing the instrument. The statistical results of errors in two different datasets are shown in the boxplots in Fig. 3(b). From the results, our proposed method achieves the best localization error less than 3 voxels.

4   Conclusion

In this paper, we have proposed a novel automatic instrument localization method for US-guided cardiac intervention therapy. In the proposed method, we design a network to provide segmentation of the instruments. With the aid of hybrid loss, the performance of the network achieved a Dice score of 69.6% and 65.8% in challenging *ex-vivo* and *in-vivo* datasets, respectively. Based on the proposed networks, the experiments show that our method obtains an instrument localization error that is less than 3 voxels without complex post-processing, which reduces the localization complexity and provides an accurate localization result.

References

1. Arif, M., Moelker, A., van Walsum, T.: Automatic needle detection and real-time bi-planar needle visualization during 3D ultrasound scanning of the liver. Med. Image Anal. **53**, 104–110 (2019)
2. Çiçek, Ö., Abdulkadir, A., Lienkamp, S.S., Brox, T., Ronneberger, O.: 3D U-Net: learning dense volumetric segmentation from sparse annotation. In: Ourselin, S., Joskowicz, L., Sabuncu, M.R., Unal, G., Wells, W. (eds.) MICCAI 2016. LNCS, vol. 9901, pp. 424–432. Springer, Cham (2016). https://doi.org/10.1007/978-3-319-46723-8_49
3. Dou, Q., Chen, H., Jin, Y., Yu, L., Qin, J., Heng, P.-A.: 3D deeply supervised network for automatic liver segmentation from CT volumes. In: Ourselin, S., Joskowicz, L., Sabuncu, M.R., Unal, G., Wells, W. (eds.) MICCAI 2016. LNCS, vol. 9901, pp. 149–157. Springer, Cham (2016). https://doi.org/10.1007/978-3-319-46723-8_18
4. Lin, T.Y., Dollár, P., Girshick, R., He, K., Hariharan, B., Belongie, S.: Feature pyramid networks for object detection. In: IEEE CVPR, pp. 2117–2125 (2017)
5. Pourtaherian, A., et al.: Medical instrument detection in 3-dimensional ultrasound data volumes. IEEE Trans. Med. Imaging **36**(8), 1664–1675 (2017)
6. Pourtaherian, A., Zanjani, F.G., Zinger, S., Mihajlovic, N., Ng, G.C., Korsten, H.H., et al.: Robust and semantic needle detection in 3D ultrasound using orthogonal-plane convolutional neural networks. IJCARS **13**(9), 1321–1333 (2018)
7. Wong, K.C.L., Moradi, M., Tang, H., Syeda-Mahmood, T.: 3D segmentation with exponential logarithmic loss for highly unbalanced object sizes. In: Frangi, A.F., Schnabel, J.A., Davatzikos, C., Alberola-López, C., Fichtinger, G. (eds.) MICCAI 2018. LNCS, vol. 11072, pp. 612–619. Springer, Cham (2018). https://doi.org/10.1007/978-3-030-00931-1_70
8. Yang, H., Shan, C., Kolen, A.F., de With, P.H.: Catheter detection in 3D ultrasound using triplanar-based convolutional neural networks. In: IEEE ICIP, pp. 371–375. IEEE (2018)
9. Yang, H., Shan, C., Pourtaherian, A., Kolen, A.F., et al.: Catheter segmentation in three-dimensional ultrasound images by feature fusion and model fitting. J. Med. Imaging **6**(1), 015001 (2019)
10. Yang, X., et al.: Towards automatic semantic segmentation in volumetric ultrasound. In: Descoteaux, M., Maier-Hein, L., Franz, A., Jannin, P., Collins, D.L., Duchesne, S. (eds.) MICCAI 2017. LNCS, vol. 10433, pp. 711–719. Springer, Cham (2017). https://doi.org/10.1007/978-3-319-66182-7_81

A Sparsely Distributed Intra-cardial Ultrasonic Array for Real-Time Endocardial Mapping

Alon Baram[1,2(✉)], Hayit Greenspan[1], and Zvi Freidman[2]

[1] Faculty of Engineering, Department of Biomedical Engineering,
Medical Image Processing Laboratory, Tel Aviv University, 69978 Tel Aviv, Israel
alontbst@gmail.com
[2] Biosense Webster (Israel) Ltd., 4 Hatnufa Street, 20692 Yokneam, Israel

Abstract. Cardiac arrhythmia is the clinical term for the family of diseases wherein the heart beats irregularly. Of these conditions, atrial fibrillation (AF) is one of the most prevalent and afflicts about 25% of the population of European descent over the age of 40. This condition leads to congestive heart failure, increases the risk of stroke five fold, impairs quality of life, causes hundreds of thousands hospitalizations in the US alone and is linked with increased mortality. Electrical pulmonary vein isolation (PVI) from the left atrial (LA) body is performed using ablation for treating AF. This and many other minimally invasive catheterizations, require real-time visualization and tracking of the LA endocardial surface. We propose a novel catheter based system incorporating ultrasound transducers mounted on a set of splines, and an algorithm capable of real time reconstruction of the chamber endocardial boundary, with almost no need for catheter movement or rotation. Unlike traditional ultrasound arrays, this catheter employs a small number of sparsely scattered transducer elements, far less than required by the Nyquist criterion, and a spherical field of view. Our concept had very little theoretical and practical known guarantees. We have developed novel methods to extract the blood pool location in space and validated them against reflecting tissue producing high contrast images of the boundary. We further validated our methods by extensive in-silico simulation studies and hardware phantom experiments. A prototype system is currently being built, following initial animal experimentation that further support the feasibility of this system in-vivo.

1 Introduction

Atrial fibrillation (AF) is the most prevalent form of cardiac rhythm disorders. It is estimated to affect 2.3 to 5.1 million people in the US alone. Due to aging of the population these numbers are expected to grow to some 5.6 to 12.1 million by 2050 [1]. AF is commonly triggered by ectopic pulses from the pulmonary veins of the left atrium (LA). Electro-anatomical mapping guided radiofrequency (RF) ablation is currently considered to be the procedure of choice to treat AF.

© Springer Nature Switzerland AG 2019
D. Shen et al. (Eds.): MICCAI 2019, LNCS 11768, pp. 272–280, 2019.
https://doi.org/10.1007/978-3-030-32254-0_31

The procedure requires percutaneous insertion of catheters into the heart and application of an alternating electrical currents in order to generate myocardial lesions for the purpose of electrical isolation of the pulmonary veins. Catheter ablation guided by electro-anatomic mapping (EAM) using CARTO or similar 3D mapping system is one of the most established, minimally invasive treatment choices for cardiac arrhythmia [4].

These systems guide the ablation by estimating and mapping the propagation of the activation wave over the endocardial surface. This is done by sampling points during the catheter's traversal of the heart's chamber, thus accumulating information sequentially point by point. After a significant number of points is gathered, a geometric reconstruction algorithm roughly estimates the endocardial surface. This process is very long, rendering the understanding of wave propagation for non-stationary rhythm disorders such as AF, which involves complex activation waves [7], difficult (Fig. 1).

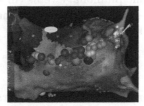 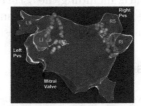

(a) LA electric propagation map

(b) LA physiology and typical ablation (red points)

Fig. 1. Clinical use of LA surface (Color figure online)

There are various other systems capable of endocardial imaging that are currently being used clinically. Of these Fluoroscopy is probably the most commonly used system for guiding cardiac procedures. Though inexpensive, it has several major disadvantages such as exposing patients and physicians to ionizing radiation, low soft tissue contrast, and providing only projections (2D) images. Other non-invasive methods include computerized tomography (CT) and magnetic resonance imaging (MRI) which provide high resolution 3D images. The former at the cost of high radiation exposure, and the latter is expensive with a limited availability in operating labs and not suitable for all patients and systems. Since the heart is not a rigid surface, its shape changes during breathing, heart beat, and the patient's pose. Thus, real time tracking of the shape is not feasible using the aforementioned devices due to their slow acquisition rate. Invasive imaging tools in the interventional laboratory include transesophageal echocardiography (TEE), intracardiac echocardiography (ICE) [3], intracardiac endoscopy [6], and EAM systems. Despite the additional risks inherent to the invasive nature of these tools, they can provide excellent real-time, detailed images that are often invaluable in guiding cardiac intervention. TEE and ICE are methods based on traditional ultrasound arrays while intracardiac endoscopy relies on fiber optics. All of those provide real time 2D and 3D images of sections from the heart chambers. The LA shape was reconstructed by sparse ICE scans in [5] using deep learning. The quality and visible areas depends on the system and method, but they always have limitations over their field of view, thus they require some catheter movement in order to see an entire chamber, or complex rotational mechanisms which makes them expensive [3]. Furthermore, due to anatomy and location restrictions not all areas can be visualized.

We have built and tested an ultrasonic system along with a novel algorithm that much more accurately maps the entire endocardial surface at a single glance. This, and the simultaneous mapping of the electrical activity at all points on the chamber surface is expected to result in a significant reduction of the overall procedural time in all scenarios including complex arrhythmias. Our proposed system is composed of a 64 elements, dual frequency ultrasonic array mounted on a "basket" spherical catheter. The array allows geometrical mapping of the entire endocardial surface, including the ostia of the pulmonary veins (in the case of the left atrium). We map the endocardial surface using a novel non-linear ellipsoidal extended Radon back-projection as described below.

2   Methods

In this section we describe our 2 dimensional basket-mounted intra-atrial ultrasonic array and develop the algorithm employed to segment the free space from the myocardium, using this array. The array consists of an ensemble Ω of N transmitting/receiving elements mounted on a spherical basket as illustrated in Fig. 5a, below. The array is operated in a synthetic aperture like mode, consisting of N transmit-receive events, in which a single element transmits followed by all elements jointly receiving. The objective is to find the locations and reflection coefficients of the scatters at the endocardial surface. Each transmitter s located at a position $x_s \in R^3$ is a source of a spherical pressure wave of the form $P_{x_s}(r,t) = p_0(t)\frac{1}{4\pi r}\delta(r - ct)$ where r is the distance from the transmitter, c is the velocity of sound in the medium, and $p_0(t)$ is the signal waveform. The wave is scattered from a point scatterer sc at x_{sc}, and received by a transducer element re at x_{re}. We denote $\Theta(el, X)$ as the angle between the normal to surface of the element $el \in \Omega$ and the vector from the element center to the point X. We denote $Dir(\Theta, ka)$ as the directivity factor which attenuates the signal as a function of Θ, wave number k and element radius a. The signal intensity measured at x_{re}. as function of the time t will be

$$S(s, sc, re) = \frac{cP_1 P_0(s)\delta(t - \frac{1}{c}(D(x_s, x_{sc}) + D(x_{sc}, x_{re})))Dir(\Theta_{s,sc}, ka)Dir(\Theta_{sc,re}, ka)}{16\pi^2 D(x_{re}, x_{sc})D(x_s, x_{sc})},$$

(1)

where $P_0(s)$ is the peak envelop ((the absolute value) of the complex envelop) of the signal transmitted from s, $P1$ is the scattering coefficient of the scatterer at sc, c is the speed of sound in the medium and $D(x, y) = \|x - y\|$ denotes the Euclidean distance between the two points x and y.

Definition 1. *For a transmitter-receiver pair* $s, re \in \Omega$ *at* $\boldsymbol{x}_s \in R^3$ *and* $\boldsymbol{x}_{re} \in R^3$, *respectively, all points* $\boldsymbol{x}_{sc} \in R^3$ *satisfying the equation* $c \cdot t_{s,sc,re} = D(\boldsymbol{x}_s, \boldsymbol{x}_{sc}) + D(\boldsymbol{x}_{sc}, \boldsymbol{x}_{re})$, *define an ellipsoid* $E \in R^3$ *such that its two foci* s *and* re *lie on its major axis of length* $c \cdot t_{s,sc,re}$.

It can be shown that:

Theorem 1. *All signals transmitted from* $\boldsymbol{x}_s$, *and scattered from all scatterers* $sc \in E(s, re, sc)$ *will be received at* $\boldsymbol{x}_{re}$ *simultaneously and coherently.*

We can now write:

Corollary 1. *The maximum signal envelop* $S(s, re, sc)$ *transmitted from* s *and received at* re *after* $t_{s,re,sc}$ *seconds, having been scattered from all reflectors* $sc \in E(s, re, sc)$ *is given by the elliptic Radon-like projection:*

$$S(s, re, sc) = \oint_{\boldsymbol{X} \in E(s, re, t_{sc})} \frac{P_1(\boldsymbol{X}) P_0(s) Dir(\Theta_{s,sc}, ka) Dir(\Theta_{sc,re}, ka) d\boldsymbol{X}}{16\pi^2 D(\boldsymbol{x}_{re}, \boldsymbol{x}_{sc}) D(\boldsymbol{x}_s, \boldsymbol{x}_{sc})},$$

(2)

where: $P_0(s)$ *is the maximum of the envelop of the signal transmitted from* s, *assumed to be positive and* s *independent and* $P_1(\boldsymbol{X})$ *is the reflection coefficient at* $\boldsymbol{X}$.

Definition 2 (Free Space). *The free space is the ensemble* F *of all points* $\boldsymbol{X}$, *for which* $P_1(\boldsymbol{X}) = 0$.

Using the fact that the entire group of transducer elements Ω is in the free-space and since the acoustic impedance of myocardial tissue is larger than that of blood it follows that for all scatterers $P_1(\boldsymbol{X}) \geq 0$. The triplets (s, re, sc); $sc \in E(s, re, sc)$; $s, re \in \Omega$ define all ellipsoids passing through the point sc whose foci are all transducer elements in Ω. Then since the integrand in Eq. 1 is non-negative it follows that

Theorem 2. *If* $S(s, re, sc) = 0$, *then* $P_1(\boldsymbol{x}_{sc}) = 0$. *so that* $sc \in F$, *or: the point* sc *is in the free space.*

Refer to Fig. 2c for an illustration. It is further easily shown that

Theorem 3. *Let* $\hat{S}(\boldsymbol{X}, s, re) = \frac{S(\boldsymbol{X}, s, re) 16\pi^2 D(\boldsymbol{x}_{re}, \boldsymbol{x}_{sc}) D(\boldsymbol{x}_s, \boldsymbol{x}_{sc})}{P_0(s) Dir(\Theta_{s,sc}, ka) Dir(\Theta_{sc,re}, ka)}$, *where* $s, re \in \Omega$ *then:* $P_1(\boldsymbol{X}) \leq \hat{S}$, *for all* $\boldsymbol{X}, s, re$.

Definition 3 (Bounding Reflection Value). *The bounding reflection value (BRV) is the defined for of all points* $\boldsymbol{X}$, *as follows*

$$\rho(\boldsymbol{X}) = \min_{s, re | \boldsymbol{X} \in E(s, re, sc); s, re \in \Omega} \hat{S}(\boldsymbol{X}, s, re).$$

(3)

The BRV is computed by segmenting a volume of $(10 \, cm)^3$ centered in the middle of the catheter and sampled using a 3 dimensional 2 mm grid. We segment the volume into a connected free space by using a region growing algorithm [2]

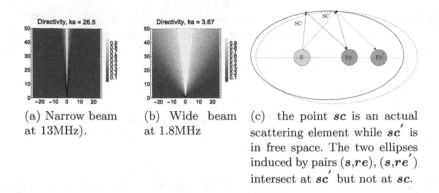

(a) Narrow beam at 13MHz).

(b) Wide beam at 1.8MHz

(c) the point sc is an actual scattering element while sc' is in free space. The two ellipses induced by pairs (s,re), (s,re') intersect at sc' but not at sc.

Fig. 2. Beam patterns and methods

with a seed at the volume center. The voxels at the perimeter of the resulting free space are referred to as the detected boundary points.

The wide beams may not be enough to distinguish between holes (PVs) and the endocardial surface, as in the case of an absence of an ellipsoid that is entirely in free space that intersects the interior of the PV, which is a common situation. Additional information about the free space can be acquired using the dependence of the emitter directivity pattern as function of the wavelength. We denote. The directivity for a piston model is proportional to $Dir(\Theta, ka) \propto \frac{2J_1(ka \sin \Theta)}{ka \sin \Theta}$, where J_1 is the first order Bessel function. Directivity can either produce wide beams suitable for the ellipsoidal back projection or narrow beams which provide a 'laser' like scan into a PV. Beams with interim width add information to the ellipsoidal back projection. Figure 2a and b shows the narrow and wide beams, respectively, which resonate in some of our newer elements. The narrow beams are used in first echo detection mode, that is, the space is free until it hits the first echo. This information is added to the wide beam scan to 'peek' inside PVs.

3   Experiments and Results

3.1   In-silico Experiment

A 64 elements transducer with a radius of 30mm radius was inserted into a left atrial model and placed at the center of a 10 cm side cube. The cube is divided into 50^3 voxels using a 2 mm 3 dimensional grid. A reflector is assigned to all grid points inside a 6 mm thick shell about the atrial boundary. Signals of a several cycles of 1.6 MHz and 7.4 MHz sine function with a Gaussian envelope, as seen in Fig. 3a were assumed. For each transducer element pair, the response for each reflector was appropriately time shifted and summed generating a simulated signal according to Eq. 1. Those were used to reconstruct volumes of wide and narrow responses as described in Sect. 2. Distances between detected boundary and simulated reflectors are shown in Fig. 3b, which describes two sided normalized distance probability. Since the distributions are skewed, we report the

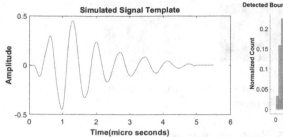
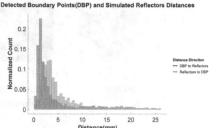

(a) Wide beam 1.6 MHz simulated signal template.

(b) Distances between detected boundary points and simulated reflectors.

Fig. 3. Simulation signal

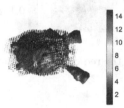
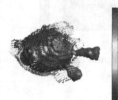
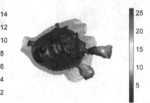

(a) Simulated reflectors to detected boundary points distances(mm) top view.

(b) Simulated Reflectors to detected boundary points distances(mm) side view.

(c) Detected boundary points to simulated reflectors distances(mm) side view.

Fig. 4. Simulation results

median and median absolute deviation (MAD) of the distances (in mm), which resulted in $1.99, 0.983$ (respectively) for the detected boundary to the reflectors and $3.377, 1.26$ (respectively) for the reflectors to boundary (Fig. 4).

3.2 In-vitro Experiments

System. A 64 element piezoelectric transducer array mounted on 12 pcb splines basket was built. Each transducer element has 2 resonance frequencies at about 1.6 MHz and 7.4 MHz, respectively. The elements were connected to an acquisition system built upon an NI platform capable of generating pulses and recording a sweep of sequential transmissions for all elements in real time. The catheter was placed in a water bath to simulate blood, enclosed in a ellipsoidal plastic enclosure, simulating the walls of a cardiac chamber.

The walls of the phantom were forced to move continuously by pumping water in and out, in order to simulate the natural cardiac wall-motion. Long time averages were then subtracted from all temporal signals in order to eliminate the constant signals caused by the reflections from the splines themselves. In all our

(a) The
catheter's
head.

(b) The
acquisition system
andphantom.

(c) Left atrium
silicon phantom.

Fig. 5. Hardware systems

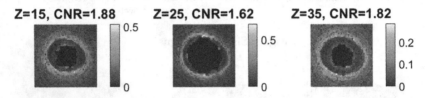

Z=15, CNR=1.88   **Z=25, CNR=1.62**   **Z=35, CNR=1.82**

Fig. 6. Slices of free space method volume along z-axis and the red detected boundary, CNR is contrast to noise ratio.

simulations we assumed that the locations of the transducers to be known. See Fig. 5a for the catheter, Fig. 5b the ellipsoid and Fig. 5c the left atrium phantoms.

Ellipsoidal Phantom Experiment. We placed the catheter in an ellipsoidal shaped phantom, having radii of 35, 32.5 and 22.5 mm, made of silicon water filled. Acquisition was performed using wide beams, as described in Sect. 2. The volume underwent dynamic range reduction using square root. An ellipsoid was fit to the boundary detected by the algorithm. Figure 6 shows slices of recorded volume with contrast to noise ratio (CNR) computed for pixel populations at 6 mm around the boundary. Figure 7 illustrates the fit and deviations of detected boundary. Note that the bottom portion is an outlier since the phantom is not a complete ellipsoid. This skews the error distribution, hence we report the median and MAD (which estimates standard deviation in a Gaussian distribution with a factor of around 1.5). Obtained radii were 36, 33.4 and 25.5, while the ellipsoid median deviation from the data is 1.4 mm and MAD is 0.6283 mm.

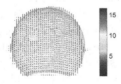

Fig. 7. Fitting an ellipsoid (in gray) to the detected boundary data. Color indicates distances from boundary points to the ellipsoidal fit (mm). Only the frontal half of the volume is shown.

Left Atrium Phantom Experiment. A silicon left atrium phantom, as shown in Fig. 5c, was scanned by our system using narrow and wide beams. The detected boundary points, along with six manually tagged points of anatomical interest were used as input to an anatomically aware, model based reconstruction algorithm [8]. We manually aligned the reconstructed anatomy with a ground truth CAD mesh and computed the difference from each vertex of the reconstruction to the ground truth mesh. Resulting mean, standard deviation, median, mad and RMS are 4.2, 4.4, 2.6, 1.77, 6.1 mm, respectively. Reconstruction result and error are depicted in Fig. 8. We see that the resulting model is close to the phantom, while the detected PVs are consistent with the CAD.

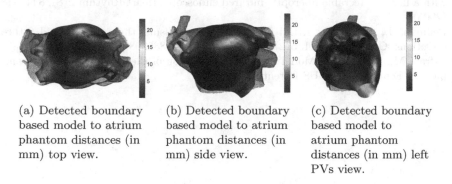

| (a) Detected boundary based model to atrium phantom distances (in mm) top view. | (b) Detected boundary based model to atrium phantom distances (in mm) side view. | (c) Detected boundary based model to atrium phantom distances (in mm) left PVs view. |

Fig. 8. Model based reconstruction

4   Conclusions

We have developed a system and method that is potentially capable of real-time detailed mapping of cardiac electrical activity. The system consists of a novel splines basket mounted multi-element sparse ultrasonic array and an algorithm for segmenting the endocardial border despite inaccuracies in element positioning. We validated the algorithm in extensive in-silico and in-vitro testings. The system will allow for the first time accurate diagnosis of complex arrhythmia in order to improve outcome of radio-frequency ablation treatment of the disorder, and reduce significantly the procedure time. The system concept and architecture are applicable for detailed study of the anatomy, perfusion, function and tissue characterization of the myocardium.

References

1. Calkins, H., et al.: 2017 HRS/EHRA/ECAS/APHRS/SOLAECE expert consensus statement on catheter and surgical ablation of atrial fibrillation. Europace **20**(1), e1–e160 (2018). 29016840[pmid]
2. Gozalez, R.C., Woods, R.E.: Digital image processing, 3rd edn. IEEE Trans. Biomed. Eng. (2013). https://doi.org/10.1109/TBME.2009.2017027

3. Kliger, C., Cruz-Gonzalez, I., Ruiz, C.E.: The present and future of intracardiac echocardiography for guiding structural heart disease interventions. Revista Española de Cardiología (English Edition) **65**(09), 791–794 (2012)
4. Knackstedt, C., Schauerte, P., Kirchhof, P.: Electro-anatomic mapping systems in arrhythmias. EP Europace **10**(suppl-3), iii28–iii34 (2008)
5. Liao, H., Tang, Y., Funka-Lea, G., Luo, J., Zhou, S.K.: More knowledge is better: cross-modality volume completion and 3D+2D segmentation for intracardiac echocardiography contouring. In: Frangi, A.F., Schnabel, J.A., Davatzikos, C., Alberola-López, C., Fichtinger, G. (eds.) MICCAI 2018. LNCS, vol. 11071, pp. 535–543. Springer, Cham (2018). https://doi.org/10.1007/978-3-030-00934-2_60
6. Nazarian, S., et al.: Direct visualization of coronary sinus ostium and branches with a flexible steerable fiberoptic infrared endoscope. Heart Rhythm **2**(8), 844–848 (2005)
7. Pellman, J., Sheikh, F.: Atrial fibrillation: mechanisms, therapeutics, and future directions. Compr. Physiol. **5**(2), 649–665 (2015). 25880508[pmid]
8. Safran, M., Bar-tal, M.: Model based reconstruction of the heart from sparse samples, 21 February 2017. US Patent 9,576,107

FetusMap: Fetal Pose Estimation in 3D Ultrasound

Xin Yang[1], Wenlong Shi[2,3], Haoran Dou[2,3], Jikuan Qian[2,3], Yi Wang[2,3],
Wufeng Xue[2,3], Shengli Li[4], Dong Ni[2,3(✉)], and Pheng-Ann Heng[1]

[1] Department of Computer Science and Engineering,
The Chinese University of Hong Kong, Hong Kong, China
[2] National-Regional Key Technology Engineering Laboratory for Medical Ultrasound,
Guangdong Key Laboratory for Biomedical Measurements and Ultrasound Imaging,
School of Biomedical Engineering, Health Science Center,
Shenzhen University, Shenzhen, China
nidong@szu.edu.cn
[3] Medical UltraSound Image Computing (MUSIC) Lab,
Shenzhen University, Shenzhen, China
[4] Department of Ultrasound, Affiliated Shenzhen Maternal and Child Healthcare,
Hospital of Nanfang Medical University, Shenzhen, China

Abstract. The 3D ultrasound (US) entrance inspires a multitude of automated prenatal examinations. However, studies about the structuralized description of the whole fetus in 3D US are still rare. In this paper, we propose to estimate the 3D pose of fetus in US volumes to facilitate its quantitative analyses in global and local scales. Given the great challenges in 3D US, including the high volume dimension, poor image quality, symmetric ambiguity in anatomical structures and large variations of fetal pose, our contribution is three-fold. (*i*) This is the first work about 3D pose estimation of fetus in the literature. We aim to extract the skeleton of whole fetus and assign different segments/joints with correct torso/limb labels. (*ii*) We propose a self-supervised learning (SSL) framework to finetune the deep network to form visually plausible pose predictions. Specifically, we leverage the landmark-based registration to effectively encode case-adaptive anatomical priors and generate evolving label proxy for supervision. (*iii*) To enable our 3D network perceive better contextual cues with higher resolution input under limited computing resource, we further adopt the gradient check-pointing (GCP) strategy to save GPU memory and improve the prediction. Extensively validated on a large 3D US dataset, our method tackles varying fetal poses and achieves promising results. 3D pose estimation of fetus has potentials in serving as a map to provide navigation for many advanced studies.

1   Introduction

Featured as real-time and radiation-free, ultrasound (US) is widely accepted in clinic for fetal health monitoring. Plenty of diagnostic biometrics can be automatically interpreted from the US images by recent researches. With broad

© Springer Nature Switzerland AG 2019
D. Shen et al. (Eds.): MICCAI 2019, LNCS 11768, pp. 281–289, 2019.
https://doi.org/10.1007/978-3-030-32254-0_32

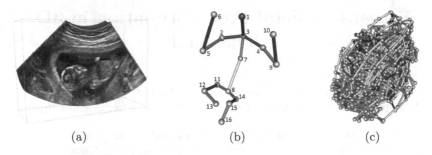

(a)   (b)   (c)

Fig. 1. 3D pose estimation of fetus in US volumes. (a) A sectional view of a fetus in US volume. (b) An instance of 3D fetal pose with 16 landmark indexes and 15 colored segments. (c) All the pose annotations of 152 fetuses in our dataset. Large variations exist when referring to (b). Better view in color version. (Color figure online)

field-of-view and low user dependency, the advent of 3D US further brings opportunities for automated solutions to attain precise descriptions of fetus [13].

However, currently, there still lacks a solution to provide structuralized descriptions for the whole fetus in 3D US. This description should facilitate not only the traditional tasks in local scale, like standard plane detection [2] and biometric measurements [11], but also the advanced analyses in global scale, like fetal movement pattern and longitudinal comparison. Therefore, we propose to approach this goal by exploring a new task dedicated to 3D pose estimation of fetus in US volumes. Specifically, as illustrated in Fig. 1(b), by localizing 16 landmarks of fetus in fully body, we aim to extract the skeleton of whole fetus and assign different segments/joints with correct torso/limb labels.

As shown in Fig. 1, estimating fetal pose in 3D US needs to tackle several challenges. *First*, the image quality of 3D US is relatively low due to the speckle noise, low resolution and acoustic shadows (Fig. 1(a)). *Second*, large variations in fetal pose, scale and orientation cause high image appearance variations, which not only generate the ambiguity in localizing symmetric landmarks but also degrade the generalization ability of automated methods (Fig. 1(b) and (c)). *Third*, accurate landmark localization heavily depends on the global context in the whole volume to suppress false positives. However, digesting the whole US volume with size about $200 \times 200 \times 200$ is very tough under limited computing resources.

Deep neural network is nowadays the dominant method for landmark detection in 3D US. A multi-task deep network was proposed in [7] for fetal eye localization in US volumes. Huang et al. exploited a semi-supervised learning method to localize 6 fetal head landmarks [5]. To use the geometric or class constraints, generative adversarial scheme was explored in [12] to regularize the landmark predictions. Although these methods are promising, the networks often suffer from their limited generalization ability, especially in our task, where fetuses have free poses with varying appearances. For 2D pose estimation, it has been well studied in computer vision field. Chen et al. proposed to learn the joint inter-connectivity prior in an adversarial scheme to refine the human pose prediction [4]. Liu et al. further distilled the articulated relationship between joints with recurrent neural network for feature boosting [6]. However, facing with the large volume and varying poses, these methods tend to be degraded as our experiments show.

In this paper, we try to tackle the challenges in 3D US for whole-body fetal pose estimation and generalize the landmark detection for large volumes. Our contribution is three-fold. (*i*) To the best of our knowledge, this is the first work about 3D pose estimation of fetus in the literature. We believe that taking the fetal pose estimation as a map, navigation can be generated to assist a series of advanced studies on automated prenatal examinations. (*ii*) We propose a self-supervised learning (SSL) framework to force the deep network to produce visually plausible pose predictions. Specifically, we leverage the landmark-based registration to effectively encode case-adaptive anatomical priors and generate evolving label proxy for supervision. The proxy is a suboptimal supervision but proves to be explicit in conveying prior knowledge for successive refinement. (*iii*) To enable our 3D deep network generate better features with higher resolution input under limited computing resource, we further adopt the gradient check-pointing (GCP) strategy to save GPU memory. With little computation overhead, GCP facilitates the training and inference of larger volumes and hence contributes to better localization performance. With extensive experiments on a large 3D US dataset, our proposed method deals with varying fetal poses and presents to be general with promising results.

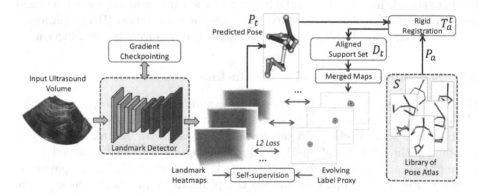

Fig. 2. Schematic view of our proposed framework for on-line refinement.

2   Methodology

Figure 2 is the overview of our proposed framework. System input is a whole US volume. A pre-trained deep network based landmark detector firstly digests the input and predicts the heatmap of 16 landmarks with an intermediate fetal pose estimation. By retrieving a support set of atlases in the pose library via rigid registration, label proxies are produced to form the self-supervision. The landmark detector is then tuned iteratively for on-line refinement. The system outputs the final pose estimation after a few number of iterations. Landmark detector is updated under the gradient checkpointing strategy in necessary.

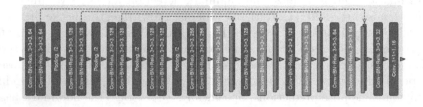

Fig. 3. Our proposed U-net like architecture for landmark detection.

2.1 Backbone of Landmark Detector

Since localizing fetal landmarks needs to consider both the global context and local details, as shown in Fig. 3, we build a 3D U-net [8] like network to simultaneously localize 16 landmarks of fetus in full body. Specifically, we deepen the network with consecutive convolutional (Conv) layers in a block and 4 pooling layers to encode high-level semantic features of the whole volume. Each Conv and deconvolutional (Deconv) is followed by a batch normalization (BN) layer and a rectified linear unit (ReLU). L2 regression loss is minimized as loss function.

2.2 Self-supervised Learning for On-Line Refinement

Due to the large variations of fetal pose, scale and orientation, deep networks for 3D fetal pose estimation in US often suffer from the low generalization ability when facing with varying and unseen fetal appearances. Anatomical prior is helpful for the problem [4,6]. However, these priors are often modeled in an indirect way and hard to take effect in our task (see Sect. 3). In this paper, as shown in Fig. 2, we propose to address the problem by producing direct shape prior for on-line refinement under a SSL scheme.

Supervising a model with the label proxy generated by the model itself and thus being annotation-free is the core idea of SSL. SSL changes classic testing fashion from simple inference to on-line learning. It fine-tunes the trained deep model with a label proxy. Strong guidance from the label proxy helps deep model update itself and generalize well to unseen cases. Recently, conditional random field [1] and interactive annotation [10] have been proposed to learn pixel-wise dependency to synthesize the label proxy in SSL. Whereas, these methods are intractable for our discrete landmark detection. Therefore, we propose to synthesize the landmark label proxy by combining the model prediction with the shape knowledge of a pose library.

$$\mathcal{D}_t = \underset{\mathcal{D}' \subset \mathcal{S}, |\mathcal{D}'|=K}{\arg \min} \sum_{a=1}^{N} \sum_{j=1}^{16} \| \mathrm{T}_a^t \times P_a^j - P_t^j \|_2, \tag{1}$$

As shown in Fig. 2, after being pre-trained on the training dataset, the landmark detector enters our SSL scheme for testing. Following the Eq. 1, for an unseen testing US volume of fetus, detector predicts its 16-channel landmark heatmaps and an intermediate 3D pose estimation P_t. Each atlas P_a in the pose library $\mathcal{S}$ is then aligned to P_t via a rigid transformation T_a^t. Since there often exist flaws in the landmarks of pose P_t, we only select a subset of landmarks P_t^j to calculate the T_a^t. Specifically, referring to Fig. 1, we choose the landmarks $j \in \{1, 2, 3, 4, 5, 7, 8, 9, 11, 14\}$ which can be robustly detected across the dataset and also have relatively small variances to fulfil the rigid registration conditions. By retrieving the top-K candidates with lowest registration errors, a support set of aligned atlas $\mathcal{D}_t$ is formed. $K = 10$ in this paper. Then, a 16-channel landmark label proxy is produced by averaging the landmark gaussian maps of the aligned atlases in $\mathcal{D}_t$. The label proxy will serve as the pseudo ground truth in iteration t to trigger the loss function. Landmark detector needs to update itself to refine its predictions and also the label proxy to minimize the loss.

Although the label proxy is initially rough, it encodes case-adaptive and strong shape prior which helps the detector to generalize to unseen US cases. The label proxy will evolve towards a suboptimal and case-specific state as the SSL iterates. Effectiveness of SSL will be elaborated in Sect. 3.

2.3   Enable Better Performance with Larger Input

Limited by GPU memory, 3D deep models often sacrifice the input size to enlarge network capacity. Plenty of content details are destroyed during the downscaling. Reducing the GPU memory consumption to break the bottleneck of input size is crucial for our task. In this work, we opt for the gradient checkpointing (GCP) strategy [3,9] to trade off the GPU memory usage with re-computation and make US volume with high resolution available for deep model.

As shown in Fig. 4, the core idea of GCP is discarding the data in some computation graph nodes after approaching a milestone node to make more GPU memory available for subsequent inference. The data of the discarded nodes will then be recovered by re-computation during backpropagation. Given an input x, data in node a is computed by the parameters of the F_1 function. Based on a and $F2$, node b is then approached. At this moment, the data in a will be discarded to release the occupied GPU memory. During the backward pass, to get the gradients of F_1 and F_2, node a will be recovered as a' by the re-computation from x and F_1. The gradient for the parameters of F_2 is calculated from a' and the gradient of b (b_grad). With a' as a transition node, the gradient for the parameters of F_1 ($F1\_paramgrad$) can be further obtained. Thus, without losing

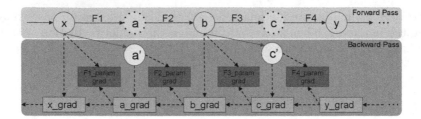

Fig. 4. Illustration of the forward pass and gradient re-computation in backward pass of the GCP. Dotted circle denotes the node in the computation graph to be emptied.

model accuracy, both the forward and backward passes can fit in the GPU. For our task, restricted by the skip connections, we manually select all the Conv layers except the Conv layers directly connected with the concatenation layer into the layer set for GCP. By using GCP to reduce GPU memory consumption, we can enable the network process US volumes with high resolution (enlarged as 1.25 times on each dimension).

3   Experimental Results

Materials and Implementation. We validate our method on a dataset of 152 fetal US volumes acquired from 152 pregnant volunteers with gestational age ranges from 10–14 weeks. Average size of volume is $220 \times 205 \times 260$. Voxel size is $0.5 \times 0.5 \times 0.5$ mm. Approved by local IRB, all volumes were anonymized and obtained by experts using a Mindray DC-8 system. Free fetal poses are allowed. An expert with 10-year experience manually annotated 16 landmarks. These 16 landmarks cover the fetal head, neck, shoulder, elbow, wrist, spine, sacra, hip joint, knee and ankle. We randomly split the dataset into 100/52 volumes for training/testing. Training set is augmented to 800 with flipping and rotation.

We implement our method in *Tensorflow*, using a standard PC with only one NVIDIA TITAN Xp GPU (12 GB). *Codes will be online available.* The original US volume is downscaled as *0.4* times before input into our basic landmark detector. *0.4* is the highest ratio allowed by the GPU for our network. With the GCP, we can enlarge the ratio to *0.5*. During the training of landmark detector on the training dataset, we update the weights with an Adam optimizer (batch size $= 1$, initial learning rate is *1e−3*, moment term is 0.5, epoch $= 20$). During the testing with SSL, initial learning rate is decreased to *5e−4*. Landmark detector runs on each testing case with SSL for 6 iterations (about 12 s in total). GCP is used for all the methods compared in this paper when it is needed. Training with GCP needs about 1.5 times of extra running time.

Quantitative and Qualitative Analysis. Two metrics are used to evaluate accuracy of pose estimation: the Euclidean distance (mm) between landmark prediction and ground truth, and the area under PCK curve (AUC, %), where PCK is the Percentage of Correct Key points, i.e., the percentage of detections with Euclidean distance below a threshold. With the basic landmark detector (Land) as backbone, we compared our SSL method with two typical refinement methods that explore the landmark dependency: (a) generative adversarial learning (GAN) [4,12] and (b) recurrent neural network (RNN) [6]. We implemented GAN by learning to classify the pair of US volume and 16-channel heatmaps, and RNN by adding a convolutional RNN layer to the last Conv layer of our landmark detector. GCP is applied to input when the downscale ratio is 0.5.

Table 1. Comparison of Euclidean distance in landmark localization

Method	Euclidean distance [mm] ↓																
	L1	L2	L3	L4	L5	L6	L7	L8	L9	L10	L11	L12	L13	L14	L15	L16	*mean*
Land-R4	1.75	6.69	2.54	7.18	8.85	11.1	2.57	3.31	9.87	13.7	4.34	9.23	7.22	3.84	6.69	6.46	*6.59*
LandGCP	1.74	8.78	2.54	5.59	6.39	6.40	2.15	2.39	11.5	11.1	2.97	6.27	5.05	2.36	5.91	4.49	*5.35*
RNN-R4	1.85	12.1	7.62	14.6	22.1	22.6	2.70	10.4	20.2	18.9	10.7	12.3	6.86	2.87	5.49	7.11	*11.14*
RNNGCP	1.76	9.47	5.93	13.5	18.1	14.9	4.45	10.4	17.1	15.0	4.41	7.27	5.56	5.33	7.11	5.35	*9.11*
GAN-R4	1.85	7.16	2.18	6.57	8.54	11.7	2.44	2.50	10.3	11.4	3.35	8.30	5.00	3.37	5.35	4.21	*5.89*
GANGCP	1.68	8.61	2.42	5.18	7.79	9.48	2.34	2.32	11.2	12.2	2.99	6.84	6.29	2.02	5.43	4.18	*5.69*
SSL-R4	1.72	5.00	2.36	4.37	6.81	13.3	2.56	3.19	8.40	10.8	3.32	6.45	7.40	2.93	4.63	4.26	*5.47*
SSLGCP	1.76	6.39	2.44	4.57	6.66	6.00	2.23	2.30	9.27	9.40	2.65	6.51	5.68	1.98	5.60	5.31	*4.92*

Table 2. Comparison of AUC in landmark localization

Method	AUC ratio [%] ↑																
	L1	L2	L3	L4	L5	L6	L7	L8	L9	L10	L11	L12	L13	L14	L15	L16	*mean*
Land-R4	81.4	56.5	75.5	50.1	47.5	32.3	72.8	74.0	48.0	28.4	63.6	27.3	44.9	61.8	48.1	49.4	*53.8*
LandGCP	82.5	48.4	74.8	61.0	65.6	51.8	78.4	75.9	45.7	35.8	70.4	46.5	49.7	76.6	51.7	55.7	*60.7*
RNN-R4	80.6	34.2	77.1	29.6	34.3	21.9	71.3	72.7	35.5	29.1	55.5	37.3	54.7	69.7	59.3	55.6	*51.2*
RNNGCP	82.8	40.3	77.3	36.5	35.5	36.2	75.5	76.0	26.6	27.5	58.1	43.9	51.3	62.4	54.0	60.0	*52.8*
GAN-R4	80.6	55.5	77.2	55.1	50.3	33.0	74.2	74.4	46.6	38.1	66.6	32.9	51.9	66.4	55.0	56.4	*57.1*
GANGCP	83.4	49.8	75.6	64.2	57.7	36.1	76.4	77.0	46.6	35.8	71.1	44.6	51.6	80.0	55.8	58.8	*60.3*
SSL-R4	81.8	61.9	75.9	65.6	56.7	22.0	73.0	75.3	56.8	37.8	65.1	46.8	42.4	70.1	63.0	57.0	*59.5*
SSLGCP	82.6	57.7	75.6	66.1	63.4	55.0	77.5	76.9	56.0	43.6	73.6	47.4	45.1	80.5	55.3	50.5	*62.9*

Table 1 presents the Euclidean distance of different methods for all the 16 landmarks. We use $R4$ to denote the model handling input with downscale ratio of 0.4, and GCP the method with GCP to handle input with larger downscale ratio of 0.5. As demonstrated in the table, almost all methods achieved lower prediction distance for all the landmarks with GCP, benefiting from its better features perceiving from higher resolution input. With this work, we are the first to prove that, GCP can improve landmark localization by enabling larger ultrasound volume input. Besides, although RNN and GAN based refinement methods bring improvements over the *Land*, they still perform obviously worse for some landmarks. With the case-adaptive label proxy as a strong prior, SSL based methods surpass the GAN/RNN and get almost the best results by achieving the top rank on 10 landmarks. The advantage of SSL can also be drawn from

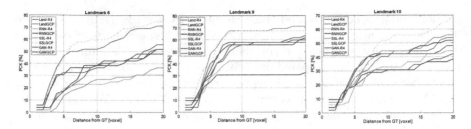

Fig. 5. PCK curves for 3 fetal landmarks. x axis is the distance threshold. *SSLGCP* (dotted green curve) gets the best results among all the competitors. (Color figure online)

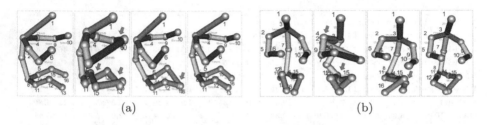

Fig. 6. Visualization of two 3D fetal pose estimations. From left to right: ground truth, *Land-R4*, *LandGCP* and *SSLGCP*. Blue digit for landmark index, green digit for length. (Color figure online)

the average prediction distance, according to which the proposed SSL achieves an average distance of 4.92 mm, and significantly outperforms the two competitors.

PCK evaluates the distribution of predicted landmarks around ground truth. Table 2 further compares the AUC of methods. Similar trends for GCP and SSL can be observed. SSL equipped with GCP (*SSLGCP*) tops the task of most landmark detections. It also achieves the highest mean AUC among all competitors. The highest improvement over the baseline *Land-R4*, about 20%, occurs on the detection of landmarks *L4, L6, L10, L12* and *L14*. Referring to Fig. 1, we can find that these are the symmetric landmarks on the limb which are hard to be differentiated by *Land, RNN* and *GAN* methods. We believe that both the strong shape prior from the evolving label proxy and the better feature input enabled by the GCP contribute to this significant improvement. We further provide the PCK curves of these landmarks from different methods in Fig. 5 for readers to check details.

In Fig. 6, we visualize two cases of fetal pose estimations to show the advantages of our method *SSLGCP*. *Land-R4* and *LandGCP* tend to be trapped by symmetric landmarks (green arrows), while our method can rectify these flaws and presents visually plausible estimations. As a byproduct of the pose estimation, the lengths of key segments of fetus are also produced in the 3D pose.

4   Conclusion

In this paper, we propose the first work about 3D fetal pose estimation in US volumes. We mainly tackle the challenges from the generalization ability with self-supervised learning and computation burden of large volumes with gradient checkpointing strategy. Extensive experiments prove the feasibility and effectiveness of our proposed method. We believe the pose estimation of fetus can serve as map and inspire the automated prenatal US image analyses.

Acknowledgments. The work in this paper was supported by the grant from Research Grants Council of Hong Kong SAR (Project No. CUHK14225616), National Natural Science Foundation of China (Project No. U1813204) and Shenzhen Peacock Plan (No. KQTD2016053112051497, KQJSCX20180328095606003).

References

1. Bai, W., et al.: Semi-supervised learning for network-based cardiac MR image segmentation. In: Descoteaux, M., Maier-Hein, L., Franz, A., Jannin, P., Collins, D.L., Duchesne, S. (eds.) MICCAI 2017. LNCS, vol. 10434, pp. 253–260. Springer, Cham (2017). https://doi.org/10.1007/978-3-319-66185-8_29
2. Baumgartner, C.F., et al.: SonoNet: real-time detection and localisation of fetal standard scan planes in freehand ultrasound. IEEE TMI **36**(11), 2204–2215 (2017)
3. Chen, T., Xu, B., Zhang, C., Guestrin, C.: Training deep nets with sublinear memory cost. arXiv preprint arXiv:1604.06174 (2016)
4. Chen, Y., Shen, C., et al.: Adversarial PoseNet: a structure-aware convolutional network for human pose estimation. In: ICCV, pp. 1212–1221 (2017)
5. Huang, R., Noble, J.A., Namburete, A.I.L.: Omni-supervised learning: scaling up to large unlabelled medical datasets. In: Frangi, A.F., Schnabel, J.A., Davatzikos, C., Alberola-López, C., Fichtinger, G. (eds.) MICCAI 2018. LNCS, vol. 11070, pp. 572–580. Springer, Cham (2018). https://doi.org/10.1007/978-3-030-00928-1_65
6. Liu, J., et al.: Feature boosting network for 3D pose estimation. IEEE TPAMI (2019)
7. Namburete, A.I., et al.: Fully-automated alignment of 3D fetal brain ultrasound to a canonical reference space using multi-task learning. MedIA **46**, 1–14 (2018)
8. Ronneberger, O., Fischer, P., Brox, T.: U-Net: convolutional networks for biomedical image segmentation. In: Navab, N., Hornegger, J., Wells, W.M., Frangi, A.F. (eds.) MICCAI 2015. LNCS, vol. 9351, pp. 234–241. Springer, Cham (2015). https://doi.org/10.1007/978-3-319-24574-4_28
9. Salimans, T., Bulatov, Y.: Saving memory using gradient-checkpointing. https://github.com/openai/gradient-checkpointing/
10. Wang, G., Li, W., et al.: Interactive medical image segmentation using deep learning with image-specific fine tuning. IEEE TMI **37**(7), 1562–1573 (2018)
11. Wu, L., et al.: Cascaded fully convolutional networks for automatic prenatal ultrasound image segmentation. In: ISBI, pp. 663–666. IEEE (2017)
12. Xu, Z., et al.: Less is more: simultaneous view classification and landmark detection for abdominal ultrasound images. In: Frangi, A.F., Schnabel, J.A., Davatzikos, C., Alberola-López, C., Fichtinger, G. (eds.) MICCAI 2018. LNCS, vol. 11071, pp. 711–719. Springer, Cham (2018). https://doi.org/10.1007/978-3-030-00934-2_79
13. Yang, X., Yu, L., et al.: Towards automated semantic segmentation in prenatal volumetric ultrasound. IEEE TMI **38**(1), 180–193 (2019)

Agent with Warm Start and Active Termination for Plane Localization in 3D Ultrasound

Haoran Dou[1,2], Xin Yang[3], Jikuan Qian[1,2], Wufeng Xue[1,2], Hao Qin[1,2],
Xu Wang[1,2], Lequan Yu[3], Shujun Wang[3], Yi Xiong[4], Pheng-Ann Heng[3],
and Dong Ni[1,2(✉)]

[1] National-Regional Key Technology Engineering Laboratory for Medical Ultrasound,
Guangdong Key Laboratory for Biomedical Measurements and Ultrasound Imaging,
School of Biomedical Engineering, Health Science Center,
Shenzhen University, Shenzhen, China
`nidong@szu.edu.cn`
[2] Medical UltraSound Image Computing (MUSIC) Lab,
Shenzhen University, Shenzhen, China
[3] Department of Computer Science and Engineering,
The Chinese University of Hong Kong, Hong Kong, China
[4] Department of Ultrasound, Luohu People's Hospital, Shenzhen, China

Abstract. Standard plane localization is crucial for ultrasound (US) diagnosis. In prenatal US, dozens of standard planes are manually acquired with a 2D probe. It is time-consuming and operator-dependent. In comparison, 3D US containing multiple standard planes in one shot has the inherent advantages of less user-dependency and more efficiency. However, manual plane localization in US volume is challenging due to the huge search space and large fetal posture variation. In this study, we propose a novel reinforcement learning (RL) framework to automatically localize fetal brain standard planes in 3D US. Our contribution is two-fold. First, we equip the RL framework with a landmark-aware alignment module to provide warm start and strong spatial bounds for the agent actions, thus ensuring its effectiveness. Second, instead of passively and empirically terminating the agent inference, we propose a recurrent neural network based strategy for active termination of the agent's interaction procedure. This improves both the accuracy and efficiency of the localization system. Extensively validated on our in-house large dataset, our approach achieves the accuracy of $3.4\,mm/9.6°$ and $2.7\,mm/9.1°$ for the transcerebellar and transthalamic plane localization, respectively. Our proposed RL framework is general and has the potential to improve the efficiency and standardization of US scanning.

1 Introduction

Acquisition of standard planes containing key anatomical structures is crucial for ultrasound (US) diagnosis. In prenatal US, typically dozens of standard planes

---

H. Dou and X. Yang—Contributed equally.

© Springer Nature Switzerland AG 2019
D. Shen et al. (Eds.): MICCAI 2019, LNCS 11768, pp. 290–298, 2019.
https://doi.org/10.1007/978-3-030-32254-0_33

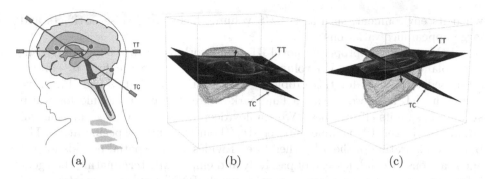

(a)   (b)   (c)

Fig. 1. Fetal brain planes in 3D US. (a) Blue lines show transthalamic (TT) and transcerebellar (TC) plane positions. Red dots (left to right) show three landmarks: genu of corpus callosum, splenium of corpus callosum, cerebellar vermis. (b)(c) Example planes from two volumes illustrate the huge search space and large fetal posture variation. (Color figure online)

are manually acquired for subsequent biometric measurements and diagnosis with a 2D US probe, such as the transthalamic (TT) and transcerebellar (TC) views for fetal brain assessment (Fig. 1). This process is very time-consuming and highly operator-dependent. In comparison, 3D US can contain multiple standard planes in just a single shot and has the inherent advantages of less user-dependency and more efficiency [7]. However, it is very challenging to manually localize standard planes in the volume due to the huge search space, the large fetal posture variability and the low image quality, as shown in Fig. 1. Therefore automatic localization of standard planes in 3D US is highly expected to improve diagnostic efficiency and decrease operator-dependency.

In recent years, some research on standard plane localization in 3D US has been conducted accordingly. Ryou et al. proposed a three-step learning method to sequentially localize the fetus, the fetal parts and detect biometry planes by classification [9]. This method narrowed the search space in the localized structures and the axial direction. Regression methods were also employed to localize cardiac planes by Random Forests [2] and the fetal abdominal plane by deep networks [10]. However, these methods tend to fail when acoustic shadow and occlusion spread in US during late pregnancy. Lorenz et al. proposed to extract the abdomen plane by detecting anatomical landmarks and aligning them to a fetal organ model [5]. The system achieved accuracy of $5.8\,mm/15.9°$ for plane localization. Although effective by using prior anatomical knowledge, the method's performance is limited by landmark detection accuracy and testing case-model difference. More recently, Li et al. proposed an iterative deep network to localize fetal brain planes in 3D US [4]. They further customized a reinforcement learning (RL) agent for view planning in MR volumes [1]. RL is promising for standard plane localization in 3D US due to its ability of mimicking experts' operation and exploring inter-plane dependency by the agent-environment interaction. However, RL may suffer from its random initialization and empirical termination when its environment, such as the US volume, has strong noise, artifacts and large appearance variations.

In this paper, we propose a novel RL framework to localize fetal brain standard planes in prenatal US volumes. We believe we are the first to employ RL-based techniques for this problem. Our contribution is two-fold. First, we equip the RL framework with a landmark-aware alignment module for warm start to ensure its effectiveness. We employ deep networks to detect anatomical landmarks in the US volume and register them to a plane-specific atlas. The plane configuration of the atlas therefore provides strong spatial bounds for RL agent actions. Second, instead of passively and empirically terminating the agent inference, we propose a recurrent neural network (RNN) based strategy for active termination of the agent's interaction procedure. The RNN-based strategy can find the optimal termination point adaptively, so it improves the accuracy and efficiency of the localization system at the same time.

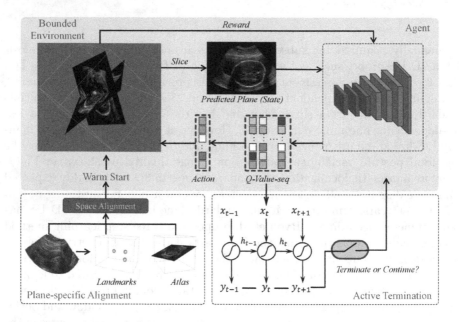

Fig. 2. Schematic view of our proposed framework.

2   Methodology

Figure 2 is the schematic view of our proposed framework. We propose to localize fetal brain standard planes in US volumes with a RL framework, which can progressively interact with the volumes and modify the search trajectory towards the final target plane. Specifically, we equipped the RL framework with (1) a landmark-aware alignment module for warm start, to ensure its effectiveness, and also (2) a recurrent neural network based strategy for active termination of the interaction procedure, to improve its accuracy and efficiency.

2.1 Deep Reinforcement Learning Framework for Plane Localization

The task of plane localization in US volumes can be well modeled under the RL framework, where an agent, in its current state s, interacts with the environments $\mathcal{E}$ by making successive actions $a \in \mathcal{A}$ that maximize the expectation of reward. Let a plane in Cartesian coordinate system be represented as $cos(\alpha)x + cos(\beta)y + cos(\phi)z + d = 0$, where $n = (cos(\alpha), cos(\beta), cos(\phi))$ is the normal, d is the distance from the plane to the volume center origin. The system will obtain the optimal plane parameters as the agent interacts with the environment.

Similar to [1], we define the action space as 8 actions, $\{\pm a_\alpha, \pm a_\beta, \pm a_\phi, \pm a_d\}$. After an action is made by the agent, the plane parameters are accordingly updated as $\alpha_t = \alpha_{t-1} + a_\alpha, \beta_t = \beta_{t-1} + a_\beta, \phi_t = \phi_{t-1} + a_\phi, d_t = d_{t-1} + a_d$. Each valid action gets its scalar reward r following the rule $r = sgn(D(P_{t-1}, P_g) - D(P_t, P_g))$, where D calculates the Euclidean distance from the predicted plane P_t to the ground truth P_g. $r \in \{+1, 0, -1\}$ indicates whether the agent is moving towards the preferred target.

With the reward signal, the agent then maximizes both the current and future rewards to obtain the action-selection policy. Following the Q-learning, Deep Q-Network [6] (DQN) can learn a state-action value function, $Q(s, a)$, via deep networks to serve as the action-selection policy. To improve the robustness of DQN against the noisy environment $\mathcal{E}$ in 3D US, we finally choose the Double DQN (DDQN) [11] as our deep agent for plane localization. The loss function for our DDQN is defined as:

$$\mathcal{L}_{DDQN}(w) = E_{s,r,a,\hat{s} \sim M}\left[\left(r + \gamma \max_{\hat{a}} Q(\hat{s}, Q(\hat{s}, a; w); \tilde{w}) - Q(s, a; w)\right)^2\right], \quad (1)$$

where $\gamma = 0.9$ is a discount factor to weight future rewards, $\hat{s}$ and $\hat{a}$ are the state and action in the next step. M is the experience replay memory to avoid frequent data sampling. w and $\tilde{w}$ are the current and target network parameters. Specifically, we select an ImageNet pre-trained $VGG-13$ as our current and target networks. Three recently predicted planes serve as the network input.

2.2 Landmark-Aware Plane Alignment for Warm Start

To ensure an effective interaction of the RL agent with the noisy 3D US environment, we propose a landmark-aware plane alignment module to leverage anatomical prior and provide a warm start for the agent. Specifically, we first detect three landmarks of fetal brain, i.e, the genu of corpus callosum, splenium of corpus callosum and cerebellar vermis, as shown in Fig. 1(a), with a customized 3D U-net [8]. Then these landmarks are used to align the testing volume with the atlas, which contains both the reference landmarks and standard plane parameters. Different from [5,7] which apply a common anatomical model to all kinds of standard planes, we propose to select specific atlas for each plane to improve

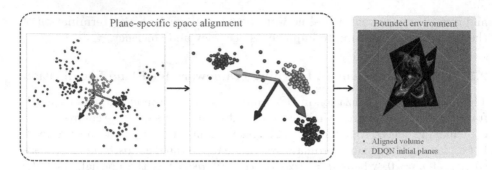

Fig. 3. Landmarks of 100 US volumes (left) aligned to a place-specific atlas space (middle) provides strong spatial bounds for RL agent actions (right). Red, green and blue dots indicate landmarks shown in Fig. 1(a). (Color figure online)

the localization accuracy. Finally, standard planes of atlas are mapped to testing volumes and serve as a warm start for our RL agent. Atlas selection for a type of standard plane P is formulated as following,

$$\mathcal{X}_P^{atl} = \min_i \sum_i^N \sum_j^N \left(\Theta(\mathrm{T}_j^i \times \boldsymbol{n}_P^j, \boldsymbol{n}_P^i) + \parallel d_P^j - d_P^i \parallel_1 \right), i \neq j. \tag{2}$$

where i, j are volume index. $\boldsymbol{n}_P^i$ is the normal of P in volume i, Θ calculates the angle between normals, d_P^i is the distance from plane P in volume i to origin. T_j^i is the transformation matrix from volume j to i, which is determined by the landmark annotation based rigid registration. Figure 3 shows the effect of our landmark alignment for 100 volumes. The accurate alignment guarantees the effectiveness of the initial point for RL agent and therefore leads to fast and improved plane localization.

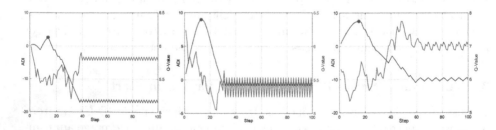

Fig. 4. Mean Q-value of 8 action candidates (yellow) and ADI (blue) on training dataset. Green point denotes the optimal termination step with maximum ADI. (Color figure online)

2.3 Recurrent Neural Network Based Active Termination

To ensure an efficient interaction of the RL agent, we propose a RNN-based active termination (AT) module to tell the agent when to stop. Usually, there is no well-defined criteria to terminate the iterative inference of RL learning. Under- and over-estimation of the termination state often degrade the final localization. Existing work makes use of a predefined maximum step, a lower Q-value [1] or oscillation of Q-value [3] as an indicator of termination. While the first one wastes a lot of computation resource if it's set to a large number, the latter two do not necessarily lead to the optimal results. As shown in Fig. 4, the optimal termination step with highest angle and distance improvement (ADI) is neither the maximum step nor the step with the lowest Q-value. This motivates us to propose a novel strategy to actively learn the optimal step. Specifically, considering the sequential characteristics of the iterative inference, as shown in Fig. 2, we formulate the mapping between the Q-value sequence and optimal step with recurrent neural networks.

The Q-values of 8 action candidates at each state serve as an input of our RNN, which then learns to output the optimal termination step with highest ADI, i.e., most significant angle and distance improvement. We train the RNN model with the inference results of the agent on our training volumes. During testing, our method terminated the iteration action of the agent according to the RNN output and get the final plane parameters. With this active termination mechanism, our agent can make efficient inference without excessive iterations.

3 Experimental Results

Materials and Implementation Details. We validate our solution on the task of localizing two standard planes (TT and TC) of fetal brain in US volumes. We built a dataset of 430 prenatal US volumes acquired from 430 healthy pregnant women volunteers. Approved by local Institutional Review Board, all volumes were anonymized and obtained by experts using a Mindray DC-9 US system with an integrated 3D probe. Free fetal poses are allowed during scanning. Gestational age ranges from 19 to 31 weeks, much broader than [4,7]. Average volume size of our dataset is $270 \times 207 \times 235$ and unified voxel size is $0.5 \times 0.5 \times 0.5 \, mm^3$. A sonographer with 5-year experience provided manual annotation of landmarks and standard planes for all the volumes. We then randomly split the dataset into 330 and 100 volumes for training and testing.

We implemented our framework in *PyTorch*, using a standard PC with a NVIDIA TITAN X(PASCAL) GPU. We trained the DDQN with Adam optimizer (learning rate $= 5e-5$) for 100 epochs (about 4 days). Replay-buffer is set as 15000. Target network copies the parameters of current network every 2000 iterations. For training RNN variants (vanilla RNN and LSTM), optimizer is Adam with L1 regression loss, batch size $= 100$, hidden size $= 64$ and epoch $= 200$ (about 15 min). The starting planes for training DDQN are randomly initialized around the ground truth plane within an angle range of $\pm25°$ and distance range of $\pm10 \, mm$. The range is determined by the average plane localization error of

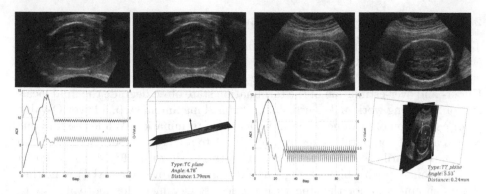

Fig. 5. TC (left) and TT (right) results. *Top row:* ground truth (left) and predicted (right) plane. *Bottom row:* left, active termination step (dotted red line) compared to optimal step in green dot, 3D visualization of ground truth and predicted plane (right). (Color figure online)

Table 1. Quantitative evaluation of our proposed framework.

Method	TC			TT		
	Ang (°)↓	Dis (mm)↓	SSIM↑	Ang (°)↓	Dis (mm)↓	SSIM↑
Regress	27.04 ± 8.40	4.10 ± 3.81	0.672 ± 0.087	24.27 ± 17.05	7.62 ± 6.00	0.507 ± 0.100
AtlasRegist	14.14 ± 7.54	3.40 ± 2.28	0.681 ± 0.148	13.43 ± 4.63	2.62 ± 1.54	0.682 ± 0.138
RegistRegress	12.44 ± 7.78	2.18 ± 2.12	0.684 ± 0.157	13.87 ± 11.77	2.80 ± 2.16	0.660 ± 0.141
DDQN-nA	31.54 ± 24.24	5.12 ± 3.67	0.685 ± 0.131	30.44 ± 24.43	5.03 ± 3.82	0.615 ± 0.132
DDQN-maxS	11.71 ± 14.32	3.53 ± 2.55	0.684 ± 0.165	12.36 ± 8.53	2.95 ± 2.94	0.694 ± 0.154
DDQN-minQ	10.68 ± 9.76	3.40 ± 2.27	0.688 ± 0.165	10.78 ± 7.62	2.62 ± 1.54	0.705 ± 0.163
DDQN-AT(FC)	10.36 ± 9.60	3.40 ± 2.28	0.689 ± 0.165	9.61 ± 5.79	2.66 ± 1.55	0.707 ± 0.161
DDQN-AT(RNN)	9.96 ± 10.19	3.41 ± 2.27	0.691 ± 0.167	9.53 ± 5.74	2.64 ± 1.62	0.709 ± 0.164
DDQN-AT(LSTM)	9.61 ± 8.97	3.40 ± 2.77	0.693 ± 0.168	9.11 ± 5.56	2.66 ± 2.06	0.709 ± 0.163

atlas based registration. For landmark detection (Adam optimizer, batch size = 1, learning rate = 0.001, moment is 0.5, epoch = 40), limited by GPU memory, US volume is resized as 0.4 times for training. Gaussian maps of landmarks are generated as ground truth. L2 loss is used for training. Iterative Closest Point algorithm is used for the rigid registration between testing case and atlas.

Quantitative and Qualitative Analysis: The efficacy of our proposed method was validated with 100 US volumes and results were demonstrated in Table 1. We adopt both spatial and content similarities to evaluate the performance, including the dihedral angle between two planes (Ang), difference of Euclidean distance to origin (Dis), and Structural Similarity Index (SSIM).

- Firstly, the proposed RL agent (DDQN-AT) has good performance on localizing two types of standard planes, and outperforms the regression-based method (Regress), the registration-based method (AtlasRegist) and their combination (RegistRegress). This can be attributed to the active interaction procedure of the agent that searches along the trajectory towards the optimal plane.

- Secondly, as can be clearly drawn from the table, when the landmark-aware space alignment module is employed on DDQNs as a warm start, they achieve significantly better performance on standard plane localization than the method without alignment (DDQN-nA). Besides, the proposed space alignment module can also be deployed in the regression model and lead to clear improvement (RegistRegress).
- Thirdly, the proposed active termination can lead to better localization with much less inference iterations. Compared to other termination policies, such as maximum step (DDQN-maxS) and minimum Q-value (DDQN-minQ), our AT based methods generally give better localization performances. Among them, DDQN-AT (LSTM) shows the best results, since it has stronger capacity in learning from the Q-value sequence. More importantly, with AT module equipped, our RL-agent requires an average of 13 steps to localize the standard planes, in comparison with 100 steps that no AT module was employed. Given the fact that such iteration steps cost most computation, the AT module will definitely improve the efficiency of the RL agent.

In Fig. 5, we visualize two testing results of DDQN-AT (LSTM) for TC and TT plane localization. Compared from image content and spatial relationship, for both tasks, our method accurately captures the plane, which is very close to the ground truth. Our active termination strategy also presents the ability to learn from the Q-value sequence and hits the optimal termination step (green dot) for large angle and distance improvement (ADI).

4   Conclusion

We proposed a general framework for standard plane localization in 3D US with a RL agent. We use a landmark-aware alignment model to exploit prior information about the standard planes from the atlas and provide the agent with an effective warm starting point. In addition, we devise a RNN-based active termination strategy to indicate the agent to stop once the optimal plane is localized, therefore improving its accuracy and efficiency. Experiments on our in-house large dataset validate the efficacy of our method and reveal its great potential for future practical applications.

Acknowledgments. The work in this paper was supported by the grant from National Natural Science Foundation of China (No. 61571304), Shenzhen Peacock Plan (No. KQTD2016053112051497, KQJSCX20180328095606003), Medical Scientific Research Foundation of Guangdong Province, China (No. B2018031) and National Natural Science Foundation of China (Project No. U1813204).

References

1. Alansary, A., et al.: Automatic view planning with multi-scale deep reinforcement learning agents. In: Frangi, A.F., Schnabel, J.A., Davatzikos, C., Alberola-López, C., Fichtinger, G. (eds.) MICCAI 2018. LNCS, vol. 11070, pp. 277–285. Springer, Cham (2018). https://doi.org/10.1007/978-3-030-00928-1_32
2. Chykeyuk, K., Yaqub, M., Alison Noble, J.: Class-specific regression random forest for accurate extraction of standard planes from 3D echocardiography. In: Menze, B., Langs, G., Montillo, A., Kelm, M., Müller, H., Tu, Z. (eds.) MCV 2013. LNCS, vol. 8331, pp. 53–62. Springer, Cham (2014). https://doi.org/10.1007/978-3-319-05530-5_6
3. Ghesu, F.C., et al.: Multi-scale deep reinforcement learning for real-time 3D-landmark detection in CT scans. IEEE TPAMI 41(1), 176–189 (2019)
4. Li, Y., et al.: Standard plane detection in 3D fetal ultrasound using an iterative transformation network. In: Frangi, A.F., Schnabel, J.A., Davatzikos, C., Alberola-López, C., Fichtinger, G. (eds.) MICCAI 2018. LNCS, vol. 11070, pp. 392–400. Springer, Cham (2018). https://doi.org/10.1007/978-3-030-00928-1_45
5. Lorenz, C., Brosch, T., et al.: Automated abdominal plane and circumference estimation in 3D US for fetal screening. In: Medical Imaging 2018: Image Processing, vol. 10574, p. 105740I (2018)
6. Mnih, V., Kavukcuoglu, K., et al.: Human-level control through deep reinforcement learning. Nature 518(7540), 529 (2015)
7. Namburete, A.I., Stebbing, R.V., Noble, J.A.: Diagnostic plane extraction from 3D parametric surface of the fetal cranium. In: MIUA, pp. 27–32 (2014)
8. Ronneberger, O., Fischer, P., Brox, T.: U-Net: convolutional networks for biomedical image segmentation. In: Navab, N., Hornegger, J., Wells, W.M., Frangi, A.F. (eds.) MICCAI 2015. LNCS, vol. 9351, pp. 234–241. Springer, Cham (2015). https://doi.org/10.1007/978-3-319-24574-4_28
9. Ryou, H., Yaqub, M., Cavallaro, A., Roseman, F., Papageorghiou, A., Noble, J.A.: Automated 3D ultrasound biometry planes extraction for first trimester fetal assessment. In: Wang, L., Adeli, E., Wang, Q., Shi, Y., Suk, H.-I. (eds.) MLMI 2016. LNCS, vol. 10019, pp. 196–204. Springer, Cham (2016). https://doi.org/10.1007/978-3-319-47157-0_24
10. Schmidt-Richberg, A., Schadewaldt, N., et al.: Offset regression networks for view plane estimation in 3D fetal ultrasound. In: Medical Imaging 2019: Image Processing, vol. 10949, p. 109493K (2019)
11. Van Hasselt, H., Guez, A., Silver, D.: Deep reinforcement learning with double q-learning. In: AAAI, pp. 1234–1241 (2016)

Learning and Understanding Deep Spatio-Temporal Representations from Free-Hand Fetal Ultrasound Sweeps

Yuan Gao$^{(\boxtimes)}$ and J. Alison Noble

Biomedical Image Analysis Group, Institute of Biomedical Engineering,
Department of Engineering Science, University of Oxford, Oxford, UK
Yuan.Gao2@eng.ox.ac.uk

Abstract. Identifying structures in nonstandard fetal ultrasound planes is a significant challenge, even for human experts, due to high variability of the anatomies in terms of their appearance, scale and position but important for image interpretation and navigation. In this work, our contribution is three-fold: (i) we model local temporal dynamics of video clips, by applying convolutional LSTMs on the intermediate CNN layers, which learns to detect fetal structures at various scales; (ii) we proposed an attention-gated LSTM, which generates spatio-temporal attention maps showing the intermediate process of structure localisation; and (iii) our approach is end-to-end trainable, and the localisation is achieved in a weakly supervised fashion i.e. with only image-level labels available during training. The proposed attention-mechanism is found to improve the detection performance substantially in terms of classification precision and localisation correctness.

Keywords: Spatial-temporal neural network · Soft attention · Weakly supervised detection · Non-standard fetal scan planes

1 Introduction

Fetal ultrasound screening requires highly experienced sonographers. This makes it difficult for a wider adoption of clinical ultrasound for pregnancy care, especially in low-and-middle-income settings, where there is a substantial lack of experienced sonographers. Therefore, automated scan plane detection algorithms would greatly assist non-expert examination. However, most published algorithms to date only consider detection of standard scan planes, and treat non-standard scan planes as background. Towards more general recognition and navigation, it is necessary to automate the detection and interpretation of contents in non-standard fetal planes. In this work, we present an automated fine-detection

Electronic supplementary material The online version of this chapter (https://doi.org/10.1007/978-3-030-32254-0_34) contains supplementary material, which is available to authorized users.

© Springer Nature Switzerland AG 2019
D. Shen et al. (Eds.): MICCAI 2019, LNCS 11768, pp. 299–308, 2019.
https://doi.org/10.1007/978-3-030-32254-0_34

system that not only recognizes the standard scan planes but also non-standard planes. This is a more challenging problem due to the need to accommodate greater variations in imaging quality, and high variability of fetal structures in terms of scale, appearance and location.

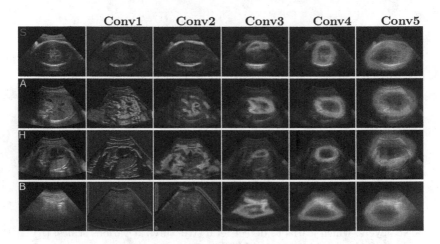

Fig. 1. Class-specific features learned at different layers of a ConvNet. Left-Right: last frame in a sequence, Conv1, Conv2, Conv3, Conv4, Conv5 layers. S: Skull, A: Abdomen, H: Heart, B: Background. (Color figure online)

Contributions: In this paper, we introduce a novel attention-gated spatio-temporal neural network (as depicted in Fig. 2), trained in a weakly supervised fashion, for detection of key fetal structures of interest (skull, abdomen and heart) in consecutive frames. (1) We apply convolutional LSTMs [1] not solely on the top layer but also on the intermediate features of a convolutional neural network (CNN), to characterise temporal dynamics of features extracted at different scales (as illustrated in Fig. 1). (2) We extend the convolutional LSTMs to be attention-gated, regularised by a doubly stochastic mechanism [2] that encourages to fully exploit spatial-temporal information, and more importantly, provides visual evidence of structures localisation. (3) Finally, we investigate the effect of global pooling (average and max) on class activation mapping.

Related Works: Recently, deep learning has become popular for analysing 2D fetal ultrasound sweeps. [3] and [4] have exhibited state-of-the-art performance in still image tasks such as classification or detection. However, such models discard temporal information that for human interpretation we know provides important cues in videos. This is a particularly significant problem for detecting cardiac views. Several recent works [5,6] and [7] have taken temporal context into account for fetal structure recognition. Chen et al. [5] proposes a recurrent network for detection of standard fetal ultrasound planes, in which they apply LSTMs built on whole image features that completely discard spatial correspondence between frames. Gao et al. [6] proposed a two stream ConvNet, learning spatio-temporal representations to detect the fetal heartbeat in ultrasound videos, which demonstrated a substantial improvement in correctly identifying heart frames. A closely related work to ours is Huang et al. [7] that incorporates a convolutional recurrent layer working at a local region level of the frames. However, and in contrast to our work, the recurrent design is only applied on the coarsest feature map extracted from the CNN. We argue that this design is more likely to focus on global appearance changes and is not well-suited to capture fine local details, which is nontrivial in our case. In addition, Schlemper et al. [8] proposed a soft attention gated network for improving ultrasound scan plane detection, which is actually an improved SonoNet [5]. However, our work is different in two distinct ways: firstly we propose a general detection framework, not only detecting different anatomies in standard scan planes but also non-standard ones, whilst [5] and [8] only detect standard scan planes and treat non-standard planes as background. Secondly, [8] focuses on aggregating spatial features with spatial attention which did not explore temporal variations and aggregation.

2 Methodology

We present the architecture of our proposed model in Fig. 2. Overall, the model consists of a CNN for extracting appearance features from consecutive frames and an Attention Gated LSTM for processing the CNN features recurrently at different locations, exploring temporal variation by selectively attending to different regions of the spatial features maps at different levels.

CNN Architecture: Inspired by a VGG very deep architecture [9], we adopt the configuration that increases CNN depth using very small convolution filters stacked with non-linearity injected in between. All convolution layers consist of 3×3 kernels, batch normalization and Rectified Linear Units. The full architecture, using shorthand notation, is $2\times$ $C(32,3,1)$-MP-$2\times$ $C(64,3,1)$-MP-$3\times$ $C(128,3,1)$-MP-$3\times$ $C(256,3,1)$-MP-$3\times$ $C(256,3,1)$-MP, where $C(d,f,s)$ indicates a convolution layer with d filters of spatial size $f \times f$, applied to the input with stride s. MP represents non-overlapping max-pooling operation with a kernel size of 2×2.

Attention Gated LSTM: The Attention Gated LSTM consists of an attention module and a convolutional LSTM, which are illustrated in Fig. 2 showing their inner structure. The max pooled convolutional maps $(X_t^l, ..., X_t^{L-1}, X_t^L)_{(t=1...T)}$, extracted form L layers (L = 5 in our CNN) at different time steps in a video, are composed of patterns with strong local correlation over time, and temporal vitiations (e.g. heart beating) tend to be smooth and restricted in a local spatial

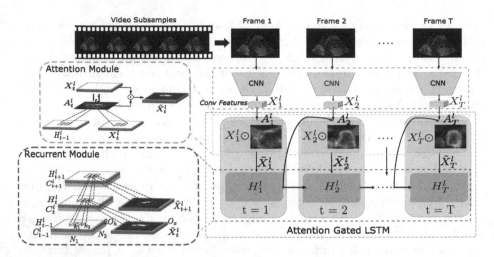

Fig. 2. Network Overview. **CNN feature maps** are fed to the **Attention Module** to generate an attention map at each time step, then the attention-warped (element-wise product) feature maps are fed to the **Recurrent Module** to update the hidden states.

neighbourhood in successive frames. Therefore, we embed such a prior in our model by replacing the fully connected LSTM gates (i.e. input gates, forget gates etc) with convolution operations. The convolutional kernels (3×3) are chosen to be significantly smaller than the intermediate convolutional map size for computational efficiency.

As noted in Fig. 2, instead of directly applying the convolutional maps to the LSTMs, we introduce a soft attention mechanism, conditioned on the convolutional maps X_t^l and their latest hidden state H_{t-1}^l, which learns to focus on salient regions over time:

$$att_t^l = W^l * tanh(W_a^l * X_t^l + U_a^l * H_{t-1}^l + b_a) \qquad (1)$$

where again the gating units are characterised by a set of small 2D-convolution kernels: $W_a^l \in \mathbb{R}^{3 \times 3 \times O_x \times O_h}$, $U_a^l \in \mathbb{R}^{3 \times 3 \times O_h \times O_h}$, $W^l \in \mathbb{R}^{3 \times 3 \times O_h \times 1}$ and bias term $b_a \in \mathbb{R}^{O_h}$. $tanh$ is non-linearity activation function. The output of this operations is a 2D map from which a normalised attention map is computed through the equation:

$$A_t^l(i,j) = p(att_{ij} | X_t^l, H_{t-1}^l) = \frac{\sigma(att_t^l(i,j))}{\sum_i \sum_j \sigma(att_t^l(i,j))} \qquad (2)$$

where $A_t^l(i,j)$ is the element of the attention map in position (i, j), *sigma* is a sigmoid unit. The attention mechanism learns to adaptively guide the LSTMs focusing on the salient(high variant) regions over time and produce the sparse hidden representation $\tilde{X}_t^l$ feeding into the LSTMs, by applying the attention map to the input Conv map with an element-wise product between each channel of the feature maps and the attention map.

Weakly Supervised Localisation: We feed the hidden states of the last time step i.e. H_T^l into the weakly supervised classification layers, which is built with two approaches: (1) 1×1 convolution is applied to mapping the feature maps down to the class score maps, and the score maps are then spatially aggregated using either a Global Max Pooling (GMP) or Global Average Pooling (GAP) operation to obtain categorical scores; (2) We aggregate the feature maps to a feature vector first with global pooling operation, then a dense layer is applied to mapping the feature vector to categorical scores. We then train the proposed model end-to-end by minimizing the objective function:

$$L = -\frac{1}{N} \sum_{n=1}^{N} \alpha_n f_n(S_c(x_n) - log \sum_{k=1}^{K} e^{S_k(X_n)}) + \lambda \sum_{i,j}(1 - \sum_{t=1}^{T} A_t(i,j)) \quad (3)$$

where the first part of L is a focal cross-entropy loss [10]: there are N training sequences x_n and K training classes ($K = 4$), S_k is the k_{th} component in the score vector $\in \mathbb{R}^K$, and **c** is the true class of x_n; α_n is a class-balanced weighting factor set by inverse class frequency; f_n is a focal modulating factor to reduce the loss contribution from well-trained examples and thus focus training on misclassified examples. The second part is a form of doubly stochastic regularization [2] to regularize the learning of spatial-temporal attention. By construction in Eq. (2), we have $\sum_{i,j} A_t(i,j) = 1$. We also encourage $\sum_t A_t(i,j) \approx 1$ by the doubly stochastic regularization, which can be interpreted as encouraging the model to pay equal attention to every frame and every part of the frame over the course of generation.

3   Experiments and Results

In this section, we evaluate the proposed model jointly for classification and localisation of the fetal structures of interest (skull, abdomen and heart) in video sequences. We compare different weakly supervised classifiers discussed above: AD-GAP (Adaptation with Global Average Pooling), AD-GMP, CAM-GAP and CAM-GMP (Class Activation Mapping with Global Max Pooling). And we also compare against their attention-gated versions: AG-AD-GAP (AG: attention gated), AG-AD-GMP, AG-CAM-GAP and AG-CAM-GMP.

Datasets: Our dataset consisted of 456 fetal ultrasound videos of healthy volunteers, with gestational ages 28 weeks or higher, which have been acquired by a number of experienced obstetricians following a simple protocol i.e. sweeping the ultrasound probe from the maternal cervix to the fundus along the longitudinal axis of the uterus. The videos have been annotated at the frame level by extracting the sequences that contain the anatomy of interest i.e. **Skull**, **Abdomen**, **Heart** and **Background**. The annotation takes both standardised and non-standardised planes into account, and there are significantly more non-standard frames than standard ones because of the simple acquisition protocol. The annotated sequences were sub-sampled with steps conditioned on their length, to create sequences consisting of five consecutive frames. A 5-fold cross-validation is prepared that each fold keeps roughly 20% of the sub-samples for validation and test, the remaining are used for training. The split is made according to the subjects identity to ensure that no samples originating from validation and test subjects were used for training. To evaluate localization, we also annotate bounding-boxes of the fetal structures on the test data. We applied several random on-the-fly data augmentation strategies during training, including (1) cropping square patches at the center of the input frames with a scaling factor randomly chosen between 0.7 to 1, and resize the crops to the size of 224×224 (input resolution); (2) rotation with an angle randomly selected within $\theta = -25°$ to 25°; (3) Random horizontal reflection i.e. flipped the frames in the left-right direction with a probability $p = 0.5$.

Implementation Details: We apply 5 recurrent modules independently on each of the convolution maps extracted from the first to fifth MP (max-pooling) layers. The number of channels of each respective hidden representations are 32, 64, 128, 256 and 256. Five hidden-representations are obtained at each time step. We feed the hidden representations of the last time-step to 5 separate classifiers. Each classifier therefore learns prediction by focusing on only one hidden representation at a specific scale. The classifier outputs are then averaged to get the final decision. All models are implemented with Tensorflow and trained from scratch (on a Nvidia GeForce GTX 1080Ti) with an Adam optimizer (learning rate: 10^{-4}, $\beta_1 = 0.5$, $\beta_2 = 0.9$ and $\epsilon = 10^{-8}$). λ in Eq. (3) is set to 1 in our experiments.

Class Activation Mapping: Examples of high level (Conv5 layer) class activation maps are illustrated in Fig. 3 for different models and different fetal structures. We find that Global Max Pooling (GMP) models, particularly the AD-GMP generates the most discriminative CAMs, localising well the target fetal structures, even in the challenging heart examples with strong acoustic shadow and highly varied appearance and location. While Global Average Pooling (GAP) models perform less superior, the AD-GAP very often failed to capture the anatomy of interest in most cases, and although CAM-GAP localise well the target structures but it tends to over-estimate its extent. We argue that this is because, averaging a feature map is prone to incorporate the global context for the classification, while GMP only accounts for the receptive field of the most discriminative unit i.e. maximally activated neuron.

Attention Analysis: Figure 4 gives examples of spatial-temporal attention captured by the AG-CAM-GMP model at different feature levels. We found that the Conv3 layer captures a rich diversity of temporal dynamics of small anatomies, for instance, the appearing and disappearing of umbilical veins, and the periodic up-down movement of atrioventricular valves. A very interesting heart example (last column), the neural network is struggling to find where the

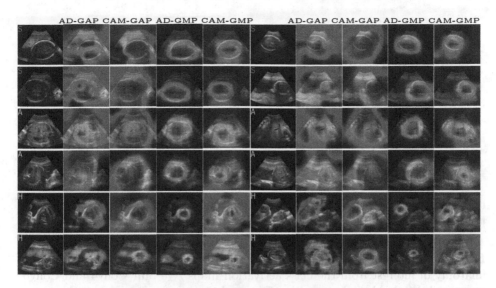

Fig. 3. Examples of the class activation maps obtained from AD-GAP, AD-GMP, CAM-GAP and CAM-GMP. The class activation maps are from Conv5 layer. S: Skull, A: Abdomen, H: Heart. (Color figure online)

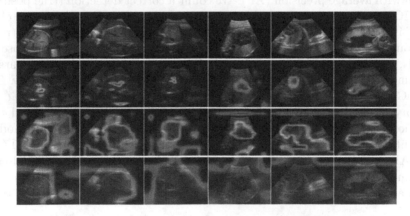

Fig. 4. Examples of multi-scale attention obtained from AG-CAM-GMP. **Row 1**: examples videos. **Row 2 to 4**: attention maps at **Conv3 to Conv5** levels, respectively (see Supplementary material). Best viewed in Adobe Reader. All videos should play automatically. (Color figure online)

heart is at the beginning but it is progressively corrected towards end of the video. Likewise, the attention is fairly random initially at Conv4, and because of the extremely large receptive field, Conv5 begin with paying attention on the whole frame, then with incorporation of contextual information, it learns to smoothly and progressively move to the structures of interest, and finally locate them. It should be noted that Conv4 finally focuses more on the anatomies inside

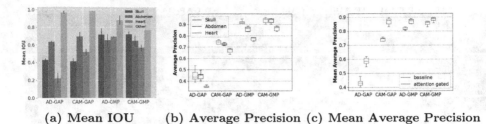

(a) **Mean IOU**   (b) **Average Precision** (c) **Mean Average Precision**

Fig. 5. Quantitative evaluation of localisation performance.

the abdomen, such as the heart, stomach bubble and umbilical vein, and Conv5 tends to focus on the whole fetal abdomen.

Evaluation Localization: We generate a bounding box and its associated anatomy of interest from the class activation maps. We blur Conv4 and Conv5 maps and threshold the lower activations, and then perform a connected component analysis to find the overlapped component, finally we fit a bounding box to the largest connected component. We jointly evaluate the classification and localisation with average precision (AP). We count a correct detection (true positive) if the IOU is above 50% of the maximum achievable IOU of its associated class, and it is a positive prediction with confidence above certain thresholds (ranging from 0.1 to 0.9). Figure 5(b) compares the categorical AP of the baseline models, in which we find the skull and abdomen category achieve comparable performance in each model, and slightly outperform the heart category. The CAM-GMP model achieves the best AP of 0.94, 0.93 and 0.85 (median) in the category of skull, abdomen and heart, respectively. In Fig. 5(c), we find that attention helps to improve the localisation performance of the baseline models. Particularly, there is a substantial improvement of the mAP (more than 10%) in the GAP models i.e. AD-GAP and CAM-GAP. Although CAMs model already perform very well but there is still a moderate increase of mAP after incorporating attention into the models.

Model Complexity: We have conducted computation complexity studies by considering two metrics: (1) the number of floating-point operations (FLOPs); (2) frame rate (speed) on a single GPU (FPS). FLOPs consist of convolution operations in the backbone (CNN) which is about 3.82 GFLOPs; Recurrent and attention modules is about 1.16GFLOPs and 0.29GFLOPs (here we only consider Conv4 and Conv5 at inference time, as we use conv4 and conv5 CAMs for the localization task); classifiers take a fractional computation that can be neglected compared to the above modules. So in total the proposed baseline model computation is about 4.98 GFLOPs (attention gated models slightly higher at 5.27GFLOPs) that is about one third the computation complexity of VGG16 [9] (15.3GFLOPs), and is comparable to SonoNet-32 [4]. We also measured the frame rates achieved on a Nvidia Geforce GTX 1080 GPU for classification and localisation combined that base-line models achieve approx. 43.2 FPS, attention-gated models are slightly slower approx. 37.5 FPS. Videos in our study were recorded at 30 FPS so all experimented models achieve real-time performance.

4 Conclusion

We have presented a general framework for detection of multiple fetal structures in free-hand ultrasound videos that it not only learns objects detection from the standardised scan planes but also dominantly from the non-standard cases (especially the abdominal and cardiac planes). Particularly, we proposed a spatial-temporal attention module that can be plug-in any feature level of a ConvNet. As result of multi-scale learning, we have demonstrated the model learns a rich diversity of spatial-temporal patterns at different Conv layers. We also found that the attention helps to improve the localisation performance significantly.

Acknowledgements. We acknowledge the ERC (ERC-ADG-2015 694581, project PULSE) the EPSRC (EP/GO36861/1, EP/MO13774/1) the CSC (DPhil Scholarship No. 201408060107) and the NIHR Biomedical Research Centre funding scheme.

References

1. Xingjian, S., Chen, Z., Wang, H., Yeung, D., Wong, W., Woo, W.: Convolutional LSTM network: a machine learning approach for precipitation nowcasting. In: NIPS (2015)
2. Xu, K., et al.: Show, attend and tell: neural image caption generation with visual attention. In: ICML (2015)
3. Chen, H., et al.: Standard plane localization in fetal ultrasound via domain transferred deep neural networks. IEEE J. Biomed. Health Inform. **19**, 1627–1636 (2015)
4. Baumgartner, C.F., Kamnitsas, K., Smith, S., Koch, L.M., Kainz, B., Rueckert, D.: SonoNet: real-time detection and localisation of fetal standard scan planes in freehand ultrasound. IEEE TMI (2017)
5. Chen, H., et al.: Automatic fetal ultrasound standard plane detection using knowledge transferred recurrent neural networks. In: Navab, N., Hornegger, J., Wells, W.M., Frangi, A.F. (eds.) MICCAI 2015. LNCS, vol. 9349, pp. 507–514. Springer, Cham (2015). https://doi.org/10.1007/978-3-319-24553-9_62
6. Gao, Y., Alison Noble, J.: Detection and characterization of the fetal heartbeat in free-hand ultrasound sweeps with weakly-supervised two-streams convolutional networks. In: Descoteaux, M., Maier-Hein, L., Franz, A., Jannin, P., Collins, D.L., Duchesne, S. (eds.) MICCAI 2017. LNCS, vol. 10434, pp. 305–313. Springer, Cham (2017). https://doi.org/10.1007/978-3-319-66185-8_35
7. Huang, W., Bridge, C.P., Noble, J.A., Zisserman, A.: Temporal HeartNet: towards human-level automatic analysis of fetal cardiac screening video. In: Descoteaux, M., Maier-Hein, L., Franz, A., Jannin, P., Collins, D.L., Duchesne, S. (eds.) MICCAI 2017. LNCS, vol. 10434, pp. 341–349. Springer, Cham (2017). https://doi.org/10.1007/978-3-319-66185-8_39

8. Schlemper, J., et al.: Attention-gated networks for improving ultrasound scan plane detection. In: MIDL (2018)
9. Simonyan, K., Zisserman, A.: Very deep convolutional networks for large-scale image recognition. In: ICLR (2014)
10. Lin, T.Y., Goyal, P., Girshick, R., He, K., Dollar, P.: Focal loss for dense object detection. In: Proceedings of ICCV (2017)

User Guidance for Point-of-Care Echocardiography Using a Multi-task Deep Neural Network

Grzegorz Toporek[1]($\boxtimes$), Raghavendra Srinivasa Naidu[1], Hua Xie[1],
Adriana Simicich[2], Tony Gades[2], and Balasundar Raju[1]

[1] Philips Research North America, Cambridge, USA
grzegorz.toporek@philips.com
[2] Philips Healthcare, Bothell, USA

Abstract. Echocardiography is a challenging sonographic examination with high user-dependence and the need for significant training and experience. To improve the use of ultrasound in emergency management, especially by non-expert users, we propose a solely image-based machine-learning algorithm that does not rely on any external tracking devices. This algorithm guides the motion of the probe towards clinically relevant views, such as an apical four-chamber or long axis parasternal view, using a multi-task deep convolutional neural network (CNN). This network was trained on 27 human subjects using a multi-task learning paradigm to: (a) detect and exclude ultrasound frames where quality is not sufficient for the guidance, (b) identify one of three typical imaging windows, including the apical, parasternal, and subcostal to guide the user through the exam workflow, and (c) predict 6-DOF motion of the transducer towards a target view i.e. rotational and translational motion. And besides that, by deploying relatively lightweight architecture we ensured the operation of the algorithm at approximately 25 frames per second on a commercially available mobile device. Evaluation of the system on three unseen human subjects demonstrated that the method can guide an ultrasound transducer to a target view with an average rotational and translation accuracy of $3.3 \pm 2.6°$ and 2.0 ± 1.6 mm respectively, when the probe is close to the target (<5 mm). We believe that this accuracy would be sufficient to find the image on which the user can make quick, qualitative evaluations such as the detection of pericardial effusion, cardiac activity (squeeze, mitral valve motion, cardiac arrest, etc.), as well as performing quantitative calculations such as ejection fraction.

Keywords: Ultrasound · Deep learning · Navigation · Echocardiography

1 Introduction

Evidence of the benefits of point-of-care ultrasound (POCUS) continues to grow. For instance, ultrasound provides emergency physicians access to real-time clinical information that can help to reduce time to diagnosis [1]. Time is always a precious resource in the emergency department. Fast and accurate ultrasound examinations, particularly examination of the heart, can help avoid severe complications or accelerate transfer of

© Springer Nature Switzerland AG 2019
D. Shen et al. (Eds.): MICCAI 2019, LNCS 11768, pp. 309–317, 2019.
https://doi.org/10.1007/978-3-030-32254-0_35

the patient to specialized departments for more thorough cardiac evaluation. Typically emergency physicians perform a focused cardiac ultrasound (FOCUS) that can be used to assess the presence of pericardial effusion and tamponade [2], left ventricular ejection, ventricular equality, exit (aortic root diameter), and entrance (inferior vena cava, diameter and respirophasic variation) [3]. Typically clinicians use one or more of three imaging windows and five views: parasternal long-axis (PLAX), parasternal short-axis (PSSA), apical four-chamber (A4C), subcostal long-axis (SCLA), and subcostal four-chamber (SC4C). Additionally, an apical two-chamber (A2C) view might be used to evaluate all parts of the myocardium. Due to time constraints in the emergency department, a diagnosis will usually be made from two out of the five views, if patient mobility and habitus allows. Finding these five target views is particularly challenging for untrained physicians; it typically requires significant training and experience.

Scanning Assistant: To assist less experienced physicians for rapid echocardiographic assessment and improve the use of ultrasound in emergency care, we propose an acquisition guidance system (Fig. 1a–b) that enables accurate placement of the ultrasound probe at the right position and orientation with respect to the heart anatomy. An intuitive user interface (Fig. 1a) provides acquisition assistance at all three commonly used imaging windows (apical, parasternal, and subcostal) and the majority of target views specified by the FOCUS protocol [1], including PLAX, PSSA, A4C, A2C and SC4C. Importantly, this navigation system is solely image-based, and does not rely on any external tracking devices.

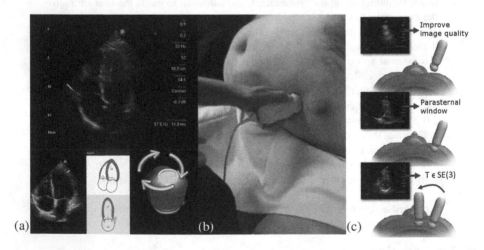

Fig. 1. User interface of a scanning assistant (a) tested on the human subject (b) using a commercially available mobile ultrasound system (Lumify, Philips). A key feature of the system is that it provides feedback in addition to probe motion (c). For instance, during scanning the physician might lose acoustic coupling or position the probe directly on the rib cage. The system informs the user that image quality needs to be improved in order to provide further guidance. Additionally, the scanning assistant detects one of the commonly used imaging windows to guide the user through the exam workflow, and adjusts imaging settings, such as penetration depth, accordingly.

Deep Learning for Ultrasound: Image-based guidance in transthoracic echocardiography is non-trivial due to the likely presence of reverberation clutter, acoustic shadow, cardiac and respiratory motion as well as patient's anatomical and physiological variability. Deep convolutional neural networks (CNN) can be trained to extract high-level features with large spatial context, making them applicable to such complex problems. Consequently, deep learning has significant advantages over standard machine learning methods. Previous methods developed for ultrasound images that required manual selection of features [4] were recently out-performed by deep learning in tasks such as view classification [5, 6] or segmentation [7].

Here we propose an fully end-to-end solution with a multi-task CNN model, which (a) assesses whether the quality of the image is sufficient for guidance, (b) identifies one of three typical imaging windows, including apical, parasternal, and subcostal, and (c) predicts motion of the transducer towards the desired imaging plane (see Fig. 1c).

Key Contributions: As far as the authors are aware, this paper is the first to propose a solely image-based user guidance system for point-of-care transthoracic echocardiography ready to be deployed on commercial mobile ultrasound scanners, such as Lumify, Philips. This fully end-to-end solution uses a multi-task deep convolutional neural network to predict relative motion of the transducer towards the diagnostically relevant views, as well as assesses image quality and identifies one of the commonly used imaging windows. The key contributions include:

- a new technique dedicated to transthoracic echocardiography to achieve entirely image-based navigation with millimeter-level accuracy,
- a method that quantitatively guides the positioning of the transducer at five target views (PLAX, PSSA, A4C, A2C, and SC4C) from three different imaging windows (apical, parasternal, and subcostal),
- a new light-weight multi-task deep convolutional neural network architecture that regresses both 3-DOF rotation and 3-DOF translation, as well as classifies ultrasound images based on the quality and imaging window,
- a solution with potential clinical deployment on a mobile device or similar hardware with limited memory and computing capabilities.

2 Methods

2.1 Data Collection and Labeling

All datasets were obtained from healthy human subjects (N = 30) using a commercial handheld, mobile, USB-based ultrasound system (Lumify, Philips) by a well-trained sonographer. Each loop consisted of a large number of frames. These frames were acquired at all three imaging windows, including apical, parasternal, and subcostal; and covered all five views defined in the FOCUS protocol [3] (i.e. PLAX, PSSA, A4C, A2C, and SC4C), see Fig. 2c. Each cardiac ultrasound frame within a dataset was automatically labelled using a custom-made data acquisition system based on optical tracking. A schematic representation of our acquisition system is shown in Fig. 2a. For

ease of annotations, each acquisition was started at one of three reference target views
(A4C, PLAX, SC4C) that implicitly defined three standardized coordinate systems at
each acoustic window. Positions of remaining frames was determined relative to this
coordinate systems. For simplicity, guidance accuracy was evaluated only for these
reference views. Remaining target views (A2C, PSSA) were identified by an expert
echocardiographer. Importantly, optical tracking was only used to collect the ground
truth data but never during the application of the system.

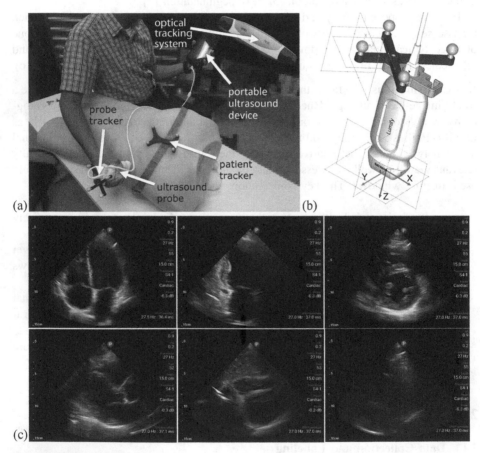

Fig. 2. (a) A schematic representation of the acquisition system. A rigid probe marker consisting
of retroreflective spheres is mounted and calibrated to an ultrasound probe. An additional patient
marker is attached to the patient's chest using an adjustable belt to account for unexpected patient
motion. Images from the portable ultrasound device are acquired and synchronized with the
optical tracking system that estimates the 6-DOF positions of both probe and patient marker;
(b) Coordinate system of the ultrasound probe; (c) Target views defined by the FOCUS protocol
towards which our algorithm can guide the user. Starting from the left: four-chamber (A4C) and
two-chamber (A2C) views from the apical imaging window, short axis (PSSA) and long axis
(PLAX) views from the parasternal imaging window, subcostal four-chamber view (SC4C). An
example of a low-quality (LQ) frame is also provided.

Two rigid markers consisting of four retroreflective spheres (NDI Medical) were attached to the ultrasound probe via a custom-made adapter as well as the patient's chest using an adjustable belt (see Fig. 2b). The transformation between probe and image ($^{\text{probe}}T_{\text{image}}$) was obtained using a custom-made wire-based ultrasound phantom, similar to the one described in [8]. A patient marker, which establishes the heart coordinate system, was used to account for unexpected motion of the heart with respect to the tracking system. Pose $T \in SE(3)$ of both probe ($^{\text{tracker}}T_{\text{probe}}$) and patient marker ($^{\text{tracker}}T_{\text{patient}}$) was estimated via a stereoscopic optical camera (Polaris Vega, NDI Medical), and synchronized with the ultrasound images acquired with the portable ultrasound device. All images were then labelled with 3D rigid transformations calculated relative to the reference image in the heart coordinate system, as listed below:

$$^{\text{patient}}T_{\text{image}} = \left(^{\text{tracker}}T_{\text{patient}}\right)^{-1} \cdot {}^{\text{tracker}}T_{\text{probe}} \cdot {}^{\text{probe}}T_{\text{image}} \tag{1}$$

Expert echocardiographer identified all low-quality (LQ) frames in each data set. We considered LQ images as those either with poor acoustic coupling or containing organs different than the heart. The remaining frames, accounting for the three different imaging windows, were considered high-quality (HQ), i.e. sufficient for our algorithm to extract features and make predictions. Stored datasets were divided into two separate sets: (a) development dataset (N = 27 subjects; 590,000 frames) from which 80% of cases were randomly chosen to train the weights of the CNN and 20% for validation, and (b) test dataset (N = 3 subjects; 21,000 frames, including: 10,000, 7,000, 1,500, and 2,500 frames for apical, parasternal, subcostal, and LQ class respectively) consisting of data points the model was not trained on. Accuracy of the algorithm was evaluated only on unseen test cases in order to determine the generalizability of the model. Tracking accuracy was evaluated only on HQ frames by calculating average absolute angular errors along each axis (rotation), and mean absolute distance (translation) to the target. Classification performance was assessed by the area under the receiver operator characteristic (ROC) curves (AUC).

2.2 Model Development

A primary feature extractor was a CNN model – broadly known as a SqueezeNet – with 8 so-called fire modules followed by one convolutional layer and global average pooling [9]. This CNN architecture was designed for limited-memory systems and to provide high energy efficiency on mobile devices [10]. This primary CNN simultaneously predicts rotation and translation for all five target views as well as classifies three acoustic windows, thus sharing features among all these tasks. For the rotation and translation tasks, we added two separate regression layers with a π *tanh* activation function after the primary feature extractor, as described in [11, 12]. For the classification task, a softmax classification layer was added after global average pooling. The total loss function was defined as:

$$\text{loss}_{\text{total}} = \lambda \cdot \text{loss}_{\text{rotation}} + \alpha \cdot \text{loss}_{\text{translation}} + \gamma \cdot \text{loss}_{\text{classification}} \tag{2}$$

$$\text{loss}_{\text{rotation}} = \cos^{-1}\left[\frac{tr(\hat{R}^T R) - 1}{2}\right] \tag{3}$$

$$\text{loss}_{\text{translation}} = \frac{1}{N}\sum_{i=1}^{N}(\hat{t}_i - t_i)^2 \left|\left\langle \frac{\hat{t}}{\|\hat{t}\|}, \frac{t}{\|t\|} \right\rangle - 1\right| \tag{4}$$

$$\text{loss}_{\text{classification}} = -\sum_{c=1}^{M} y_c \log(p_c) \tag{5}$$

where λ, α, γ are hyperparameters used to balance between the rotation, translation, and classification loss respectively; $R \in SO(3)$ stands for a rotation matrix; $t = [t_i \ldots t_N]^T$, and $N = 3$, stands for translation vector; $\langle \cdot \rangle$ represents inner product of two vectors and $\text{loss}_{\text{classification}}$ is a cross entropy loss for multi-classification task, $M = 4$.

The model was trained in TensorFlow using RMSprop optimizer with a batch size of 32, an initial learning rate of 0.0001, and decayed every 4.7M iterations with an exponential rate of 0.5. Batch normalization, weight decay of 0.0005, early stopping criteria were used as regularization techniques. All loss function hyperparameters $(\lambda, \alpha, \gamma)$ were set to 1. Ultrasound images were converted from Cartesian to Polar space and randomly augmented during the training using various ultrasound-specific techniques, including injection of a reverberation clutter, alteration of penetration depth, change of gain and aspect ratio as well as post-modification of TGC curve.

3   Results

In the vicinity of the target views (see Fig. 2c), the average absolute angular accuracy was $2.5 \pm 1.4°$, $2.4 \pm 1.8°$, and $5.5 \pm 5.0°$ around the x, y, z axes respectively (see Table 1).

The average absolute translation accuracy was 2.0 ± 1.6 mm. The overall accuracy decreased when the distance to the target position increased. For instance, the predicted translational inaccuracy measured at the distance above 20 mm from the target view was significantly higher (p-value < 0.0001, unpaired, two-tailed t test) than below 5 mm, 5.6 ± 4.7 mm vs. 2.0 ± 1.6 mm respectively. The average classification accuracy was 98% and 89% for imaging window identification and low-quality frame detection respectively (see Fig. 3b–c). ROC curves with associated AUCs are shown in Fig. 3a.

Table 1. Accuracy of the system as a function of distance d and angle a_i around each axis (x, y, z), where $i \in \{1\ldots3\}$; $\bar{a}$ represents the average absolute angular error, and $\bar{d}$ represents the absolute translation error with respect to three target views: A4C, PLAX, and SC4C.

Gap from the target view	Angular accuracy	Translational accuracy
$\forall i, a_i < 5°, d < 5$ mm	$\bar{a}_1 = 2.0 \pm 1.4°$	$\bar{d} = 2.0 \pm 1.6$ mm
	$\bar{a}_2 = 2.4 \pm 1.8°$	
	$\bar{a}_3 = 5.5 \pm 5.0°$	
$\forall i, a_i < 10°, d < 10$ mm	$\bar{a}_1 = 3.0 \pm 2.2°$	$\bar{d} = 2.7 \pm 2.0$ mm
	$\bar{a}_2 = 2.5 \pm 1.9°$	
	$\bar{a}_3 = 4.9 \pm 3.9°$	
$\forall i, a_i < 15°, d < 15$ mm	$\bar{a}_1 = 3.2 \pm 2.3°$	$\bar{d} = 3.6 \pm 2.2$ mm
	$\bar{a}_2 = 3.0 \pm 2.2°$	
	$\bar{a}_3 = 6.3 \pm 4.7°$	
$\forall i, a_i < 20°, d < 20$ mm	$\bar{a}_1 = 3.3 \pm 2.6°$	$\bar{d} = 4.8 \pm 4.0$ mm
	$\bar{a}_2 = 3.1 \pm 2.3°$	
	$\bar{a}_3 = 6.8 \pm 4.9°$	
$\forall i, a_i > 20°, d > 20$ mm	$\bar{a}_1 = 3.5 \pm 2.8°$	$\bar{d} = 5.6 \pm 4.7$ mm
	$\bar{a}_2 = 4.2 \pm 3.1°$	
	$\bar{a}_3 = 8.5 \pm 6.6°$	

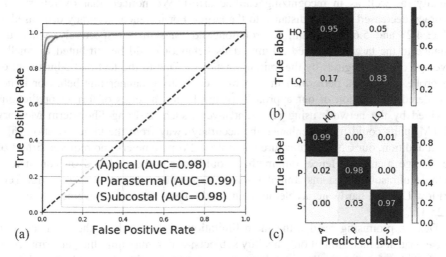

Fig. 3. (a) Pairwise comparison of receiver operating characteristic (ROC) curves for classification tasks i.e. each class is shown with respect to other classes. The ROC curves are similar with AUCs ranging from 0.98 to 0.99 for apical (A), subcostal (S) and parasternal (P) respectively (mean 0.97); (b) A confusion matrix for identification of low-quality (LQ) frames with respect to high-quality (HQ) frames shows accuracy ranging from 83% to 95% for LQ and HQ, respectively, where HQ represents apical, parasternal, and subcostal views; (c) A confusion matrix for imaging window classification shows the accuracy ranging from 0.97% to 0.99% for subcostal (S), parasternal (P), and apical (A) views respectively. The confusion matrix was normalized by the number of cases in each class. Inclusion threshold was set to 0.5.

4 Conclusion and Future Work

A solely image-based scan guidance system for point-of-care transthoracic echocardiography was developed and evaluated on unseen independent in vivo datasets. Our deep learning-based algorithm was trained using a multi-task learning paradigm. A single neural network was used to (a) detect and exclude ultrasound frames where quality is not sufficient for the guidance, (b) identify one of three typical imaging windows, including the apical, parasternal, and subcostal, to guide the user through the exam workflow, and (c) predict 6-DOF motion of the transducer towards clinically-relevant views, such as the four-chamber or long-axis views. To begin with, finding an optimal acoustic window to image the heart can be challenging, especially for technically difficult patients. Our system could possibly accelerate this phase of the examination by providing an objective measure of image quality; herein we demonstrated 95% accuracy for high-quality image classification. Moreover, it was demonstrated that the ultrasound probe could be guided to three pre-defined reference target views with an average rotational accuracy of $3.3 \pm 2.6°$, when the probe was close to the target (<5 mm). The lowest rotation accuracy was shown around the z-axis; mostly because angles for this axis have the largest span, ranging from 0 to π. This accuracy may be sufficient to perform all assessments relevant in the acute/emergency setting, including presence of a pericardial effusion, left ventricular ejection, ventricular equality, as well as in recognizing cardiac arrest. We noticed that overall system accuracy decreased with the distance to the target. For instance, accuracy decreased to $5.4 \pm 4.2°$ and 5.6 ± 4.7 mm, for rotation and translation respectively, when the distance to the target exceeded 20 mm. This behavior could be attributed to smaller coverage of these regions by the training instances. Due to the fact that adjustment of the probe position is performed in a step-wise iterative manner this behavior is not considered a limitation of our approach. In the future, a series of former predictions provided by the network using recurrent layers, such as Long Short-term Memory (LSTM) units could further enhance the accuracy away from the target location [6].

In addition, our CNN architecture had only 1.2M parameters and required 5 MB of the storage memory. Hence, our method could be readily deployed on commercial portable ultrasound systems. Initial tests on a premium mobile device – with TensorFlow Lite and hardware acceleration enabled – demonstrated an average frame rate of 25 Hz.

Despite promising results, the main limitation of this study is the small training dataset size and inclusion of only healthy subjects, which may limit the performance of the algorithm for technically difficult patients or patients with abnormal physiological conditions. Further work would include adding data from a larger number of subjects, including patients with impaired cardiac function.

References

1. American College of Emergency Physicians: Ultrasound guidelines: emergency, point-of-care, and clinical ultrasound guidelines in medicine. Ann. Emerg. Med. **69**, e27–e54 (2017). https://doi.org/10.1016/j.annemergmed.2016.08.457
2. Plummer, D., Brunette, D., Asinger, R., Ruiz, E.: Emergency department echocardiography improves outcome in penetrating cardiac injury. Ann. Emerg. Med. **21**, 709–712 (1992). https://doi.org/10.1016/S0196-0644(05)82784-2
3. Kennedy Hall, M., Coffey, E.C., Herbst, M., et al.: The "5Es" of emergency physician-performed focused cardiac ultrasound: a protocol for rapid identification of effusion, ejection, equality, exit, and entrance. Acad. Emerg. Med. **22**, 583–593 (2015). https://doi.org/10.1111/acem.12652
4. Lempitsky, V., Verhoek, M., Noble, J.A., Blake, A.: Random forest classification for automatic delineation of myocardium in real-time 3D echocardiography. In: Ayache, N., Delingette, H., Sermesant, M. (eds.) FIMH 2009. LNCS, vol. 5528, pp. 447–456. Springer, Heidelberg (2009). https://doi.org/10.1007/978-3-642-01932-6_48
5. Madani, A., Arnaout, R., Mofrad, M.: Fast and accurate view classification of echocardiograms using deep learning. Nat. Digit. Med. 1–8 (2018). https://doi.org/10.1038/s41746-017-0013-1
6. Van Woudenberg, N., et al.: Quantitative echocardiography: real-time quality estimation and view classification implemented on a mobile android device. In: Stoyanov, D., et al. (eds.) POCUS/BIVPCS/CuRIOUS/CPM -2018. LNCS, vol. 11042, pp. 74–81. Springer, Cham (2018). https://doi.org/10.1007/978-3-030-01045-4_9
7. Leclerc, S., Smistad, E., Pedrosa, J., et al.: Deep learning for segmentation using an open large-scale dataset in 2D echocardiography. IEEE Trans. Med. Imaging 1 (2019). https://doi.org/10.1109/TMI.2019.2900516
8. Chen, T.K., Abolmaesumi, P., Thurston, A.D., Ellis, R.E.: Automated 3D freehand ultrasound calibration with real-time accuracy control. In: Larsen, R., Nielsen, M., Sporring, J. (eds.) MICCAI 2006. LNCS, vol. 4190, pp. 899–906. Springer, Heidelberg (2006). https://doi.org/10.1007/11866565_110
9. Iandola, F.N., Han, S., Moskewicz, M.W., et al.: SqueezeNet: AlexNet-level accuracy with 50x fewer parameters and <0.5 MB model size, pp. 1–13. arXiv:160207360v4 (2017)
10. Sehgal, A., Kehtarnavaz, N.: Guidelines and benchmarks for deployment of deep learning models on smartphones as real-time apps, pp. 1–10. arXiv:190102144 (2019)
11. Toporek, G., Wang, H., Balicki, M., Xie, H.: Autonomous image-based ultrasound probe positioning via deep learning. In: Hamlyn Symposium on Medical Robotics (2018)
12. Mahendran, S., Ali, H., Vidal, R.: 3D pose regression using convolutional neural networks. In: 2017 IEEE Conference on Computer Vision and Pattern Recognition Workshops (CVPRW) (2017)

Integrating 3D Geometry of Organ for Improving Medical Image Segmentation

Jiawen Yao[1], Jinzheng Cai[2], Dong Yang[3], Daguang Xu[3(✉)],
and Junzhou Huang[1]

[1] Department of Computer Science and Engineering,
The University of Texas at Arlington, Arlington, TX 76019, USA
[2] Department of Biomedical Engineering, University of Florida,
Gainesville, FL 32611, USA
[3] NVIDIA Corporation, Bethesda, USA
daguangx@nvidia.com

Abstract. Prior knowledge of organ shape and location plays an important role in medical imaging segmentation. However, traditional 2D/3D segmentation methods usually operate as pixel-wise/voxel-wise classifiers where their training objectives are not able to incorporate the 3D shape knowledge explicitly. In this paper, we proposed an efficient deep shape-aware network to learn 3D geometry of the organ. More specifically, the network uses a 3D mesh representation in a graph-based CNN which can handle the shape inference and accuracy propagation effectively. After integrating the shape-aware module into the backbone FCNs and jointly training the full model in the multi-task framework, the discriminative capability of intermediate feature representations is increased for both geometry and segmentation regularizations on disentangling subtly correlated tasks. Experimental results show that the proposed network can not only output accurate segmentation, but also generate smooth 3D mesh simultaneously which can be used for further 3D shape analysis.

1 Introduction

Automatic 3D organ segmentation on CT [2,13] and MRI [12,14] is an important topic in computer-assisted diagnosis (CAD), which implies a broad range of applications. In recent years, 3D deep neural networks [4,8,15] have been widely applied to this area which largely improve the performance of conventional segmentation approaches. Though being able to capture the volumetric contexts, 3D network usually suffers from the lack of pre-trained models and large memory consumption requirement. More important, the voxel-wise prediction cannot characterize the plausible anatomical shape of an organ as the organ is usually locally smooth and single-connected. Recently, models which used shape priors are proposed [9,12]. ACNN [9] is one of the pioneering works that introduced

---

J. Yao—Work mainly done during an internship at NVIDIA.

© Springer Nature Switzerland AG 2019
D. Shen et al. (Eds.): MICCAI 2019, LNCS 11768, pp. 318–326, 2019.
https://doi.org/10.1007/978-3-030-32254-0_36

shape priors based on Stacked Auto-Encoders but it is trained in two separate stages and not in the unified manner.

The emergence of neural networks in 3D geometry provides a new means for learning the shape information of objects [3,10]. Although showing promising results, most of the networks only focus on CAD synthesis images. Their effects on more challenging medical datasets have not been investigated yet. Moreover, segmentation tasks in medical datasets usually don't provide 3D points for training but only the masks annotated on 2D slices. When generating points from such stacked 2D masks, it is not easy to have well-distributed 3D points without noise. Things could be more severe as those networks are sensitive to sharp features on 3D objects, making it challenging for an accurate organ shape reconstruction.

In this paper, we proposed the *shape-aware* network that can efficiently learn the 3D geometry of an organ and avoid the under-sampling effects by considering the neighboring vertices information and measuring the shape consistency constraints in lower dimension space. More specifically, the *shape-aware* network learns to deform a mesh to fit the target organ geometry. Motivated by [11], the deformation is performed by a graph-based convolutional network (GCN) using coarse-to-fine strategy. To further solve the issue of under-sampling, we measure the shape- and details-consistency from different viewpoints using 2D projections [7]. 2D projections of 3D points will reduce the under-sampling effects and enforce the network to follow 3D geometry of the target better than [11]. After incorporation of multi-task regularization during training, the discriminative capability of intermediate features can be further improved and hence the segmentation performance. Experimental results show that the segmentation models trained with the proposed *shape-aware* network can achieve better performance and robustness. The proposed network is independent of the network architecture and can be combined with any 3D segmentation FCN backbones.

2   Methodology

Figure 1 shows the pipeline of the whole approach. The proposed *shape-aware* network is combined with a 3D FCN backbone for joint end-to-end training. It takes an initial mesh and the multi-scale contexual feature maps from 3D FCN as inputs. Different from other point clouds learning approaches [10], vertices locations and hidden layer features are updated using the information from neighboring vertices by graph convolutions. The output of shape-aware network is the predicted point clouds that fit the ground-truth points from mesh. We formulate it as a multi-task learning to explore the complementary information, which can infer the results of organ segmentation and shape simultaneously.

Shape-Aware Network. The shape-aware network is designed to learn 3D shape of the target organ. A coarse-to-fine strategy [11] is adopted to start from an initial mesh with fewer vertices and add more only when necessary using graph unpooling layer which will reduce memory costs and produce stable deformations for different levels. The initial mesh contains vertices, associated

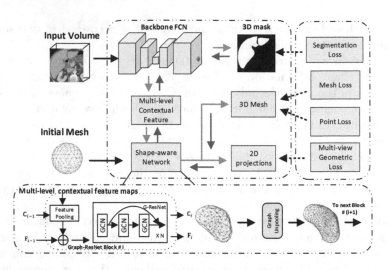

Fig. 1. The overall pipeline of the proposed method.

edge, and triangle information to identify neighbour vertices. It can be denoted as $\mathcal{M} = (\mathcal{V}, \mathcal{E}, \mathbf{F})$, where $\mathcal{V}$ means the set of vertices, $\mathcal{E}$ is the set of edges which each one connecting two vertices, and $\mathbf{F}$ are feature vectors attached on vertices.

The basic component of shape-aware network is the Graph-ResNet block and graph unpooling layer from [11] (we show one example in Fig. 1). In the i-th Graph-ResNet block, the inputs are locations of vertices C_{i-1} and vertex features F_{i-1} from previous $(i-1)$-th block. In the first block, the input is only vertices C_0 from the initial mesh. In each Graph-ResNet block, feature pooling layer is used to pool multi-level contextual features of vertices C_{i-1} from backbone FCN. 3D FCNs takes a volume as input and outputs the probability map directly. Its architecture basically contains the down-sampling and up-sampling path. We concatenate features in different levels of down-sampling and up-sampling path together to produce multi-level contextual feature maps which represent different levels of contextual information, i.e., intensities appearance in various sizes of receptive fields. Given the 3D coordinate of a vertex, we can get the corresponding feature vector from feature maps. The pooled feature is then concatenated with the 3D shape feature F_{i-1} attached to the same vertex from previous block.

After the concatenation, feature vectors and associated vertices are fed into a series of graph convolutions based ResNet (G-ResNet). A G-ResNet includes a series of graph convolutional layers with residual connections. A graph-based convolutional layer [1] is used to apply deformation on irregular graph and update the features as $f_i^{l+1} = w_0 f_i^l + \sum_{j \in \mathcal{N}(i)} w_1 f_j^l$, where $f_i^l \in \mathbb{R}^{d_l}, f_i^{l+1} \in \mathbb{R}^{d_{l+1}}$ are the feature vectors on vertex i before and after graph convolution, $\mathcal{N}(i)$ is the neighboring vertices of i and can be found in $\mathcal{E}$. w_0, w_1 are trainable parameter matrices that are applied to all vertices. The G-ResNet will produce the new coordinates (C_i) and 3D shape feature (F_i) for each vertex. Graph-ResNet block will not change the number of vertex but only update their locations and attached features. The followed graph unpooling layer [11] is designed to increase the number of vertex. This layer will add a vertex at the center of each edge and connect it with the two end-points of this edge. If three new vertices are added to the same triangle, it will also connect them together. The 3D feature for newly added vertex is set as the average of its two neighbors. The new up-sampled vertices and features will pass into the next Graph-ResNet block and the final one will only predict final locations C_{out}.

Measure Consistency Constraints in 2D Projections. To measure consistency between predicted points C_{out} and GT points, the most popular choice is Chamfer distance [6,11]. However, medical datasets are different from CAD synthesis images in which GT points in medical data might be under-sampled from stacked 2D masks, Chamfer distance does not guarantee predictions follow the geometric shape and will be easily biased by noisy points. To reduce effects from under-sampling issue, one good way is to project points to 2D plane and then compare multi-view 2D consistencies in lower dimension [7].

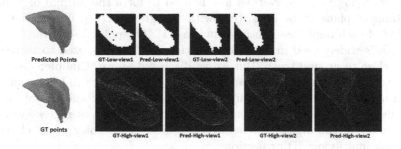

Fig. 2. Illustration of shape- and details-consistency from low and high resolution images in two views. 'Low' and 'High' refer to 'Low-resolution' and 'High-resolution', respectively.

Following the projection camera intrinsic matrix in [7], we can produce 2D projection images from 3D points as shown in Fig. 2. Camera intrinsic matrix of view camera can be estimated by projected image height h and width w. Therefore, by controlling the projected image size (h, w), images can keep more or less details. From the figure, we can see if we set h, w to large values (512), the projected images could contain details of the organ. In comparison, if h, w are set to small values (48), rough shape information is observed without fine details. Based on high and low resolution 2D projections, we can measure the details- and shape-consistency between prediction and GT images. First, denote I_{pred}^L, I_{gt}^L as low resolution images. The shape-consistency is measured for each view v as $\mathcal{L}_v^L = \sum_i \|I_{pred}^L(i) - I_{gt}^L(i)\|_2^2$. High resolution images preserve details and we can measure the details-consistency [7] by only using the non-zero pixels in prediction projected image I_{pred}^H and then checking the corresponding position in I_{gt}^H and search its neighbors for non-zeros. The error is only accumulated if all neighbors are zeros. This consistency constraint can reduce the influence of projection errors. More formally, it can be defined as $\mathcal{L}_v^H = \sum_{I_{pred}^H(i)==1} \|I_{pred}^H(i) - \max_{j \in \mathcal{N}(i)} I_{gt}^H(j)\|_2^2$. The total multi-view geometric loss is then defined by combining both consistency constraints in high and low resolution images, denoted as

$$\mathcal{L}_{mv} = \sum_v (\mathcal{L}_v^L + \mathcal{L}_v^H). \tag{1}$$

Joint End-to-End Training Loss. We define four kinds of losses in total (see Fig. 1) to constrain the segmentation outputs and the mesh deformation procedure. The segmentation loss is the Dice loss [8] which performs robustly with imbalanced training data. The mesh loss is used to make stable deformation and produce nice 3D mesh in coarse-to-fine strategy. It includes: Laplacian loss, edge length loss and normal loss. Laplacian loss encourages neighboring vertices to have the same movement which acts like a local detail preserving operator. It will be added before and after each Graph-ResNet block. Edge length loss is to penalize flying vertices. Normal loss is used to force the normal of a locally fitted tangent plane to be consistent with the ground-truth observation. The definition of each mesh loss can be found in [11]. The point loss is the Chamfer loss which is widely used in 3D reconstruction [10,11]. It is used to regress the vertices close to ground-truth. But as we discussed above, Chamfer loss is not sufficient to preserve geometric shape of ground-truth and it will lose accuracy in medical imaging as the ground-truth points are not perfect and contain noises. The multi-view geometric loss is added to make the vertices regression follow the geometry of the organ and reduce the effects from noisy point clouds by performing multi-view 2D projections.

3   Experimental Results

In this section, we conducted extensive experiments to explore the performances of our proposed shape-aware network on segmentation and shape reconstruction. Three state-of-the-art 3D F-CNN architectures are chosen, including 3D U-Net [4], V-Net [8] and DenseVoxNet [15].

Data Preparation: All experiments are conducted based on the Liver task of Medical Segmentation Decathlon (MSD) challenge. There are in total 131 3D Liver CT scans and we reported results using 3 fold cross-validation. As experiments are performed to evaluate the effectiveness of shape-aware network module, liver ROIs will be cropped first and then all data are re-sampled to $128 \times 128 \times 128$ as the input volumes of backbone 3D FCNs. Points are sampled from ground truth masks using the open-source blender python package and each case will have around 2,000 points. The initial mesh is initialized as a sphere with 162 vertices and 480 edges using MeshLab [5].

Model Training: The network is implemented in Tensorflow and Adam optimizer with weight decay 1e−5 is used. The batch size is set to 1 and the total number of training epoch is 500. The view number v is set to 9. Learning rate is initialized as 1e−4 and drops to 1e−5 after 300 epochs. All the experiments were conducted on an NVIDIA TITAN X GPU.

Quantitative Results: For 3D mesh reconstruction, we report the Chamfer distance (CD) and Earth Mover's distance (EMD) following Fan *et al.* [6]. For segmentation performance, we report Dice score. In experiments, we train three backbone FCNs without our shape-aware module and will highlight them as "No shape-aware" in the following tables. Then we add the proposed shape-aware network and jointly train the model only excluding multi-view geometric loss (described as "+ shape-aware w/o mv"). The full models with multi-view geometric loss function are emphasized in "+ shape-aware" columns.

Table 1 shows results from CD and EMD and the smaller the better. Models trained with multi-view geometric loss outperform models without it and results demonstrate the effectiveness of constraining geometric shape across different viewpoints in lower 2D projections.

Table 1. Mean and standard deviation of CD and EMD scores from different models.

Networks	+ shape-aware w/o mv		+ shape-aware	
	CD	EMD	CD	EMD
3D U-Net [4]	1.6271 ± 0.2132	0.8681 ± 0.0140	$\mathbf{1.5099 \pm 0.1531}$	$\mathbf{0.8231 \pm 0.0414}$
V-Net [8]	1.5968 ± 0.1289	0.9235 ± 0.2102	$\mathbf{1.5662 \pm 0.1197}$	$\mathbf{0.8962 \pm 0.1088}$
DenseVoxNet [15]	1.4311 ± 0.2374	0.8912 ± 0.0927	$\mathbf{1.3176 \pm 0.1597}$	$\mathbf{0.8646 \pm 0.0349}$

Table 2 lists the mean and standard deviation of Dice scores on three test folds. From Table 2, one can see the performance with a significant increase compared with the baseline models without 3D geometry knowledge. Models with multi-view geometric loss can produce overall best results.

Table 2. Mean and standard deviation of the global Dice scores (%) from different models.

Networks	No shape-aware	+ shape-aware w/o mv	+ shape-aware
3D U-Net [4]	93.7485 ± 1.4291	95.8369 ± 0.4349	$\mathbf{95.8390 \pm 0.3995}$
V-Net [8]	95.3204 ± 0.2828	95.9178 ± 0.5823	$\mathbf{95.9856 \pm 0.4845}$
DenseVoxNet [15]	96.0948 ± 0.7026	96.3738 ± 0.7249	$\mathbf{96.4782 \pm 0.5794}$

Qualitative Results: Figure 3 shows the predicted point cloud on one testing case using DenseVoxNet [15] backbone. When trained with multi-view geometric loss, the network fits the geometry of the liver from different views better and could preserve details and correct geometric appearance as much as possible. One can see from red boxes in Fig. 3 that the geometric shape of predicted liver point cloud from the proposed shape-aware is more accurate. Figure 4 presents the visualizations of testing cases from each fold. We only show the input scan, ground-truth, DenseVoxNet segmentation along with the proposed shape-aware module trained without and with multi-view geometric loss. It can be shown that the segmentation branch can benefit from 3D geometry learning to refine its boundary by incorporating the shape-aware module. Furthermore, the geometric consistency loss makes the shape-aware network approximate liver's shape better by regularizing the segmentation branch to follow the 3D geometric of the organ. The shape-aware network is equipped with powerful Graph CNN based residual blocks in a very deep architecture. Moreover, advanced 3D geometry learning techniques are used to guide shape reconstruction. With those techniques, the proposed model is able to learn very complex geometry of organ.

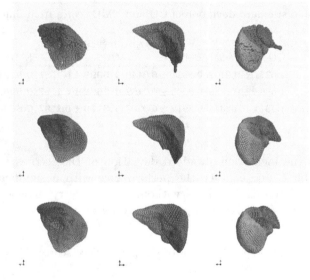

Fig. 3. Point clouds visualization for one testing case. From top to bottom row: GT point cloud (PC), predicted PC from "+shape-aware", and PC from "w/o mv" (Color figure online)

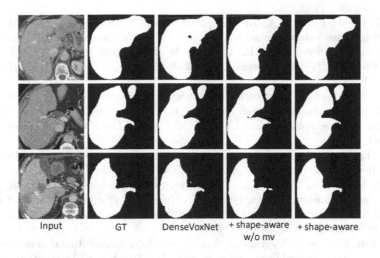

| Input | GT | DenseVoxNet | + shape-aware w/o mv | + shape-aware |

Fig. 4. Segmentation results on testing cases from each fold.

4 Conclusion

In this paper, we investigated how 3D geometry can be incorporated explicitly into classical 3D FCNs for better organ segmentation. To solve the undersampling issue from medical masks, the proposed shape-aware network deforms the mesh using information from multi-level contextual features, and measures the consistency constraints in 2D projections. Results and analysis in the experiment section show that the model trained with our shape-aware network achieves better performance on Liver segmentation tasks than others. It can also generate precise 3D mesh for future organ shape analysis. In the future, we plan to extend the proposed network to segmentation of other organs.

Acknowledgements. This work was also partially supported by US National Science Foundation IIS-1718853 and the NSF CAREER grant IIS-1553687.

References

1. Bronstein, M.M., Bruna, J., LeCun, Y., Szlam, A., Vandergheynst, P.: Geometric deep learning: going beyond Euclidean data. IEEE Signal Process. Mag. **34**(4), 18–42 (2017)
2. Cai, J., Lu, L., Zhang, Z., Xing, F., Yang, L., Yin, Q.: Pancreas segmentation in MRI using graph-based decision fusion on convolutional neural networks. In: Ourselin, S., Joskowicz, L., Sabuncu, M.R., Unal, G., Wells, W. (eds.) MICCAI 2016. LNCS, vol. 9901, pp. 442–450. Springer, Cham (2016). https://doi.org/10.1007/978-3-319-46723-8_51
3. Choy, C.B., Xu, D., Gwak, J.Y., Chen, K., Savarese, S.: 3D-R2N2: a unified approach for single and multi-view 3D object reconstruction. In: Leibe, B., Matas, J., Sebe, N., Welling, M. (eds.) ECCV 2016. LNCS, vol. 9912, pp. 628–644. Springer, Cham (2016). https://doi.org/10.1007/978-3-319-46484-8_38

4. Çiçek, Ö., Abdulkadir, A., Lienkamp, S.S., Brox, T., Ronneberger, O.: 3D U-Net: learning dense volumetric segmentation from sparse annotation. In: Ourselin, S., Joskowicz, L., Sabuncu, M.R., Unal, G., Wells, W. (eds.) MICCAI 2016. LNCS, vol. 9901, pp. 424–432. Springer, Cham (2016). https://doi.org/10.1007/978-3-319-46723-8_49

5. Cignoni, P., Callieri, M., Corsini, M., Dellepiane, M., Ganovelli, F., Ranzuglia, G.: MeshLab: an open-source mesh processing tool. In: Scarano, V., Chiara, R.D., Erra, U. (eds.) Eurographics Italian Chapter Conference. The Eurographics Association (2008)

6. Fan, H., Su, H., Guibas, L.J.: A point set generation network for 3D object reconstruction from a single image. In: IEEE CVPR, pp. 605–613 (2017)

7. Jiang, L., Shi, S., Qi, X., Jia, J.: GAL: geometric adversarial loss for single-view 3D-object reconstruction. In: Ferrari, V., Hebert, M., Sminchisescu, C., Weiss, Y. (eds.) ECCV 2018. LNCS, vol. 11212, pp. 820–834. Springer, Cham (2018). https://doi.org/10.1007/978-3-030-01237-3_49

8. Milletari, F., Navab, N., Ahmadi, S.A.: V-net: fully convolutional neural networks for volumetric medical image segmentation. In: 2016 Fourth International Conference on 3D Vision (3DV), pp. 565–571. IEEE (2016)

9. Oktay, O., Ferrante, E., Kamnitsas, K., et al.: Anatomically constrained neural networks (ACNNS): application to cardiac image enhancement and segmentation. IEEE Trans. Med. Imaging 37(2), 384–395 (2018)

10. Qi, C.R., Su, H., Mo, K., Guibas, L.J.: PointNet: deep learning on point sets for 3D classification and segmentation. In: IEEE CVPR, pp. 652–660 (2017)

11. Wang, N., Zhang, Y., Li, Z., Fu, Y., Liu, W., Jiang, Y.-G.: Pixel2Mesh: generating 3D mesh models from single RGB images. In: Ferrari, V., Hebert, M., Sminchisescu, C., Weiss, Y. (eds.) ECCV 2018. LNCS, vol. 11215, pp. 55–71. Springer, Cham (2018). https://doi.org/10.1007/978-3-030-01252-6_4

12. Wu, J., et al.: A deep Boltzmann machine-driven level set method for heart motion tracking using cine MRI images. Med. Image Anal. 47, 68–80 (2018)

13. Yang, D., et al.: Automatic liver segmentation using an adversarial image-to-image network. In: Descoteaux, M., Maier-Hein, L., Franz, A., Jannin, P., Collins, D.L., Duchesne, S. (eds.) MICCAI 2017. LNCS, vol. 10435, pp. 507–515. Springer, Cham (2017). https://doi.org/10.1007/978-3-319-66179-7_58

14. Yao, J., Xu, Z., Huang, X., Huang, J.: An efficient algorithm for dynamic MRI using low-rank and total variation regularizations. Med. Image Anal. 44, 14–27 (2018)

15. Yu, L., et al.: Automatic 3D cardiovascular MR segmentation with densely-connected volumetric ConvNets. In: Descoteaux, M., Maier-Hein, L., Franz, A., Jannin, P., Collins, D.L., Duchesne, S. (eds.) MICCAI 2017. LNCS, vol. 10434, pp. 287–295. Springer, Cham (2017). https://doi.org/10.1007/978-3-319-66185-8_33

Estimating Reference Bony Shape Model for Personalized Surgical Reconstruction of Posttraumatic Facial Defects

Deqiang Xiao[1], Li Wang[1], Hannah Deng[2], Kim-Han Thung[1],
Jihua Zhu[1,3], Peng Yuan[2], Yriu L. Rodrigues[2], Leonel Perez Jr.[4],
Christopher E. Crecelius[4], Jaime Gateno[2,5], Tiansku Kuang[2],
Steve G. F. Shen[6], Daeseung Kim[2], David M. Alfi[2,5],
Pew-Thian Yap[1], James J. Xia[2,5(✉)], and Dinggang Shen[1(✉)]

[1] BRIC and Department of Radiology, University of North Carolina
at Chapel Hill, Chapel Hill, USA
dgshen@med.unc.edu
[2] Department of Oral and Maxillofacial Surgery, Houston Methodist Hospital,
Houston, TX, USA
jxia@houstonmethodist.org
[3] School of Software Engineering, Xi'an Jiaotong University, Xi'an, China
[4] Department of Oral and Maxillofacial Surgery, Walter Reed National Military
Medical Center, Bethesda, MD, USA
[5] Department of Surgery (Oral and Maxillofacial Surgery), Weill Medical
College, Cornell University, New York, NY, USA
[6] Department of Oral and Craniofacial Surgery, Shanghai 9th Hospital,
Shanghai Jiaotong University College of Medicine, Shanghai, China

Abstract. In this paper, we introduce a method for estimating patient-specific reference bony shape models for planning of reconstructive surgery for patients with acquired craniomaxillofacial (CMF) trauma. We propose an automatic bony shape estimation framework using pre-traumatic portrait photographs and post-traumatic head computed tomography (CT) scans. A 3D facial surface is first reconstructed from the patient's pre-traumatic photographs. An initial estimation of the patient's normal bony shape is then obtained with the reconstructed facial surface via sparse representation using a dictionary of paired facial and bony surfaces of normal subjects. We further refine the bony shape model by deforming the initial bony shape model to the post-traumatic 3D CT bony model, regularized by a statistical shape model built from a database of normal subjects. Experimental results show that our method is capable of effectively recovering the patient's normal facial bony shape in regions with defects, allowing CMF surgical planning to be performed precisely for a wider range of defects caused by trauma.

Keywords: Craniomaxillofacial (CMF) · Trauma · Surgical planning · Simulation · Facial bone estimation · Three-dimensional facial reconstruction · Sparse representation · Adaptive-focus deformable shape model (AFDSM)

© Springer Nature Switzerland AG 2019
D. Shen et al. (Eds.): MICCAI 2019, LNCS 11768, pp. 327–335, 2019.
https://doi.org/10.1007/978-3-030-32254-0_37

1 Introduction

In routine clinical practice of craniomaxillofacial (CMF) surgical planning using computer-aided surgical simulation (CASS), a three-dimensional (3D) bone model is reconstructed from a computed tomography (CT) or cone beam computed tomography (CBCT) scan of patient's head. (Note: We will use CT to represent both CT and CBCT in the following text). After that, a surgeon simulates the surgery by virtually cutting the 3D model into multiple bony segments and moving them individually to their desired positions. This is mainly achieved based on 3D cephalometric analysis, in which the patient's clinical examination and cephalometric values are compared to the normative values derived from normal subjects [1]. The cephalometric analysis is a group of anatomical landmark-based linear and angular measurements of the skeleton and face. While cephalometric analysis works reasonably well in correcting straight-forward jaw deformities, it is inadequate in treating patients with complex CMF defects (e.g. trauma). Instead of relying on population-averaged measurements, patient-specific reference anatomy is needed for high-precision planning of complex reconstructive surgery. Ideally, the pre-traumatic CT scan of the patient can be used to construct a reference shape model for surgical planning. Unfortunately, such pre-traumatic CT scan usually does not exist. Therefore, the purpose of this article is to estimate a patient-specific reference bony shape model for planning the surgical correction of post-traumatic CMF defects.

There are several methods proposed in the past decade for CMF skeleton reconstruction. The most commonly used method is the mirror-imaging mapping [2], which is realized by mapping the normal facial skeleton side to the defected side. Since it is based on the hypothesis of absolute symmetric human facial structure, this method is very limited and cannot handle the cases losing normal structures on both sides (e.g. bilateral defects). Statistical shape model (SSM) is another common method applied for normal facial skeleton estimation [3]. In this method, a set of facial bone shapes from normal subjects are first acquired, and then the principal component analysis (PCA) is applied on these shapes to construct a SSM [4]. By fitting the established SSM onto the remaining normal parts of patient's facial bone, the patient's normal bone shape is estimated. A main limitation of the SSM-based method is its weak generalization capability, because the SSM is constructed on a small available dataset of normal subjects. Recently, the method of using geometric deformation was proposed to estimate the normal facial bone [5, 6]. The main idea of this method is to deform the patient's defected facial bone with an estimated deformation field to obtain its normal version. The deformation field can be calculated using the surface interpolating techniques of thin plate spline (TPS) or Laplacian surface editing [7] based on the two sets of landmarks, which are the landmarks located on the patient's bone and the corresponding normal bone landmarks estimated, respectively. The geometric deformation-based method is able to produce an accurate normal bone estimation relative to other conventional methods. However, it cannot be used for the patients with large defects, for which only a limited number of landmarks located on the remaining structures would cause the deformation field estimation to fail. Bottom line, all abovementioned methods only work on certain types of defects, they cannot be generalized to all types of CMF defects. Thus, there is an urgent need, from clinicians, to develop a generalized method of using reference shape model.

Our hypothesis is that the patient's (casual) portrait photographs, taken prior to the trauma, can be utilized to restore the "normal" bony shape in the areas with traumatic defects. Our approach involves three steps. First, we reconstruct the patient's 3D facial surface from pre-trauma two-dimensional (2D) portrait photographs. Second, we generate an initial estimate of the patient's normal bony shape via sparse representation [8] based on a database of paired facial and bony shape models. Third, we refine the initial estimate of the bony shape by registering it to the post-traumatic bony shape (i.e., the post-traumatic 3D CT model). The deformable registration is regularized by a SSM constructed from the bony shape surfaces of normal subjects.

The contribution of this study is that we applied the 2D portrait photographs and 3D post-traumatic CT for patient-specific reference model estimation, with an initialization from a correction model and the refinement from a deformable shape model. Clinically, this approach makes a paradigm shift on the way that surgeon used to plan reconstructive surgeries. Instead of using linear and angular measurements and surgeon's imagination, a patient-specific reference bony shape model can accurately guide surgeons to plan the reconstructive surgery in treating patients with post-traumatic CMF defects.

2 Method

The proposed method, summarized in Fig. 1, consists of three major steps: (1) reconstruction of pre-traumatic 3D facial surface, (2) estimation of initial reference bony shape model, and (3) refinement of the bony shape model.

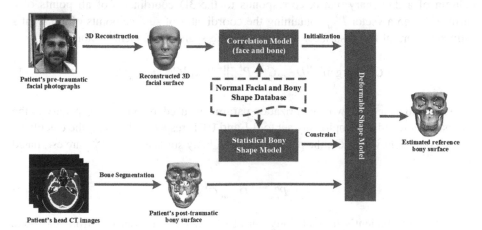

Fig. 1. Overview of our proposed approach.

2.1   Reconstruction of Pre-traumatic 3D Facial Surface

A 3D facial surface is estimated based on the patient's pre-traumatic 2D portrait photographs. This is achieved by matching a set of 68 3D facial key-points, which are reconstructed from a photograph using a convolutional neural network (CNN) based method [9], with the corresponding key-points on the mean face of the Basel Face Model (BFM) [10]. For each photograph, the mean face is warped using a dense deformation field generated by TPS interpolation. Finally, all warped surfaces are merged into a single 3D facial surface using the method described in [11].

2.2   Estimation of Initial Reference Bony Shape Model

We construct a model that relates facial and bony surfaces, both of which are obtained with head CT scans of a group of normal subjects. An initial estimation of the patient's normal bony structure is obtained by feeding the patient's 3D facial surface to this model.

Normal Facial and Bony Shape Database. 3D facial and bony surfaces are generated using marching cubes for each normal subject after CT bone segmentation. The facial and bony surfaces of different subjects are rigidly aligned using the landmarks extracted using the method described in [12]. In order to establish correspondences for the extracted surfaces across the different subjects, we non-rigidly map a template surface onto each aligned surface using coherent point drift (CPD) algorithm. The template surface is defined as one of the aligned surfaces, and its shape is the closest to the averaged shape of the entire set of surfaces.

Correlation Model. The initial bone shape model is estimated using sparse representation technique with paired face and bone dictionaries, D_{Face} and D_{Bone}. Each column of a dictionary matrix corresponds to the 3D coordinates of all points of a surface. Given a vector P_{Est}^F containing the coordinates of surface points of a patient's estimated normal facial surface, we solve for the sparse coefficient vector C:

$$C^* = \arg\min_{C} \left\| D_{Face}C - P_{Est}^F \right\|^2 + \lambda_1 \|C\|_1 + \lambda_2 \|C\|_2, \tag{1}$$

where λ_1 and λ_2 are the two regularization parameters used to control the sparsity of the representation and are empirically set to 0.1 and 0.01, respectively. With the calculated sparse coefficient vector C^*, the patient's normal bony surface points P_{Est}^B are estimated by

$$P_{Est}^B = D_{Bone}C^*. \tag{2}$$

Finally, the patient's normal bony surface model can be derived from the bone template surface based on the estimated surface points.

Initial Normal Bony Shape Estimation. We first map the patient's normal facial surface onto the imaging space of the CT facial template using iterative closest point (ICP) algorithm. Then, the corresponding points on the mapped facial surface are extracted by non-rigid surface matching between the mapped facial surface and the normal facial template surface using the CPD algorithm. Finally, we achieve an initial normal bony shape estimation by inputting the corresponding points into the correlation model.

2.3 Refinement of the Initially-Estimated Reference Model

To refine the initially-estimated reference bony shape, we utilize the adaptive-focus deformable shape model (AFDSM) [13] to deform the initial estimation onto the patient's post-traumatic bony surface. The AFDSM-based non-rigid surface matching is realized by first defining an attribute vector on each vertex. The neighboring vertexes of each vertex V_i are organized into different layers on the surface mesh, where each neighboring vertex $V_{i,j}^k$ in the kth layer is connected to V_i by k edges. After that, the attribute vector F_i of vertex V_i is defined as follows,

$$F_i = \frac{\left[f_{i,1}f_{i,2}f_{i,3}\cdots f_{i,R}\right]^T}{\sum_{i=1}^{N}\sum_{k=1}^{R}\left|f_{i,k}\right|}, f_{i,k} = \begin{vmatrix} x_i & x_{i,1}^k & x_{i,2}^k & x_{i,3}^k \\ y_i & y_{i,1}^k & y_{i,2}^k & y_{i,3}^k \\ z_i & z_{i,1}^k & z_{i,2}^k & z_{i,3}^k \\ 1 & 1 & 1 & 1 \end{vmatrix}, \tag{3}$$

where $f_{i,k}$ denotes the determinant of a matrix that contains position information of vertex V_i and its three nearest neighboring vertexes within the kth layer, R denotes the number of neighboring layers for V_i ($R = 6$), and N is the total number of vertexes on the surface mesh. Based on the attribute vector F_i, the energy function is defined as follows,

$$E = \sum_{i=1}^{N}\left(E_i^{model} + E_i^{data}\right), \tag{4}$$

where E_i^{model} denotes the degree of attribute vector difference between the initial and deformed shapes for vertex V_i, and E_i^{data} denotes the degree of attribute vector difference between the deformed and target shapes for vertex V_i. The initial and target shapes are defined as the initially-estimated bony surface and the patient's post-traumatic bony surface, respectively. We applied a greedy deformation algorithm to minimize the energy function E in Eq. (4) based on affine transformation.

To guarantee the normality of the deformed shape after each optimization iteration, the deformation procedure is further regularized within a statistical normal shape. A SSM of the bony shape is constructed from the normal bony shape database (see Sect. 2.2) via PCA, as given below,

$$S_{SSM}^i = \bar{S} + W^i P, \tag{5}$$

where S_{SSM}^i denotes the reconstructed bony shape by applying the SSM on S^i, and S^i denotes the bony shape at the i-th iteration, $\bar{S}$ denotes the mean bony shape from the normal bony shape database, W^i is a coefficients vector, and P is a matrix of principal components. The S_{SSM}^i is used to constrain the optimization as follows,

$$S^i_{updated} = \alpha_i S^i_{SSM} + (1 - \alpha_i)S^i, \tag{6}$$

where $S^i_{updated}$ is the corresponding updated bony shape, and α_i is a hyperparameter that determines the weight between S^i_{SSM} and S^i, and is gradually reduced so that the last deformed shape is closer to the target shape ($\alpha_i \epsilon [0.60, 0.95]$). At the end of each iteration, the deformed shape is updated and used as input for the next iteration.

3 Experiments and Results

3.1 Materials and Methods

A set of CT scans of 30 normal subjects were used to construct the normal facial and bony shape database. These de-identified CT data were collected in an unrelated project [14]. For each subject, the CT scans were segmented for generating 3D models. Following the clinical routine, 51 anatomic landmarks were digitized.

We first simulated synthetic patient data from CT images of normal subjects for evaluation. For each testing synthetic sample, synthetic 2D portrait photographs were first generated. The BFM mean facial surface was deformed onto the testing subject's facial CT surface using the CPD algorithm. A statistical facial texture model [10] was then applied to assign a color value on each surface vertex of the deformed BFM surface. The deformed facial surface was then rendered in 3D space, and multiple screen shots of the 3D face were taken to mimic 2D portrait photographs. Afterward, synthetic post-traumatic bony shape was generated. An experienced CMF surgeon manually edited the normal CT bony surface, mimicking a unique type of common realistic CMF trauma on the testing subject.

To perform evaluation on synthetic patient data, each subject was used in turn as the testing sample, while the remaining 29 subjects were used to construct a normal facial and bony shape database. Each synthetic patient data was fed into our proposed framework to estimate the reference bony shape. Then, the quantitative evaluation was completed by measuring the distances between the corresponding landmarks on the estimated and original bony surfaces. The qualitative evaluation was completed by a different CMF surgeon, who ranked the similarity of the two surfaces using a 1–3 visual analog score (VAS, 1: the same, 2: similar but not the same, and 3: different).

Finally, our approach was tested on three real patients who suffered from severe facial trauma due to traffic accidents and gunshot wounds. Each patient had undergone multiple surgeries to reconstruct their facial defects. We used the patient's pre-traumatic 2D portrait photographs and post-traumatic CT scans to estimate a reference model with our proposed approach. The predicted reference shape models were compared to their actual postoperative CT models after final reconstructive surgery.

3.2 Results

The quantitative results for synthetic data are summarized in Table 1. The averaged distance between the estimated and the actual surface was 3.7 mm, which is a high degree of accuracy for post-traumatic reconstructive planning. The qualitative results of synthetic data also showed: same (26/30), similar (4/30), and different (0/30). Figure 2 shows the results of eight randomly selected synthetic testing subjects. In addition, the CMF surgeon was satisfied with all the results that he would use them clinically as a reference model to guide reconstructive surgery.

Table 1. Facial bone estimation error (in mm) on synthetic data with our proposed approach.

Mean	Standard deviation	Median	Minimum	Maximum
3.68	0.43	3.66	2.91	4.90

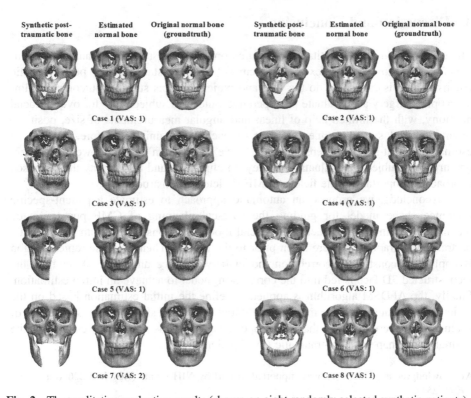

Fig. 2. The qualitative evaluation results (shown on eight randomly selected synthetic patients).

We also successfully estimated the reference models for real patients. According to the CMF surgeon after visual inspection of the results, our estimated bony shape models for the real patients were clinically acceptable. Figure 3 illustrates the comparison of the original trauma, the estimated reference bony shape model, and the postoperative outcome of a representative patient. Please note: His surgery was planned using conventional CASS method. Therefore, the postoperative outcome was not necessarily a ground truth.

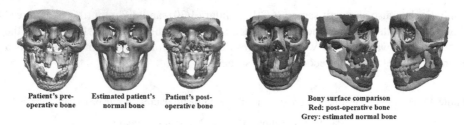

| Patient's pre-operative bone | Estimated patient's normal bone | Patient's post-operative bone | Bony surface comparison
Red: post-operative bone
Grey: estimated normal bone |

Fig. 3. A comparison of the original trauma, the estimated reference bony shape model, and the postoperative outcome of a real patient.

4 Discussion and Conclusion

There is no definitive quantitative measures on the success of post-traumatic reconstruction due to its complexity. The current clinical standard for post-traumatic reconstruction is "surgeons do the best and patient accepts surgical outcomes". Clinicians plan surgery and evaluate postoperative outcomes subjectively for overall facial harmony, with the limited help of linear and angular measurements of size, position, orientation and symmetry measurement of each facial unit. Therefore, without an estimated patient-specific reference model as we proposed in this study, we have to rely on surgeon's subjective evaluation as they do clinically, and this is why the proposed approach is important in the field of CMF skeleton reconstruction.

To conclude, we propose an automatic approach to estimate a patient-specific reference shape model for guiding the surgical planning of CMF post-traumatic reconstruction. In this approach, a 3D facial model is reconstructed from the patient's portrait photographs that were taken prior to the trauma. Then, a sparse representation is applied to construct a correlation model between face and bone. After that, the reconstructed 3D face is fed into the correlation model to achieve an initial estimation. Finally, the AFDSM algorithm is applied to refine the initial estimation based on the patient's post-traumatic bone model and a statistical normal shape model. The results of evaluations have confirmed that our proposed approach is capable of estimating the normal bony shape of post-traumatic CMF patients.

Acknowledgment. This work was supported in part by NIH grants (R01 DE022676 and R01 DE027251).

References

1. Xia, J., et al.: Algorithm for planning a double-jaw orthognathic surgery using a computer-aided surgical simulation (CASS) protocol. Part 2: three-dimensional cephalometry. Int. J. Oral Maxillofac. Surg. **44**(12), 1441–1450 (2015)
2. Gellrich, N.C., et al.: Computer assisted oral and maxillofacial reconstruction. J. Comput. Inf. Technol. **14**(1), 71–77 (2006)
3. Anton, F.M., et al.: Virtual reconstruction of bilateral midfacial defects by using statistical shape modeling. J. Oral Maxillofac. Surg. **47**(7), 1054–1059 (2019)

4. Heimann, T., Meinzer, H.: Statistical shape models for 3D medical image segmentation: a review. Med. Imag. Anal. **13**(4), 543–563 (2009)
5. Wang, L., et al.: Estimating patient-specific and anatomically correct reference model for craniomaxillofacial deformity via sparse representation. Med. Phys. **42**(10), 5809–5816 (2015)
6. Xie, S., Leow, W.K., Lim, T.C.: Laplacian deformation with symmetry constraints for reconstruction of defective skulls. In: Felsberg, M., Heyden, A., Krüger, N. (eds.) CAIP 2017. LNCS, vol. 10425, pp. 24–35. Springer, Cham (2017). https://doi.org/10.1007/978-3-319-64698-5_3
7. Sorkine, O., et al.: Laplacian surface editing. In: Proceedings of Eurographics/ACM SIGGRAPH Symposium on Geometry Processing, pp. 175–184 (2004)
8. Donoho, D.L.: For most large underdetermined systems of linear equations the minimal l_1-norm solution is also the sparsest solution. Commun. Pure Appl. Math. **59**(6), 797–829 (2006)
9. Bulat, A., Tzimiropoulos, G.: How far are we from solving the 2D & 3D face alignment problem? (and a dataset of 230,000 3D facial landmarks). In: Proceedings of IEEE International Conference on Computer Vision, vol. 1, p. 8 (2017)
10. Blanz, V., Vetter, T.: Face recognition based on fitting a 3D morphable model. IEEE Trans. Pattern Anal. Mach. Intell. **25**(9), 1063–1074 (2003)
11. Piotraschke, M., Blanz, V.: Automated 3D face reconstruction from multiple images using quality measures. In: Proc. IEEE Conference on Computer Vision and Pattern Recognition, pp. 3418–3427 (2016)
12. Zhang, J., et al.: Automatic craniomaxillofacial landmark digitization via segmentation-guided partially-joint regression forest model and multiscale statistical features. IEEE Trans. Biomed. Eng. **63**(9), 1820–1829 (2016)
13. Shen, D., Davatzikos, C.: An adaptive-focus deformable model using statistical and geometric information. IEEE Trans. Pattern Anal. Mach. Intell. **22**(8), 906–913 (2000)
14. Yan, J., et al.: Three-dimensional CT measurement for the craniomaxillofacial structure of normal occlusion adults in Jiangsu, Zhejiang and Shanghai Area. China J. Oral Maxillofac. Surg. **8**, 2–9 (2010)

A New Approach of Predicting Facial Changes Following Orthognathic Surgery Using Realistic Lip Sliding Effect

Daeseung Kim[1], Tianshu Kuang[1], Yriu L. Rodrigues[1],
Jaime Gateno[1,3], Steve G. F. Shen[2], Xudong Wang[2], Han Deng[1],
Peng Yuan[1], David M. Alfi[1,3], Michael A. K. Liebschner[4(✉)],
and James J. Xia[1,3(✉)]

[1] Department of Oral and Maxillofacial Surgery,
Houston Methodist Research Institute, Houston, TX, USA
jxia@houstonmethodist.org
[2] Department of Oral and Craniomaxillofacial Surgery, Shanghai Ninth People's
Hospital, Shanghai Jiaotong University College of Medicine, Shanghai, China
[3] Department of Surgery (Oral and Maxillofacial Surgery), Weill Medical
College, Cornell University, New York, NY, USA
[4] Department of Neurosurgery, Baylor College of Medicine, Houston, TX, USA
mall@bcm.edu

Abstract. Accurate prediction of facial soft-tissue changes following orthognathic surgery is crucial for improving surgical outcome. However, the accuracy of current prediction methods still requires further improvement in clinically critical regions, especially the lips. We develop a novel incremental simulation approach using finite element method (FEM) with realistic lip sliding effect to improve the prediction accuracy in the area around the lips. First, lip-detailed patient-specific FE mesh is generated based on accurately digitized lip surface landmarks. Second, an improved facial soft-tissue change simulation method is developed by applying a lip sliding effect in addition to the mucosa sliding effect. The soft-tissue change is then simulated incrementally to facilitate a natural transition of the facial change and improve the effectiveness of the sliding effects. A preliminary evaluation of prediction accuracy was conducted using retrospective clinical data. The results showed that there was a significant prediction accuracy improvement in the lip region when the realistic lip sliding effect was applied along with the mucosa sliding effect.

1 Introduction

Orthognathic surgery is a bony surgical procedure specially designed to correct jaw deformities. Although facial soft-tissue is not directly operated on, it naturally follows the movements of underlying bony segments. Due to the complex nature of facial anatomy, orthognathic surgery requires extensive surgical planning. To date, surgeons can accurately plan bony surgeries by virtually cutting deformed jaws into pieces and repositioning them individually to a desired position. However, they are still unable to predict soft tissue changes following the bony procedure because of complex facial anatomy, physical interaction of the facial structures, and inaccurate prediction results.

Current methods of predicting three-dimensional (3D) facial changes according to the bony movements are convoluted [1–4]. Among them, finite element method (FEM) is reported to be the most common and accurate method [4]. However, prediction accuracy in the clinically critical regions, i.e., the lips, is beyond the acceptable range [3]. Lip geometry, especially the lower lip, is one of the most prominent features determining facial aesthetics. However, in patients with jaw deformity, the lower lips are often severely deformed (strained, Fig. 1). After orthognathic surgery, the shape and position of the upper and lower lips are changed individually, and the strained lower lip is automatically restored to its relaxed status. In the past, we have made significant progress on developing FEM prediction methods using a realistic mucosa sliding effect in order to improve the accuracy in clinically critical regions [1]. While adding the mucosa sliding effect had significantly improved the prediction accuracy of the facial changes including the lips [1], we treated the upper and lower lips as a whole. The prediction accuracy in the lip, especially the lower lip, thus still requires further improvement. This is especially true for patients with severe jaw deformities and asymmetry [1].

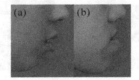

Fig. 1. Strained lip in (a) mandibular hypoplasia, (b) mandibular hyperplasia.

In this study, we hypothesize that the simulation of the lip sliding is a key factor for the improvement of soft-tissue-change prediction accuracy in the lip regions. Therefore, we propose the following approach: (1) lip-detailed patient-specific FE mesh generation, and (2) incremental FEM simulation method that incorporates the realistic lip sliding effect along with the mucosa sliding effect. Our method was quantitatively evaluated using clinical datasets. The contribution of our new method is the advancement in the FE mesh modeling and the simulation method to improve facial change prediction accuracy, which can innovate the surgical planning procedure for orthognathic surgery.

2 Methods

Our new facial change prediction approach consists of two stages. In the first stage, a lip-detailed patient-specific mesh is generated to further improve our previously developed patient-specific mesh generation method. In the second stage, facial soft-tissue change is predicted using incremental FEM simulation method with the realistic sliding effect of the lip and the mucosa. Both are described below in detail.

2.1 Lip-Detailed Patient-Specific FE Mesh Generation

The initial patient-specific and anatomically-detailed hexahedral FE mesh is generated using our previously developed method, which has been proven efficient and accurate [5]. The lip region of the initial FE mesh is further detailed, and the upper and lower lips are separated by the following steps: (1) digitization of lip surface points, (2) selection of lip nodes to be modified, and (3) generation of detailed lip nodes.

Digitization of Lip Surface Points. Digitization of lip surface points was necessary because the image quality in the lip regions is generally poor, e.g., the lip inner surface along the labial surface of the teeth is difficult to detect on CT images due to orthodontic braces and artifacts of amalgam fillings. To overcome this challenge, CT parasagittal views are generated along and perpendicular to the dental arch between the labial commissure (the two lip-end points). Surgeons then manually digitize a group of points along the cross section of the upper and lower lip surfaces, respectively, to form smooth lip contours (Fig. 2).

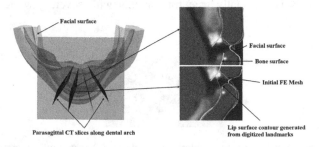

Fig. 2. Digitization of lip surface points on the parasagittal CT slices. Contours for upper and lower lip surfaces are generated based on the digitized points (red). (Color figure online)

Selection of Lip Nodes to Be Modified. Once the points on the upper and lower lip surfaces are digitized, the mesh nodes corresponding to the inner and outer surfaces of each lip are selected in 2-manifold. Each mesh node is then assigned with a 2D grid coordinate (l_u_i, l_v_j) (Fig. 3a). To select the mesh nodes to be modified in the lip region (Fig. 4a), a digitized lip boundary is defined as the contour enclosing the digitized lip points (black dots in Fig. 3b and c). Among the selected lip nodes, the ones inside of the digitized lip boundary are the nodes to be modified based on the digitized lip points (Fig. 3b). The mesh nodes outside of the lip boundary will remain unchanged and designated as the reference points for the lip surface modification next.

Generation of Detailed Lip Nodes. The nodes inside of the digitized lip boundary is modified based on the digitized points. However, the digitized points cannot directly be used for the mesh because the numbers and locations of the points are not correlated to the exact numbers and locations of the existing mesh grids. Generating mesh nodes directly from the digitized lip points can cause invalid or severely distorted mesh elements. Therefore, lip-detailed mesh needs to be generated while preserving original structure of the initial FE mesh. This is achieved by following procedure. First, 2D grid

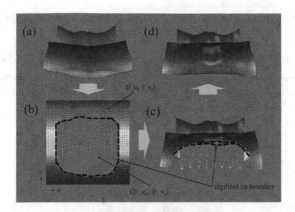

Fig. 3. Lip surface mesh generation based on the digitized landmarks (illustrated by upper lip). (a) Frontal view of lip surface extracted from FE mesh. Lip outer surface (blue) and lip inner surface (red). (b) Lip surface and the digitized landmark represented in the grid coordinate system. Digitized lip boundary is shown in black dots. (c) Detailed lip nodes represented in 3D Cartesian coordinate system. (d) Final lip-detailed mesh surface (Color figure online)

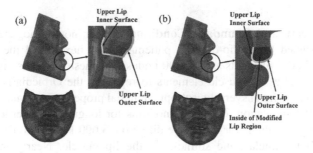

Fig. 4. An example of lip-detailed mesh. (a) Initial mesh without lip-detailed geometry. (b) Lip-detailed mesh with lip opening.

coordinates of the digitized lip points (lp_u, lp_v) are interpolated using 3D Cartesian and 2D grid coordinates of the neighboring mesh nodes. As explained above, the grid coordinates of the digitized lip points (lp_u, lp_v) are not aligned with the existing mesh grid pattern (Fig. 3b). Second, given the coordinates (3D Cartesian and the 2D grid) of the digitized lip points and the reference points, the detailed lip nodes are acquired by approximating 3D Cartesian coordinates of the lip nodes on the existing mesh grid pattern using thin plate splines (TPS). The lip nodes inside of the digitized lip boundary are then modified by replacing them with the acquired detailed lip nodes (Fig. 3c and d and, green and orange in Fig. 4). Finally, to complete the detailed lip mesh generation, the mesh nodes inside of the modified lip region (Fig. 4b) are also modified according to the lip surface modification using TPS. The modification is completed for the upper and lower lips, respectively. The area of the detailed-lip improvement is limited to the lip region without harming the geometrical accuracy of the initial FE mesh.

2.2   Incremental Simulation of Facial Changes with the Realistic Sliding Effect

The facial soft-tissue change is predicted incrementally using realistic sliding effect of the lips and the mucosa. First, material property and boundary condition are defined for the lip-detailed patient-specific FE mesh. Second, facial soft-tissue change simulation is performed using FEM according to the surgical plan.

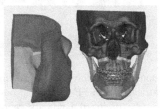

Fig. 5. The boundary condition (represented on bony surface and FE mesh for illustration purpose. Red: fixed nodes; Green: moving nodes; Pink: sliding nodes; and Green-blue: free nodes. (Color figure online)

Material Property and Boundary Condition. Linear non-homogeneous material property is assigned to the lip-detailed patient-specific hexahedral mesh, a total of approximately 40,000 elements and 50,000 nodes. The mesh elements inside of the lip regions are selected as lip muscle elements to represent the Orbicularis Oris muscle. They are assigned with transversely isotropic material property to maintain the shape of the lip during the simulation. (Young's modulus for longitudinal (vertical) direction: 9,000 Pa, Young's modulus for transverse direction: 3,000 Pa, Poisson's ratio for both direction: 0.47) to simulate the stiffness of the lip muscle. Nearly incompressible isotropic linear properties (Young's modulus: 3,000 Pa, Poisson's ratio: 0.47) are applied to the rest of the FE mesh elements. Three different types of boundary nodes are defined on the mesh innermost surface; fixed, moving, and sliding nodes (Fig. 5). Fixed nodes (in red) are defined in the region which is not altered during the surgery. Moving nodes (in green) are nodes that are assumed to be attached to the bone and move together with the bone. They are located on the superior part of the maxillary segment and the inferior part of the mandibular segment to simulate the bony movements during the surgery. Sliding nodes (in pink) are defined around the regions which slide along the bone surface, i.e., the lips and the intraoral mucosa. Unlike the other boundary nodes that are defined on the mesh innermost surface, the lip sliding nodes are defined on the upper and lower lip surfaces. Assignment of boundary nodes is patient-specific and manual. The rest of the nodes are free nodes (in green-blue), and their movement is unconstrained. We assumed the postoperative face is fully relaxed. Therefore, the movement of the free nodes is determined by FEM.

Incremental Facial Change Simulation. The incremental facial change simulation is performed with the mucosa and lip sliding effects using FEM [1]. The incremental simulation is implemented to facilitate a natural transition of the facial change and to enhance the effectiveness of the lip and mucosa sliding movements. It is achieved by evenly dividing the entire bony movement (the surgical plan) into 3 increments, in which each bony segment is moved from its preoperative position to the postoperative one in 3 increments. The acquired incremental bony movement is applied as a boundary condition for the moving nodes. The results of the previous incremental simulation serve as the input for the next incremental simulation, till all 3 are completed. For each incremental simulation, the stiffness matrix and the lip sliding nodes are updated accordingly.

Each incremental simulation is implemented in 2 steps. In the first step, facial change according to the incremental bony movements is simulated with nodal force constraint on the mucosa sliding nodes. The mucosa sliding effect is applied by forcing the mucosa sliding nodes to move along the bony surface by considering only the tangential components of the nodal force of the mucosa sliding nodes [1, 2]. In addition, the lip sliding effect is applied along with the mucosa sliding effect, by allowing the upper and lower lip sliding nodes to move freely according to the bony movements without penetrating each other. This is implemented by a master-slave approach [6] which constrains degrees-of-freedom (DOF) of the movement of the lip sliding nodes. The collisions between the upper and lower lip sliding nodes are detected by point-wise collision detection algorithm (threshold: 0.2 mm). This is to ensure the upper and lower lips does not collide to each other during the vertical movement, while the movements in other directions are not constrained. As a result, the upper and lower lips slide against each other and move independently without penetration. No friction is assumed. However, the result of the first step may include a geometrical mismatch between the bone surface and the mucosa sliding nodes, which is unrealistic [1].

In the second step, this geometrical mismatch is resolved by applying the nodal displacement boundary condition, which is acquired by finding the closest point from each mucosa sliding node to the postoperative bony surface, for the mucosa sliding nodes [1]. No bony movements are applied in the second step. The lip sliding effect is also applied as described above. As a result, the mucosa sliding nodes are ensured to match with the bony surface. In this study, FEM simulation is implemented with our in-house code using Matlab.

3 Experiment and Results

We evaluated our lip-detailed facial change prediction method on five randomly selected patients who are suffered from jaw deformity, underwent an orthognathic surgery, and had complete sets of pre- and postoperative CT data (3 females and 2 males with 21 ± 2.5 years old) from our digital archive [IRB0413-0045]. The facial change prediction was performed using three different simulation methods. Method #1 was the traditional FEM simulation approach without sliding effect [1]. All FE mesh nodes contacting the bony segments were assumed to be fixed to the bony segments. Method #2 was our previously developed three-stage FEM simulation with the mucosa sliding effect using nodal spatial constraint [1]. The sliding effect was applied only to the intraoral mucosa, in which the upper and lower lips were treated as a whole. In both methods, high-quality patient FE meshes were generated using our previous method described in [5]. Method #3 is our incremental simulation with the new lip-detailed FE mesh, and the realistic lip and the mucosa sliding effects developed in this study.

Both pre- and postoperative CT scans were segmented, and 3D models were reconstructed. Postoperative CT models were registered to corresponding preoperative ones based on surgically unaltered regions, i.e., cranium, and served as a "blueprint". Virtual osteotomies were performed on the preoperative model, and the movement vectors of each bony segment, from pre- to postoperative positions, were computed based on the blueprint. Each acquired movement vector was applied to the corresponding moving nodes as a boundary condition to predict the facial soft-tissue changes.

Since the accuracy improvement was mainly in the lip region, only the prediction error of the upper and lower lips was evaluated in this experiment. The upper and lower lips were defined by the anatomical landmarks: subnasale, cheilion, and labiomental fold. The surface deviation error was measured using an average of absolute Euclidean distances between the predicted and the postoperative outcome. Friedman test with Wilcoxon Signed-Rank test was used to detect whether there was a statistically significant difference in accuracy among the three methods.

Table 1. Prediction accuracy evaluation of three different simulation methods using surface deviation error. * Significantly greater than 1 mm ($P < 0.05$), ** Significant improvement compared with Method #1 and #2.

Region	Prediction method			Improvement over method #2 (%)
	Method#1	Method#2	Our approach	
Upper lip	1.11	0.99	0.84	14
Lower lip	1.53*	1.57*	0.85**	46**

The results showed that the prediction accuracy in the lip region was improved with our method. Specifically, the results of Wilcoxon Signed-Rank test showed that using our method, the prediction accuracy of the lower lip was statistically significantly improved ($P < 0.05$). (Table 1 and Fig. 6). Our method achieved a 46.0% of accuracy improvement over Method #2 (Table 1 and Fig. 6). In addition, the lower lip prediction accuracy achieved sub-millimeter accuracy (0.85 mm), while the other two methods showed error significantly greater than 1 mm (Method #2: 1.53 mm; Method #2: 1.57 mm) according to Wilcoxon Signed-Rank test ($p < 0.05$). Finally, although it was not statistically significantly different, the prediction accuracy for the upper lip also showed a trend of 14% of improvement over Method #2 (Table 1 and Fig. 6).

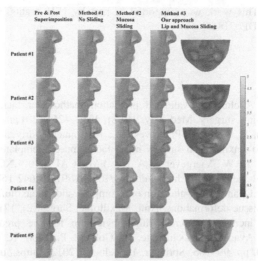

Blue: preoperative face; Red: postoperative face; Green: prediction results

Fig. 6. Prediction results using three different methods: Traditional method without sliding effect (Method #1); Mucosa sliding effect only (Method #2); Our approach (Method #3) with lip and mucosa sliding effect. Color-coded surface deviation errors between the postoperative face and the prediction results using our approach are in the rightmost column. (Color figure online)

4   Discussion and Conclusion

We have significantly improved our previous FEM simulation method with the addition of realistic lip sliding effect to predict the facial soft-tissue change following orthognathic surgery. The evaluation results also confirmed our hypothesis that the application of lip sliding effect can improve the prediction accuracy in the lip region.

The realistic lip sliding effect plays a major role in the facial change prediction in addition to the mucosa sliding effect. The inaccurate prediction are mainly occurred in the lip region, especially in patients with severe jaw deformity, which the low lips are severely deformed [3]. While the mucosa sliding effect improves the prediction accuracy [1, 2], the upper and lower lip movements are still treated as a whole and not simulated independently. In our proposed method, the FE mesh of the upper and lower lips are detailed and separated, allowing to simulate the upper and the lower lip changes individually. Finally, the sliding effect was effectively enhanced by applying the incremental bony movements, facilitating a smooth and natural soft-tissue change.

In the future, our method will be investigated with an extended number of patients for more intensive validation. The prediction accuracy also needs to be evaluated with qualitative evaluation method that reflects clinician's visual evaluation because current quantitative evaluation, i.e., surface deviation error, does not fully reflect the clinician's qualitative assessment [1]. In addition, the manual generation of the lip-detailed mesh can prevent clinicians from adopting it to daily clinical use, and this needs to be addressed in the future.

Acknowledgment. This work was supported in part by NIH grants (R01 DE022676, R01 DE027251 and R01 DE021863).

References

1. Kim, D., et al.: A clinically validated prediction method for facial soft-tissue changes following double-jaw surgery. Med. Phys. **44**(8), 4252–4261 (2017)
2. Kim, H., Jürgens, P., Nolte, L.-P., Reyes, M.: Anatomically-driven soft-tissue simulation strategy for cranio-maxillofacial surgery using facial muscle template model. In: Jiang, T., Navab, N., Pluim, J.P.W., Viergever, M.A. (eds.) MICCAI 2010. LNCS, vol. 6361, pp. 61–68. Springer, Heidelberg (2010). https://doi.org/10.1007/978-3-642-15705-9_8
3. Nadjmi, N., et al.: Quantitative validation of a computer-aided maxillofacial planning system, focusing on soft tissue deformations. Ann. Maxillofac. Surg. **4**(2), 171–175 (2014)
4. Pan, B., et al.: Incremental kernel ridge regression for the prediction of soft tissue deformations. In: Ayache, N., Delingette, H., Golland, P., Mori, K. (eds.) MICCAI 2012. LNCS, vol. 7510, pp. 99–106. Springer, Heidelberg (2012). https://doi.org/10.1007/978-3-642-33415-3_13
5. Zhang, X., et al.: An eFTD-VP framework for efficiently generating patient-specific anatomically detailed facial soft tissue FE mesh for craniomaxillofacial surgery simulation. Biomech. Model. Mechanobiol. **17**(2), 387–402 (2018)
6. Muñoz, J.J., Jelenić, G.: Sliding contact conditions using the master–slave approach with application on geometrically non-linear beams. Int. J. Solids Struct. **41**(24), 6963–6992 (2004)

An Automatic Approach to Reestablish Final Dental Occlusion for 1-Piece Maxillary Orthognathic Surgery

Han Deng[1], Peng Yuan[1], Sonny Wong[2], Jaime Gateno[1,3],
Fred A. Garrett[2], Randy K. Ellis[2], Jeryl D. English[2], Helder B. Jacob[2],
Daeseung Kim[1], and James J. Xia[1,3(✉)]

[1] Department of Oral and Maxillofacial Surgery,
Houston Methodist Research Institute, Houston, TX, USA
jxia@houstonmethodist.org
[2] Department of Orthodontics, University of Texas Houston Health Science
Center Dentistry School, Houston, TX, USA
[3] Department of Surgery (Oral and Maxillofacial Surgery),
Weill Medical College, Cornell University, New York, NY, USA

Abstract. Accurately establishing a desired final dental occlusion of the upper and lower teeth is a critical step in orthognathic surgical planning. Traditionally, the final occlusion is established by hand-articulating the stone dental models. However, this process is inappropriate to digitally plan the orthognathic surgery using computer-aided surgical simulation. To date, there is no effective method of digitally establishing final occlusion. We propose a 3-stage approach to digitally and automatically establish a desired final dental occlusion for 1-piece maxillary orthognathic surgery, including: (1) to automatically extract points of interest and four key teeth landmarks from the occlusal surfaces; (2) to align the upper and lower teeth to a clinically desired Midline-Canine-Molar relationship by minimization of sum of distances between them; and (3) to finely align the upper and lower teeth to a maximum contact with the constraints of collision and clinical criteria. The proposed method was evaluated qualitatively and quantitatively and proved to be effective and accurate.

1 Introduction

Dentistry is going digital, and so is orthognathic surgery. In the last decade, computer-aided surgical simulation (CASS) becomes the standard of care for planning orthognathic surgery [1]. An important step in CASS orthognathic surgery planning is to establish a desired dental occlusion (called "final occlusion") between the upper and lower teeth. Traditionally, surgeons hand-articulate upper and lower stone dental models. The instant tactile response and cognitive insight help them to quickly achieve a desired position of the stone models, i.e., midline alignment, Class I canine and molar relations, and a maximized contact between the upper and lower teeth. However, it is

---

H. Deng and P. Yuan—Contribute Equally.

© Springer Nature Switzerland AG 2019
D. Shen et al. (Eds.): MICCAI 2019, LNCS 11768, pp. 345–353, 2019.
https://doi.org/10.1007/978-3-030-32254-0_39

completely different in the digital world. The digital upper and lower dental models are represented by point clouds or triangulated surfaces that have a lack of tactile response. When they are in contact, they can still be moved towards and penetrate into each other. Therefore, in the current CASS clinical protocol, surgeons still need to hand-articulate the stone models to the final occlusion and use CBCT scanner to scan them together into the computer. It takes at least an hour in the office. If the digital dental models are generated using an intraoral scanner, it will take additional 4 h to 3D print the teeth models for hand articulation. This process is convoluted, time-consuming and cost-inefficient, and may introduce unpredicted inaccuracy into the planning.

There are reports on digital dental occlusion [2, 3]. However, they either require moving the models together manually or are computationally inefficient, and thus have not been used clinically. In the past, we have developed a method of digitally articu-lating the upper and lower dental models into maximum intercuspation (MI) [4–6]. However, this method is problematic and only used in the laboratory setting. It only considers MI relationship, which is an occlusion that simply maximizes the contacting areas between the upper and lower teeth without considering the other important clinical criteria. Thus, most of time, the results cannot be used in clinical practice. In addition, it requires manually extracting the occlusal surface by removing the braces and the gums from the digital models. Moreover, it is computationally inefficient. Even after the models are manually prepared, it takes more than an hour to complete the computation. Due to these problems, we can only utilize it in the laboratory.

In this project, we propose a three-stage approach to automatically articulate the upper and lower dental models to the final occlusion for 1-piece maxillary orthognathic surgery. In the first stage, points of interest (POI) and four key teeth landmarks (each landmark appears on both left and right side) are automatically extracted from the teeth occlusal surfaces. In the second stage, the upper and lower teeth are aligned to a clinically desired Midline-Canine-Molar (M-C-M) relationship. In the third stage, the upper and lower teeth are finely aligned to a best possible maximum contact, i.e., the best option among many possibilities of making contacts between the upper and lower teeth with the constraints of clinical criteria and collision.

The contributions of this proposed approach are that: (1) the approach jointly considers the clinical criteria and a maximized contact between the upper and lower teeth to seek the best possible final dental occlusion; (2) it is a fully automatic approach without labor-intensive manual manipulation, which is a mandatory step in our pre-vious method; and (3) it is computationally efficient.

2 Method

Our automatic dental articulation is completed in three stages to: (1) extract POI and four key landmarks that are not digitized in regular clinical routine, (2) establish a clinically desired M-C-M relationship, and (3) seek a maximum contact with the constraints of collision and clinical criteria. During the articulation, the lower teeth remains static while the upper teeth articulates onto the lower teeth. Since the digital articulation is a part of CASS planning, all the teeth landmarks, except four, have already been digitized following the clinical routine [7, 8]. Our approach is described below in details.

2.1 POI Extraction

Each dental model consists of thousands of points. During the articulation, only the points on the upper and lower occlusal surfaces are occluded. We refer the points on the occlusal surfaces that form the edges, cusps and grooves as POI – the points of interest. They are automatically extracted in the following four steps.

Occlusal Surface Extraction: Orthodontic braces and gums interfere with the digital dental articulation. Therefore, it is necessary to extract the occlusal surfaces from the teeth models. First, a 200-point fitting curve is created using seven already digitized teeth landmarks (Fig. 1a, Table 1). A plane (called PCA plane) is created by principle component analysis (PCA) using the same landmarks. The distance h_v between each vertex v on the model and the PCA plane is calculated. Then, the fitting curve and the vertices of the entire teeth model are projected onto the PCA plane. The distance r_v between each projected vertex and the projected fitting curve is calculated. We set a threshold H empirically, e.g., 15, since the height of the tooth crown is usually within 10 mm. For each vertex u belongs to model vertex set $\{v\}$ such that $h_u < H$, we define a parameter ϕ_u as $\alpha \cdot h_u + (1 - \alpha) \cdot r_u$, where α is coefficient (empirically set as 0.2) that controls the relative influence of h_u and r_u. Then k-means clustering algorithm is performed using ϕ_u to extract a "clean" surface for the next step (Fig. 1b).

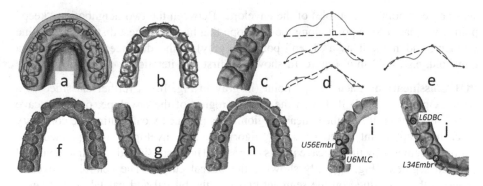

Fig. 1. Points-of-Interest (POI) extraction and landmark detection (Note: the diameter of all the landmarks/points are intentionally enlarged for illusion purpose). (Color figure online)

Envelope Simplification: Across-sectional plane of the teeth is created for each point of the fitting curve (Fig. 1c), forming 200 planes for the entire teeth model. An envelope is calculated based on the intersectional line of each cross-sectional plane and the occlusal surface (brown curve in Fig. 1c). Each envelop is then simplified using Douglas-Peucker algorithm to extract key geometric feature points. As shown in Fig. 1d, a line segment is iteratively formed by connecting the two neighboring "keep" points on the envelope. In the first iteration, the two neighboring "keep" points are the

Table 1. Teeth landmarks used in our proposed approach (1: used for POI extraction; 2: used for M-C-M alignment; * automatically detected landmark)

	Upper teeth landmark	Predefined name	Corresponding lower teeth landmark	Predefined name
Midline	Midpoint of central incisors	$U0^{1,2}$	Midpoint of central incisors	$L0^{1,2}$
Canine	Canine cusp	$U3C^{1,2}$	Embrasure between canine and 1st premolar	$L34Embr^{2,*}$
	–	–	Canine cusp	$L3C^{1}$
Molar	Embrasure between 2nd premolar and 1st molar	$U56Embr^{2,*}$	Mesiobuccal cusp of 1st molar	$L6MBC^{1,2}$
	Mesiobuccal cusp of 1st molar	$U6MBC^{1}$	–	–
	Mesiolingual cusp of 1st molar	$U6MLC^{2,*}$	Central fossa of lower 1st molar	$L6CF^{2}$
	Central fossa of 1st molar	$U6CF^{2}$	Distobuccal cusp of 1st molar	$L6DBC^{2,*}$
	Mesiobuccal cusp of 2nd molar	$U7MBC^{1}$	–	–
	–	–	Mesiobuccal cusp of 2nd molar	$L7MBC^{1}$

start and end points (in purple) of the envelope. Between the two neighboring "keep" points, we search for a point along the envelope that has the largest distance to the line segment, and mark it as a "keep" point (in gray) if the distance is larger than a threshold, e.g., 0.02 mm. Figure 1d shows the first two iterations.

POI Classification: Each "keep" point (in gray in Fig. 1e) is further classified as a "convex point" (in red) if it is in the convex region of the envelope, or a "concave point" (in green) if it is in the concave region. This is done by calculating the concavity of each "keep" point based on Javis' algorithm. All envelopes are separated into multiple segments by the concave points (Fig. 1f). The cusps (in red) are first identified on each segment (Fig. 1g, only showing the buccal cusps). The central groove (in green) is then identified on the segment between the buccal and palatal/lingual cusps (Fig. 1h).

Landmark Detection: The classified cusp points are used together with the already digitized landmarks to detect two pairs of un-digitized but required landmarks for the upper and lower teeth, respectively (Table 1). The distances between each cusp point and the PCA plane are calculated, which are used to seek peaks and valleys among the cusp points (in red, Fig. 1g). Finally, the names and the locations of already digitized landmarks are used in conjunction to extract our desired peak and valley points for upper (U6MLC and U56Embr, Fig. 1i) and lower (L6DBC and L34Embr, Fig. 1j) teeth.

2.2   Midline-Canine-Molar Alignment

The purpose of M-C-M alignment is to align the "mobile" upper teeth to the "static" lower teeth based on the clinical criteria. The detailed process is described below.

Local Coordinate System. In order to incorporate the clinical criteria (dental midline alignment, and canine and molar relationships) into the algorithm, a local coordinate system is established for each of the key landmarks on the "static" lower teeth, respectively (Table 1, Fig. 2). First, the lower occlusal plane is created using PCA based on the nine key teeth landmarks. The direction of the normal vector Z of the lower occlusal plane is from the teeth root towards the crown. Next, each landmark is projected to the lower occlusal plane. A new fitting curve is then formed based on the projected landmarks. The local coordinate system is defined as follows: the z-axis for all the landmarks is the normal vector Z; the x-axis for each landmark is the tangent line of the fitting curve, pointing from the left side to the right; and the y-axis is orthogonal to the x- and z-axis, pointing from the labial/buccal side to the lingual (Fig. 2c).

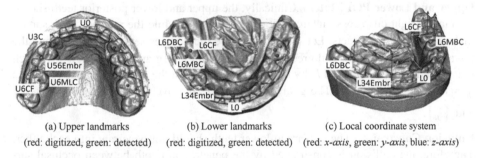

(a) Upper landmarks   (b) Lower landmarks   (c) Local coordinate system
(red: digitized, green: detected)   (red: digitized, green: detected)   (red: x-axis, green: y-axis, blue: z-axis)

Fig. 2. Landmarks and local coordinate systems (Color figure online)

Minimization of Sum of Distances. In this step, we jointly consider the clinical requirements on midline, canine, and molar. Each upper landmark l_u has a corresponding lower landmark l_l. We rotate and translate upper teeth using a transformation matrix M. Thus, each upper dental landmark l_r has a new position $M \cdot l_r$. The following distances between the paired upper and lower landmarks are calculated: (1) d_{mi}^x is the distance between midline landmarks (U0 and L0) along local x-axis, where d_{mi} is a vector from L0 to U0; (2) d_c^x is the distance between each pair of canine landmarks (U3C and L34Embr) along local x-axis, where d_c is a vector from L34Embr to U3C; and (3) d_{mo}^E is the *Euclidean* distance between each pair of the molar landmarks (U56Embr and L6MBC, U6MLC and L6CF, U6CF and L6DBC), where d_{mo} is the vector from lower molar landmark to the corresponding upper molar landmark.

It is also important to ensure the upper dental arch is on the labial/buccal side (outside) of the lower dental arch. To ensure that the directions of both vectors d_{mi} and d_c are from the lingual to the labial side, we need $y_{mi} \cdot d_{mi} < 0$ and $y_c \cdot d_c < 0$, where y_{mi} and y_c are the local y-axis of L0 and L34Embr, respectively. Similarly, we use d_{mo} to ensure the upper molar is above the lower molar by $z \cdot d_{mo} > 0$, where z is the local z-axis. In order to apply the above constraints, we add a penalty function by using a large coefficient Ω ($\Omega \to \infty$) for d_{mi}, d_c, and d_{mo}. Thus, the objective function for finding the transformation matrix M of the upper teeth is:

$$
Min\ \{d_{mi}^x + \sum_{canine} d_c^x + \sum_{molar} d_{mo}^E
$$
$$
+\Omega[\mathbb{1}(\,y_{mi} \cdot d_{mi}) + \sum_{canine} \mathbb{1}\,(y_c \cdot d_c) + \sum_{molar} \mathbb{1}(-z \cdot d_{mo})]\},
\tag{1}
$$

where $\mathbb{1}$ is indicator function so that $\mathbb{1}(x) := \begin{cases} 1, & if\ x > 0 \\ 0, & if\ x \le 0 \end{cases}$.

2.3   Fine Alignment

The purpose of the third stage is to iteratively seek a maximum contact between the upper and lower teeth, while keeping the constraints of collision and clinical criteria (the M-C-M relationship). The details are described below.

Upper and Lower POI Match. Clinically, the upper and lower posterior teeth should maintain a tight cusp-fossa intercuspation relationship, while the anterior teeth should make a maximum contacts. Let $\{u_i\}$ and $\{l_j\}$ be the vertices sets of the upper and the lower POIs (the red peak and green valley points in Fig. 1g and h), respectively. Each u_i is paired with a lower POI l_{j_i} by finding the vertex with the closest distance to u_i, i.e., $l_{j_i} = argmin_{l \in \{l_j\}} \|u_i - l\|$. The goal is to minimize the overall distance between $\{u_i\}$ and $\{l_{j_i}\}$.

Collision Constraint. The upper and lower teeth should not penetrate into each other. Therefore, the collision is constrained by the penetration depth between occlusal surfaces of the upper and lower teeth. Based on our clinical observation, a 0.1 mm of penetration depth is allowed because it is deemed to be an error of the constructed STL model. The upper and lower vertices on occlusal surfaces are paired using the same method for point match. For each pair, the penetration depth is calculated as the distance of upper vertex v_{upper} and lower vertex v_{lower} along the normal direction of the lower vertex n_{lower}. They should not be greater than 0.1 mm. In addition, to reduce the computational complexity, we only compute the penetration depth when the Euclidean distance between a pair of vertices is smaller than a certain threshold ϵ, i.e., 1.0 mm. The constraint is $(Rv_{upper} + t - v_{lower}) \cdot n_{lower} + \epsilon \ge 0$, where R is rotation matrix and t is translation matrix.

Clinical Criteria Constraint. During the POI-based fine alignment, the M-C-M relationship must be maintained. Therefore, we set a threshold for constraining the distances between the landmarks U0 and L0 along the local x, y, and z-axes (Fig. 2c). The movement and resulted position of U0 is constrained by the clinical criteria and normative values, i.e., the distance along the x-axis is within 1.5 mm for midline deviation; the distance along the y-axis is within the normal range of 1.5–3.0 mm for overjet; and the distance along the z-axis is within the normal range of 2.0–4.0 mm for overbite (the deeper the better). We believe that such a small amount of the movement will not disrupt the canine and molar relationships established by M-C-M alignment.

Transformation Matrix Update. During each iteration, a rotational center of the upper teeth model is calculated and updated based on the distance between the upper and the lower POIs. A weight is assigned to each vertex on the upper POI according to its distance to the closest vertex on the lower POI as $w_i = \frac{1}{e^{|u_i - l_i|}}$. The rotation center is calculated as weighted center of upper POI, i.e., $\tilde{o} \leftarrow \frac{\sum_i w_i u_i}{\sum_i w_i}$.

The transformation of the upper teeth is calculated by solving the optimization problem of minimizing the distance between current paired $\{u_i\}$ and $\{l_{j_i}\}$ subject to the above collision and clinical constraints. The objective function is written as

$$Min \sum_{i=1}^{n} \left\| R(u_i - \tilde{o}) + \tilde{o} + t - l_{j_i} \right\|^2 \tag{2}$$

where R is rotation matrix and t is translation matrix.

The upper teeth model is thus translated and rotated to a new position. In the following iteration, we re-match upper and lower POI and repeat the above steps. The process is stopped when the difference between overall distances yield from two consecutive iterations is small than a certain threshold δ (i.e., 0.05 mm) or when the total number of iterations exceeds 30.

3   Experiments and Results

The accuracy and efficiency of our approach was evaluated using 5 sets of patient dental models qualitatively and quantitatively [IRB# Pro00003644]. First, each pair of the upper and lower stone dental models were scanned separately using a cone-beam computed tomography scanner, forming a set of independent upper and lower digital models in STL format. The models are reconstructed by standard marching cubes and Laplacian-based surface smoothing. Each model contains about 700 thousand triangles (1.8 million vertices). The quality of the models is adequate in CASS practice for designing surgical splints. Next, the final occlusion of the upper and lower stone models were hand-articulated by two experienced orthodontists, and scanned together using the same scanner, forming a final occlusal template. The corresponding individually scanned models were then registered to the template, resulting in the upper and lower teeth at their final occlusion (control group – the ground truth). Third, our three-stage approach was used to automatically articulate the upper and lower models to the final occlusion (experimental group). The code was written using Matlab and run on a regular office personal computer (i7 CPU and 16 GB memory). Finally, the computer-generated occlusions were compared to the hand-articulated ones.

During the qualitative evaluation, the corresponding computer- and hand-articulated dental models were randomly assigned as the first or second set. Two orthodontists, blinded from the articulation method, together evaluated results on a 27" monitor. A 3-scale visual analog scale (VAS, 1: the first set was better; 2: they were equal; and 3: the first set was worse) was used. The evaluation criteria included: midline alignment, Class I canine relation, Class I molar relationship, and maximum contact. During the quantitative evaluation, we calculated the distances of midline and canines deviating from their ideal positions along their local x-axis using corresponding midline and canine key landmarks (Table 1). We also calculate the *Euclidian* distances between molar key landmarks. Finally, Wilcoxon Signed Rank tests were performed.

The results showed that all the upper and lower dental models were successfully aligned to the desired final occlusion using our approach. The computational time for each set of the articulation was within 3 min. The qualitative results showed that all 5 sets of computer-articulated models were as good as the hand-articulated ones (Fig. 3). The quantitative results showed that except one, there was no statistically significant difference between the computer- and hand-articulated final occlusions. The distance of the left molar relationship generated by our approach was statistically smaller than the ground truth, indicating the computer-generated occlusions were better than the hand-articulated ones (Table 2).

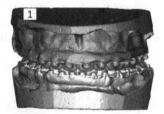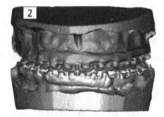

Fig. 3. Results of a randomly selected case (1: hand-articulated; 2: computer-generated)

Table 2. Measurement comparison

	Hand-articulated		Computer-articulated		
	Median	Range	Median	Range	P value
Midline deviation	0.04	−0.49	0.41	0.35	−0.52	0.44	0.87
Right canine relation	1.37	0.27	2.53	0.95	0.56	2.53	0.98
Left canine relation	−1.44	−1.93	−0.88	−1.23	−1.84	−0.57	0.96
Right molar relation	2.12	1.37	3.23	2.15	1.64	3.76	0.11
Left molar relation	2.87	1.91	4.38	2.35	1.64	4.11	0.02

4   Discussion and Conclusion

Previously proposed methods of digital dental articulation either were ineffective, convoluted, or required labor-intensive interaction. Our proposed three-stage approach is able to effectively, accurately and full automatically articulate the upper and lower teeth into a desired final dental occlusion for one-piece maxillary orthognathic surgery. In the first stage, the POI of occlusal surface and four key landmarks that are not digitized in clinical routine are automatically extracted from the teeth models. In the second stage, the upper and lower teeth are aligned to fulfill a clinically desired M-C-M relationship by minimization of sum of distances between them. In the third stage, the upper and lower teeth are finely articulated to a maximum contact with the collision and clinical criteria constraints. In the future, we will validate the approach ultimately using a larger sample size. We will also expand our approach to multi-piece maxillary orthognathic surgery.

Acknowledgment. This work was supported in part by NIH grants (R01 DE022676 and R01 DE027251).

References

1. Xia, J.J., et al.: Algorithm for planning a double-jaw orthognathic surgery using a computer-aided surgical simulation (CASS) protocol. Part 1: planning sequence. Int. J. Oral Maxillofac. Surg. **44**(12), 1431–1440 (2015)
2. Nadjmi, N., et al.: Virtual occlusion in planning orthognathic surgical procedures. Int. J. Oral Maxillofac. Surg. **39**(5), 457–462 (2010)
3. Wu, W., et al.: Haptic simulation framework for determining virtual dental occlusion. Int. J. Comput. Assist. Radiol. Surg. **12**(4), 595–606 (2017)
4. Chang, Y.-B., et al.: An automatic and robust algorithm of reestablishment of digital dental occlusion. IEEE Trans. Med. Imaging **29**(9), 1652–1663 (2010)
5. Chang, Y.-B., et al.: In vitro evaluation of new approach to digital dental model articulation. J. Oral Maxillofac. Surg.: Official J. Am. Assoc. Oral Maxillofac. Surg. **70**(4), 952–962 (2012)
6. Xia, J.J., Chang, Y.-B., Gateno, J., Xiong, Z., Zhou, X.: Automated digital dental articulation. In: Jiang, T., Navab, N., Pluim, J.P.W., Viergever, M.A. (eds.) MICCAI 2010. LNCS, vol. 6363, pp. 278–286. Springer, Heidelberg (2010). https://doi.org/10.1007/978-3-642-15711-0_35
7. Li, J., et al.: New approach to establish an object reference frame for dental arch in computer-aided surgical simulation. Int. J. Oral Maxillofac. Surg. **46**(9), 1193–1200 (2017)
8. Xia, J.J., et al.: Algorithm for planning a double-jaw orthognathic surgery using a computer-aided surgical simulation (CASS) protocol. Part 2: three-dimensional cephalometry. Int. J. Oral Maxillofac. Surg. **44**(12), 1441–1450 (2015)

MIC Meets CAI

A Two-Stage Framework for Real-Time Guidewire Endpoint Localization

Rui-Qi Li[1,2], Guibin Bian[1,2], Xiaohu Zhou[1,2], Xiaoliang Xie[1,2],
ZhenLiang Ni[1,2], and Zengguang Hou[1,2,3(✉)]

[1] State Key Laboratory of Management and Control for Complex Systems,
Institute of Automation, Chinese Academy of Sciences, Beijing 100190, China
zengguang.hou@ia.ac.cn
[2] University of Chinese Academy of Sciences, Beijing 100049, China
[3] CAS Center for Excellence in Brain Science and Intelligence Technology,
Beijing 100190, China

Abstract. The ability of real-time instrument tracking is a stepping stone to various computer-assisted interventions. In this paper, we introduce a two-stage framework for real-time guidewire endpoint localization in fluoroscopy images during the percutaneous coronary intervention. In the first stage, in order to predict all bounding boxes that contain a guidewire, a YOLOv3 detector is applied, and following the detector, a post-processing algorithm is proposed to refine the bounding boxes produced by the detector. In the second stage, an SA-hourglass network modified on stacked hourglass network is proposed, to predict dense heatmap of the guidewire endpoints that may be contained in each bounding box. Although our SA-hourglass network is designed for endpoint localization of guidewire, in fact, we believe the network can be generalized to the keypoint localization task of other surgical instruments. In order to prove our view, SA-hourglass network is trained not only on a guidewire dataset but also a retinal microsurgery dataset, and both achieve the state-of-the-art localization results.

Keywords: Guidewire · Keypoint localization · Surgical instrument

1 Introduction

The keypoint localization of surgical instruments is one of the key components of computer-assisted interventions. From the localization results, we can estimate the pose of the instruments and infer the use status of the instruments. For percutaneous coronary intervention (PCI), the most important surgical instrument is the guidewire which is navigated under real-time fluoroscopy images during the

---

Electronic supplementary material The online version of this chapter (https://doi.org/10.1007/978-3-030-32254-0_40) contains supplementary material, which is available to authorized users.

D. Shen et al. (Eds.): MICCAI 2019, LNCS 11768, pp. 357–365, 2019.
https://doi.org/10.1007/978-3-030-32254-0_40

intervention, as shown in Fig. 1. Real-time keypoint (i.e. endpoint) localization of guidewire in the fluoroscopy images is of great significance. It can be used in technical skills assessment [1]. More importantly, it could be applied in computer-assisted interventions to help the computer understand the real-time situation.

As far as we know, there is a few research focus on this specific task. Most of research about interventional guidewires focus on guidewire segmentation [2] and the fitting curve [3,4] of the guidewire. Although the endpoint's position of the guidewire can be easily inferred from the segmentation results or the fitting curve results, however, these methods pay more attention to the main body of the guidewire rather than the endpoints. From the results in [2], we can see a median centerline distance error of 0.2 mm but a median endpoint distance error of 0.9 mm. Essentially, the guidewire is a kind of surgical instruments. There has been a lot of research concentrate on the keypoint localization of the surgical instruments used in laparoscopic surgery and retinal surgery [5–7]. Compared with these instruments, the guidewire presents more difficulties so that these methods cannot be applied directly:

1. **Small size of visible part:** Only a small portion of the guidewire is visible, while the main body of the guidewire is almost invisible.
2. **Simple appearance of the endpoint:** Simple appearance seems like an advantage for localization, but it also means there will be more similar structures in the fluoroscopy images, which have a low signal-to-noise ratio.
3. **Non-rigid body:** Not like other surgical instruments, the guidewire is not a rigid body. Therefore, under the premise of a low frame rate (8FPS), the shape of guidewire varies significantly from frame to frame.

To address the above difficulties, a detection stage is proposed before the localization stage inspired by [8]. The overall framework is shown in Fig. 1. In both stages, a method based on deep convolutional neural network (CNN) is proposed. CNN is extremely powerful in extracting local features and performing good predictions utilizing a large receptive field.

Our contributions are as follows. (1) We introduce a cascade framework for guidewire endpoint localization. (2) A post-processing algorithm is proposed in the first stage to deal with the false positives and false negatives of the detections. (3) We also propose a SA-hourglass network in the second stage which can be applied in keypoint localization of other instruments as well. Besides, our framework can achieve real-time localization at an inference rate of approximately 10FPS (fluoroscopy image is about 8FPS).

2   Method

2.1   Stage 1: Guidewire Detection

Our task is to predict a bounding box for each guidewire in consecutive fluoroscopy images. It is different from the detection task which only needs to detect the objects in a single image, also different from the tracking task which needs

Workflow:

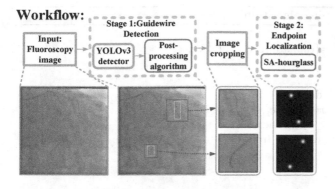

Fig. 1. The overall framework for guidewire endpoint localization. In the first stage, detect the location (white box) of all guidewires. Then crop the corresponding patch (red box) from the image. In the second stage, the localization network predicts the heatmaps of two endpoints. The post-processing algorithm and SA-hourglass in green boxes are newly proposed by us. (Color figure online)

Fig. 2. Demonstrations of two types of attention maps generated by segmentation labels and endpoint positions respectively

to track a class agnostic object. Therefore, a detector can be applied to produce accurate candidates (bounding boxes) of the guidewire, then the constraint relationships between frames can be used to reselect these candidates.

Choosing a Detector: Currently, there are two popular architectures of object detection: one-stage architectures represented by YOLO [9], and two-stage architectures represented by Faster-RCNN [10]. One-stage detectors perform better on speed, while two-stage detectors perform better on accuracy. In order to select an appropriate detector, we train YOLOv3 and Faster-RCNN respectively using our guidewire dataset. Experimental results show that the detection accuracy of YOLOv3 is slightly lower than that of Faster-RCNN (96.4% vs. 98.4% in mAP), but YOLOv3 performs much better than Faster-RCNN in time efficiency (0.05 s vs. 0.12 s). In order to meet the real-time requirement, YOLOv3 is chosen as the detector of our framework. The outputs of the detector are several candidate boxes, each with a confidence score. We only select candidates with scores larger than a given threshold, which is hard to set, as the final outputs.

Post-processing Algorithm: In a continuous sequence of images, there are two primary constraints between two consecutive frames: (1) The distance between the same object in two consecutive frames could not be too far. (2) Existing objects do not suddenly disappear, and objects could not suddenly appear where there was no object before. These two constraints can be used to judge whether the candidate is correct, with the objects existing in the previous frame.

Based on these conditions, a post-processing algorithm is proposed to refine the output candidates of the YOLOv3 detector. Instead of using a single threshold, inspired by the Canny edge detector, all candidates are reselected into two

---

Algorithm 1. Post-processing algorithm

Initialize: $O^t = \emptyset$, $O_{temp}^t = \emptyset$
Input: $C_H^t = \{c_0, ..., c_N\}$, $C_L^t = \{c_0, ..., c_M\}$, O^{t-1}, O_{temp}^{t-1}
1: **if** t==1 **then** $O^t = C_H^t$
2: **else**
3:    **for** $o_i \in \{O^{t-1}, O_{temp}^{t-1}\}$ **do**
4:       $c_{best} = c_j$ where max(S-IOU(c_j, o_i)),$c_j \in \{C_H^t, C_L^t\}$
5:       **if** S-IOU(c_{best}, o_i) $\geq \sigma_{IOU}$ **then**
6:          add c_{best} to O^t; delete o_i from O^{t-1} or O_{temp}^{t-1}; delete c_j from C_H^t or C_L^t
7:    **for** $o_i \in O^{t-1}$ **do**
8:       add o_i to O_{temp}^t
9:    **for** $c_i \in C_H^t$ **do**
10:       add c_i to O_{temp}^t
11: **return** O^t,O_{temp}^t

---

candidate lists (C_H and C_L) using two thresholds (th_H and th_L, $th_H > th_L$). If the candidate's confidence score is larger than th_H, the candidate is considered highly likely to contain a guidewire and will be put into the list C_H. If the score is less than th_H but larger than th_L, the candidate is considered likely to contain a guidewire and will be put into the list C_L. Two output lists O^t, O_{temp}^t will be created at each timestep t: O^t is used to store the output candidates which already confirmed to contain a guidewire at time t; O_{temp}^t is used to store the temporary output candidates which need to be confirmed in the next timestep. The algorithm is actually to select candidates from two candidate lists C_H and C_L to two output lists O^t and O_{temp}^t at each timestep t with the help of O^{t-1} and O_{temp}^{t-1}. Details can be seen in Algorithm 1. All candidates in O^t and O_{temp}^t are the outputs of the algorithm, also the outputs of the first stage.

Since the shape of the guidewire is variable, a new S-IOU (Intersection over Union) is applied in algorithm: first enlarge each box to a square box by extending the height or width of the box, and then calculate the IOU of two square boxes.

2.2   Stage 2: Guidewire Endpoint Localization

The guidewire endpoint localization component in our framework predicts the heatmaps of two guidewire endpoints, given each bounding box produced by the first stage, as shown in Fig. 1. Because these two endpoints have a similar appearance, we serve both endpoints as the same type of keypoint and predict them in one heatmap. The ground truth of the heatmap is still created by applying a Gaussian kernel to the endpoint's ground truth position as in [7].

Image Cropping: Directly cropping the image by the bounding box and resizing it to the input resolution of the localization network will change the aspect ratio of the guidewire. To keep the aspect ratio of the guidewire, each bounding box is enlarged to a square box by extending either their height or their width.

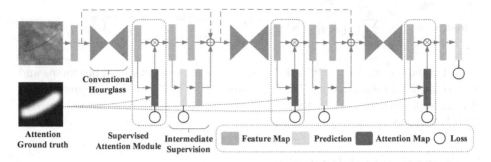

Fig. 3. The proposed SA-hourglass architecture, newly added supervised attention module is shown in the blue boxes. (Color figure online)

The square box is further enlarged with a factor during training and evaluation. During training, a random rescaling factor between 1.1 and 1.3 is applied for data augmentation. During the evaluation, a factor of 1.2 is applied to compensate for possible offsets in the detection results, as shown in Fig. 1.

SA-Hourglass: Stacked hourglass [11] is one of the most popular architectures in human pose estimation. We modify the stacked hourglass by adding a Supervised-Attention (SA) module following the output feature maps of each hourglass and name it as SA-hourglass, as shown in Fig. 3.

Also, some configurations are modified to meet the need of endpoint localization of the guidewire. First, in order to increase the localization accuracy, the first max pooling layer is removed for enlarging the output heatmap size. Second, only three hourglasses are applied in our network. For guidewire and other medical instruments, there is no complex spatial relationships need to learn, so only three hourglasses are applied to reduce the inference time.

Supervised-Attention Module: Our attention module is similar to conventional soft attention in [12]. Following the output feature map of each hourglass, two 3×3 and a 1×1 convolutional layers are applied to generate the attention map. Then the attention map is applied to the feature map which generates it, as shown in Fig. 3. In general, attention mechanism in CNN is used to add a non-linear operation in feature extraction. Since there is no supervision to attention modules, the attention maps learned by the network may not be the results we want. Especially in the heatmap regression, the attention map is supposed to pay more attention around the keypoints, however, because of the pixel-wise distribution of the heatmap is imbalanced, the gradient is dominated by the majority background pixels. As a result, the attention around the keypoints is suppressed, and the focus of attention shifts to the background.

After giving the ground truths to attention maps, SA-hourglass network can be regarded as a multi-task learning network. We propose two methods to generate the ground truth of the attention maps: (1) the same as the ground truth of heatmaps but using a larger Gaussian kernel; (2) additional segmentation labels after several Gaussian filtering. Demonstrations are shown in Fig. 2. Mean-square error (MSE) loss is used in both the attention part and the hourglass part:

$$loss = \frac{1}{wh}(\sum_{x=1}^{w}\sum_{y=1}^{h}(S(x,y) - S^*(x,y))^2 + \lambda \sum_{x=1}^{w}\sum_{y=1}^{h}(A(x,y) - A^*(x,y))^2) \quad (1)$$

In this equation, $S \in \mathbb{R}^{w*h}$ and $A \in \mathbb{R}^{w*h}$ are the predictions of heatmaps and attention maps respectively. $S^* \in \mathbb{R}^{w*h}$ and $A^* \in \mathbb{R}^{w*h}$ are the ground truths of heatmaps and attention maps respectively. λ is for balancing the influence of both loss terms

3   Experimental Results

3.1   Datasets

Two datasets are made to validate our post-processing algorithm and SA-hourglass network respectively. All the images in the two datasets are from in-vivo PCI. And a public dataset is applied to verify the generalization of our SA-hourglass.

Dataset1 consists of 1238 fluoroscopy images with a size of 512*512 (each image contains only one guidewire). All images are randomly divided into the training set (653 images) and the testing set (585 images). We manually label each guidewire's bounding box, segmentation label, and two endpoints' positions.

Dataset2 consists of 10 in-vivo fluoroscopy sequences, with a total of 367 images with a size of 512*512 (contain 609 guidewires in all). Only the bounding box of each guidewire is manually labeled. It should be pointed out that there is no duplicate image between Dataset1 and Dataset2.

The Retinal Microsurgery (RM) dataset [6] contains three video sequences with 1171 images, each with a resolution of 640*480 pixels. Each image contains a single instrument with 4 annotated joints (start shaft, end shaft, left tip and right tip). Analogously to [6], the first 50% of all three sequences is for training and the rest is for testing.

3.2   Implementation Details

For post-processing algorithm, we set σ_{IOU} to 0.3, th_H to 0.3, th_L to 0.01. These two thresholds are obtained through experiments, and they are not difficult to find. We suggest that th_H should not exceed 0.5 and th_L should not exceed 0.1. For SA-hourglass, in data augmentation, random flip, random rotation $[-20°, 20°]$, random grayscale adjustment $[-20, 20]$ and random contrast ratio $[0.8, 1.2]$ are adopted for Dataset1, while only random rotation $[-10°, 10°]$ is adopted for RM dataset. The sigma of Gaussian used in the heatmap's ground truth is 3 for Dataset1 and 7 for RM dataset. λ in loss function is 0.5. The network is implemented using Tensorflow, and for optimization, rmsprop optimizer is applied with a learning rate of 2.5e−4 and batch size of 4. Training takes about 13 h on an NVIDIA Titan XP for 500 epochs.

3.3 Detection Experiments

Evaluation Metric: The evaluation metric used in detection experiments is simple: to count the number of true positives (correct), false positives and false negatives (miss) in all frames in test sequences. The correct is defined as the S-IOU score between the detection result and the ground truth exceeds 0.3.

Results: YOLOv3 detector with and without post-processing algorithm are compared in the experiments. The detector has been trained by Dataset1, and Dataset2 is used for evaluation. As shown in Table 1, the results illustrate that the YOLOv3 detector alone works well, but problems remain. And the introduction of our algorithm can significantly reduce the number of false positives and misses in the outputs. From the results, we can also see that it is tough for us to set a single threshold for the detector.

Table 1. Detection results on Dataset2

Detector	Correct	Miss	False positive
YOLO with post-processing ($th_H = 0.3$, $th_L = 0.01$)	604	5	1
YOLO without post-processing (threshold $= 0.1$)	580	29	26
YOLO without post-processing (threshold $= 0.3$)	522	87	6
YOLO without post-processing (threshold $= 0.01$)	608	1	246

3.4 Localization Experiments

Evaluation Metric: Percentage of Correct Keypoints (PCK) metric is used to measure the localization results. PCK reports the percentage of localization results that fall within a distance of the ground truth.

Results: Two state-of-the-art methods on surgical tool keypoint localization are applied for comparison: CSL [7] and in SRPEI [5]. In all, five models are evaluated on both Dataset1 and RM dataset: (1) CSL, (2) SRPEI, (3) Stacked hourglass (3-stack), (4) SA-hourglass with segmentation attention, (5) SA-hourglass with keypoint attention. The results are illustrated in Fig. 4.

From the results, we can see that stacked hourglass's accuracy is significantly improved after SA modules are added (become SA-hourglass). We attribute this improvement to the idea of coarse-to-fine implicitly used in SA-hourglass. Our SA module is designed to generate the coarse attention maps which can eliminate many useless areas of the input. Therefore, we can get more precise results by using a small sigma of Gaussian in the ground truth of output heatmaps. SA module can also be seen as another intermediate supervision with special usage.

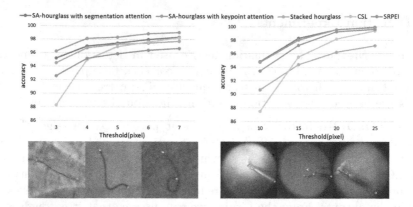

Fig. 4. Average PCK of all keypoints of PCI guidewires (upper left) and RM instruments (upper right). (below) Some localization examples, yellow and green points represent the ground truth and the localization result respectively (Color figure online)

Two kinds of SA-hourglass both achieve the state-of-the-art localization results on both datasets. SA-hourglass with keypoint attention performs best on Dataset1, reaching an accuracy of 96.24% (for threshold = 3), and SA-hourglass with segmentation attention performs best on RM Dataset, reaching an accuracy of 94.82% (for threshold = 10). Besides, the average inference time of our SA-hourglass is about 0.05 s, which fully meets the real-time requirement of fluoroscopy images (8FPS) after adding the detection time.

4   Conclusion

We propose a two-stage framework to localize the guidewire endpoints in real-time fluoroscopy or a fluoroscopy video. For the detection stage, a YOLOv3 detector is applied as a proposal mechanism, and a post-processing algorithm is introduced to refine the bounding boxes produced by the detector. For the localization stage, an SA-hourglass is designed and achieves the state-of-the-art localization results on two datasets. Our framework could be applied to the localization task of other small objects in medical images. As for larger objects, the SA-hourglass network could be directly used without detection stage.

Acknowledgments. This work was supported in part by the National Natural Science Foundation of China (Grants 61533016, U1713220, U1613210), by the National Key Research and Development Program of China under Grant 2017YFB1302704, by the Strategic Priority Research Program of CAS under Grant XDBS01040100.

References

1. Mazomenos, E.B., et al.: A survey on the current status and future challenges towards objective skills assessment in endovascular surgery. J. Med. Robot. Res. **01**(03), 1640010 (2016)
2. Ambrosini, P., Ruijters, D., Niessen, W.J., Moelker, A., van Walsum, T.: Fully automatic and real-time catheter segmentation in X-Ray fluoroscopy. In: Descoteaux, M., Maier-Hein, L., Franz, A., Jannin, P., Collins, D.L., Duchesne, S. (eds.) MICCAI 2017. LNCS, vol. 10434, pp. 577–585. Springer, Cham (2017). https://doi.org/10.1007/978-3-319-66185-8_65
3. Vandini, A., Glocker, B., Hamady, M., Yang, G.Z.: Robust guidewire tracking under large deformations combining segment-like features (SEGlets). Med. Image Anal. **38**, 150–164 (2017)
4. Heibel, H., Glocker, B., Groher, M., Pfister, M., Navab, N.: Interventional tool tracking using discrete optimization. IEEE Trans. Med. Imaging **32**(3), 544–555 (2013)
5. Kurmann, T., et al.: Simultaneous recognition and pose estimation of instruments in minimally invasive surgery. In: Descoteaux, M., Maier-Hein, L., Franz, A., Jannin, P., Collins, D.L., Duchesne, S. (eds.) MICCAI 2017. LNCS, vol. 10434, pp. 505–513. Springer, Cham (2017). https://doi.org/10.1007/978-3-319-66185-8_57
6. Sznitman, R., Ali, K., Richa, R., Taylor, R.H., Hager, G.D., Fua, P.: Data-driven visual tracking in retinal microsurgery. In: Ayache, N., Delingette, H., Golland, P., Mori, K. (eds.) MICCAI 2012. LNCS, vol. 7511, pp. 568–575. Springer, Heidelberg (2012). https://doi.org/10.1007/978-3-642-33418-4_70
7. Laina, I., et al.: Concurrent segmentation and localization for tracking of surgical instruments. In: Descoteaux, M., Maier-Hein, L., Franz, A., Jannin, P., Collins, D.L., Duchesne, S. (eds.) MICCAI 2017. LNCS, vol. 10434, pp. 664–672. Springer, Cham (2017). https://doi.org/10.1007/978-3-319-66185-8_75
8. Papandreou, G., et al.: Towards accurate multi-person pose estimation in the wild. In: Proceedings of the IEEE Conference on Computer Vision and Pattern Recognition, pp. 4903–4911 (2017)
9. Redmon, J., Farhadi, A.: YOLOv3: an incremental improvement. arXiv preprint arXiv:1804.02767 (2018)
10. Ren, S., He, K., Girshick, R., Sun, J.: Faster R-CNN: towards real-time object detection with region proposal networks. IEEE Trans. Pattern Anal. Mach. Intell. **39**(6), 1137–1149 (2016)
11. Newell, A., Yang, K., Deng, J.: Stacked hourglass networks for human pose estimation. In: Leibe, B., Matas, J., Sebe, N., Welling, M. (eds.) ECCV 2016. LNCS, vol. 9912, pp. 483–499. Springer, Cham (2016). https://doi.org/10.1007/978-3-319-46484-8_29
12. Chu, X., Yang, W., Ouyang, W., Ma, C., Yuille, A.L., Wang, X.: Multi-context attention for human pose estimation. In: Proceedings of the IEEE Conference on Computer Vision and Pattern Recognition, pp. 5669–5678 (2017)

Investigating the Role of VR in a Simulation-Based Medical Planning System for Coronary Interventions

Madhurima Vardhan[1], Harvey Shi[1], John Gounley[2], S. James Chen[3], Andrew Kahn[4], Jane Leopold[5], and Amanda Radles[1(✉)]

[1] Department of Biomedical Engineering, Duke University, Durham, USA
amanda.randles@duke.edu
[2] Computational Science and Engineering Division, Oak Ridge National Laboratory, Oak Ridge, USA
[3] Department of Medicine/Cardiology, University of Colorado, Boulder, USA
[4] Division of Cardiovascular Medicine, University of California San Diego, San Diego, USA
[5] Division of Cardiovascular Medicine, Brigham and Women's Hospital, Boston, USA

Abstract. Virtual reality (VR) based computational fluid dynamics (CFD) simulations are emerging as a viable solution to guide complex surgical or invasive procedures, such as percutaneous coronary intervention (PCI), as they enable a realistic first-person experience of underlying patient anatomy and physiology. Realistic VR experience can be assessed by immersion, an objective VR property. However, it remains unclear how immersion influences virtual PCI procedures and what level of immersion is required. This study answers both these questions by evaluating the application of a CFD-based VR system and comparing semi-immersive and fully immersive VR displays. Nine patient-specific arterial models were simulated using CFD and used to conduct a quantitative user evaluation (n = 31) with both types of VR displays. The findings of this study reveal that VR immersion significantly improves the accuracy of simulated stent placement in complex arterial geometries, relative to traditional desktops with no immersion ($p < 0.05$). Higher accuracy is noted by the use of semi-immersive VR display, which offers higher display fidelity as compared to the fully immersive VR display ($p < 0.05$). Interestingly, CFD data mapped on to arterial geometries strongly influences the location of stent placement. This finding is demonstrated by the lack of significant accuracy deviation between the two immersive displays when CFD data is shown. This study provides compelling evidence that a CFD-based VR system rendered on semi-immersive displays can enable more accurate and efficient stent placement.

Keywords: Virtual reality · Computational fluid dynamics · Stent

Supported by Sigma Xi grant, Duke Theo Pilkington Fellowship and the Office of the Director, National Institutes Of Health under Award Number DP5OD019876.

D. Shen et al. (Eds.): MICCAI 2019, LNCS 11768, pp. 366–374, 2019.
https://doi.org/10.1007/978-3-030-32254-0_41

1   Introduction

Treatment planning is currently witnessing a paradigm shift towards the integration of virtual reality (VR) to address the spatial complexity associated with interventional procedures [5,6]. VR allows 3D viewing and direct interaction with medical imaging data that have traditionally been confined to two-dimensional (2D) desktops [5]. However, current VR platforms are limited to anatomic viewing and modification as they typically rely only on the imaging data. Imaging data by itself does not reveal the underlying patient physiology, which is often the key to clinical decision-making [5]. Physiological flow assessment can be achieved by applying computational fluid dynamics (CFD) simulations to patient-specific arterial geometries [10,12], and can enhance understanding of the relationship between disease progression and patient physiology [7]. By allowing concurrent visualization of anatomy and personalized simulation results treatment planning can be significantly enhanced. However, CFD mappings further result in an added layer of complexity to anatomically complex arterial geometries. Such complex 3D personalized CFD simulations are especially ripe for the application of immersive displays. This work proposes a CFD-based medical planning system that leverages VR technology and personalized physiological flow simulations to enable more accurate, robust, and efficient placement of intravascular stents.

Percutaneous coronary intervention (PCI) is an invasive medical procedure guided by 2-dimensional X-ray images where a mesh-like structure, known as a stent, is implanted to restore normal flow in coronary arteries [4]. PCI treatment planning can be difficult due to: (1) the complex three-dimensional structure of the vasculature (2) minimal physiological flow knowledge [4,8,11]. These challenges incentivize the creation of a VR-based simulation for providing an immersive first-person physiological viewing experience to physicians. VR devices offer high immersion, a key VR metric measured by display and interaction fidelity, allowing for improved spatial judgment and arterial annotation, respectively. Immersion is an intrinsic property of virtual environments, describing the degree to which a user engages with the environment and perceives it as realistic. However, with the advent of commercial-grade VR devices, there is no consensus as to optimal level of immersion that maybe best suited for virtual PCI.

The first goal of this study is to evaluate the influence of immersion and the optimal level of immersion required for accurate stent placement. Immersion depends on rendering software application and display technology of the device [1]. The use of a unified software platform that supports three display devices ensures that any deviations in stent placement from a single user were due to differences in the display technology. Three different immersion levels are considered in this study: (1) traditional desktop which has no immersion, (2) zSpace a semi-immersive VR display (3) HTC Vive a fully VR immersive display.

The second goal of this study is to use VR-based CFD platform to assess whether knowledge of physiological flow factors, such as wall shear stress (WSS), influence preferred stent placement. WSS is the hemodynamic force exerted by blood on the vessel wall. Evaluation of WSS is important because it captures the underlying coronary physiology as described by local hemodynamics and can be used to examine the consequences of impaired blood flow and plaque development [7]. A quantitative user evaluation (n = 31) was performed using the proposed VR-CFD platform. The findings of the user study provide compelling evidence that using the proposed CFD/VR-based platform, physiological assessment of the entire coronary arterial network can enable a rational approach in the diagnosis and treatment of coronary artery disease.

2   Methods

Patient-Specific Arterial Reconstructions and Simulations. Nine de-identified CT angiographic datasets were obtained with Institutional Review Board approval. 3D left and right coronary artery (LCA and RCA) geometries were reconstructed using Mimics commercial software (Materialise, Leuven, Belgium) and evaluated by two experienced cardiologists to confirm accuracy of the reconstructions with respect to vessel size, length, and stenosis. The 9 reconstructed models were used as input to HARVEY, a massively parallel CFD application that has been validated using *in vitro* experiments [3,10]. To ensure that realistic physiological flow behavior was captured, averaged patient data was used with a transient velocity waveform as the inlet boundary condition and resistance outlet boundary conditions [12]. Two types of 3D rendering of each geometry were created: one showing the anatomy without flow results and one with WSS data mapped on the surface of the arterial geometries (shown in Figs. 1 and 2).

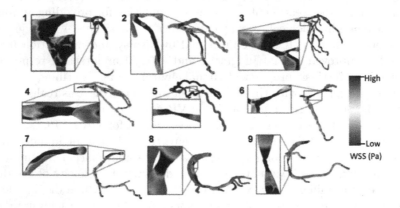

Fig. 1. The nine coronary artery geometries used in this study, with insets showing the regions of coronary stenoses, related to the location of stent placement. Low WSS (0–2 Pa) and High WSS (3–5 Pa). 1–6 are left coronary arteries. 7–9 are right coronary arteries.

Rendering Arterial Geometries with WSS and Without WSS on VR Platform. Arterial geometries were rendered on VR devices using Harvis. Harvis is a software platform for hemodynamic visualization built using the Unity Engine, a 3D framework for graphical applications. Harvis supports three types of displays: 2D desktops, semi-immersive zSpace 3D displays and fully immersive HTC Vive head-mounted display (HMD). In this study, the following display specification were employed: (1) 2D desktop—21-inch diagonal 1920 by 1080 pixel monitor, (2) semi-immersive zSpace display—23.6-inch diagonal 1920 by 1080 pixel monitor with stylus controller (3) fully immersive HTC Vive HMD—1080 by 1200 pixel displays for each eye, with two controllers (Fig. 2).

Quantitative User Study and Tasks. In this work, 31 participants (18 males and 13 females) were recruited for the user evaluation based on power analysis using Wilcoxon signed-rank test. In order to participate in the study, participants were required to have normal-to-corrected vision and expertise in medicine or physical science. We believe such professional expertise is representative of the target audience for end usage and tool development, respectively.

Participants were not required to have prior experience with VR and 25% of users had no prior experience, 55% used VR once or twice, and 6% used VR more than 5 times. Prior to starting the study, participants received a brief standardized tutorial about PCI and stenting procedures and the relationship between WSS and coronary disease (included in supplemental material). All participants completed the user study with all devices on the same day. Upon completion of the study all participants received monetary compensation.

Experimental Task—All users were assigned the task of stent placement for 3 arterial geometries, sampled randomly from the total pool of 9. Users specified preferred stent location by adding two dots marking the start and end of the stent (Fig. 2). The geometries were displayed with and without WSS maps, on all three devices (Figs. 1 and 2), resulting in 6 total tasks per device. Therefore, between the 3 devices (2D desktop, zSpace and Vive HMD) and 31 participants, 558 total trials were collected. An intra-observer comparison between devices was drawn for each unique trial-participant pair.

Quantitative Metrics and Statistical Analysis—The correct stent endpoints for each LCA and RCA case were determined by an experienced interventional cardiologist. These two points were treated as the ground truth and the summed distance deviation with respect to the user-placed points was computed. The lower the distance deviation, the higher the accuracy of placement. Duration is reported as the completion time of each stent placement trial. A paired t-test was used to evaluate statistical differences, with significance assumed for $p < 0.05$.

Bias Minimization—Several measures were taken to reduce any bias. First, before starting the task of stent placement, users were familiarized with the use of each device and the study task using short, required tutorials that were consistent for all users. Second, all stent placement with geometries with and without WSS were randomized for each user. Of the total 9 geometries, 3 were randomly chosen for every participant. Third, device randomization among users was also undertaken to prevent any learning effects. Fourth, all quantitative measurements were recorded by the software with no manual recording. Finally, to prevent fatigue and strain from the use of VR, the device duration was kept reasonable (between 5–7 min) and users were asked to report any fatigue experienced at the end of the study.

3   Results and Discussion

The primary goal was to determine the influence of immersion on stent placement and to identify the optimal level of immersion. To assess whether immersion influences stent placement, user accuracy on the semi-immersive VR display was compared to a traditional 2D desktop with no immersion. The semi-immersive VR display was used to evaluate the influence of immersion since the fish-tank VR setup is more similar to traditional 2D desktop pattern and offers higher display fidelity than fully immersive displays. Figure 3 shows the accuracy results for 2D desktop and semi-immersive VR display, quantified as the summed distance deviation between the user-placed endpoints and stent endpoints placed by an experienced cardiologist. It is noted that the semi-immersive device has significantly lower distance deviation compared to 2D desktop (25.74 ± 2.56 mm vs. 31.25 ± 2.95 mm, $p < 0.05$) and thus offers greater accuracy. This distance deviation (6 mm) is about 50% of the mean length for a coronary lesion and is thus clinically significant. This result underscores the notion that immersive virtual environments improve user accuracy for identifying stent location relative to that of the 2D display.

   To determine the optimal level of immersion, the results from the semi-immersive zSpace display were compared to those from the fully immersive HTC Vive. Among the two VR displays, zSpace has the higher display fidelity despite a lower resolution screen, as the HMD suffers from the screen-door effect—more noticeable gaps between pixels due to closeness of the display [2]. Figure 3 shows

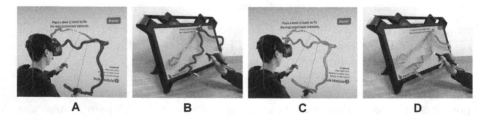

Fig. 2. The two types of arterial models and two VR devices used in this study. **A** and **B** show the geometry with WSS data displayed on the HTC Vive HMD (fully immersive) and zSpace monitor (semi-immersive), respectively. **C** and **D** show the arterial geometry without WSS on the same two devices. Each image shows two blue dots marking the endpoints of a placed stent.

that semi-immersive VR has lower distance deviation compared to fully immersive VR display (25.74 ± 2.56 mm vs. 31.96 ± 2.94 mm, $p < 0.05$) and therefore demonstrates higher accuracy. This finding can be explained by the following reasons: the semi-immersive zSpace (1) offers higher display fidelity, (2) has a simpler setup relative to the HMD, and (3) includes both outside visual context and geometric overview, which are important factors for viewing complex geometries. On the other hand, while the fully immersive HTC Vive HMD has higher interaction fidelity due to its larger field of view, the stent placement task does not require the large degree of interaction with the geometry that one might encounter with a task such as geometric modification. We note that differences in the accuracy could potentially result from the combination of the VR display and controllers; however, the same wand-style interaction setup was used for both VR devices to minimize the effect of controller differences. Therefore, display fidelity overrides interaction fidelity in this context. Similar findings have also been reported by Qi *et al.* when comparing the zSpace to an HMD device for volume visualization problems [9].

The secondary goal was to determine whether the inclusion of physiological flow data influenced stent placement. To ascertain this goal, accuracy data for 2D desktop, semi-immersive and fully immersive devices was compared using the presence and absence of WSS data (Fig. 3). Previous studies have suggested WSS to be an important indicator for the development and progression of plaque in coronary arteries [7], so this quantity was chosen as the representative flow parameter. The results show significant differences in accuracy for fully immersive, semi-immersive and the 2D desktop when no WSS data is included (33.11 ± 4.53 mm, 22.89 ± 3.49 mm, 30.67 ± 4.4 mm, $p < 0.05$). However, no significant differences in accuracy for fully immersive, semi-immersive and 2D desktop were noted when WSS data was mapped on arterial geometries (30.80 ± 3.76 mm, 28.59 ± 3.74 mm, 31.82 ± 3.96 mm, $p > 0.05$). These findings suggest that participants use physiological flow information, such as WSS, for marking stent location independent of the device platform.

To further investigate the additional complexity of simulation data and its impact on optimal immersion-level, the internal displacement between stent

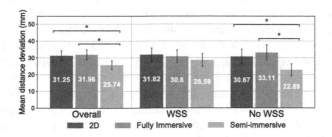

Fig. 3. Overall mean distance deviation, broken down by WSS and no WSS data for 2D desktop, fully immersive, and semi-immersive devices. Brackets $= p < 0.05$. Error bars $=$ SE.

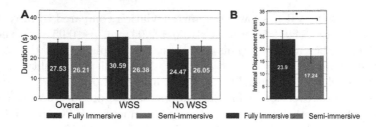

Fig. 4. Influence of physiological flow. (A) Task duration with WSS and without WSS displayed, and for overall (combined) results. (B) User-controlled stent displacement between task with and without WSS display. Brackets = p < 0.05. Error bars = SE.

locations by a user for geometries with and without simulation data displayed was calculated individually on both the semi-immersive and fully immersive devices (Fig. 4B). Here internal displacement is calculated as the distance in dot placement by that user (serving as their own control) on the geometry with overlaid flow data vs. without. Displacement was found to be significantly different between devices (17.24 ± 2.88 mm vs. 23.90 ± 3.43 mm, p < 0.05). The results show that with the inclusion of personalized flow data, users were more accurate on semi-immersive display compared to fully immersive display. This finding reinforces the influence of display fidelity on accurate stent placement, regardless of the presence of WSS results.

No significant differences were noted for duration of stent placement task on each of the displays. As shown in Fig. 4A, time comparison for the fully immersive and semi-immersive devices when WSS was displayed (30.59 ± 3.05 s vs. 26.38 ± 2.79 s) and when it was not displayed (24.47 ± 2.08 s vs. 26.05 ± 2.47 s). This highlights the fact that despite adding complex WSS maps on arterial geometries, the duration of task completion remained relatively unchanged.

As shown in Fig. 1, the LCA has a more complex vascular geometry compared to the RCA due vessel tortuosity and branching patterns. Therefore, placement accuracy was further analyzed by dividing the WSS and no WSS results each into data for LCA and RCA geometries (Fig. 5). With WSS there were no significant differences between the accuracy of the fully immersive (FI) and semi-immersive (SI) devices, as previously discussed. This trend carries over to the LCA, despite it being a more complex vasculature, (FI = 34.09 ± 4.86 mm, SI = 33.21 ± 5.02 mm, p < 0.05) and RCA (FI = 24.22 ± 5.65 mm, SI = 19.36 ± 4.71 mm, p < 0.05) results with simulation data. However, without WSS data, there were significant differences in accuracy, which are also reflected in both the LCA (FI = 33.88 ± 5.39 mm, SI = 26.87 ± 4.74 mm, p < 0.05) and RCA (FI = 31.58 ± 8.37 mm, SI = 14.93 ± 4.16 mm, p < 0.05). These results demonstrate that stent placement accuracy remains unaltered by spatial complexity as long as the WSS maps are included.

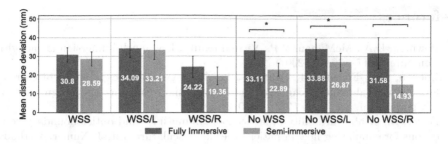

Fig. 5. Complexity differences and distance deviation, showing LCA (**L**) and RCA (**R**) results with WSS and without WSS. Brackets = p < 0.05. Error bars = SE.

4   Conclusion

In this study, we assessed how differing levels of VR immersion influence treatment planning when viewing both anatomic and flow data. The semi-immersive display provided significantly greater accuracy compared to a traditional 2D desktop. The findings reported here suggest that immersion, as determined by display fidelity, is the overriding VR property that yields higher accuracy for participants to identify the location for stent placement. When compared with two different levels of immersion, the results demonstrate that higher display fidelity of the semi-immersive device significantly improves accuracy compared to fully immersive displays. Furthermore, the findings reported here suggest that WSS, a hemodynamic risk factor computed from CFD simulations, can guide users where to implant a stent. When presented with WSS data, participants were able to determine where to implant a stent with similar accuracy in both the semi and fully immersive virtual environments.

This study constitutes the first necessary step to evaluate the VR technology best suited for PCI using CFD-simulated real patient data on multiple VR displays. The conclusions reported in this work are generalizable to other devices, users and context in several ways. First, the VR displays used were chosen to be representative of common immersive technology formats that are readily available. The fully immersive HTC Vive is similar to many other head-mounted displays from Oculus, HTC, and Dell; the zSpace family of displays is also well established and allows us to represent fish-tank VR experiences. Second, this study serves as a prototype setup for building relevant cohorts that span domain and VR experience. Finally, while the results obtained in this study focus on PCI, these findings are applicable to other clinical interventions for peripheral and cerebral diseases, which also involve the placement of intravascular stents.

Overall, a unified rehearsal training platform, such as that proposed in this work, would enhance training and diminish subjectivity arising from differences in procedural skill sets. This study demonstrates that a simulation-based VR treatment planning platform can enable personalized learner objective performance feedback for medical training and the practice of complex procedures.

References

1. Bowman, D.A., McMahan, R.P.: Virtual reality: how much immersion is enough? Computer **40**(7), 36–43 (2007)
2. Coburn, J.Q., Freeman, I., Salmon, J.L.: A review of the capabilities of current low-cost virtual reality technology and its potential to enhance the design process. J. Comput. Inf. Sci. Eng. **17**(3), 031013 (2017)
3. Feiger, B., et al.: Suitability of lattice Boltzmann inlet and outlet boundary conditions for simulating flow in patient-specific vasculature. Int. J. Numer. Methods Biomed. Eng. **35**, e3198 (2019)
4. Gallagher, A., Cates, C.: Approval of virtual reality training for carotid stenting: what this means for procedural-based medicine. JAMA **292**(24), 3024–3026 (2004)
5. Gosling, R.C., Morris, P.D., Soto, D.A.S., Lawford, P.V., Hose, D.R., Gunn, J.P.: Virtual coronary intervention: a treatment planning tool based upon the angiogram. JACC: Cardiovasc. Imaging **12**(5), 865–872 (2019)
6. Hajek, J., et al.: Closing the calibration loop: an inside-out-tracking paradigm for augmented reality in orthopedic surgery. In: Frangi, A.F., Schnabel, J.A., Davatzikos, C., Alberola-López, C., Fichtinger, G. (eds.) MICCAI 2018. LNCS, vol. 11073, pp. 299–306. Springer, Cham (2018). https://doi.org/10.1007/978-3-030-00937-3_35
7. Koskinas, K.C., Chatzizisis, Y.S., Baker, A.B., Edelman, E.R., Stone, P.H., Feldman, C.L.: The role of low endothelial shear stress in the conversion of atherosclerotic lesions from stable to unstable plaque. Curr. Opin. Cardiol. **24**(6), 580–590 (2009)
8. Laver, K., Lange, B., George, S., Deutsch, J., Saposnik, G., Crotty, M.: Virtual reality for stroke rehabilitation. Stroke **49**(4), 160–161 (2018)
9. Qi, W., Taylor II, R.M., Healey, C.G., Martens, J.B.: A comparison of immersive HMD, fish tank VR and fish tank with haptics displays for volume visualization. In: Proceedings of the 3rd Symposium on Applied Perception in Graphics and Visualization, pp. 51–58. ACM (2006)
10. Randles, A., Kale, V., Hammond, J., Gropp, W., Kaxiras, E.: Performance analysis of the lattice Boltzmann model beyond Navier-stokes. In: 2013 IEEE 27th International Symposium on Parallel & Distributed Processing (IPDPS), pp. 1063–1074. IEEE (2013)
11. Seymour, N., et al.: Virtual reality training improves operating room performance: results of a randomized, double-blinded study. Ann. Surg. **236**(4), 458 (2002)
12. Taylor, C.A.: The HeartFlow concept combining angiographic imaging and non-invasive hemodynamic lesion assessment: technology description. In: Transcatheter Cardiovascular Therapeutics (TCT) Conference (2010)

Learned Full-Sampling Reconstruction

Weilin Cheng[1], Yu Wang[2], Ying Chi[2], Xuansong Xie[2], and Yuping Duan[1(✉)] (iD)

[1] Center for Applied Mathematics, Tianjin University, Tianjin 300072, China
{chengwl,yuping.duan}@tju.edu.cn
[2] Alibaba Group, Hangzhou, China
{tonggou.wangyu,xinyi.cy}@alibaba-inc.com, xingtong.xxs@taobao.com

Abstract. X-ray computed tomography (CT) reconstruction with sparse projection views was proposed to reduce both the radiation dose and scan time. However, lacking of sufficient projection views may lead to severe artifacts for analytical reconstruction method such as the filtered back projection (FBP). Although the projection data is incomplete, we can generate the full-sampling system matrices according to the sufficient-sampling conditions [5]. Thus, we propose a novel iterative reconstruction model to fit the target images and the corresponding high resolution measurements in Radon domain by the full-sampling system matrices. Our proposed model is solved by the learned alternating minimization method, which accounts for a forward operator in deep neural network by the unrolling strategy. Numerical results demonstrate that the proposed approach outperforms some latest learning based reconstruction methods for the sparse-view CT problems.

Keywords: Sparse-view · CT reconstruction · Full sampling · CNN

1 Introduction

Image reconstruction from down-sampled or limited measurements, e.g., low dose and limited angle CT, are examples of ill-posed inverse problems, which can be formulated as estimating the image $u \in X$ from the measurement $g \in Y$,

$$g = Au + n, \tag{1}$$

where the reconstruction space X and data space Y are typically Hilbert space, $A : X \rightarrow Y$ is the projection matrix for sparse CT, and $n \in Y$ is the random noises generated during the imaging processes. The goal of CT reconstruction is to recover the image u from the set of acquired projection data g. For the sparse-view CT, the system matrix, denoted by A_S, has fewer rows than columns so that there is a nontrivial nullspace and has infinity many solutions. Even if the solution of the inverse problem exists and is unique, the linear operator A_S may

---

The work is supported by NSFC 11701418, Major Science and Technology Project of Tianjin 18ZXRHSY00160 and Recruitment Program of Global Young Expert.

© Springer Nature Switzerland AG 2019
D. Shen et al. (Eds.): MICCAI 2019, LNCS 11768, pp. 375–384, 2019.
https://doi.org/10.1007/978-3-030-32254-0_42

still be ill-conditioned such that the condition number $\|A\|\|A^{-1}\|$ is large and the linear system (1) is sensitive to the perturbations in data.

One way for the ill-posed inverse problem is to introduce certain regularity into the problem to guarantee the existence, uniqueness and stability of the solution. The general regularization method gives the following energy minimization problem

$$\min_{u \in X} \mathcal{D}(Au, g) + \mathcal{R}(u), \tag{2}$$

where $\mathcal{D}(Au, g)$ is the data fidelity term and $\mathcal{R}(u)$ is the regularization. Thus, the task of solving (2) mainly includes: (1) how to define the data fidelity to describe the interrelationship between g and u; and (2) how to model the regularization according to the prior information of u. In case of additive Gaussian noise and u being piecewise constant, we can obtain the well-known total variation minimization model for CT reconstruction [7]. Although TV regularization improves the reconstruction quality compared to analytical reconstruction such as filtered back-projection (FBP) method, it is still not judicious to choose the data fidelity and regularization in such a sophisticated way.

Due to the development of deep convolutional neural networks (CNN) in a broad range of computer vision tasks, deep learning techniques are being actively used in medical imaging community. The pioneer work of Yang *et al.* [8] reformulated an ADMM algorithm for compressive sensing MR imaging into a deep network by learning the parameters end-to-end in the training phase. Jin *et al.* [4] used the deep CNN as a post-processing step after the reconstruction of FBP to mitigate noises and artifacts. Adler and Öktem [1] proposed the learned primal dual algorithm for CT reconstruction by unrolling the proximal primal-dual optimization method and replacing the proximal operators with CNNs. Liu, Kuang and Zhang [6] used a deep learning regularization structure to learn the data consistence from the observed data. Dong, Li and Shen [3] proposed a joint spatial-Radon domain reconstruction (JSR) model for sparse view CT imaging, and was recently reformulated into the feed-forward deep network [9]. Learning-based models have been already proven efficient for image reconstruction problems.

In this work, we aim to reconstruct the sparse-view CT by making using of the full-sampling system matrix, which is called as the learned full sampling reconstruction (FSR). Instead of modeling the data fidelity term according to the noise distribution and the regularization term based on the prior information, we take the advantages of deep CNN to learn the interrelationship between observed data and reconstruction image and the prior information directly from the data. As we can obtain the full sampling system-matrix according to the sufficient sampling conditions in [5], we introduce another fidelity term to enforce the closeness of the reconstructed image and the full sampling projection data. In this way, we can learn the prior information of the completed Radon domain data from the training data, which is then applied to approximate the full-sampling projection in the testing. We use the alternating direction method to achieve an iterative scheme, and find the best update in each iteration using the CNN.

Numerical experiments demonstrate that the proposed FSR-net achieves better performance in sparse-view CT reconstruction.

2   Our Approach

In CT reconstruction, the system matrix A reflects the relationship between the projections on detector and the reconstructed objects. For the circular fan-beam CT, the dimensions of the system matrix A are $M \times N_{\text{pix}}$, where N_{pix} denotes the total number of pixels and M is the number of ray integrations defined by

$$M = N_{\text{views}} \times N_{\text{bins}}$$

with N_{views} being the number of views (i.e., 2π arc is divided into N_{views} equally spaced angular intervals) and N_{bins} being the number of bins on the detectors (i.e., the detector is equally divided into N_{bins}). Before we discuss the sparse-view CT, we define the full sampling based on the four sufficient-sampling conditions (SSCs) in [5], which is obtained by setting the sampling parameters N_{views} and N_{bins} for given N_{pix} to characterize the invertibility and stability of the system matrix. The first pair of the SSCs characterizes invertibility of A, that is

$$\text{SSC1}: M \geq N_{\text{pix}} \quad \text{and} \quad \text{SSC2}: \sigma_{\min} \neq 0,$$

where $\sigma_{\min}$ is the smallest singular value of A. The other pair of the SSCs characterizes the numerical stability for inversion of A, which is defined as

$$\text{SSC3}: \frac{\kappa(A)}{\kappa_{DC}} < r_{\text{samp}} \quad \text{and} \quad \text{SSC4}: N_{\text{views}} = N_{\text{bins}} = 2N,$$

where $\kappa(A) = \frac{\sigma_{\max}}{\sigma_{\min}}$, $\kappa_{DC} = \lim\limits_{\substack{N_{\text{bins}} \to \infty \\ N_{\text{views}} \to \infty}} \kappa(A)$, r_{samp} is a finite ratio parameter greater than 1, and N is the length of the field-of-view (ROV) of the detector. The relationship between N and N_{pix} is $N_{\text{pix}} \approx \frac{\pi}{4}N^2$ and we simply let $N \approx \sqrt{N_{\text{pix}}}$. Both the SSC1 and SSC4 are simple to evaluate, which will be used in our work.

When the N_{views} is not large enough to meet the SSCs for the fixed N_{bins}, it can be regarded as the sparse-view CT problem. Our goal is to develop efficient reconstruction methods for such ill-posed inverse problem. Since the full-sampling system matrix can be constructed according to the SSCs, we directly bridge the completed Radon domain data $f \in Z$ and the reconstructed image $u \in X$ through a full-sampling system matrix such that

$$f = A_F u,$$

where $A_F : X \to Z$ is the full-sampling projection matrix and Z is a Hilbert space. Therefore, we propose the following minimization model to jointly reconstruct the spatial and Radon domain data for sparse-view CT

$$\min_{u \in X, f \in Z} \mathcal{D}(A_S u, g) + \mathcal{R}(u) + \mathcal{F}(A_F u, f), \tag{3}$$

where $\mathcal{F}(A_F u, f)$ is used to measure the distance between $A_F u$ and f. Since the unknown u and f are coupled together in (3), we introduce a new variable $\tilde{u}$ and rewrite (3) by adding a fitting term $\|\tilde{u} - u\|^2$ as follows

$$\min_{u \in X, f \in Z, \tilde{u} \in X} \mathcal{D}(A_S \tilde{u}, g) + \mathcal{R}(\tilde{u}) + \mathcal{F}(A_F u, f) + \frac{1}{2r} \|\tilde{u} - u\|_X^2, \qquad (4)$$

where r is a positive parameter used to measure the trade-off between the under-sampling data g and a full-sampling projected data f. The first term in (4) contains the linear operator A_S, which can be reformulated based on the Legendre-Fenchel conjugate [2]

$$\min_{u \in X, f \in Z, \tilde{u} \in X} \max_{p \in Y} \langle A_S \tilde{u}, p \rangle - \mathcal{D}^*(p, g) + \mathcal{R}(\tilde{u}) + \mathcal{F}(A_F u, f) + \frac{1}{2r} \|\tilde{u} - u\|_X^2, \quad (5)$$

where $\mathcal{D}^*$ denotes the conjugate of $\mathcal{D}$. The classical alternating direction method can be used to obtain an efficient algorithm for the multiple variable minimization problem (5), which gives

$$\begin{cases} p^{k+1} = \arg \min_{p \in Y} \quad \mathcal{D}^*(p, g) - \langle A_S \tilde{u}^k, p \rangle + \frac{1}{2\tau} \|p - p^k\|_Y^2, \\ \tilde{u}^{k+1} = \arg \min_{\tilde{u} \in X} \quad \mathcal{R}(\tilde{u}) + \langle A_S \tilde{u}, p^{k+1} \rangle + \frac{1}{2r} \|\tilde{u} - u^k\|_X^2, \\ f^{k+1} = \arg \min_{f \in Z} \quad \mathcal{F}(A_F u^k, f) + \frac{1}{2\sigma} \|f - f^k\|_Z^2, \\ u^{k+1} = \arg \min_{u \in X} \quad \mathcal{F}(A_F u, f) + \frac{1}{2r} \|u - \tilde{u}^{k+1}\|_X^2, \end{cases} \qquad (6)$$

where τ and σ are positive parameters. As shown, the proximal method is adopted for the subproblem with respect to p and f in case the likelihood functional $\mathcal{D}(\cdot, \cdot)$ and $\mathcal{F}(\cdot, \cdot)$ are non-smooth. The solutions to each subproblem can be expressed as follows

$$\begin{cases} p^{k+1} = (\mathcal{I} + \tau \partial \mathcal{D}^*)^{-1}(p^k, \tau A_S \tilde{u}, g), \\ \tilde{u}^{k+1} = (\mathcal{I} + r \partial \mathcal{R})^{-1}(u^k, r A_S^* p^{k+1}), \\ f^{k+1} = (\mathcal{I} + \sigma \partial \mathcal{F})^{-1}(f^k, \sigma A_F u^k), \\ u^{k+1} = (\mathcal{I} + r \partial \mathcal{F})^{-1}(\tilde{u}^{k+1}, r A_F^* f^{k+1}). \end{cases} \qquad (7)$$

Guided by the success of deep learning, we use CNN for unrolled iterative scheme such that the network can learn how to combine the variables in the object functional, which accounts for a deep feed-forward neural network by using CNNs to approximate the inverse operators in (7). The alternating direction algorithm with I iterations is outlined as Algorithm 1.

Remark 1. In the algorithm, we assume the constraint $\tilde{u} = u$ holds unconditionally. Therefore, f^{k+1} is calculated based on $A_F \tilde{u}^{k+1}$ rather than $A_F u^k$ as $\tilde{u}^{k+1}$ was already updated in the previous step. Besides, instead of selecting specific values for τ, σ and r, we let the network learn the appropriate value by itself.

Algorithm 1. Learned Full Sampling Reconstruction (FSR)

1: Initialize u^0, f^0, p^0, $\tilde{u}^0$
2: **for** $k = 0, \ldots, I$, **do**
3:      $p^{k+1} \leftarrow \Gamma_{\theta^p}(p^k, A_S u^k, g)$
4:      $\tilde{u}^{k+1} \leftarrow \Lambda_{\theta^{\tilde{u}}}(u^k, A_S^* p^{k+1})$
5:      $f^{k+1} \leftarrow \Pi_{\theta^f}(f^k, A_F \tilde{u}^{k+1})$
6:      $u^{k+1} \leftarrow \Xi_{\theta^u}(\tilde{u}^{k+1}, A_F^* f^{k+1})$
7: **return** u^I, f^I

3 Experiments and Results

In this section, we evaluate the proposed algorithm on both the ellipse data [1] and a piglet data[1] by comparing with the state-of-the-art work, i.e., FBP-Unet denoising [4] and Leaned Primal-Dual network (PD-net) [1].

3.1 Implementation

The methods are implemented in Python using Operator Discretization Library (ODL) and TensorFlow. We let the number of data that persists between the iterates be $N_u = N_{\tilde{u}} = 6$ and $N_p = N_f = 7$. The convolution are all 3×3 pixel size, and the numbers of channels in each iteration are p of $9 \rightarrow 32 \rightarrow 32 \rightarrow 7$, $\tilde{u}$ of $7 \rightarrow 32 \rightarrow 32 \rightarrow 6$, f of $8 \rightarrow 32 \rightarrow 32 \rightarrow 7$ and u of $7 \rightarrow 32 \rightarrow 32 \rightarrow 6$. The network structure of one iteration is illustrated in Fig. 1, where totally 10 iterations are contained in our network. As shown, each iteration involves four 3-layer that is the depth of network is 120 layers. Our FSR-net has approximately 4.9×10^5 parameters, while FBP-Unet and PD-net have 10^7 and 2.4×10^5 parameters, respectively.

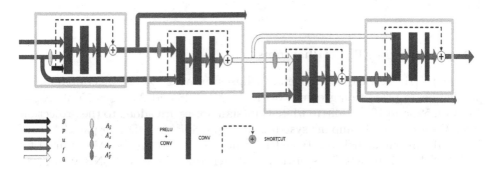

Fig. 1. Network architecture to solve the tomography problem. Each box corresponds to one variable, which are all of the same architecture.

---

[1] http://homepage.usask.ca/~xiy525/.

We use the Xavier initialization scheme to initialize the convolution param-
eters, and initialize all biases to zero. Let $\Theta = \{\theta^p, \theta^{\tilde{u}}, \theta^f, \theta^u\}$ and $\mathcal{T}^\dagger$ be the
pseudo-inverse of the minimization process (3) defined as

$$\mathcal{T}^\dagger_\Theta(g) \approx (u_{\text{true}}, f_{\text{true}}) \quad \text{for data } g \text{ satisfying (1)},$$

Suppose $(\mathcal{T}_\Theta(u), \mathcal{T}_\Theta(f)) = \mathcal{T}^\dagger_\Theta(g)$ and $(g_1, u_1^*), (g_2, u_2^*), \ldots, (g_L, u_L^*)$ be L
training samples. We apply the ADAM optimizer in TensorFlow to minimize
the following empirical loss function

$$\mathcal{L}(\Theta) = \frac{1}{2L} \sum_{i=1}^{L} \left(\|\mathcal{T}_\Theta(u_i) - u_i^*\|_X^2 + \|\mathcal{T}_\Theta(f_i) - A_F u_i^*\|_Z^2 \right). \tag{8}$$

Most parameters are set the same as the PD-net in [1]. We use 2×10^5 batches on
each problem and a learning rate schedule according to cosine annealing, i.e., the
learning rate at step t is $\eta^t = \frac{\eta^0}{2}\left(1 + \cos(\pi \frac{t}{t_{max}})\right)$, where the initial learning rate
is set as $\eta^0 = 10^{-3}$ for the ellipse data and $\eta^0 = 10^{-4}$ for the piglet phantom.
We let the parameter β_2 of the ADAM optimizer to 0.99 and limit the gradient
norms to 1 to improve training stability. The batch size is set as 5 and 1 for the
ellipse data and piglet phantom, while the epoch is set as 22 for both datasets.

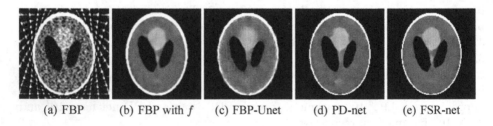

(a) FBP   (b) FBP with f (c) FBP-Unet   (d) PD-net   (e) FSR-net

Fig. 2. Reconstruction comparison on the ellipse data, where the window is set to [0.1,
0.4].

3.2   Results on Ellipse Phantoms

Similar to [1], we randomly generate ellipses on a 128×128 pixel domain by
parallel beam projection geometry with $N_{\text{bins}} = 128$ and $N_{\text{views}} = 15$, $N_{\text{views}} =$
30. Both 5% and 10% additive white Gaussian noises are added to the projection
data. We use the full sampling system matrix provided by ODL for parallel beam
CT as A_F in our model (3). Table 1 presents the PSNR and SSIM obtained by
the CNN based models. It is obviously shown that the best PSNR values are
always achieved by our FSR-net and PD-net ranks the second position, both
of which are significantly better than the Unet based post-processing method.
Especially, the advantage of our FSR-net over PD-net becomes more convincing
for $N_{\text{views}} = 15$ and 5% Gaussian noise, giving an improvement exceeding 1 dB,
which demonstrates the effectiveness of our model in sparse-view reconstruction.

The comparison of the PSNR and SSIM between the FBP with g and FBP using the reconstructed projection data f from our model in Table 1 also demonstrates that our model can recover the Radon domain data to certain qualities. We display the reconstruction results of the sparse 15 views with 5% Gaussian noise in Fig. 2, which shows that our reconstruction preserves the geometry and details better than the other two methods.

Table 1. Comparison results for the ellipse phantom in terms of PSNR, SSIM and Runtime.

N_{views}	Noises	Methods	PSNR	SSIM	Time	FBP (PSNR)	FBP (SSIM)
30	5%	FBP-Unet	28.1693	0.9346	**1.5**	19.7216	0.5938
		PD-net	39.2301	0.9860	4.6		
		FSR-net	**39.6588**	**0.9897**	6.6	**21.5168**	**0.8930**
	10%	FBP-Unet	26.2985	0.9250	**1.5**	19.1199	0.5073
		PD-net	31.9033	**0.9707**	4.6		
		FSR-net	**32.1213**	0.9695	6.6	**21.2971**	**0.8881**
15	5%	FBP-Unet	19.8411	0.7224	**1.4**	16.1378	0.4217
		PD-net	30.3615	**0.9719**	4.4		
		FSR-net	**32.0468**	0.9707	6.4	**21.3333**	**0.8607**
	10%	FBP-Unet	19.4893	0.7370	**1.4**	15.5722	0.3394
		PD-net	25.1603	**0.9301**	4.4		
		FSR-net	**25.9528**	0.9238	6.4	**20.8019**	**0.8470**

Moreover, we apply the model trained by the sparse 30 views and 5% Gaussian noise to test data with different sparsity, i.e., g obtained by $N_{views} = 30, 25, 20$. We compare the results with the learned PDHG net, primal-net and PD-net from [1] in terms of PSNR and SSIM in Table 2. As shown, our model performs more stable in adapting with different testing data, which is because our model minimizes the distance between the reconstructed image and the full-sampling projection data.

3.3 Results on Piglet Phantom Data

We test the proposed model on simulated CT data of a deceased piglet, which is scanned from a 64-slice multi-detector CT scanner (Discovery CT750 HD, GE Healthcare) using $100 \, \text{kV}$ and $0.625 \, \text{mm}$ slice thickness. We use 896 images of size 512×512 as the ground truth for training and 10 for evaluation. We adopt the fan-beam geometry with $N_{bins} = 512$ and $N_{bins} = 1024$, source to axis distance $500 \, \text{mm}$ and axis to detector distance $500 \, \text{mm}$. The number of views is set as follows

- For $N_{bins} = 512$, the observed data g is generated by 64 uniformly distributed views over 2π arc with two different Poisson noises of 10^4 and 5×10^5 incident photons per pixel before attenuation. The full-sampling system matrix A_F is constructed according to SSC1, i.e., $N_{\text{views}} = 512$;

- For $N_{\text{bins}} = 1024$, the observed data g is generated with either 120 views or 60 views and Poisson noise of 10^4 incident photons. The full-sampling system matrix A_F is defined according to SSC4, i.e., $N_{\text{views}} = 1024$. Because $N_{\text{views}} = 1024$ gives too much computational burden, we use $N_{\text{views}} = 720$ in practice.

As shown in Tables 3 and 4, our model outperforms other methods in reconstruction quality. Especially when we use the parameters trained by $N_{\text{views}} = 64$ to reconstruct the sparse data such as $N_{\text{views}} = 32, 28, 24$, our model achieves a PSNR 0.5~3 dB higher than PD-net. Both the reconstructed images and the error maps are displayed in Fig. 3, the first column displays the FBP reconstruction of observed data g (1st row) and our estimated full-sampling measurement f (2nd row). It is obviously shown that our model can well inpaint the Radon domain data and improve the reconstruction quality.

Table 2. Reconstruction comparison on the piglet phantom for different sparsities.

N_{views}	30		25		20	
	PSNR	SSIM	PSNR	SSIM	PSNR	SSIM
PDHG-net	29.6762	0.9111	27.4642	0.8602	22.8205	0.6866
Primal-net	37.2040	0.9848	35.4175	0.9812	33.1559	0.9655
PD-net	39.2301	0.9860	36.4508	0.9757	34.6969	0.9365
FSR-net	**39.6588**	**0.9897**	**38.6696**	**0.9853**	**35.8236**	**0.9769**

Table 3. Comparison results for the piglet phantom in terms of PSNR, SSIM and Runtime.

N_{bins}	N_{views}	Noises	Methods	PSNR	SSIM	time	FBP(PSNR)	FBP(SSIM)
512	64	5×10^5	FBP-Unet	32.165	0.992	**5.2**	27.02	0.832
			PD-net	36.202	0.997	5.3		
			FSR-net	**36.875**	**0.997**	6.6	**27.423**	**0.9222**
	64	10^4	FBP-Unet	28.917	0.9853	**5.2**	22.7613	0.4196
			PD-net	29.999	0.9887	5.3		
			FSR-net	**30.564**	**0.9903**	6.6	**27.3457**	**0.9182**
1024	120	10^4	FBP-Unet	30.8926	0.9898	**5.3**	20.5832	0.3023
			PD-net	32.382	0.9933	5.4		
			FSR-net	**33.084**	**0.9941**	6.7	**27.3967**	**0.921**
	60	10^4	FBP-Unet	28.192	0.9793	**5.5**	18.0077	0.1658
			PD-net	31.263	0.9913	5.6		
			FSR-net	**31.763**	**0.9921**	7	**27.3917**	**0.9198**

Table 4. Reconstruction comparison on the piglet phantom for different sparsities.

N_{views}	32		28		24	
	PSNR	SSIM	PSNR	SSIM	PSNR	SSIM
FBP-Unet	23.44	0.9513	20.1502	0.9008	18.9658	0.855
PD-net	25.27	**0.9761**	21.0392	0.9453	18.333	0.906
FSR-net	**25.86**	0.973	**23.0581**	**0.9534**	**21.1436**	**0.9304**

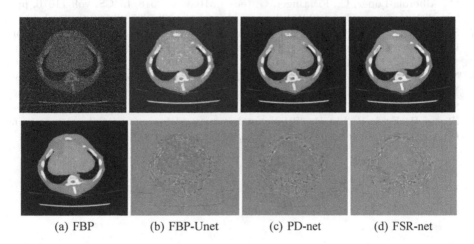

    (a) FBP   (b) FBP-Unet   (c) PD-net   (d) FSR-net

Fig. 3. Reconstruction comparison of a piglet phantom with $N_{views} = 64$ and $N_{bins} = 512$.

4   Conclusion

We proposed a novel iterative reconstruction model by fitting the reconstructed image with its corresponding measurements in Radon domain through the full-sampling system matrices. This new algorithm is in the family of deep learning based iterative reconstruction schemes. The application on sparse-view CT image reconstruction demonstrates the effectiveness of the proposed model and it is also clearly shown that the proposed method can be applied to other applications such as limited-angle CT reconstruction and compressed-sensing MR reconstruction.

References

1. Adler, J., Öktem, O.: Learned primal-dual reconstruction. IEEE Trans. Med. Imaging **37**(6), 1322–1332 (2018)
2. Chambolle, A., Pock, T.: A first-order primal-dual algorithm for convex problems with applications to imaging. J. Math. Imaging Vis. **40**(1), 120–145 (2011)
3. Dong, B., Li, J., Shen, Z.: X-ray CT image reconstruction via wavelet frame based regularization and radon domain inpainting. J. Sci. Comput. **54**(2–3), 333–349 (2013)

4. Jin, K.H., McCann, M.T., Froustey, E., Unser, M.: Deep convolutional neural network for inverse problems in imaging. IEEE Trans. Image Process. **26**(9), 4509–4522 (2017)
5. Jorgensen, J.S., Sidky, E.Y., Pan, X.: Quantifying admissible undersampling for sparsity-exploiting iterative image reconstruction in X-ray CT. IEEE Trans. Med. Imaging **32**(2), 460–473 (2013)
6. Liu, J., Kuang, T., Zhang, X.: Image reconstruction by splitting deep learning regularization from iterative inversion. In: Frangi, A.F., Schnabel, J.A., Davatzikos, C., Alberola-López, C., Fichtinger, G. (eds.) MICCAI 2018. LNCS, vol. 11070, pp. 224–231. Springer, Cham (2018). https://doi.org/10.1007/978-3-030-00928-1_26
7. Sidky, E.Y., Jørgensen, J.H., Pan, X.: Convex optimization problem prototyping for image reconstruction in computed tomography with the chambolle-pock algorithm. Phys. Med. Biol. **57**(10), 3065 (2012)
8. Yang, Y., Sun, J., Li, H., Xu, Z.: Deep ADMM-Net for compressive sensing MRI. In: Proceedings of the 30th International Conference on Neural Information Processing Systems, pp. 10–18 (2016)
9. Zhang, H., Dong, B., Liu, B.: JSR-Net: a deep network for joint spatial-radon domain CT reconstruction from incomplete data. arXiv preprint arXiv:1812.00510 (2018)

A Deep Regression Model for Seed Localization in Prostate Brachytherapy

Yading Yuan$^{(\boxtimes)}$, Ren-Dih Sheu, Luke Fu, and Yeh-Chi Lo

Department of Radiation Oncology, Icahn School of Medicine at Mount Sinai,
New York, NY 10029, USA
yading.yuan@mssm.edu

Abstract. Post-implant dosimetry (PID) is an essential step of prostate brachytherapy that utilizes CT to image the prostate and allow the location and dose distribution of the radioactive seeds to be directly related to the actual prostate. However, it a very challenging task to identify these seeds in CT images due to the severe metal artifacts and high-overlapped appearance when multiple seeds are clustered together. In this paper, we propose an automatic and efficient algorithm based on a 3D deep fully convolutional network for identifying implanted seeds in CT images. Our method models the seed localization task as a supervised regression problem that projects the input CT image to a map where each element represents the probability that the corresponding input voxel belongs to a seed. This deep regression model significantly suppresses image artifacts and makes the post-processing much easier and more controllable. The proposed method is validated on a large clinical database with 7820 seeds in 100 patients, in which 5534 seeds from 70 patients were used for model training and validation. Our method correctly detected 2150 of 2286 (94.1%) seeds in the 30 testing patients, yielding 16% improvement as compared to a widely-used commercial seed finder software (VariSeed, Varian, Palo Alto, CA).

Keywords: 3D deep fully convolutional network · Seed localization · Prostate brachytherapy

1 Introduction

With estimated 174,650 new cases and 31,620 deaths in 2019, prostate cancer remains the most common type of cancer diagnosed in men in the US [1]. Seed implant brachytherapy, which involves permanent implantation of radioactive sources (seeds) within the prostate gland, is the standard option for low and intermediate risk prostate cancer [2]. Despite various improvements in planning and seed delivery, the actual radiation dose distribution may deviate from the plan due to various factors such as needle positioning variations, prostate deformation, seed delivery variations and seed migration. Therefore, post-implant dosimetry (PID) is recommended to assure the quality of the implantation and

© Springer Nature Switzerland AG 2019
D. Shen et al. (Eds.): MICCAI 2019, LNCS 11768, pp. 385–393, 2019.
https://doi.org/10.1007/978-3-030-32254-0_43

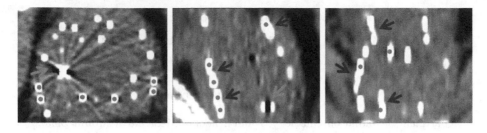

Fig. 1. An example of seed appearance in CT images in axial (left), sagittal (middle) and coronal (right) view, respectively. Yellow arrows indicate the metal artifacts and red dots represent mannually annotated seed locations. Clustered seeds can be clearly seen in saggital and coronal views, as indicated by the blue arrows. (Color figure online)

to establish the relationship between radiation dose and clinical outcomes [3]. PID is typically performed at day 30 following implantation that utilizes CT to image the implanted area, from which prostate and surrounding organs at risk (OARs) are outlined and seed locations are identified.

Accurate localization of implanted seeds is essential to quantify the dose distribution to those organs. However, manual identification of these seeds is time consuming given a large number of seeds implanted, typically taking 10 – 20 min to identify 60 to 100 seeds per patient. Therefore, accurate and automated methods for seed localization are of great demand. While the radio-opaque seeds appear with high contrast on the CT images, automatic seed localization is in practice a challenging task due to the following two unique characteristics, as shown in Fig. 1 (Note that not all the seeds are marked on the same 2D view). Firstly, the presence of fiducial markers introduces severe metal artifacts on CT images, which significantly increases the complexity of seed identification. Secondly, due to seed delivery variations and seed migration, some implanted seeds are very close to each other to form seed clusters. This highly-overlapped appearance makes it hard to identify individual seed on CT images.

Several automatic approaches have been developed to localize seeds in CT images such as the geometry-based recognition method [4] and Hough transform [5]. Recently, Nguyen et al. [6] proposed a cascaded method that involves thresholding and connected component analysis as initial detection of seed candidates, and followed by a modified k-means method to separate groups of seeds based on a priori intensity and volume information. Zhang et al. [7] employed canny edge detection and an improved concave points matching to separate touching seeds after gray-level-histogram based thresholding. All these methods use hand-crafted features that require specialized domain knowledge. Meanwhile, sophisticated pre- and post-processing steps are usually introduced to facilitate the seed localization procedure. As a result, the evaluation of these methods was mainly conducted with physical phantom or small amount of clinical cases.

Recently, deep convolutional neural networks (CNNs) have become popular in medical image analysis [8] and have achieved state-of-the-art performance in various medical image computing tasks such as lung nodule detection [9],

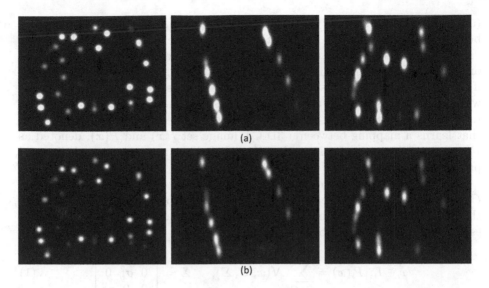

Fig. 2. (a) The target probability maps created from the dot manual annotations in Fig. 1. (b) The corresponding predicted probability maps inferred from the proposed deep regression network.

gland instance segmentation in histology images [10], liver and tumor segmentation [11], skin lesion segmentation [12] and classification [13]. Due to the capability of learning hierarchical features directly from raw image data, CNNs usually yield better generalization performance especially when evaluating on a large scale of dataset.

Enlightened by the latest advances in deep learning research, we propose a novel framework based on deep CNNs to automatically localize the implanted seeds in 3D CT images. Our contributions in this paper are three fold. Firstly, we model seed localization as a regression problem and introduce a fully automated solution by leveraging the discriminative power of deep CNNs. To the best of our knowledge, this is the first attempt of using deep neural networks to tackle this challenging task. Secondly, instead of directly predicting the seed coordinates in 3D space, we design a probability map of seed locations to account for the uncertainty of manual identification, which improves the robustness of model prediction. Finally, we evaluated the proposed method on a large clinical database with 7820 seeds in 100 patients, and compared the results with a commercial seed finder software (VariSeed, Varian, Palo Alto, CA).

2   Methodology

2.1   Deep Regression Model

As shown in Fig. 1, the ground truth is provided as dot annotations, where each dot corresponds to one seed. However, considering the seed has a finite dimension (about 0.8 mm in diameter and 4.5 mm in length), any dot annotation should be considered as correct as long as it's located on the seed. As a result, a large variation can be observed in the ground truth in terms of the annotation positions on the seeds, which makes it unnecessarily challenging and prone to overfitting if the exact annotation positions are directly used as learning target. Instead, we convert the discrete dot annotations into a continuous probability map $P(\boldsymbol{x})$ ($\boldsymbol{x} \in R^3$) and cast the seed localization task as a supervised regression problem that learns a mapping between a 3D CT image set $I(\boldsymbol{x})$ and $P(\boldsymbol{x})$, denoted as $\hat{P}(\boldsymbol{x}, \boldsymbol{w}) = F(I(\boldsymbol{x}), \boldsymbol{w})$ for $\hat{P}(\boldsymbol{x})$ the inferred probability map and $\boldsymbol{w}$ the learned parameters (weights).

For each training image $I_i(\boldsymbol{x})$ that is annotated with a set of 3D points $C_i = \{C_1, \ldots, C_{N(i)}\}$, where $N(i)$ is the total number of seeds annotated by the user, we define the ground truth probability map to be a kernel density estimation based on the provided points:

$$\forall \boldsymbol{x} \in I_i, \; P_i(\boldsymbol{x}) = \sum_{C \in C_i} \mathcal{N}(\boldsymbol{x}; C, \Sigma), \qquad \Sigma = \begin{bmatrix} \sigma_x^2 & 0 & 0 \\ 0 & \sigma_y^2 & 0 \\ 0 & 0 & \sigma_z^2 \end{bmatrix}. \tag{1}$$

Here $\boldsymbol{x}$ denotes the coordinates of any voxel in image I_i, and $\mathcal{N}(\boldsymbol{x}; C, \Sigma)$ is the normalized 3D Gaussian kernel evaluated at $\boldsymbol{x}$, with the mean at the user annotation C and a diagonal covariance matrix Σ. Considering the physical seed dimension and the magnification effect during CT imaging, we empirically set $\sigma_x = \sigma_y = 1$ mm and $\sigma_z = 2$ mm in our study. Figure 2(a) shows several examples of the probability map that are created from the dot manual annotations in Fig. 1, and (b) are the corresponding predicted maps inferred from the proposed deep regression model.

We train a deep regression network (DRN) to map the input CT images to the probability map using a symmetric convolutional encoding-decoding structure, as shown in Fig. 3. Convolution and max-pooling are employed to aggregate contextual information of CT images in the encoding pathway, and transpose convolution is used to recover the original resolution in the decoding pathway. Each convolutional layer is followed by batch normalization and rectified linear unit (ReLU) to facilitate gradient back-propagation. Long-range skip connections, which bridge across the encoding blocks and the decoding blocks, are also created to allow high resolution features from encoding pathway be used as additional inputs to the convolutional layers in the decoding pathway. By explicitly assembling low- and high-level features, DRN benefits from local and global contextual information to reconstruct more precise probability map of seed locations. Considering the target probability map is non-negative, we use *softplus* as the activation function in the last convolutional layer to ensure a positive output of DRN, which approximates the ReLU function as:

$$softplus(x) = \frac{1}{\beta} \cdot log(1 + exp(\beta \cdot x)). \tag{2}$$

In this study, we set $\beta = 1$. The convolutional kernel size is fixed as 3 and stride as 1, except for transpose convolution where we set both kernel size and stride

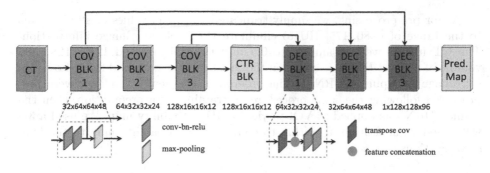

Fig. 3. Architecture of the proposed deep regression network (DRN). DRN is a fully 3D model that employs convolution and max-pooling to aggregate contextual information, and uses transpose convolution and long-range skip connection for better determination of seed locations. The numbers under each block represent the dimensions of its output, in which the first dimension denotes the feature channel.

as 2 for upscaling purpose. Zero-padding is used to ensure the same dimension during convolution. All the operations are performed in 3D space.

Training DRN is achieved by minimizing a loss function between the predicted probability map $F((I\boldsymbol{x}), \boldsymbol{w})$ and the target map $P(\boldsymbol{x})$. Since the majority of voxels in the target probability map belongs to background, DRN tends to focus more on learning background rather than the Gaussian-shaped seed annotations. In order to account for this imbalance between background and seed annotations, we use a weighted Mean Squared Error (MSE) as the loss function, with the weight as the target map $P(\boldsymbol{x})$:

$$L(\boldsymbol{w}) = \frac{1}{N} \cdot \sum_{n=1}^{N} [P(\boldsymbol{x}_n) \cdot (P(\boldsymbol{x}_n) - \hat{P}(\boldsymbol{x}_n, \boldsymbol{w}))^2], \tag{3}$$

where N is the total number of voxels in the training mini batch.

2.2 Implementation

Our DRN was implemented with Python using Pytorch (v.0.4) package. Training DRN took 500 iterations from scratch using Adam stochastic optimization method with a batch size of 4. The initial learning rate was set as 0.003, and learning rate decay and early stopping strategies were utilized when validation loss stopped decreasing. In order to reduce overfitting, we randomly flipped the input volume in left/right, superior/inferior, and anterior/posterior directions on the fly for data augmentation. We used seven-fold cross validation to evaluate the performance of our model on the training dataset, in which a few hyper-parameters were also experimentally determined via grid search. All the experiments were conducted on a workstation with four Nvidia GTX 1080 TI GPUs. The average training time was about 70 s per iteration.

As for pre-processing, we simply truncated the voxel values of all CT scans to the range of $[-80, 175]$ HU to eliminate the irrelevant image information. The CT images were resampled to 0.5 mm isotropically and $128 \times 128 \times 96$ volume of interest (VOI) centered on the prostate was extracted from the entire CT image as input to DRN. During inference, the new CT images were pre-processed following the same procedure as training data preparation, then the trained DRN was applied to VOI to yield a 3D probability map. We used a 3D watershed segmentation algorithm to convert the probability map to the final seed locations.

3   Experiments

We assembled a database of 100 prostate cancer patients treated with seed implant brachytherapy from 2008 to 2019 in our institution. The number of implanted seeds (Palladium 103) ranged from 48 to 156. Seventy patients with 5534 seeds were randomly selected for model training and validation, while the remaining 30 patients with 2286 seeds were reserved for independent testing. A CT scan was performed on each patient 30 days after implantation, with in-plane resolution ranging from 0.6×0.6 to 1.4×1.4 mm and slice thickness from 2.5 to 3.0 mm.

The ground truth was obtained by a semi-automatic procedure, in which VariSeed seed finder algorithm was first used to search implanted seeds near prostate region in the CT images. Since this automatic procedure usually results in a few erroneous seed placements, user intervention was required to correct these errors based on the seed locations in the CT images. The seed localization as well as the reconstructed radiation dose distribution were finally approved by a radiation oncologist.

We evaluated the performance of the proposed method by comparing the pair-wise distance between the predicted seed locations and the ground-truth locations. For a seed obtained from the automated method and one from ground truth, if their distance was the shortest among the list of seeds that needed to be paired, they were considered as a pair and removed from the list. If a pair-wise distance was not larger than 3 mm, the corresponding ground truth seed was considered as being correctly identified by the automated method.

Figure 4 shows two examples of PID study in CT images in axial, sagittal and coronal views, respectively, in which 77 seeds were implanted in patient (a) and 143 seeds in (b). Also shown are the corresponding DRN predictions of the probability map. It clearly shows that the metal artifacts and seed overlap appearance are significantly suppressed, which makes the seed localization much easier. The plots on the right show the 3D distributions of the ground truth and the seeds identified by DRN. Overall, it took about 60 s for DRN to recover the number of implanted seeds on 30 testing patients. The median pair-wise distance was 0.70 mm $[25\% - 75\%: 0.36 - 1.28$ mm$]$.

Table 1 details the comparison between DRN and VariSeed seed finder in seed detection, in which the first and fourth rows list the number of implanted seeds.

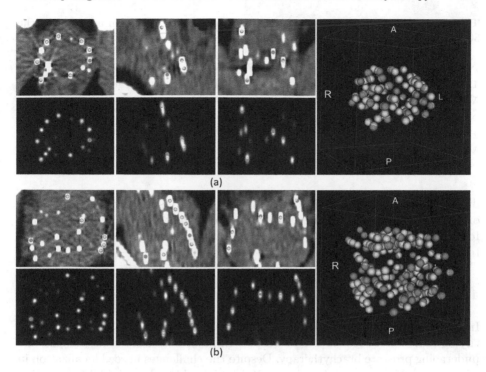

Fig. 4. Two examples of PID study in CT images in axial, sagittal and coronal views. The second and fourth rows are the corresponding probability maps generated by the proposed DRN model. The right column shows the overall 3D distributions of the ground truth and seeds identified by DRN. In each figure, the red dots represent the ground truth while the cyan dots are seed locations identified by DRN. (Color figure online)

For a large range of number of implanted seeds (from 48 to 143), the proposed DRN outperformed VariSeed by a big margin on almost every patient. Overall, DRN correctly identified 2150 out of 2286 seeds (94.1%) in 30 testing patients, achieving 16% improvement as compared to VariSeed (81.0%).

Because there is no common platform available for comparing different automatic algorithms of seed localization in prostate brachytherapy, we only compared the proposed DRN model with VariSeed, which occupies over 50% market share in prostate brachytherapy software business. While it can be challenging to fully implement algorithms from other research projects, it would be interesting to compare the proposed DRN model with some of the previously mentioned methods in the future. Meanwhile, since DRN model was able to yield a much more distinct probability distribution in axial view, as shown in Fig. 4, we found the majority of seed mismatch occurred in z direction. As a result, we set the threshold as 3 mm to allow the paired seeds can only be offset by one image slice. Considering the seed diameter is much smaller than its length, an anisotropic thresholding strategy will be explored in our future work. At last,

Table 1. Comparison between DRN and VariSeed in seed detection accuracy on the 30 testing patients. Bold values are the numbers of implanted seeds in each patient.

No. of seeds	48	50	52	52	58	58	60	62	66	66	66	69	69	71	71
DRN (%)	95.8	92.0	96.2	98.1	94.8	87.9	91.7	91.9	86.4	97.0	97.0	94.2	91.3	93.0	95.8
VariSeed (%)	79.2	48.0	42.3	65.4	79.3	77.6	76.7	69.4	75.8	81.8	90.9	84.1	79.7	74.6	91.5
No. of seeds	72	72	74	77	78	79	82	84	88	95	99	100	108	117	143
DRN (%)	94.4	93.1	91.9	96.1	94.9	94.9	93.9	97.6	95.5	90.5	94.0	92.0	90.7	100.0	95.8
VariSeed (%)	77.8	90.3	79.7	87.0	67.9	87.3	100.0	76.2	84.1	81.1	85.9	73.0	85.2	94.0	92.3

due to the availability of radioactive materials in our institute, our study focused on Palladium-103. To generalize the DRN model to other type of seeds, such as Iodine-125, one way is to adjust the standard deviation of the Gaussian kernel to account for the difference of the seed dimension.

4   Conclusion

In this paper, we pioneered the application of deep learning in the task of identifying radioactive seeds in CT-based post-implant dosimetry study for patients undergoing prostate brachytherapy. Despite the challenges in seed localization in CT images, the proposed deep regression model achieved much higher detection accuracy as compared to a widely-used commercial software on a large clinical database. Also, our model was found to be very efficient, taking about 2 s on average for a new test case. Instead of manually drawing 3D bounding box or mask on each seed, our method only requires dot annotations as ground truth for model training, which greatly simplifies the data labelling procedure. This weakly-supervised learning framework can be easily generalized to other object detection tasks such as fiducial marker tracking in 2D/3D real-time imaging and source/catheter positioning in high dose rate (HDR) brachytherapy.

Acknowledgment. This work is partially supported by grant UL1TR001433 from the National Center for Advancing Translational Sciences, National Institutes of Health, USA.

References

1. Siegel, R.L., et al.: Cancer statistics, 2019. Cancer J. Clin. **69**, 7–34 (2019)
2. Chin, J., et al.: Brachytherapy for patients with prostate cancer: American society of clinical oncology/cancer care ontario joint guideline update. J. Clin. Oncol. **35**, 1737–43 (2017)
3. Stock, R., et al.: Importance of post-implant dosimetry in permanent prostate brachytherapy. Eur. Urol. **41**, 434–439 (2002)
4. Liu, H., et al.: Automatic localization of implanted seeds from post-implant CT images. Phys. Med. Biol. **48**(9), 1191–1203 (2003)

5. Holupka, E.J., et al.: An automatic seed finder for brachytherapy CT postplans based on the Hough transform. Med. Phys. **31**(9), 2672–2679 (2004)
6. Nguyen, H.G., et al.: Automatic 3D seed location and orientation detection in CT image for prostate brachytherapy. In: IEEE ISBI 2014, pp. 1320–1323 (2014)
7. Zhang, G., et al.: Automatic seed picking for brachytherapy postimplant validation with 3D CT images. Int. J. CARS. **12**, 1985–1993 (2017)
8. Litjens, G., et al.: A survey on deep learning in medical image analysis. Med. Imaging Anal. **42**, 60–88 (2017)
9. Setio, A., et al.: Validation, comparison, and combination of algorithms for automatic detection of pulmonary nodules in computed tomography images: the LUNA16 challenge. Med. Imaging Anal. **42**, 1–13 (2017)
10. Xu, Y., et al.: Gland instance segmentation using deep multichannel neural networks. IEEE Trans. Med. Imaging **64**(12), 2901–2912 (2017)
11. Bilic, P., et al. : The liver tumor segmentation benchmark (LiTS). arXiv preprint arXiv:1901.04056 (2019)
12. Yuan, Y., et al.: Automatic skin lesion segmentation using deep fully convolutional networks with Jaccard distance. IEEE Trans. Med. Imaging **36**(9), 1876–1886 (2017)
13. Yu, L., et al.: Automated melanoma recognition in dermoscopy images via very deep residual networks. IEEE Trans. Med. Imaging **36**(4), 994–1004 (2017)

Model-Based Recommendations for Optimal Surgical Placement of Epiretinal Implants

Michael Beyeler[1,2,3(✉)], Geoffrey M. Boynton[1], Ione Fine[1,2], and Ariel Rokem[2,3]

[1] Department of Psychology, University of Washington, Seattle, WA 98195, USA
{mbeyeler,gboynton,ionefine}@uw.edu
[2] Institute for Neuroengineering (UWIN), University of Washington, Seattle, WA 98195, USA
[3] eScience Institute, University of Washington, Seattle, WA 98195, USA
arokem@uw.edu

Abstract. A major limitation of current electronic retinal implants is that in addition to stimulating the intended retinal ganglion cells, they also stimulate passing axon fibers, producing perceptual 'streaks' that limit the quality of the generated visual experience. Recent evidence suggests a dependence between the shape of the elicited visual percept and the retinal location of the stimulating electrode. However, this knowledge has yet to be incorporated into the surgical placement of retinal implants. Here we systematically explored the space of possible implant configurations to make recommendations for optimal intraocular positioning of the electrode array. Using a psychophysically validated computational model, we demonstrate that better implant placement has the potential to reduce the spatial extent of axonal activation in existing implant users by up to ∼55%. Importantly, the best implant location, as inferred from a population of simulated virtual patients, is both surgically feasible and is relatively stable across individuals. This study is a first step towards the use of computer simulations in patient-specific planning of retinal implant surgery.

Keywords: Retinal implant surgery · Axonal stimulation · Computational model

1 Introduction

Argus II (Second Sight Medical Products, Inc., https://secondsight.com) is currently the only retinal prosthesis system to receive approval from both the US Food & Drug Administration and the Conformité Européenne Mark. For successful implantation of the device, surgeons are instructed to place the electrode array parafoveally over the macula, approximately diagonal at −45° to the horizontal meridian (see Surgeon Manual [10], p. 29), for reasons of surgical ease.

© Springer Nature Switzerland AG 2019
D. Shen et al. (Eds.): MICCAI 2019, LNCS 11768, pp. 394–402, 2019.
https://doi.org/10.1007/978-3-030-32254-0_44

However, instead of seeing focal spots of light, patients implanted with epiretinal electronic implants report seeing highly distorted percepts that range in description from 'blobs' to 'streaks' and 'wedges' [8]. Electrophysiological evidence from *in vitro* preparations of rat and rabbit retina suggests that these distortions may arise from incidental stimulation of passing axon fibers in the optic fiber layer (OFL) [5,6,11]. Although there is believed to be a systematic relationship between the severity of distortions due to axonal stimulation and the retinal location of the stimulating electrode [2–4], this knowledge has yet to be incorporated into the patient-specific planning of retinal implant surgery [1], or surgical recommendations for intraocular positioning of the electrode array.

The contributions of this paper are three-fold. First, we present a strategy to optimize the intraocular placement of epiretinal implants, based on a psychophysically validated computational model of the vision provided by Argus II. Second, we validate this strategy on three Argus II patients and a population of virtual patients. Third, we recommend an optimal intraocular location that is both surgically feasible and relatively consistent across individuals.

2   Methods

Prior work suggests a dependence between the shape of a visual percept generated by an epiretinal implant and the retinal location of the stimulating electrode [4,5]. Because retinal ganglion cells (RGCs) send their axons on highly stereotyped pathways to the optic nerve [7], an electrode that stimulates nearby axonal fibers would be expected to antidromically activate RGC bodies located

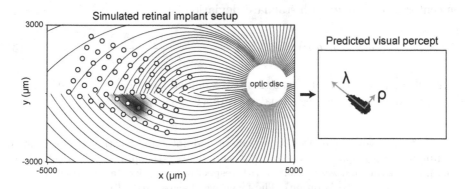

Fig. 1. A simulated map of retinal NFBs (*left*) can account for visual percepts (*right*) elicited by epiretinal implants. *Left*: Electrical stimulation (red circle) of a NFB (black lines) could antidromically activate retinal ganglion cell bodies peripheral to the point of stimulation, leading to tissue activation (black shaded region) elongated along the NFB trajectory away from the optic disc (white circle). *Right*: The resulting visual percept appears elongated as well; its shape can be described by two parameters, λ (spatial extent along the NFB trajectory) and ρ (spatial extent perpendicular to the NFB). See [4] for more information. (Color figure online)

peripheral to the point of stimulation, leading to percepts that appear elongated in the direction of the underlying nerve fiber bundle (NFB) trajectory (Fig. 1, *right*) [4]. As can be seen in (Fig. 1, *left*), electrodes near the horizontal meridian are predicted to elicit circular percepts, while other electrodes are predicted to produce elongated percepts that will differ in angle based on whether they fall above or below the horizontal meridian.

Reference [4] used a simulated map of NFBs in each subject's retina to accurately predict the shape of percepts elicited by the Argus system, assuming that:

i. An axon's sensitivity to electrical stimulation decays exponentially with decay constant ρ as a function of distance from the stimulation site (x_{stim}, y_{stim}).
ii. An axon's sensitivity to electrical stimulation decays exponentially with decay constant λ as a function of distance from the soma (x_{soma}, y_{soma}), measured as path length along the axon.

This allowed for percept shape to be described as a 2-D intensity profile, $I(x, y)$:

$$I(x, y) = f(x, y; x_{soma}, y_{soma}, \lambda) \, g(x, y; x_{stim}, y_{stim}, \rho), \tag{1}$$

where f modeled an exponential fall-off along the axon, with maximal sensitivity close to the cell body:

$$f(x, y; x_{soma}, y_{soma}, \lambda) = \exp\left(-\frac{d^2(x, y, x_{soma}, y_{soma})}{2\lambda^2} \right), \tag{2}$$

using path length $d(x, y, x_{soma}, y_{soma})$ measured between a point (x, y) on the axon and the soma (x_{soma}, y_{soma}); and g was a two-dimensional Gaussian function centered over (μ, ν) with standard deviation σ:

$$g(x, y; \mu, \nu, \sigma) = \exp\left(-\frac{(x - \mu)^2 + (y - \nu)^2}{2\sigma^2} \right). \tag{3}$$

The resulting intensity profile was then thresholded to arrive at a binary image, which served as the predicted visual percept (Fig. 1, *right*).

Table 1. Model parameters. Device placement and optic disc location were estimated from fundus photographs, whereas ρ and λ were fit to psychophysical data (see [4] for details). Device rotation was measured with respect to the horizontal meridian (positive angles: counter-clockwise rotation). The fovea was located at $(0,0)$.

Subject ID	Device center $(x,y; \mu m)$	Device rotation (deg)	Optic disc center $(x, y; \text{deg})$	ρ (μm)	λ (μm)
1	$(-1331, -850)$	-28	$(16.2, 1.4)$	352	299
2	$(-467, 206)$	-26	$(14.0, 1.2)$	91	659
3	$(-1807, 401)$	-22	$(16.3, 2.4)$	414	1383

This model was previously validated on psychophysical data from three Argus II patients with severe retinitis pigmentosa [4]. Electrical stimulation was delivered to a number of pre-selected electrodes in random order, and subjects were asked to outline perceived percept shape on a touch screen. The images predicted by the model were then compared to the drawings, and the best-fitting values for ρ and λ were determined for each subject in a cross-validation procedure. Note that a single value of ρ and λ was fitted for each subject, and then used for all electrodes in that subject's array (see Table 1).

To determine the optimal intraocular positioning of Argus II for Patients 1–3, we performed a grid search over the space of feasible implant configurations and used the model described in [4] to estimate average percept size. We limited the search to a region of the retina where the model was deemed valid [7]. This included array centers located in the range $x \in [-2000\,\mu\mathrm{m}, 400\,\mu\mathrm{m}]$ and $y \in [-1200\,\mu\mathrm{m}, 1200\,\mu\mathrm{m}]$, which we sampled at $200\mu\mathrm{m}$ resolution. We considered implantation angles in the range $[-90°, 90°]$ with a $5°$ step size.

Since ρ and λ were fixed for each subject, the size of each predicted percept was closely related to the amount of axonal stimulation. Moreover, since visual outcomes in epiretinal implants depend crucially on the ability of the device to generate localized percepts, average percept size serves as a simple proxy for the quality of the generated visual experience.

3   Experiments and Results

3.1   Optimal Implant Placement: Three Argus II Patients

Results are shown in Fig. 2. Percept predictions for the actual implant configuration are shown in the leftmost column, where each percept is overlaid over the corresponding electrode in a schematic of each patient's implant.

Consistent with the psychophysical data described in [4], electrodes located in close proximity to the horizontal meridian elicited more focal percepts than more eccentric electrodes. One could therefore reduce average percept size without changing the location, simply by rotating the array so that as many electrodes as possible lie close to the horizontal meridian (second column, labeled "rotation only"); a strategy that worked especially well for Patient 2.

On the other hand, if one were free to place the implant at any parafoveal location oriented at any angle in $[-90°, 90°]$, average percept size could be even further reduced (third column, labeled "rotation + translation").

The possible reduction in percept size is quantified in the rightmost column. In the case where the implant location was fixed, but a rotation of the device was allowed, mean percept size could be reduced by up to 20%. When both location and angle were allowed to vary the mean percept size could be reduced by up to 55%. Interestingly, Fig. 2 suggests that all three patients could have benefited from a similar intraocular positioning of the device, a roughly $90°$ shift from the currently recommendation location.

Figure 3 further quantifies the effect of array positioning on mean percept size. Heat maps in the left column show the effect of altering the array location.

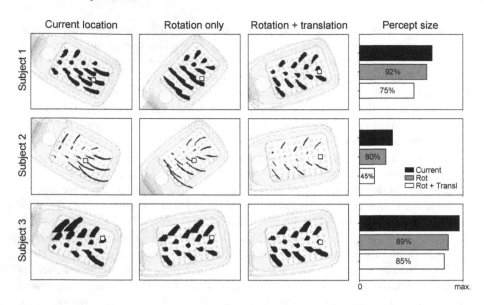

Fig. 2. Model predictions of percept shape for different electrodes, overlaid over a schematic of each patient's implant. Predictions for the actual implant configurations (leftmost column) are contrasted with optimized arrangements, either where the device location is the same but device orientation is adjusted to minimize the spatial extent of axonal activation (second column), or where both device location and orientation are optimized (third column). Mean percept size for the three configurations are shown in the rightmost column. Small squares indicate the location of the fovea.

At each location, the implant was rotated to find the angle that minimized average percept size. These corresponding rotation angles are shown in the right column. Thus, for Patient 1, the ideal location would be $x = -2000$, $y = 0$, at a rotation of $\sim 20°$. For all three patients, the ideal location lay close to $x = -2000$, $y = 0$. Indeed, by happenstance, Patient 3's device lay close to the optimal implant location. However, due to specifications by the device manufacturer, all three patients had the array implanted at negative angles almost $45°$ away from the optimal angle. Our simulations suggest that positive angles (reddish colors) would be preferable for most implant locations.

3.2   Optimal Implant Placement: Virtual Patients

To investigate whether these findings would generalize to other Argus II users, we simulated a population of 90 virtual patients, each with randomly assigned values for ρ (in the range $[50\,\mu\text{m}, 500\,\mu\text{m}]$) and λ (in the range $[200\,\mu\text{m}, 1600\,\mu\text{m}]$). These two model parameters are thought to capture important individual differences across patients, and might serve as a phenomenological description of both neuroanatomical parameters as well as drawing preferences [4]. We then repeated the experiment described above to determine the optimal implant location and orientation for each individual in the population.

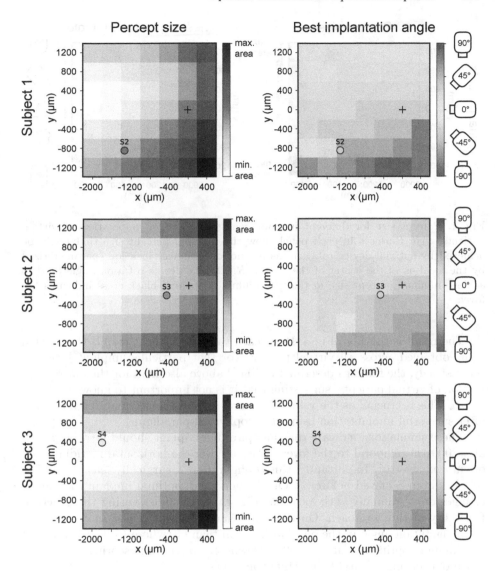

Fig. 3. Percept size for different implant configurations for Patients 1–3. *Left*: Surfaces in each panel show the minimal percept size that could be achieved by optimal device rotation, as a function of device location (i.e., center of the array). Small circles depict actual device locations for Patients 1–3, with the color indicating the empirically measured percept size. *Right*: The corresponding device rotation angle used to achieve minimal percept size in the left column, with the color of the small circles indicating the actual device rotation for Patients 1–3. Note that due to the symmetry of the electrode grid in Argus II, 90° and −90° are two technically equivalent configurations. The small black cross indicates the fovea. (Color figure online)

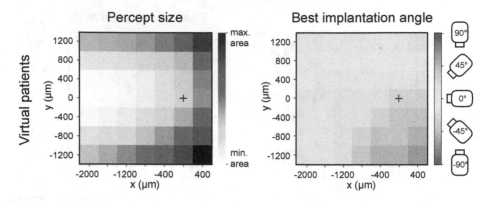

Fig. 4. Percept size for different implant configurations in a population of virtual patients. *Left*: Surfaces in each panel show the minimal percept size that could be achieved by optimal device rotation, as a function of device location (parameterized by the location of the center of the array). *Right*: The device rotation angle used to achieve minimal percept size in the left column. The small black cross indicates the fovea.

The result is shown in Fig. 4. Here, each value in the heat map is the median value obtained across all virtual patients for that particular implant location. Interestingly, the findings described in Fig. 2 above also hold for the entire population of virtual patients, suggesting that it is not important to know ρ and λ a *priori*. This is crucial, as the values for ρ and λ can currently only be measured after successful implantation using psychophysical paradigms.

These simulations indicate that an epiretinal implant should best be placed at ~2000 μm temporal to the fovea, centered over the horizontal meridian, and orientated at ~10°. Importantly, this configuration is surgically feasible, and in fact has been achieved before [1]. On the one hand, optimal implantation angle changes only gradually with location (Fig. 4, *right*), underscoring the practical feasibility of this approach. On the other hand, percept size is more sensitive to implantation angle in the optimal location than elsewhere (full width at half maximum in optimal location: ~60°, elsewhere: ~90°), underscoring the importance of choosing a suitable implantation angle.

4   Conclusion

This preliminary study is a first step towards the use of computer simulations in the patient-specific planning of retinal implant surgery. We show here that the visual outcome of epiretinal implant surgery might be substantially improved by guiding the intraocular positioning of the electrode array using a patient-specific computational model of the spatial layout of the OFL. Our findings suggest that optimized array placement could reduce the spatial extent of axonal activation in existing Argus II users by up to ~55%. Importantly, predicted percept sizes are robust to small deviations from the optimal location and orientation of the array, as well as to small deviations of the model parameters that predict the shape of the percept.

The optimal implant location, as inferred from a population of virtual patients, is ~2000 μm temporal to the fovea, centered over the horizontal meridian, and orientated at ~10° with respect to the meridian. Importantly, this placement is surgically feasible. Our method requires *a priori* knowledge about the location of the fovea and horizontal meridian, but these can be estimated presurgically based on anatomical landmarks in fundus images. Moreoever, intraoperative op-tical coherence tomography (OCT) can be used to guide the placement of the array [9].

Acknowledgments. Supported by the Washington Research Foundation Funds for Innovation in Neuroengineering and Data-Intensive Discovery (M.B.), by an award from the Gordon and Betty Moore Foundation (Award #2013-10-29) and the Alfred P. Sloan Foundation (Award #3835) to the University of Washington eScience Institute (A.R.), and by the National Institutes of Health (NIH K99 EY-029329 to M.B., EY-12925 to G.M.B., and EY-014645 to I.F.).Research credits for cloud computing were provided by Amazon Web Services.

References

1. Ahuja, A.K., Behrend, M.R.: The $Argus^{TM}$ II retinal prosthesis: factors affecting patient selection for implantation. Prog. Retinal Eye Res. **36**, 1–23 (2013). https://doi.org/10.1016/j.preteyeres.2013.01.002
2. Beyeler, M., Boynton, G.M., Fine, I., Rokem, A.: pulse2percept: a Python-based simulation framework for bionic vision. In: Huff, K., Lippa, D., Niederhut, D., Pacer, M. (eds.) Proceedings of the 16th Science in Python Conference, pp. 81–88 (2017). https://doi.org/10.25080/shinma-7f4c6e7-00c
3. Beyeler, M.: Biophysical model of axonal stimulation in epiretinal visual prostheses. In: 2019 9th International IEEE/EMBS Conference on Neural Engineering (NER), pp. 348–351 (2019). https://doi.org/10.1109/NER.2019.8716969
4. Beyeler, M., Nanduri, D., Weiland, J.D., Rokem, A., Boynton, G.M., Fine, I.: A model of ganglion axon pathways accounts for percepts elicited by retinal implants. Sci. R. **9**(1), 9199 (2019). https://doi.org/10.1038/s41598-019-45416-4
5. Fine, I., Boynton, G.M.: Pulse trains to percepts: the challenge of creating a perceptually intelligible world with sight recovery technologies. Philos. Trans. R. Soc. Lond. B Biol. Sci. **370**(1677), 20140208 (2015). https://doi.org/10.1098/rstb.2014.0208
6. Fried, S.I., Lasker, A.C.W., Desai, N.J., Eddington, D.K., Rizzo, J.F.: Axonal sodium-channel bands shape the response to electric stimulation in retinal ganglion cells. J. Neurophysiol. **101**(4), 1972–1987 (2009). https://doi.org/10.1152/jn.91081.2008
7. Jansonius, N.M., et al.: A mathematical description of nerve fiber bundle trajectories and their variability in the human retina. Vis. Res. **49**(17), 2157–2163 (2009). https://doi.org/10.1016/j.visres.2009.04.029
8. Luo, Y.H., Zhong, J.J., Clemo, M., da Cruz, L.: Long-term repeatability and reproducibility of phosphene characteristics in chronically implanted argus(R) II retinal prosthesis subjects. A. J. Ophthalmol. (2016). https://doi.org/10.1016/j.ajo.2016.07.021

9. Rachitskaya, A.V., Yuan, A., Marino, M.J., Reese, J., Ehlers, J.P.: Intraoperative OCT imaging of the argus II retinal prosthesis system. Ophthalmic Surg. Lasers Imaging Retina **47**(11), 999–1003 (2016). https://doi.org/10.3928/23258160-20161031-03

10. Second Sight Medical Products: Argus II Retinal Prosthesis System Surgeon Manual (2013). https://www.accessdata.fda.gov/cdrh_docs/pdf11/h110002c.pdf

11. Weitz, A.C., et al.: Improving the spatial resolution of epiretinal implants by increasing stimulus pulse duration. Sci. Transl. Med. **7**(318), 318ra203 (2015). https://doi.org/10.1126/scitranslmed.aac4877

Towards Multiple Instance Learning and Hermann Weyl's Discrepancy for Robust Image-Guided Bronchoscopic Intervention

Xiongbiao Luo[1(✉)], Hui-Qing Zeng[2], Yan-Ping Du[2], and Xiao Cheng[2]

[1] Department of Computer Science, Xiamen University, Xiamen, China
xiongbiao.luo@gmail.com
[2] Zhongshan Hospital, Xiamen University, Xiamen, China

Abstract. This paper proposes an advantageous approach that introduces multiple instance learning (MIL) and Hermann Weyl's discrepancy (HWD) to improve image-guided bronchoscopic intervention. Numerous 2D-3D registration methods used for bronchoscopic navigation suffer from problematic bronchoscopic video images (e.g., bubbles and collision) that easily collapse the registration optimization since these images remain challenging to precisely calculate the similarity between bronchoscopic real images and virtual renderings generated from CT slices, resulting in inaccurate bronchoscopic navigation. To address this limitation, we develop a new navigation framework that employs a MIL-driven image classification strategy to remove problematic frames and then performs a HWD-enhanced 2D-3D registration procedure. We validate our framework on patient data. The experimental results demonstrate that our effective and accurate navigation method outperforms others approaches. In particular, the average navigation accuracy of position and orientation was improved from (6.8, 18.0) to $3.5\,\mathrm{mm}$, $9.4°$).

1 Introduction

Image-guided bronchoscopic navigation systems provide much useful information such as continuous position and orientation of a bronchoscope in the preoperative image space to assist interventions (e.g., transbronchial lung biopsy) to diagnose and treat lung cancer. However, these systems have difficulty in precisely estimating the bronchoscope motion using current image- and sensor-based navigation methods that have their disadvantages [1–4]. Image-based bronchoscopic navigation, which is an active topic and is also the topic of this paper, usually define an image intensity-based similarity measure to minimize the pixel difference between bronchoscopic video images and virtual renderings generated from preoperative imaging modality (e.g., CT). Unfortunately, bronchoscopic image artifacts or uncertainties (Fig. 1) are the most challenging problem in image-based navigation methods, which impede image-based navigation methods to continuously and accurately track the bronchoscope movement. Even although numerous research papers have been published in the literature [4–7], these image uncertainties or problematic images remain a tough proposition

© Springer Nature Switzerland AG 2019
D. Shen et al. (Eds.): MICCAI 2019, LNCS 11768, pp. 403–411, 2019.
https://doi.org/10.1007/978-3-030-32254-0_45

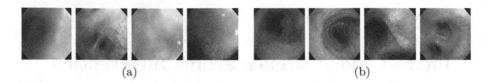

Fig. 1. Examples of typical bronchoscopic video images. The left four in (a) show problematic or uninformative frames due to specular- or inter-reflection, bubbles, and so on, and the others in (b) display informative images without any artifacts.

in navigated bronchoscopy. Therefore, a more effective method to tackle these image uncertainties is still intensively expected for robust bronchoscopic navigation.

This work seeks for an accurate and robust image-based navigation framework. We propose a new navigation approach with two strategies to tackle bronchoscopic image artifacts. First, an image categorization strategy is performed to recognize these problematic images before an intensity-based optimization process. We employ multiple instance learning (MIL) to classify bronchoscopic images [8]. On the other hand, an intensity-based similarity measure plays an essential role in the 2D-3D registration during optimization. Image-based bronchsocopic navigation requires a robust similarity function to precisely characterize the intensity difference and adapt itself successfully to image changes (uncertainties) due to nonlinear illumination, specular- or inter-reflection, bubbles, motion blurring, or collision with the bronchial walls in bronchoscopy. To this end, we introduces Hermann Weyl's discrepancy (HWD) in this study, which was proved to be a powerful similarity characterization approach [9].

The contribution of this work is summarized in the following aspects. First, we propose a new HWD-driven similarity measure for 2D-3D registration and demonstrate its effectiveness and robustness to track the bronchoscope during bronchoscopic navigation. While we extend a new application of HWD in computer assisted intervention (CAI), we also believe such a similarity measure has the potential to resolve the problem of image registration in computer aided diagnosis (CAD). Next, we present a MIL-based image artifact classification method to boost bronchoscope tracking and navigation. Additionally, we introduce the concept of the MIL-HWD driven bronchoscopic navigation, which should be also suitable to other endoscopic navigation procedures (e.g., colonoscopy).

2   Approaches

Our approach (Fig. 2) to track or navigate the bronchoscope (i.e., estimate six degrees of freedom position and orientation of the bronchoscope) consists of three main steps: (1) MIL-based image classification, (2) HWD-based similarity characterization, and (3) video-CT (2D-3D) registration. While the first step is to classify uncertain or uninformative images before the similarity computation, the second step uses HWD to characterize the similarity between the bronchoscopic real and CT-based virtual images before the optimization in the final step (3).

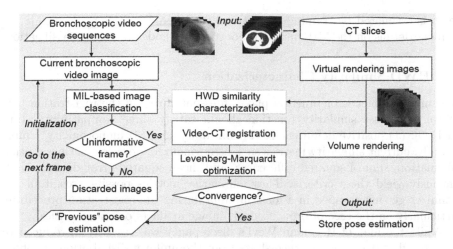

Fig. 2. Flowchart of our proposed method based on MIL and HWD

2.1   MIL-Based Image Classification

MIL was introduced for natural image classification by Maron et al. [10]. We use MIL to classify uninformative images to enhance bronchoscopic navigation.

Suppose that we divide the bronchoscopic real image $\mathcal{I}_i^R$ at time or frame i into a set of overlapping patches (instances) $\mathcal{I}_i^R = \{\mathbf{I}_{ij}^R\}_{j=1}^N$, where N is the number of patches. After constructing a binary MIL classifier by a set of training data $\{(\mathcal{I}_i^R, y_i)\}_{i=1}^M$ (M is the number of frames and $y_i \in \{0, 1\}$ is a bag of labels), an unknown patch or instance $\mathbf{I}_{ij}^R$ in the bag $\mathcal{I}_i^R$ can be labeled to y_i by

$$y_i = \max_j(y_{ij}), \quad y_{ij} = \mathcal{F}(\mathbf{I}_{ij}^R), \tag{1}$$

where $\mathcal{F}(\cdot)$ is a sum of weighted weak classifiers. To solve the MIL problem (Eq. 1), we employ the MIL boosting method to classify the bronchoscopic image $\mathcal{I}_i^R$ by maximizing its likelihood over all the labeled bags $\{(\mathcal{I}_i^R, y_i)\}$ [8,11]:

$$\mathcal{P} = \prod_i (p(y_i|\mathcal{I}_i^R))^{y_i} (1 - p(y_i|\mathcal{I}_i^R))^{1-y_i}, \tag{2}$$

where the probability $p(y_i|\mathcal{I}_i^R)$ of the bronchoscopic image or bag $\mathcal{I}_i^R$ being positive is computed by the Noisy-OR model [11]:

$$p(y_i|\mathcal{I}_i^R) = 1 - \prod_{j \in N} (1 - p(y_{ij}|\mathbf{I}_{ij}^R)), \tag{3}$$

which is associated with the probability $p(y_{iJ}|\mathbf{I}_{ij}^R)$ of the positive instance $\mathbf{I}_i^R$. We calculate $p(y_{iJ}|\mathbf{I}_{ij}^R)$ by the standard logistic function:

$$p(y_{ij}|\mathbf{I}_{ij}^R) = \frac{1}{1 + exp(-y_{ij})}, \tag{4}$$

which is estimated by training an instance classifier. We refer readers to [8,11] for more details on the MIL and MIL boosting methods for image classification.

2.2 HWD Similarity Characterization

The similarity metric or function plays an essential role in the registration procedure. A robust similarity function should satisfy three compatibility standards [9]: (1) positive definiteness, (2) continuity, and (3) monotonicity. Unfortunately, current similarity metrics such as normalized cross correlation, mutual information, sum of squared differences, and mean squared error do not simultaneously yield these criteria. These similarity metrics possibly result in the optimizer getting trapped in a local minima during the registration procedure, particularly on the case of bronchoscopic image artifacts or uncertainties.

While the idea of Hermann Weyl's discrepancy was initially introduced to evaluate what degree a sequence shifts from the uniform distribution, a robust similarity function can be defined by extending the concept of HWD [9]

$$\|S\|_{\mathcal{A}}^d = \sup_{a \in \mathcal{A}} \left| \int_a S dx \right|, \tag{5}$$

where S is a multi-dimensional function of x: $\{S \in \mathcal{L}(\mathbb{R}^d, x) | d \in \mathbb{N}\}$, d is the dimension of x, sup denotes the supremum of a set, and $\mathcal{A}$ indicates a set of the connected area a in $\mathbb{R}^d$. To efficiently calculate such a discrepancy, i.e., operation $O(n^2) \Longrightarrow O(n)$, a set of integral images is defined as

$$\mathcal{G}_S^{\mathbf{v}} = \left\{ \int_{\mathbf{T_u(B_v)}} S dx | \mathbf{u} \in \Re^d \right\}, \tag{6}$$

where $\mathbf{T_u(B_v)}$ represents transform: $S \Longrightarrow S \circ \mathbf{T_u}$, $\mathbf{T_u(B_v)} = \{\mathbf{t} - \mathbf{u} | \mathbf{t} \in \mathbf{B_v}\}$, and $\mathbf{B_v} = \{(\lambda_1 b_1, \cdots, \lambda_d b_d)^T | \lambda_1 > 0, \cdots, \lambda_d > 0\}$, $\mathbf{v} = (b_1, \cdots, b_d) \in \{-1, 1\}^d$. Therefore, for all $d \in \mathbb{N}$ and nonnegative $S \in \mathcal{L}(\mathbb{R}^d, x)$, $S \geq 0$, a new alignment or similarity function $\Delta_{\mathcal{A}}[S](\mathbf{u})$ is formulated in accordance with HWD

$$\Delta_{\mathcal{A}}[S](\mathbf{u}) = \psi(S, S \circ \mathbf{T_u}) = \|S - S \circ \mathbf{T_u}\|_{\mathcal{A}}^d = \max_{\mathbf{v} \in \{-1,1\}^d} \left\{ \sup \mathcal{G}_{S - S \circ \mathbf{T}}^{\mathbf{v}} \right\}, \tag{7}$$

which was demonstrated to achieve the following properties [9]

$$nonnegativity: \int \|S\| dx \geq 0 \Rightarrow \Delta_{\mathcal{A}}[S](\mathbf{u}) = 0 \Longleftrightarrow \mathbf{u} = 0, \tag{8}$$

$$Continuity: \Delta_{\mathcal{A}}[S](\mathbf{u}) \leq \Delta_x[S](\mathbf{u}) \|S\|_\infty, \tag{9}$$

$$Monotonicity: 0 \leq \lambda_1 \leq \lambda_2 \Longrightarrow \Delta_{\mathcal{A}}[S](\lambda_1 \mathbf{u}) \leq \Delta_{\mathcal{A}}[S](\lambda_2 \mathbf{u}). \tag{10}$$

Hence, $\Delta_{\mathcal{A}}[S](\mathbf{u})$ is a robust similarity metric for 2D or 3D data registration.

2.3   Video-CT Registration

Bronchoscopic navigation requires an accurate video-CT registration procedure with a robust similarity function. The HWD-based similarity function (Eq. 7) can enhance the 2D-3D registration procedure. Therefore, our similarity function $\mathcal{S}_{\mathcal{M}}$ between the classified real image $\mathcal{I}_i^R$ and virtual image $\mathcal{I}^v$ is defined as

$$\mathcal{S}_{\mathcal{M}}\left(\mathcal{I}_i^R,\mathcal{I}^v(\mathbf{Q}_i)\right) = \|\mathcal{I}_i^R - \mathcal{I}^v(\mathbf{Q}_i)\|_{\mathcal{A}}^2 = \max_{\mathbf{v}\in\{-1,1\}^2}\left\{\sup \mathcal{G}_{\mathcal{I}_i^R-\mathcal{I}^v(\mathbf{Q}_i)}^{\mathbf{v}}\right\}, \quad (11)$$

where $\mathbf{Q}_i$ is a six-dimensional vector to describe the position and orientation (three Euler angles) of the bronchoscope along the $x-$, $y-$, and $z-$axis in the 3D CT image space and $\mathcal{A}$ is a set of patches divided from the real image $\mathcal{I}_i^R$.

Finally, bronchoscopic navigation (i.e., continuously estimate the position and orientation of the bronchoscope) can be formulated an deterministic optimization procedure to search for the optimal estimate $\tilde{\mathbf{Q}}_i$ by maximizing the similarity $\mathcal{S}_{\mathcal{M}}\left(\mathcal{I}_i^R,\mathcal{I}^v(\mathbf{Q}_i)\right)$ between $\mathcal{I}_i^R$ at frame i and $\mathcal{I}^v$ with respect to $\mathbf{Q}_i$

$$\tilde{\mathbf{Q}}_i = arg \max_{\mathbf{Q}_i} \mathcal{S}_{\mathcal{M}}\left(\mathcal{I}_i^R,\mathcal{I}^v(\mathbf{Q}_i)\right), \quad (12)$$

which is solved by the Levenberg-Marquardt method in our implementation [12].

3   Validation

Bronchoscopic video images generally contain three main categories: (1) uninformative images shown in Fig. 1(a), (2) inter-bronchus images with or without folds, e.g., the left two images in Fig. 1(b), and (3) intra-bronchus images, e.g., the right two images in Fig. 1(b). We tested five datasets (three of them for training) in MIL. Each dataset includes bronchoscopic images more than 800 frames. We manually collect 100 images for each category from three videos to train the MIL boosting classifier. Each image was divided into 10 instances (Harr-like features were extracted), i.e., the set $\mathcal{A}$ contains 10 patches.

We compare several image-based methods in this work: (1) MoMSE: a modified mean squared error based method [1], (2) NMI: a normalized mutual information based method, (3) HWD: only HWD based navigation, (4) MIL+HWD: our method discussed in Sect. 2. We evaluate these methods on these five datasets with bronchoscopic video images and their corresponding CT slices. Three experts used a typical software to manually generate ground truth datasets, respectively, and their average was used as the final ground truth.

4   Results

Table 1 quantifies the navigation accuracy of the compared methods. The average position and orientation errors of our method were 3.5 mm and 9.4°, which are much better than those of the previous published methods that had average

Table 1. The navigation accuracy of the compared methods by computing the position and orientation errors between the estimates and ground truth

Datasets	MoMSE	NMI	HWD	MIL+HWD
Case A	28.8 ± 20.3 mm	17.7 ± 13.3 mm	13.5 ± 13.2 mm	6.8 ± 7.5 mm
	$30.6 \pm 29.2°$	$31.2 \pm 20.3°$	$28.8 \pm 16.5°$	$8.8 \pm 7.6°$
Case B	7.2 ± 6.5 mm	8.0 ± 6.5 mm	5.2 ± 3.2 mm	1.8 ± 0.8 mm
	$22.8 \pm 20.3°$	$17.4 \pm 14.5°$	$15.6 \pm 13.5°$	$3.8 \pm 1.2°$
Case C	4.5 ± 3.2 mm	6.9 ± 5.2 mm	4.2 ± 2.8 mm	3.6 ± 2.2 mm
	$11.5 \pm 6.6°$	$11.9 \pm 8.5°$	$10.3 \pm 5.6°$	$7.8 \pm 5.2°$
Case D	14.8 ± 12.2 mm	10.3 ± 10.3 mm	6.3 ± 8.5 mm	3.2 ± 2.8 mm
	$38.6 \pm 26.8°$	$23.9 \pm 27.6°$	$18.9 \pm 20.8°$	$14.0 \pm 12.8°$
Case E	12.6 ± 8.8 mm	7.7 ± 5.8 mm	4.8 ± 4.2 mm	2.0 ± 3.2 mm
	$21.6 \pm 17.5°$	$18.7 \pm 16.4°$	$16.4 \pm 12.5°$	$12.4 \pm 22.5°$
Average	13.6 ± 10.2 mm	10.1 ± 8.2 mm	6.8 ± 6.4 mm	3.5 ± 3.3 mm
	$25.0 \pm 20.1°$	$20.6 \pm 17.5°$	$18.0 \pm 13.8°$	$9.4 \pm 9.9°$

errors of at least 6.8 mm and 18.0°. We also manually and visually inspect the tracked results generated the virtual images if they resemble bronchoscopic real images. Table 2 shows the successfully tracked frames in terms of visual inspection, which also demonstrates the effectiveness of our method.

Figure 3 displays examples of the bronchosocpic real images and corresponding virtual images generated from the tracked results from the different methods. While Fig. 3 demonstrates the robustness of HWD working well on severe image artifacts, it also shows that MIL+HWD outperforms HWD. Based on our experimental results, while MIL+HWD and HWD have quite similar results on clear views, MIL+HWD generally works better than HWD on problematic views. Also note that the average accuracy of MIL-based uninformative image classification was about 87% of the experimental bronchoscopic images. Our future work will further improve the accuracy of bronchoscopic uninformative image classification by introducing deep learning convolutional neural networks such as VGG16[1].

Additionally, the current processing time of our proposed method is about 0.4 seconds per frame without any acceleration devices (e.g., GPU) or code optimization, all of which can speed our method up to real-time requirement.

5   Discussion

This work aims to deal with bronchoscopic image uncertainties and develop a robust video-CT registration method to enhance image-based bronchoscopic navigation. Several interesting aspects of this work are clarified in the following.

---

[1] https://neurohive.io/en/popular-networks/vgg16/.

Table 2. A quantitative comparison of the number and percentage of the bronchoscopic images tracked successfully by the different methods

Datasets	MoMSE	NMI	HWD	MIL+HWD
Case A	55.9%	61.0%	70%	79.1%
(1600)	(875)	(976)	(1030)	(1185)
Case B	52.0%	50.8%	78.2%	87.3%
(1220)	(634)	(620)	(954	(1065)
Case C	59.8%	53.7%	69.9%	78.9%
(1306)	(781)	(701)	(913)	(1031)
Case D	59.0%	63.3%	68.8%	73.0%
(1675)	(988)	(1060)	(1152)	(1223)
Case E	52.3%	71.7%	74.7%	88.5%
(850)	(446)	(609)	(635)	(752)
Total	56.0%	59.6%	69.9%	79.1%
(6651)	(3724)	(3966)	(4654)	(5256)

First, the MIL-based classifiers are employed to remove image artifacts before the video-CT registration to improve the performance of bronchoscopic navigation. By classifying and discarding bronchoscopic video images with artifacts, the optimizer avoids getting trapped in a local minima in the registration procedure. Next, a robust similarity metric on the basis of Hermann Weyl's discrepancy was proposed for 2D-3D registration. HWD is an unique function that simultaneously satisfies positive definiteness and monotonicity in general optimization environments. In particular, the monotonicity of HWD leads to converge only one optimal solution during optimization. In addition, we believe that such a HWD-based similarity metric is also applicable to computer aided diagnosis.

Although our method works well for bronchoscopic navigation, it still fails to track all the video frames. The proposed method has several limitations. First, MIL possibly fails to classify uninformative images, resulting in incorrect registration. It is also difficult to properly determine the number of patches on the bronchosocpic image in MIL. Deep learning-based image classification methods are a promising way to classify uninformative bronchoscopic video images. Next, one hard assumption is that CT-driven virtual rendering images can be always generated to correspond to any real bronchoscopic video images, i.e., the CT-derived anatomical model can fully reconstruct the bronchial tree. Unfortunately, the bronchial tree is not well reproduced in the virtual images due to the low resolution of the CT images. Additionally, while patients are usually asked to fully inhale or exhale and hold their breath during the CT scanning, they are breathing and deforming regularly during bronchoscopy. In general, these limitations remain challenging to robust video-CT registration that still gets trapped in a local minima during image-based bronchoscopic navigation.

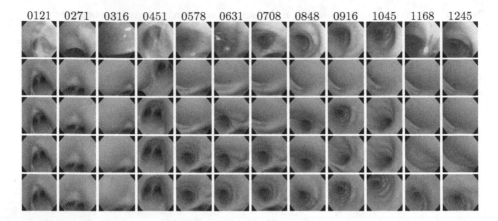

Fig. 3. Visual comparison of the navigation results of Case C. The first row shows selected frame numbers and the second row their corresponding real images. The third to sixth rows display the virtual images generated from the pose estimates of using the methods of MoMSE, NMI, HWD, and MIL+HWD, respectively. Our proposed MIL+hwd approach shows the best performance.

6   Conclusion

This paper proposes a new bronchoscopic navigation strategy that employs multiple instance learning and develops a robust similarity metric on the basis of Hermann Weyl's discrepancy to boost the video-CT registration procedure. We seek to solve the problems of bronchoscopic image uncertainties and inaccurate characterization of the similarity between the bronchoscopic real and CT-based virtual rendering images during navigated bronchoscopy. With the MIL-based uninformative image removal and HWD-based similarity function, our method evaluated on patient datasets was demonstrated to be more effective and accurate than other approaches, especially the average navigation accuracy of position and orientation was improved from (6.8, 18.0) to (3.5 mm, 9.4°).

Acknowledgment. This work was partly supported by the Fundamental Research Funds for the Central Universities (No. 20720180062) and National Natural Science Foundation of China (No. 61971367).

References

1. Deguchi, D., et al.: Selective image similarity measure for bronchoscope tracking based on image registration. MedIA **13**(4), 621–633 (2009)
2. Soper, T.D., Haynor, D.R., Glenny, R.W., Seibel, E.J.: In vivo validation of a hybrid tracking system for navigation of an ultrathin bronchoscope within peripheral airways. IEEE TBME **57**(3), 736–745 (2010)
3. Luo, X., Feuerstein, M., Deguchi, D., Kitasaka, T., Takabatake, H., Mori, K.: Development and comparison of new hybrid motion tracking for bronchoscopic navigation. MedIA **16**(3), 577–596 (2012)

4. Luo, X., Wan, Y., He, X., Mori, K.: Observation-driven adaptive differential evolution and its application to accurate and smooth bronchoscope three-dimensional motion tracking. MedIA **24**(1), 282–296 (2015)
5. Hofstad, E.F., et al.: Intraoperative localized constrained registration in navigated bronchoscopy. Med. Phys. **44**(8), 4204–4212 (2017)
6. Shen, M., Giannarou, S., Shah, P.L., Yang, G.-Z.: BRANCH: bifurcation recognition for airway navigation based on structural characteristics. In: Descoteaux, M., Maier-Hein, L., Franz, A., Jannin, P., Collins, D.L., Duchesne, S. (eds.) MICCAI 2017. LNCS, vol. 10434, pp. 182–189. Springer, Cham (2017). https://doi.org/10.1007/978-3-319-66185-8_21
7. Byrnes, P.D., Higgins, W.E.: Efficient bronchoscopic video summarization. IEEE TBME **66**(3), 848–863 (2018)
8. Babenko, B., Yang, M.-H., Belongie, S.: Robust object tracking with online multiple instance learning. IEEE TPAMI **33**(8), 1619–1632 (2011)
9. Moser, B.A.: A similarity measure for image and volumetric data based on Hermann Weyl's discrepancy. IEEE TPAMI **33**(11), 2321–2329 (2011)
10. Maron, O., Ratan, A.L.: Multiple-instance learning for natural scene classification. Proc. ICML **1998**, 341–349 (1998)
11. Viola, P., Platt, J.C., Zhang, C.: Multiple instance boosting for object detection. Proc. NIPS **2005**, 1417–1426 (2005)
12. Gavin H.: The Levenberg-Marquardt method for nonlinear least squares curve-fitting problems. Technical report, Duke University, USA (2011)

Learning Where to Look While Tracking Instruments in Robot-Assisted Surgery

Mobarakol Islam[1,2], Yueyuan Li[2,3], and Hongliang Ren[2(✉)]

[1] NUS Graduate School for Integrative Sciences and Engineering (NGS),
National University of Singapore, Singapore, Singapore
[2] Department of Biomedical Engineering, National University of Singapore,
Singapore, Singapore
`mobarakol@u.nus.edu, ren@nus.edu.sg`
[3] University of Michigan-Joint Institute, Shanghai Jiao Tong University,
Shanghai, China
`rowena_lee@sjtu.edu.cn`

Abstract. Directing of the task-specific attention while tracking instrument in surgery holds great potential in robot-assisted intervention. For this purpose, we propose an end-to-end trainable multitask learning (MTL) model for real-time surgical instrument segmentation and attention prediction. Our model is designed with a weight-shared encoder and two task-oriented decoders and optimized for the joint tasks. We introduce batch-Wasserstein (bW) loss and construct a soft attention module to refine the distinctive visual region for efficient saliency learning. For multitask optimization, it is always challenging to obtain convergence of both tasks in the same epoch. We deal with this problem by adopting 'poly' loss weight and two phases of training. We further propose a novel way to generate task-aware saliency map and scanpath of the instruments on MICCAI robotic instrument segmentation dataset. Compared to the state of the art segmentation and saliency models, our model outperforms most of the evaluation metrics.

1 Introduction

Robot-assisted minimally invasive surgery (RMIS) has a variety of advantages such as higher surgeon dexterity, enhanced patient safety and shorter stay period. Moreover, 3D visualization and remote control option on systems such as Da Vinci Xi robot [13] enable operating precision with depth perception. However, there remain challenges in image cognition because surgeries take place in a complicated environment with shadows, specular reflection, partial occlusion, and body fluid. Therefore, real-time instruments tracking and segmentation can enhance the context awareness of surgeons and provides extensive control in intervention. In robotic surgery, it is further expected the system to identify and

This work supported by the Singapore Academic Research Fund under Grant R-397-000-297-114 and NMRC Bedside & Bench under grant R-397-000-245-511.

locate the most important instrument and process it with autofocusing priority as human visual perception.

Recently, the convolutional neural network (CNN) has been extensively utilized in semantic image segmentation and tracking. There several works on surgical tool detection, segmentation and pose estimation. Most of the approaches [1,2,6,7,18] deploy tracking by segmentation as it is faster and accurate localization. Other models [3,20] use tracking by detection technique. However, the inference time of the detection is higher and the rectangular box is unable to define the exact shape of the instrument.

Saliency map is worthy of more attention in surgical instrument segmentation. Incorporating attention with segmentation enable the model to direct where to focus and which order. The recent works on visual attention including SalGAN [15], DSCLRCN [10] utilize combined loss function of binary cross entropy (BCE) and adversarial loss to predict attention map. However, most of the saliency model predict natural visual attention. A task-specific saliency approach commenced in the field autonomous driving [14], but the application in image-guided robotic surgery is still lack of development. In addition, although some efforts to embed segmentation into multitask learning (MTL) has been made [4,12], the parallel processing of segmentation and attention remains a problem. Therefore, our motivation in this paper is to prove the feasibility of proceeding learning in multitasks, segmentation and scan path prediction, on real-time surgical images.

Our contributions are summarized as follows:

- We propose an MTL model with a weight-shared encoder and dual task-aware decoders.
- We introduce a batch Wasserstein loss to extract the dissimilarity between ground truth and prediction saliency with lower time-cost. We also adopt two phases of learning for multitask optimization.
- Our model has a novel design of decoders, attention module, and boundary refinement module which boost up the model performance.
- We come up with an innovative way to generate task-oriented saliency map and scanpath based on MICCAI robotic instrument segmentation dataset [1] to get the priority of focus on surgical instruments. Our model achieves impressive results and surpasses the existing state-of-the-art model with the dice accuracy of 94.3%, 66.9% for binary and type segmentation and AUC of saliency is 92.9% with the speed of 127 frames per second (FPS).

2   Proposed Approach

We propose an MTL model using a shared encoder and two task-specific decoders. We introduce batch Wasserstein loss for the saliency task optimization. To get real-time performance, we design light and efficient decoder with attention module (AM), Boundary Refinement (BR) module and spatial and channel "Squeeze & Excitation" (scSE) [17].

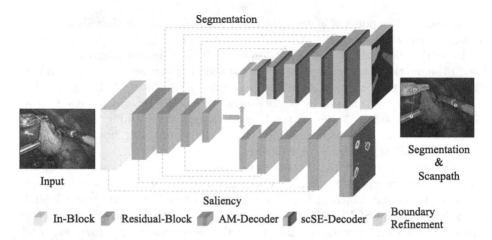

Fig. 1. Our proposed MTL model. It has shared encoder and task-oriented decoders for the segmentation and saliency prediction.

2.1   Attention Module (AM)

We design a light attention module to suppress irrelevant regions and emphasize salient features. It contains global pooling layer followed by convolution block and sigmoid layer to extract the global features and multiplies with original input to refine the feature maps (as shown in Fig. 2c). The size of all the filters in this module consider 1 to reduce computational cost.

2.2   AM Decoder

Decoder with attention module (AM) is designed to recover the saliency map from lower dimensional feature maps. Decoder forms with 3 blocks of convolution (conv), deconvolution (deconv) and convolution followed by batch-normalization (BN) and ReLU layers (see Fig. 2d). It fuses low-level feature from corresponding encoder block to capture the fine-grained information distorted by convolution and pooling. AM block helps to filter the attentive features from decoder feature maps.

2.3   scSE Decoder

Decoder with scSE module builds to retrieve the feature maps for segmentation from low-resolution encoder feature maps. It consists of Concatenation, conv (3×3), Inplace Adaptive BN (ABN) and deconv (4×4) as shown in Fig. 2a. In a decoder, scSE unit alternates the direction of the feature maps and signify the meaningful features.

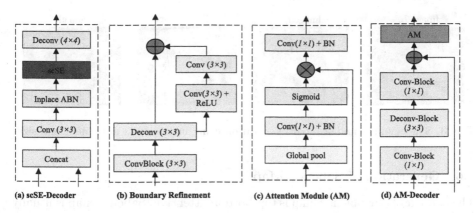

Fig. 2. Proposed modules such as (a) scSE-decoder, (b) Boundary refinement (BR), (c) Attention module, (d) AM-decoder

2.4   Network Architecture

Our multitask model forms of the shared encoder and task-oriented decoders as illustrated in Fig. 1. The encoder forms of In-Block and light-weight residual block of Resnet18. In-Block consists of conv-block (conv-bn-relu) followed by pooling layer. Feature maps of the encoder are used in task-specific decoders such as scSE-decoder and AM-decoder for segmentation and saliency prediction respectively. Boundary refinement module builds of residual structure (Fig. 2b) is used to predict and refine the segmentation score maps. LogSoftmax and Sigmoid layers are used to predict final segmentation and saliency maps.

2.5   Loss Function

We design a loss function for the saliency optimization using *Wasserstein distance* [5]. It calculates the dissimilarity for the probability distribution. To reduce computation cost, we design batch-Wasserstein loss (L_{bW}) which squeezes a batch into a vector instead of the individual image for measurement. The ground-truth and prediction maps are down-sample to half to improve to efficiency. Finally, we combine the binary cross entropy (L_{bce}) loss and batch-Wasserstein loss (L_{bW}) with weight factor of α ($\alpha = 0.3$ after tuning). Therefore, the fused loss function for the saliency can be written as $\mathcal{L}_{sal} = \alpha L_{bW} + (1 - \alpha)L_{bce}$.

The total loss is made up of two parts, the cross-entropy loss for segmentation and the fused saliency loss for saliency prediction. Because two different loss functions are merged together, a dynamically adjusted weight λ has to be assigned to the final loss function [12].

$$\mathcal{L}_{total} = \lambda_{seg}\mathcal{L}_{seg} + \lambda_{sal}\mathcal{L}_{sal} \tag{1}$$

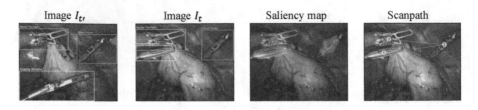

| Image $I_{t'}$ | Image I_t | Saliency map | Scanpath |

Fig. 3. Saliency map and scanpath generation using instruments movement and size

2.6   Generation of Saliency Map

The context of our saliency map is top-bottom attention. Saliency map is usually generated from fixation map which is manually annotated by eye tracker [9] or mouse click [8]. We simulate the clicking process by locating fixation points only in the wrist and clasper parts of instruments. A temporal weight of every instrument is assigned based on the movement and formulated by deformation and displacement. The movement of the instrument part is assumed to be a Markov process. Then for attention map of image I_t, only one previous image $I_{t'}(t' = t - \Delta t)$ would be taken as reference (see Fig. 3. Denote the size of this part i at time t, t' as s_{it}, $s_{it'}$. The deformation μ_i is defined as $\max\{s_{it}, s_{it'}\}/\min\{s_{it}, s_{it'}\}$. λ_{de} and λ_{di} are the weights of the deformation and displacement ($\lambda_{de} = 0.5$, $\lambda_{di} = 0.5$). The displacement d_i is the Euclidean distance between the centers of part i at t and t'. The weight w_i is obtained by merging these two variables after normalization and weighted.

$$w_i = \lambda_{\text{de}} \frac{\mu_i}{\min\{\mu_1, \mu_2, \dots\}} + \lambda_{\text{di}} \log\left(\frac{2d_i}{\min\{d_1, d_2, \dots\}}\right) \tag{2}$$

3   Experiments

3.1   Dataset

We use the robotic instrument segmentation dataset [1] to conduct all the experiments. There are in total eight types of da Vinci's surgical instruments whose names are *Large Needle Driver, Prograsp Forceps, Monopolar Curved Scissors, Vessel Sealer, Fenestrated Bipolar Forceps and Grasping Retractor*. We take six sequences (1, 2, 3, 5, 6, 8) for training and the rest for testing. The ground truth of the saliency map is generated according to the method mentioned in Sect. 2.6.

3.2   Implementation Details

Optimizing a multitask learning (MTL) model is always challenging as it has to converge two tasks with different loss functions. We observe that the best model for each task is in different epochs. Therefore, we propose multi-phase learning for our model. In phase I, we assign the loss factors to 1 for both saliency and

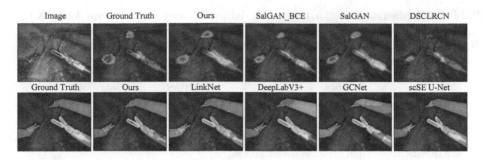

Fig. 4. Input, ground truth annotations, saliency map and type segmentation generated by our model and other models of the same image are shown.

segmentation as in Eq. 1. In phase II, we fine-tune the earliest converged model for a task by emphasizing the loss of the remaining task. To do this, we reduce the loss factor (λ_{seg} or λ_{sal}) of the converged task by using 'poly' learning rate policy [11].

$$\lambda_{\text{seg}} \text{ or } \lambda_{\text{sal}} = (1 - \frac{iter}{max\_iter})^{power} \tag{3}$$

For other hyper-parameters, we use Adam optimizer with an initial learning rate 0.001 and 'poly' learning rate with the power of 0.9 to update it. The momentum and weight decay set constant to 0.99 and 10^{-4} respectively. We implement the proposed model in Python and Pytorch. All the experiments are conducted with three Nvidia GTX 1080 Ti GPUs.

3.3 Results

Quantitative Result. As is shown in Table 1, we take four evaluation metrics for saliency map and two for segmentation. Our model achieves the best performance in saliency metrics of BCE, NSS, and AUC-B. It has the highest dice in type segmentation and highest dice and Hausdorff distance in binary segmentation. SalGAN and DeepLabV3+ have the competitive results, but they are for single task. TernausNet11 achieves the best performance in FPS, but as a multitask network, the efficiency of our model is already high enough for real-time guidance.

Qualitative Results. The visualized comparison of different models is shown in Fig. 4. Obviously, our saliency map has the most similar distribution to ground truth and our type segmentation has the smallest false positive area. Figure 5a shows that our prediction of binary segmentation is more similar to ground truth with dice accuracy of 94.3%. Figure 5b shows that our model is competitive in scanpath prediction as it is better than SalGAN [15] models.

Table 1. Evaluation score for the testing dataset. Binary cross entropy loss (BCE), similarity (Sim.), normalized scan path saliency (NSS), area under curve-Borji (AUC-B), dice and Hausdorff distance (Hausd.). The best values of each metric are boldened. The values better than ours are underlined.

Model	Saliency				Type Seg.		Binary Seg.		
	BCE ↓	Sim ↑	NSS ↑	AUC-B ↑	Dice ↑	Hausd ↓	Dice ↑	Hausd ↓	FPS ↑
†Ours	**0.056**	0.571	**4.04**	**0.929**	**0.669**	10.96	**0.943**	**10.12**	127
SalGAN_BCE	0.071	0.534	3.86	0.846	-	-	-	-	<u>233</u>
SalGAN [15]	0.064	0.508	3.62	0.883	-	-	-	-	-
DSCLRCN [10]	0.220	**0.582**	4.02	0.830	-	-	-	-	-
LinkNet	-	-	-	-	0.532	13.24	0.919	10.83	<u>177</u>
DUpsampling [19]	-	-	-	-	0.510	13.43	0.847	13.52	126
ERFNet	-	-	-	-	0.522	12.36	0.901	11.78	121
DeepLabV3+	-	-	-	-	0.660	11.01	0.924	10.94	58
MobileNetV2	-	-	-	-	0.475	16.71	0.864	12.88	51
Peng et al. [16]	-	-	-	-	0.601	12.28	0.932	10.89	105
scSE U-Net	-	-	-	-	0.520	**10.80**	0.922	10.92	<u>131</u>
TernausNet11	-	-	-	-	0.430	11.79	0.904	11.45	**351**
BiSeNet	-	-	-	-	0.482	12.28	0.920	10.99	60

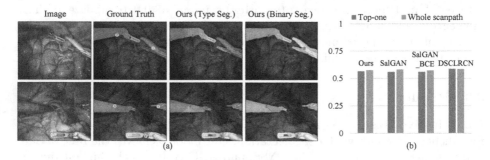

Fig. 5. (a) Visualization of type and binary segmentation. (b) Diagram of the accuracy of the top-one scanpath and whole scanpath prediction.

4 Discussion and Conclusion

In this work, we present a real-time multitask learning model to predict segmentation and scanpath of the surgical instruments during surgery. We introduce and generate task-oriented attention guidance to train the system where to look during robotic surgery. We propose batch-Wasserstein loss, a novel loss function for the saliency prediction. Our model can train end-to-end and optimize for both problems with shared encoder and task-specific decoders. There are still scopes to improve the model with temporal information as scanpath depends on the instrument movement of the consecutive frames. Nonetheless, the extensive evaluation of our model demonstrates the efficiency and stability in real-time robotic surgery.

References

1. Allan, M., et al.: 2017 robotic instrument segmentation challenge. arXiv preprint arXiv:1902.06426 (2019)
2. Chaurasia, A., Culurciello, E.: LinkNet: exploiting encoder representations for efficient semantic segmentation. In: 2017 IEEE Visual Communications and Image Processing (VCIP), pp. 1–4. IEEE (2017)
3. Chen, Z., Zhao, Z., Cheng, X.: Surgical instruments tracking based on deep learning with lines detection and spatio-temporal context. In: 2017 Chinese Automation Congress (CAC), pp. 2711–2714. IEEE (2017)
4. Dvornik, N., Shmelkov, K., Mairal, J., Schmid, C.: BlitzNet: a real-time deep network for scene understanding. In: Proceedings of the IEEE International Conference on Computer Vision, pp. 4154–4162 (2017)
5. Frogner, C., Zhang, C., Mobahi, H., Araya, M., Poggio, T.A.: Learning with a Wasserstein loss. In: Advances in Neural Information Processing Systems, pp. 2053–2061 (2015)
6. García-Peraza-Herrera, L.C., et al.: ToolNet: holistically-nested real-time segmentation of robotic surgical tools. In: 2017 IEEE/RSJ International Conference on Intelligent Robots and Systems (IROS), pp. 5717–5722. IEEE (2017)
7. Islam, M., Atputharuban, D.A., Ramesh, R., Ren, H.: Real-time instrument segmentation in robotic surgery using auxiliary supervised deep adversarial learning. IEEE Robot. Autom. Lett. 4, 2188–2195 (2019)
8. Jiang, M., Huang, S., Duan, J., Zhao, Q.: SALICON: saliency in context. In: Proceedings of the IEEE Conference on Computer Vision and Pattern Recognition, pp. 1072–1080 (2015)
9. Judd, T., Ehinger, K., Durand, F., Torralba, A.: Learning to predict where humans look. In: 2009 IEEE 12th International Conference on Computer Vision, pp. 2106–2113. IEEE (2009)
10. Liu, N., Han, J.: A deep spatial contextual long-term recurrent convolutional network for saliency detection. IEEE Trans. Image Process. 27(7), 3264–3274 (2018)
11. Liu, W., Rabinovich, A., Berg, A.C.: ParseNet: looking wider to see better. arXiv preprint arXiv:1506.04579 (2015)
12. Nekrasov, V., Dharmasiri, T., Spek, A., Drummond, T., Shen, C., Reid, I.: Real-time joint semantic segmentation and depth estimation using asymmetric annotations. arXiv preprint arXiv:1809.04766 (2018)
13. Ngu, J.C.Y., Tsang, C.B.S., Koh, D.C.S.: The da Vinci Xi: a review of its capabilities, versatility, and potential role in robotic colorectal surgery. Robot. Surg.: Res. Rev. 4, 77–85 (2017)
14. Palazzi, A., Abati, D., Calderara, S., Solera, F., Cucchiara, R.: Predictingthe driver's focus of attention: the DR (eye) VE project. IEEE Trans. Pattern Anal. Mach. Intell. 41, 1720–1733 (2018)
15. Pan, J., et al.: SalGAN: visual saliency prediction with generative adversarial networks. arXiv preprint arXiv:1701.01081 (2017)
16. Peng, C., Zhang, X., Yu, G., Luo, G., Sun, J.: Large kernel matters-improve semantic segmentation by global convolutional network. In: Proceedings of the IEEE Conference On Computer Vision and Pattern Recognition, pp. 4353–4361 (2017)

17. Roy, A.G., Navab, N., Wachinger, C.: Concurrent spatial and channel 'squeeze & excitation' in fully convolutional networks. In: Frangi, A., Schnabel, J., Davatzikos, C., Alberola-López, C., Fichtinger, G. (eds.) MICCAI 2018. LNCS, vol. 11070, pp. 421–429. Springer, Cham (2018). https://doi.org/10.1007/978-3-030-00928-1_48
18. Shvets, A.A., Rakhlin, A., Kalinin, A.A., Iglovikov, V.I.: Automatic instrument segmentation in robot-assisted surgery using deep learning. In: 2018 17th IEEE International Conference on Machine Learning and Applications (ICMLA), pp. 624–628. IEEE (2018)
19. Tian, Z., Shen, C., He, T., Yan, Y.: Decoders matter for semantic segmentation: data-dependent decoding enables flexible feature aggregation. arXiv preprint arXiv:1903.02120 (2019)
20. Zhao, Z., Voros, S., Weng, Y., Chang, F., Li, R.: Tracking-by-detection of surgical instruments in minimally invasive surgery via the convolutional neural network deep learning-based method. Comput. Assist. Surg. **22**(sup1), 26–35 (2017)

Efficient Soft-Constrained Clustering for Group-Based Labeling

Ryoma Bise[1(✉)], Kentaro Abe[1], Hideaki Hayashi[1], Kiyohito Tanaka[2], and Seiichi Uchida[1]

[1] Kyushu University, Fukuoka City, Japan
bise@ait.kyushu-u.ac.jp
[2] Kyoto Second Red Cross Hospital, Kyoto, Japan

Abstract. We propose a soft-constrained clustering method for group-based labeling of medical images. Since the idea of group-based labeling is to attach the label to a group of samples at once, we need to have groups (i.e., clusters) with high purity. The proposed method is formulated to achieve high purity even for difficult clustering tasks such as medical image clustering, where image samples of the same class are often very distant in their feature space. In fact, those images degrade the performance of conventional constrained clustering methods. Experiments with an endoscopy image dataset demonstrated that our method outperformed various state-of-the-art methods.

1 Introduction

Collecting a large number of labeled images as training data is required in machine learning classification tasks because deep neural networks require sufficient training data to learn discriminative features for robust classification. In general object image recognition tasks, crowdsourcing services (e.g., Amazon MechanicalTurk) have been widely used for labeling images efficiently and quickly by using workers from all over the world. However, we cannot use such services for medical images because most annotators of the services cannot attach appropriate labels due to a lack of biomedical knowledge. Considering the large diversity of recent classification tasks of medical images, there is a huge demand for systems that reduce the labeling effort.

To label data efficiently, several *group-based labeling* methods [1–3] have been proposed, where the data is first clustered and then the images of each cluster are labeled by an expert, as shown in Fig. 1(a). If the purity of each cluster is high enough (i.e., if each cluster is mostly comprised of the images from the same class), group-based labeling is far more effective than instance-based (i.e., one-by-one) labeling. Imagine a situation that all images of a cluster are listed in a file viewer and an expert observes them. If the expert finds that all of them belong to the same class, she/he can attach the same label to them at once. Even when a cluster contains a small number of images from different classes, it is still easy to find and exclude them before labeling; this is because those images will be *visually salient* in the list.

D. Shen et al. (Eds.): MICCAI 2019, LNCS 11768, pp. 421–430, 2019.
https://doi.org/10.1007/978-3-030-32254-0_47

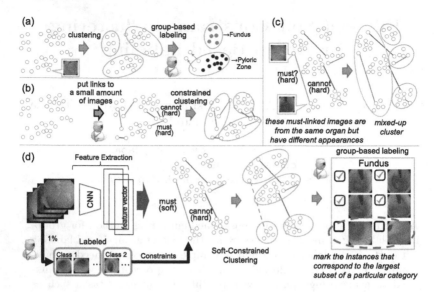

Fig. 1. (a) Group-based labeling with clustering. (b) Hard-constrained clustering. (c) An unexpected result by hard-constrained clustering; the middle of the mixed-up cluster is better to belong to another cluster. (d) The proposed soft-constrained clustering for group-based labeling.

In order to increase the purity of each cluster for higher efficiency of group-based labeling, *constrained clustering*, such as [4,5], is a reasonable choice. As shown in Fig. 1(b), an expert selects a small number of samples from the dataset and put links to them before clustering. If a pair of two samples must (cannot) belong to the same cluster, they are linked by a must-link (cannot-link). Then a clustering is performed while satisfying the constraints indicated by the links. A small effort of putting the links will greatly help to increase the purity of the resulting clusters.

If a class is unimodal and thus the samples belong to the class can be grouped by a single cluster, the conventional constrained clustering will work well without any side-effect; however, if a class is not unimodal, the must-link constraints may adversely affect clustering. As shown in Fig. 1(c), a must-link for distant samples causes a mixed-up cluster in order to satisfy the constraint by the must-link. Such an undesired must-link is not avoidable, especially for medical image applications. The appearance of a medical image often changes even in the same class due to huge appearance variations, different shooting angles, etc., and the class distribution often becomes multimodal whose components are distant to each other.

In this paper, we propose a novel soft-constrained clustering method for medical image labeling tasks. Different from the conventional constrained clustering methods, we allow the violation of must-link constraints to deal with the classes with multimodal (scattered) distributions, as shown in Fig. 1(d). Specifically, must-links are evaluated as penalties while cannot-links are still treated as hard constraints. In addition, the proposed method is formulated as a single optimization problem, whereas the conventional soft-constrained clustering methods first solve the hard-constrained problem and then modify the cluster assignment. We have evaluated the performance of the proposed method in the task to put 20 labels to about 12,000 endoscopic images collected from several hospitals. Specifically, the proposed method achieved higher performance measurements (purity and recall of the clusters) than state-of-the-art clustering methods under different numbers of clusters and rates of links (i.e, constraints).

2   Related Work

The most famous constrained clustering method is COP-Kmeans [4], which modifies the assignment step of K-means to satisfy must/cannot-link constraints. It performs hard-constrained clustering and thus is not suitable for medical images. Soft-constraint clustering methods, such as CVQE [6] and LCVQE [7] have been proposed to relax the hard constraints to a penalty evaluation. For example, CVQE penalizes violation of must-link constraints by adding a penalty of the distance between the two nearest cluster centers of these two points. LCVQE improves the computational costs by modifying the penalty term in the objective function of CVQE. Similar to these methods, PCK-means [8] and MPCK-means [9] methods design the penalty function as 0/1-Loss. Those soft-constrained clustering algorithms first solve the hard-constrained problem and then update the cluster assignment of each sample. This two-step organization is reasonable for discarding a small number of erroneous constraints but not for dealing with multimodal distributions; this is because as shown in Fig. 1(c) the must-links under multimodal distributions may disturb the first step. Recently, Le et al. [5] proposed a Binary Optimization for Constrained K-means (BOCK) where the optimization problem formulated as a single binary linear programming problem. Although it uses not a two-step formulation, it performs hard-constrained clustering and thus is not suitable for medical images.

Our soft-constrained clustering method is formulated as a single optimization problem while dealing with the must-constraints in a penalty term. As shown in the later experimental result, this formulation is very suitable for medical image labeling tasks because the multimodal distribution of medical images will give many undesired must-links and thus the typical two-step optimization will fail. To the authors' best knowledge, any soft-constrained clustering method like ours has been neither proposed nor applied to medical images.

3   Efficient Labeling

Figure 1(d) shows the overview of our labeling scheme including the proposed clustering method. In this scheme, features are first extracted for each image by DenseNet [10] pre-trained by ImageNet.[1] An expert attaches labels to a very few

---

[1] We selected one of the most famous networks as a feature representation network.

samples (1%). From the attached label, must-link and cannot-link constraints are defined; must-link (cannot-link) for a pair of samples from the same class (different classes). Next, the proposed soft-constrained clustering method is applied by using the must-link as a penalty and the cannot-link as a hard constraint. Then, the images in the "prominent" cluster, which contains the most labeled samples among all clusters, is shown to an expert and the expert attaches the labels to all samples. If the cluster only contains samples from the same class, the expert can attach the same class label to them at once. Even if the cluster contains several samples from different classes, the expert can do the same just after discarded those samples. The remaining samples (the discarded samples and the samples in other clusters) are fed to the clustering at the next round. Finally, this process is repeated until all samples have been labeled.

4 Soft-Constrained Clustering

4.1 Problem Setting

The formulation of our soft-constrained clustering method can be started from that of the K-means clustering. Given N samples $\mathcal{X} = \{\boldsymbol{x}_j \in \mathbb{R}^D\}_{j=1}^N$, where D is the dimension of the feature vector, the goal of K-Means is to find a set $\mathcal{C}$ containing K cluster's centroids $\mathcal{C} = \{\boldsymbol{c}_i \in \mathbb{R}^D\}_{i=1}^K$ and assign each sample $\boldsymbol{x}_j$ to one of non-overlapping clusters. The optimal clustering minimizes the within cluster sum of squares (WCSS). According to [5], it is formulated as:

$$\min_{\mathbf{C},\mathbf{S}} \|\mathbf{X} - \mathbf{SC}\|_F^2, \quad \text{s.t. } s_{ij} \in \{0,1\} \ \forall i,j, \quad \sum_{i=1}^K s_{ij} = 1 \ \forall j = 1,\dots,N, \quad (1)$$

where $\mathbf{X} \in \mathbb{R}^{D \times N}$ is the matrix whose the j-th column corresponds to $\boldsymbol{x}_j \in \mathbb{R}^D$, and $\mathbf{C} \in \mathbb{R}^{D \times K}$ is a cluster centroid matrix whose i-th column corresponds to the centroid $\boldsymbol{c}_i$. $\mathbf{S} \in \mathbb{R}^{K \times N}$ is a cluster assignment matrix, where its (i,j)-th element s_{ij} has the value of 1 if the sample $\boldsymbol{x}_i$ is assigned to the j-th cluster and 0 otherwise. The first constraint restricts $\mathbf{S}$ to be a binary assignment matrix and the second constraint represents each sample to be assigned to only one cluster. The j-th column of $\mathbf{SC}$ indicates the centroid of the cluster to which the j-th sample $\boldsymbol{x}_j$ is assigned. $|\cdot|_F$ denotes the Frobenius norm of a matrix.

In the constrained clustering task, we need to specify must-links and cannot-links. A must-link will be attached to a sample pair that need to belong to the same cluster. A cannot-link will be attached to a pair that cannot belong to the same cluster. Here, we assume that an expert attaches correct labels to a small number of samples for each class ($i = 1,\dots,N_c$), where N_c is the number of classes. Denoting $\mathcal{L}_i$ as the set of labeled samples for class i, $\boldsymbol{x}_j \in \mathcal{L}_i$ indicates that the j-th sample belongs to the i-th class. Using the labeled samples, we then generate the must-link and cannot-link constraints. A pair of samples is registered to the must-link set $\mathcal{M}$ if these labels are the same, and to the cannot-link set $\mathcal{D}$ if different.

The proposed soft-constrained clustering method also tries to optimize the set of K cluster centroids C and the cluster assignments that minimize the sum of the WCSS distortion. The main difference from (1) is that the cannot-links $\mathcal{D}$ are imposed as hard constraints. Another, more important difference is that the must-links are evaluated as penalties; must-link constraints can be violated but penalized. This non-consistent treatment for the cannot-link and must-link comes from the property of medical images; as we noted, must-links are often too hard to satisfy for the class with a multimodal (scattered) distribution.

Consequently, the proposed method is formulated as:

$$\min_{C,S} \|X - SC\|_F^2 + \omega \sum_{(x_p, x_q) \in \mathcal{M}} \sum_{i=1}^{K} |s_{ip} - s_{iq}|_1, \tag{2}$$

$$s.t. \ s_{ij} \in \{0, 1\} \ \forall i, j, \quad \sum_{i=1}^{K} s_{ij} = 1 \ \forall j = 1, \ldots, N, \tag{3}$$

$$s_{ip} + s_{iq} \leq 1, \ \forall i = 1, \ldots, K \ \forall (x_p, x_q) \in \mathcal{D}, \tag{4}$$

where (4) represents the cannot-link constraints. If two samples x_p and x_q are paired by a cannot-link (i.e, $(x_p, x_q) \in \mathcal{D}$) and they try to belong to the same cluster i, $s_{ip} + s_{iq} = 1 + 1 \nleq 1$; consequently, this situation violates the constraint and is not allowed. The second term of the objective function (2) represents soft-constraints of the must-link. If two samples x_p and x_q are paired by a must-link (i.e., $(x_p, x_q) \in \mathcal{M}$) and they try to belong to different clusters, it becomes $s_{ip} - s_{iq} = 1 > 0$ and thus penalizes the objective function by ω, which is a positive constant.

4.2 Optimization for Soft-Constraints Clustering

To minimize (2) with constraints (3) and (4), we take an alternating optimization approach that alternatively updates the cluster centroid matrix C and the assignment matrix S until convergence, which is similar to the original K-means optimization approach (EM algorithm). In the update step for C by fixing S, we can ignore the constraints and the second penalty term of the objective function. We update C by solving the regularized least square problem to avoid numerical issues for large-scale problems [11]:

$$\min_{C} \|X - SC\|_F^2 + \lambda \|C\|_F^2, \tag{5}$$

where λ is the regularization parameter and we set λ to be 10^{-4} in our experiments. The problem is a convex quadratic optimization problem and it can be solved in closed-form.

$$C = XS^T(SS + \lambda I)^{-1}, \tag{6}$$

where $(SS + \lambda I)$ is guaranteed to be full-rank.

Next, we update S by fixing C. Let $Y \in \mathbb{R}^{K \times N}$ be a matrix whose (i, j)-th element y_{ij} is the squared distance from x_j to its centroid c_i; namely, $y_{ij} =$

Table 1. 20 classes defined for stomach endoscope images. BD, UP, MD, LO, LD, and LU stand for (stomach) body, upper, middle, lower, (camera) look-down, and look-up, respectively.

Fundus	Fundus on UP BD/LU	UP BD/LU	UP BD/LD
UP-MD BD/LU	UP-MD BD/LD	MD BD/LU	MD BD/LD
MD-LO BD/LU	MD-LO BD/LD	LO BD/LD	Angular Incisure LO BD/LD
AntralZone on LO BD/LD	Angular Incisure	Angular Incisure-Antral Zone	Antral Zone
Pyloric Antral	Pyloric Zone	Pylorus	Junction

Table 2. Quantitative performance evaluation by purity and recall. Larger is better.

Metric	Conditions	KM	BOCK [5]	MPCK [9]	LCVQE [7]	Proposed w/o must link	Proposed
Purity	$K=100$, $R=1\%$	0.602	0.627	0.421	0.573	0.658	**0.715**
	$K=100$, $R=3\%$	0.726	0.673	0.544	0.660	0.712	**0.789**
	$K=100$, $R=5\%$	0.681	0.716	0.494	0.587	**0.747**	0.747
	$K=50$, $R=1\%$	0.623	0.549	0.369	0.616	0.517	**0.660**
	$K=50$, $R=3\%$	0.668	0.648	0.521	0.636	0.651	**0.727**
	$K=50$, $R=5\%$	0.637	0.694	0.498	0.643	0.662	**0.702**
Recall	$K=100$, $R=1\%$	0.132	0.138	0.109	0.122	0.147	**0.159**
	$K=100$, $R=3\%$	0.156	0.167	0.147	0.155	0.158	**0.179**
	$K=100$, $R=5\%$	0.162	0.169	0.170	0.159	**0.174**	0.174
	$K=50$, $R=1\%$	0.254	0.230	0.170	0.230	0.218	**0.270**
	$K=50$, $R=3\%$	0.287	0.281	0.263	0.269	0.273	**0.310**
	$K=50$, $R=5\%$	0.262	0.296	0.258	0.279	0.295	**0.297**

$\|c_i - x_j\|_2^2$. By using $\mathbf{Y}$, the first term of (2) can be written as $\langle \mathbf{Y}, \mathbf{S} \rangle$, which represents Frobenius inner product of $\mathbf{Y}$ and $\mathbf{S}$.

By rewriting the second term with KM variables $\gamma_{i,(p,q)}$, which is defined for each pair of p and q which satisfies $(x_p, x_q) \in \mathcal{M}$, the updating problem of $\mathbf{S}$ becomes:

$$\min_{\mathbf{S}, \gamma} \ \langle \mathbf{Y}, \mathbf{S} \rangle + \omega \sum_{(x_p, x_q) \in \mathcal{M}} \sum_{i=1}^{K} \gamma_{i,(p,q)}, \tag{7}$$

$$\text{s.t. } s_{ij} \in \{0, 1\} \ \forall i, j, \quad \sum_{i=1}^{K} s_{ij} = 1 \ \forall j = 1, \ldots, N, \tag{8}$$

$$s_{ip} + s_{iq} \leq 1, \ \forall i = 1, \ldots, K \ \forall (x_p, x_q) \in \mathcal{D}, \tag{9}$$

$$s_{ip} - s_{iq} \leq \gamma_{i,(p,q)}, \ -s_{ip} + s_{iq} \leq \gamma_{i,(p,q)}, \ \forall i \ \forall (x_p, x_q) \in \mathcal{M}, \tag{10}$$

where the set $\gamma = \{\gamma_{i,(p,q)}\}$. This problem is a mixed binary linear programming; that is, the combination of the binary programming problem for $\mathbf{S}$ and the linear programming problem for γ. We solve this problem by the branch-and-

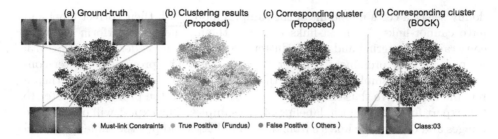

Fig. 2. Clustering result examples at $K = 50$ and $R = 0.03$. tSNE is used for these two-dimensional visualizations. (a) Distribution of samples whose true label is "Fundus." Green dots indicate unlabeled samples and red indicate labeled samples that were used as must-link constraints. (b) Clustering results from our method. (c) Results of proposed methods and (d) results of BOCK [5]. In (c) and (d), magenta dots indicate samples from other classes. (Color figure online)

bound optimization technique. In our experiments using over 10,000 images, the convergence time is about 30 s for this step. These two steps for updating **C** and **S** are alternatively iterated until convergence.

5 Experimental Results

In this section, we conducted experiments to evaluate the capability of the proposed method to support efficient ground-truth annotation for endoscopic image clustering. The endoscopy images were collected from several hospitals, including 11,599 stomach images captured by endoscopy. In the clustering task, these stomach images captured were classified into 20 classes listed in Table 1, according to the part in stomach and two camera capturing angles (look-down/look-up) for several parts.

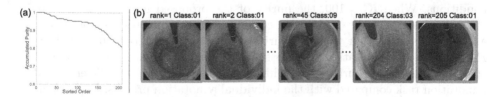

Fig. 3. (a) Accumulated purity curve with distance from the centroid of the cluster, where the cluster corresponds with the one in Fig. 2(c). The vertical axis indicates accumulated purity, and horizontal axis indicates sorted order by distance from centroid. (b) Images in cluster. Images were sorted by distance from centroid from left to right. "rank" shows the order by the distance in the cluster and rank = 1 is the closest. "Class" is a true label of the image (e.g., Class:01 is "Fundus.")

We designed the performance metrics that fit the situation where clustering is used for the actual labeling process. In the evaluation scenario, we randomly select a certain amount of the samples along with their correct label and have cannot-links and must-links by using them. Then, we perform our soft-constrained clustering and get K clusters. Among them, as described in Sect. 3, we pick up the "prominent" cluster for each class. The prominent cluster contains the most samples labeled by the expert with a certain class and thus a reliable cluster. We thus show the images belonging to the prominent cluster to the expert for finalizing the labeling of the samples. The expert will observe the images and discard the images from different classes and put the same class label to all the remaining images. Consequently, we need to have high purity and high recall at the prominent cluster to reduce this finalizing operation. The purity for each class is the number of true positives divided by the number of unlabeled samples in the prominent cluster. The recall for each class is the number of true positives in the prominent cluster divided by the total number of the samples of the class. In the later result, these measurements are averaged over all classes.

The performance of the proposed method was compared with several clustering methods: K-Means (KM) that is non-constrained clustering and the Binary Optimization approach for Constrained K-means (BOCK) that is hard-constrained clustering. Metric-based Pairwise Constrained K-means (MPCK) [9] and Linear-time Constrained Vector Quantization Error (LCVQE) [7] that are state-of-the-art soft-constrained clustering[2]. As discussed in Sect. 2, both soft-constrained clustering methods were designed to discard a small number of erroneous constraints. In addition, we evaluated the proposed method without using must link as an ablation study. The parameter ω was set to 50 for all experiments. To demonstrate the robustness for the rate of labeled samples over the total data R and the number of clusters K, we evaluated the performance under several conditions: $K = 50$, 100 and $R = 1\%$, 3%, 5%, where the labeled samples were randomly picked up, and then the must-link and cannot-link constraints were generated on the basis of the labeled data. When $R = 1\%$, the average number of labeled data in each class is about 29.

As shown in Table 2, our method achieved the best performance under all conditions. When $K = 100$, the purity of the proposed method was over 0.7. Here, we note that the purity was computed using only the unlabeled data, and thus it could occur that the purity with $R = 5\%$ is better than that with $R = 10\%$. In the annotation task for separating a set of images to a particular class and others, this purity value is high enough to improve the efficiency of the annotation task compared with the individual annotation process. In particular, in the case where the number of labeled data was low (1%), the purity of the proposed method is the highest and shows 8% ($=0.715 - 0.627$) improvement compared with the second best, BOCK. Our method also achieved the best recall.

Figure 3 shows the image examples in a cluster corresponding with class "Fundus." To analyze the relationship the distance from the centroid and the class

---

[2] A most popular hard-constrained clustering, COP-Kmeans [4] has not been compared; it did not work due to its heavy computational complexity for our large dataset.

label of the sample, we sorted the data by distances from the cluster centroid. Figure 3(a) shows the accumulated purity curve. In this plot, the samples near the centroid tend to have the same label as the labeled samples in the cluster.

The average running time for clustering over 10,000 images was 14s, 1119s, 10s, 1824s, and 130s by KM, BOCK, MPCK, LCVQE, and the proposed method, respectively. Our method was much faster than the other state-of-the-arts, BOCK and LCVQE, and its speed is acceptable for the group-based labeling scheme.

6   Conclusion

We proposed a soft-constrained clustering suitable for group-based labeling. The proposed method performs clustering by using must-links for penalties instead of hard-constraints by considering that the class distribution of medical images is often not unimodal but multimodal whose components are distant to each other. The advantage of our method is that we formulate the soft-constrained clustering problem as a single optimization problem rather than a typical two-step optimization where the problem is solved as a hard-constrained problem and then update the result. Our method achieved higher purity and recall than several state-of-the-art clustering methods under various conditions with different numbers of clusters and rates of the must/cannot-links.

Acknowledgments. This work was supported by JSPS KAKENHI Grant Number JP19K22895 and AMED Grant Number JP18lk1010028.

References

1. Biswas, A., Jacobs, D.: Active image clustering: seeking constraints from humans to complement algorithms. In: Proceedings of CVPR, pp. 2152–2159 (2012)
2. Galleguillos, C., McFee, B., Lanckriet, G.: Iterative category discovery via multiple kernel metric learning. IJCV **108**(1–2), 115–132 (2014)
3. Bruce, M.W., Draper, A., Beveridge, J.R.: Efficient label collection for unlabeled image datasets. In: Proceedings of CVPR, pp. 4594–4602 (2015)
4. Wagstaff, K., Cardie, C., Rogers, S., Schrodl, S.: Constrained k-means clustering with background knowledge. In: Proceedings of ICML, pp. 577–584 (2001)
5. Le, H.M., Eriksson, A., Do, T.-T., Milford, M.: A binary optimization approach for constrained k-means clustering. In: Jawahar, C.V., Li, H., Mori, G., Schindler, K. (eds.) ACCV 2018. LNCS, vol. 11364, pp. 383–398. Springer, Cham (2019). https://doi.org/10.1007/978-3-030-20870-7_24
6. Davidson, I., Ravi, S.S.: Clustering with constraints: feasibility issues and the k-means algorithm. In: Proceedings on SIAM Data Mining (2005)
7. Pelleg, D., Baras, D.: K-means with large and noisy constraint sets. In: Kok, J.N., Koronacki, J., Mantaras, R.L., Matwin, S., Mladenič, D., Skowron, A. (eds.) ECML 2007. LNCS (LNAI), vol. 4701, pp. 674–682. Springer, Heidelberg (2007). https://doi.org/10.1007/978-3-540-74958-5_67
8. Basu, S., Banerjee, A., Mooney R.J.: Active semi-supervision for pairwise constrained clustering. In: Proceedings of SIAM on Data Mining, pp. 333–344 (2004)

9. Bilenko, M., Basu, S., Mooney, R.J.: Integrating constraints and metric learning in semi-supervised clustering. In: Proceedings of ICML, pp. 81–88 (2004)
10. Huang, G., Liu, Z., Maaten, L., Weinberger, K.Q.: Densely connected convolutional networks. In: Proceedings of CVPR (2017)
11. Rifkin, R.M., Lippert, R.A.: Notes on regularized least squares, Technical report, MIT-CSAIL (2007)

Leveraging Other Datasets for Medical Imaging Classification: Evaluation of Transfer, Multi-task and Semi-supervised Learning

Hong Shang[1], Zhongqian Sun[1], Wei Yang[1], Xinghui Fu[1], Han Zheng[1], Jia Chang[2], and Junzhou Huang[1(✉)]

[1] Tencent AI Lab, Shenzhen, China
joehhuang@tencent.com
[2] Tencent AIMIS, Shenzhen, China

Abstract. To address the data scarcity challenge in developing deep learning based medical imaging classification, a widely-used strategy is to leverage other available datasets in training. Three machine learning algorithms belong to this concept, namely, transfer learning (TL), multi-task learning (MTL) and semi-supervised learning (SSL). TL and MTL bring another labeled dataset usually from different categories, while SSL utilizes an unlabeled dataset from the same category. Each has proven useful for medical imaging tasks. In this work, we unified these three algorithms into one framework, to directly compare individual contribution and combine them to extract extra performance. For SSL, state-of-the-art consistency based methods were evaluated, including Π-Model and virtual adversarial training. Experiments were done on classifying gastric diseases given endoscopic images trained with various amount of data. It was observed that individually TL has the most while SSL has the least performance gain. When used together, their contribution build up constructively leading to further improved performance especially with larger capacity network. This work helps guide applying each or combination of TL/MTL/SSL for other medical applications.

Keywords: Machine learning · Computer-aided diagnosis

1 Introduction

A well known challenge for developing computer-aided diagnosis using the powerful tool of deep convolutional neural network (CNN) is the lack of large labeled medical data. Learning from limited medical data is critical, as both data acquisition and its annotation is costly. A widely-used strategy is to leverage other available datasets in training. Three machine learning algorithms belong to this concept, namely, transfer learning (TL), multi-task learning (MTL) and semi-supervised learning (SSL). TL and MTL bring other labeled dataset usually

© Springer Nature Switzerland AG 2019
D. Shen et al. (Eds.): MICCAI 2019, LNCS 11768, pp. 431–439, 2019.
https://doi.org/10.1007/978-3-030-32254-0_48

from different categories, while SSL utilizes unlabeled dataset from the same category. Though each has proven useful for medical tasks, it remains unanswered: how their effect compare with each other, and whether they can be combined. Reviewing separate studies cannot provide direct comparison, due to mismatched dataset and implementation details. In this work, we unified these three algorithms into one framework, to not only directly compare individual contribution, but also combine them to extract extra performance. Rigorous experiments were done with an application of classifying gastric diseases given endoscopic images.

2   Related Work

TL uses pretrained network either as a feature extractor, or as a starting point for further training on target task (fine-tuning) [8]. Initialization matters as training deep CNNs is a non-convex optimization problem. TL, especially fine-tuning, is becoming standard practice for medical image analysis [4]. A still in debate question is the choice of source data, natural images with large size [13] or medical images with more similarity, an overview of which refers to [3].

Different from TL done sequentially, MTL works in parallel by training multiple related tasks simultaneously with a shared representation, increasing effective data size and regularization power [2]. MTL implementation in deep learning is an active research topic [9,12], however, the 20-year old hard parameter sharing is still the most commonly used approach [17]. It shares all the layers except the last fully connect (FC) layer.

SSL assumes data of each class lie in a cluster or manifold, and that unlabeled data helps to illustrate such structure, thus better estimate the decision boundary between classes [18]. An overview of SSL (mostly not deep learning based) on medical applications refers to [3]. Here we focus on state-of-the-art, deep learning compatible, SSL methods, which sharing an assumption that realistic perturbations of unlabeled data should not alter model prediction. These methods differ by how to generate the second prediction with potential difference: Π-Model uses stochastic data augmentation and dropout [7], Temporal Ensembling averages predictions over training steps [7], Mean Teacher averages model weights instead [15], Virtual Adversarial Training (VAT) takes adversarial perturbation optimized to deviate from current prediction [10]. Besides achieving competing performance, these methods are simple to integrate, as only additional loss term is involved without changing model structure or training process.

3   Unified Framework

The challenge of unifying TL/MTL/SSL is to merge MTL and SSL, as TL deals with initialization independently. We adopt commonly used fine-tuning with a model pretrained on ImageNet for TL, hard parameter sharing for MTL, and state-of-the-art Π-Model and VAT for SSL. The unified framework is shown in Fig. 1, where (x_0, y_0) is a labeled dataset for the target task, (x_1, y_1) is another

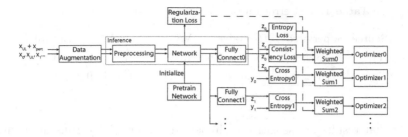

Fig. 1. Structure of the unified framework

labeled dataset for an auxiliary task in MTL, (x_{UL}) is an unlabeled dataset for SSL. x_0, x_1, x_{UL} all go through data augmentation, preprocessing, and a CNN to cast raw image pixels into a feature vector. Cross entropy loss is used for target task given y_0 and prediction z_0 from FC0, and for auxiliary task given y_1 and prediction z_1 from FC1.

For SSL, x_{UL} goes through the network twice to generate another prediction. Note SSL shares the last FC layer with the target task, while MTL has its own. These two predictions could differ due to stochastic process such as data augmentation and added perturbation, x_{pert}. To minimize such difference, the consistency loss is defined as mean squared error between two prediction probabilities for Π-Model [7], or KL divergence for VAT [10]. The difference between Π-Model and VAT is mainly on x_{pert}, random noise for Π-Model, while adversarial perturbation for VAT. A ramp up function is applied on consistency loss [7]. Besides, entropy is minimized (EntMin), as a reasonable model should produce confident prediction for realistic input [10]. Each loss is weighted and combined with regularization loss before applying an optimizer. The regularization loss applies to shared parameters and unique parameters in FC layer.

This framework can be trained end-to-end with each dataset fed alternatively, implemented in TensorFlow [1]. In each step, a batch contains data from one task, and the corresponding optimizer is called to update all shared parameters and this task's unique parameters. Compared to summing individual loss and applying one optimizer, this method allows each task to be manipulated separately and flexibly, thus easily scaled for arbitrary number of tasks, either MTL or SSL. Note that TL/MTL/SSL only affect training not inference, which is shown within the blue box in Fig. 1.

4   Experiments and Results

4.1   Evaluation Strategy

To get unbiased and realistic evaluation, we face challenges as follows: (1) the lack of widely-accepted baseline for tasks on private medical dataset, (2) comparison confounded by implementation variations, such as model structure, data augmentation, etc, (3) even with shared implementation, a notorious fact in deep

Table 1. Test error rates on SSL benchmark of CIFAR-10

Source	Supervised	Π-Model	VAT	VAT + EntMin
[11]	20.26 ± 0.38	16.37 ± 0.63	13.86 ± 0.27	13.13 ± 0.39
Ours	17.7 ± 0.1	14.6 ± 0.2	13.2 ± 0.2	12.9 ± 0.1

learning that results are sensitive to hyperparameters (HP), thus different HP tuning budget could lead to unfair comparison.

To alleviate issue 1, we firstly verified our SSL implementation, a prone to error component of the unified framework, on standard benchmark CIFAR-10 [6]. Issue 2 is already addressed with our unified implementation. To address issue 3, we designed the HP tuning strategy as follows, considering both fair comparison and limited training budget. Shared HP are determined based on baseline, such as batch size, to get conservative estimate of performance improvement. For TL, only learning rate is tuned. For SSL and MTL, only unique HP are tuned, such as coefficient for additional loss, repeated for each training data size. If network is replaced, all HP stay the same, with results biased towards the original network.

4.2 Semi-supervised Learning Reproduction

To verify our SSL implementation, we conducted experiments on benchmark of CIFAR-10 (4000/41000 images for labeled/unlabeled training data), and compared to a previous study, which systematically compared several SSL algorithms within a common framework [11]. Experimental setup was matched with [11], including data augmentation, preprocessing, regularization and network structure, which is a Wide ResNet [16] with depth of 28 and width of 2. However, we used Nesterov momentum optimizer with momentum of 0.9, initial learning rate of 0.1, annealed by a factor of 0.1 at epoch 500, 750 and 875 (1000 in total). Test error was reported at the point of lowest validation error, averaged over 4 run, each with 2 GPUs. Each of our results, shown in Table 1, outperformed the corresponding result in [11], however, the gap over fully-supervised baseline is smaller due to our improved baseline.

4.3 Medical Datasets and Baseline

A real world application was evaluated, classifying gastric endoscopic images into normal, benign and cancer, with 61491/24708/2679 images correspondingly in a dataset collected by our collaborating hospitals. The auxiliary task in MTL was chosen as identifying current examining organs during endoscopy, namely esophagus, stomach and duodenum, using data from the same source as above with 67684/143093/49686 images correspondingly. Disease labels were biopsy-proven, while organ was labeled by gastroenterologists. Both datasets were split into training, validation and testing randomly with ratio of 8:1:1, without overlap between testing and either task's training data. Samples are shown in Fig. 2. For

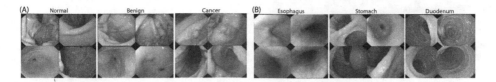

Fig. 2. Endoscopic image samples for classifying (A) gastric diseases, (B) organs.

studying SSL, we randomly sampled the training dataset (1%, 4%, 20%) with the rest treated as unlabeled, to emulate a practical setting where all the data were available from records, however, the following annotation is time consuming, or cannot be completed with limited resource. Validation set shrank together with training set to avoid unfair comparison [11]. Testing set stayed the same. When splitting data, we ensured all the images of one patient were not split, as similar images may exist from the same patient with different viewpoints.

DenseNet with 121 layers (DenseNet121) was chosen, a widely-used choice achieving competing performance with efficient feature reuse [5]. It was trained with Nesterov momentum optimizer, with momentum of 0.9, batch size of 64, learning rate of 0.002, weight decay of 0.0001. For data augmentation, an image was first resized to have its shorter side of 240, from which a 224×224 crop was sampled and randomly flipped. For preprocessing, mean value per each channel was subtracted. Validation set was used to choose a point by evaluating mean of each class's F_1 score (instead of accuracy due to unbalanced class). Test F_1 for each class was reported, averaged over 4 run, each with 4 GPUs. A baseline was created for each training data size (1%, 4%, 20%, 100%), as shown in Fig. 3(A). When data size increases exponentially, performance improves almost linearly, similar as a previous study [14].

4.4   Individual Improvement

Individually applying TL/SSL/MTL can improve performance, as shown in Fig. 3(A). For SSL, Π-Model results were reported (comparison with VAT see Sect. 4.6). Note when 100% training data is used, SSL is not applicable due to the lack of unlabeled data with our experimental setting. Our results showed that TL has the most while SSL has the least performance gain. SSL comes with the highest training cost, including more HP to tune and longer training duration with dual forward calculation per step. Besides, TL/MTL is free to choose data from other categories, thus can choose data already available in large size, while SSL does not have such flexibility. Previous study on CIFAR-10 reach similar conclusion that TL outperformed SSL [11]. Note the performance gap between TL/SSL/MTL and baseline is decreasing with data size increasing.

4.5   Combined Improvement

As shown in Fig. 3(B) (TL+MTL, TL+SSL), MTL or SSL (Π-Model) on top of TL can further improve performance over the new baseline of TL only,

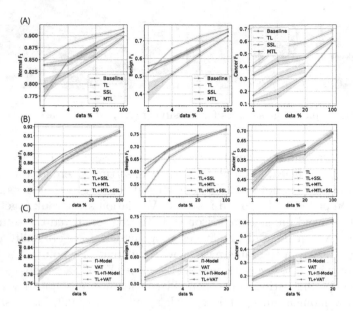

Fig. 3. F_1 score for the class of normal (left), benign (center), cancer (right), comparing (A) baseline and individually applying TL/SSL/MTL, (B) SSL and/or MTL on top of TL, (C) Π-Model and VAT. X-axis represents percentage of labeled training data (logarithmic scale). Shaded regions indicate standard deviation over 4 run.

however, the extent varies for different data size. For small dataset (1% data with 750 images, or 4% data with 3267 images), MTL and SSL led to significant and similar amount of improvement. For larger dataset (20% with 16000 images), SSL contributed more than MTL. When the entire dataset was used (100% with 79806 images), MTL improvement was not differentiable. It seems conflicting that MTL helps more than SSL individually, however, has lower contribution on top of TL for larger dataset. The possible explanation is that MTL comes with a side effect, a discrepancy between training (two tasks) and testing data (only caring target task), which is not an issue for SSL. When overfitting is moderate, benefit from additional regularization cannot overcome the side effect. Therefore, MTL is better fit for small dataset, while SSL is more likely to continuously improve over a relatively good baseline. Combining TL/SSL/MTL together, as shown in Fig. 3(B) (TL+MTL+SSL), we got the best performance for each amount of data, indicating TL/SSL/MTL contributes from different perspective and can be combined constructively, therefore should be used for developing new applications where the extent of data scarcity is unknown. Above all, the best performance with 20% data cannot compete with simply TL with 100% data, suggesting there is a limit on what can be achieved with TL/SSL/MTL and more labeled data are always desired.

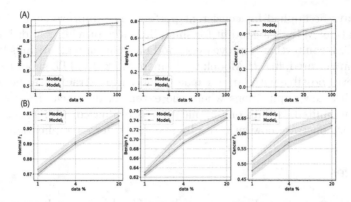

Fig. 4. Similar as Fig. 3 but comparing different model capacity (A) with TL, (B) with combined TL/MTL/SSL.

4.6   Semi-supervised Learning Comparison

Π-Model was chosen for SSL in previous sections, as it achieved slightly better performance than VAT both with and without TL, as shown in Fig. 3(C). In opposite, VAT won on CIFAR-10 benchmark, where we noticed VAT is more sensitive to its specific HP. Therefore, VAT could benefit from the unrealistically large validation set on CIFAR-10 for HP tuning [11].

4.7   Network Capacity

Network capacity, a crucial component of any deep learning system, remains the same in experiments so far. To study how results above generalize to other networks, we conducted experiments after replacing network to Wide ResNet with depth of 50 and width of 2 (WRN-50-2), increasing total parameters from 8.0 Million to 68.9 Million, also with a better ImageNet pretrained model [5, 16]. DenseNet with more parameters was not chosen as its inference speed is not acceptable. Results comparing DenseNet121 ($Model_s$) and WRN-50-2 ($Model_L$) are shown in Fig. 4 with TL (A), and with combined TL/SSL/MTL (B). With less regularization (TL only), WRN-50-2 performance dropped dramatically for small data size with strong overfitting. However, with additional regularization of SSL/MTL, WRN-50-2 always outperformed DenseNet121. Therefore, it is recommended to combine TL/SSL/MTL whenever possible and use large capacity network with better feature representation to extract extra performance. When SSL and MTL cannot be applied, a smaller network reduces overfitting risk.

5   Conclusion

In this work, we unified TL/SSL/MTL into one framework to leverage additional datasets for training. Rigorous experiments were done on a gastric diseases classifier to study individual and combined contribution. Our results suggest: TL should always be applied for consistent performance improvement with simple implementation; MTL is a good fit for small data size providing additional regularization; SSL can further improve over good baseline, and algorithms less sensitive to HP are desired, like Π-Model; Combined TL/SSL/MTL should always be used whenever possible with larger capacity model to extract extra performance for developing new applications where the extent of data scarcity is unknown. This work is limited as only one application is evaluated. More tasks need be studied to demonstrate how such results generalize across applications.

References

1. Abadi, M., et al.: TensorFlow: large-scale machine learning on heterogeneous systems (2015). https://www.tensorflow.org/. Software available from tensorflow.org
2. Caruana, R.: Multitask learning. Mach. Learn. **28**(1), 41–75 (1997)
3. Cheplygina, V., de Bruijne, M., Pluim, J.P.: Not-so-supervised: a survey of semi-supervised, multi-instance, and transfer learning in medical image analysis. Med. Image Anal. **54**, 280–296 (2019)
4. Hoo-Chang, S., et al.: Deep convolutional neural networks for computer-aided detection: CNN architectures, dataset characteristics and transfer learning. IEEE Trans. Med. Imaging **35**(5), 1285 (2016)
5. Huang, G., Liu, Z., Van Der Maaten, L., Weinberger, K.Q.: Densely connected convolutional networks. In: CVPR, vol. 1, p. 3 (2017)
6. Krizhevsky, A., Hinton, G.: Learning multiple layers of features from tiny images. Technical report. Citeseer (2009)
7. Laine, S., Aila, T.: Temporal ensembling for semi-supervised learning. In: Proceedings International Conference on Learning Representations (ICLR) (2017)
8. Litjens, G., et al.: A survey on deep learning in medical image analysis. Med. Image Anal. **42**, 60–88 (2017)
9. Misra, I., Shrivastava, A., Gupta, A., Hebert, M.: Cross-stitch networks for multi-task learning. In: Proceedings of the IEEE Conference on Computer Vision and Pattern Recognition, pp. 3994–4003 (2016)
10. Miyato, T., Maeda, S.I., Ishii, S., Koyama, M.: Virtual adversarial training: a regularization method for supervised and semi-supervised learning. IEEE Trans. Pattern Anal. Mach. Intell. **41**, 1979–1993 (2018)
11. Oliver, A., Odena, A., Raffel, C.A., Cubuk, E.D., Goodfellow, I.: Realistic evaluation of deep semi-supervised learning algorithms. In: Advances in Neural Information Processing Systems, pp. 3239–3250 (2018)
12. Ruder, S.: An overview of multi-task learning in deep neural networks. arXiv preprint arXiv:1706.05098 (2017)
13. Russakovsky, O., et al.: ImageNet large scale visual recognition challenge. Int. J. Comput. Vis. (IJCV) **115**(3), 211–252 (2015). https://doi.org/10.1007/s11263-015-0816-y
14. Sun, C., Shrivastava, A., Singh, S., Gupta, A.: Revisiting unreasonable effectiveness of data in deep learning era. In: Proceedings of the IEEE International Conference on Computer Vision, pp. 843–852 (2017)
15. Tarvainen, A., Valpola, H.: Mean teachers are better role models: weight-averaged consistency targets improve semi-supervised deep learning results. In: Advances in Neural Information Processing Systems, pp. 1195–1204 (2017)

16. Zagoruyko, S., Komodakis, N.: Wide residual networks. In: Richard, C., Wilson, E.R.H., Smith, W.A.P. (eds.) Proceedings of the British Machine Vision Conference (BMVC), pp. 87.1–87.12. BMVA Press, September 2016. https://doi.org/10.5244/ C.30.87, https://dx.doi.org/10.5244/C.30.87
17. Zhang, Z., Luo, P., Loy, C.C., Tang, X.: Facial landmark detection by deep multi-task learning. In: Fleet, D., Pajdla, T., Schiele, B., Tuytelaars, T. (eds.) ECCV 2014. LNCS, vol. 8694, pp. 94–108. Springer, Cham (2014). https://doi.org/10. 1007/978-3-319-10599-4_7
18. Zhou, Z.H.: A brief introduction to weakly supervised learning. Natl. Sci. Rev. **5**(1), 44–53 (2017)

Incorporating Temporal Prior from Motion Flow for Instrument Segmentation in Minimally Invasive Surgery Video

Yueming Jin[1(✉)], Keyun Cheng[1], Qi Dou[2], and Pheng-Ann Heng[1,3]

[1] Department of Computer Science and Engineering,
The Chinese University of Hong Kong, Hong Kong, China
ymjin@cse.cuhk.edu.hk
[2] Department of Computing, Imperial College London, London, UK
[3] T Stone Robotics Institute, The Chinese University of Hong Kong,
Hong Kong, China

Abstract. Automatic instrument segmentation in video is an essentially fundamental yet challenging problem for robot-assisted minimally invasive surgery. In this paper, we propose a novel framework to leverage instrument motion information, by incorporating a derived temporal prior to an attention pyramid network for accurate segmentation. Our inferred prior can provide reliable indication of the instrument location and shape, which is propagated from the previous frame to the current frame according to inter-frame motion flow. This prior is injected to the middle of an encoder-decoder segmentation network as an initialization of a pyramid of attention modules, to explicitly guide segmentation output from coarse to fine. In this way, the temporal dynamics and the attention network can effectively complement and benefit each other. As additional usage, our temporal prior enables semi-supervised learning with periodically unlabeled video frames, simply by reverse execution. We extensively validate our method on the public 2017 MICCAI EndoVis Robotic Instrument Segmentation Challenge dataset with three different tasks. Our method consistently exceeds the state-of-the-art results across all three tasks by a large margin. Our semi-supervised variant also demonstrates a promising potential for reducing annotation cost in the clinical practice.

1 Introduction

With advancements of robot-assisted minimally invasive surgery, enhancing automatic context awareness of the surgical procedure is important for improving surgeon performance and patient safety. Segmentation of the surgical instrument plays a fundamental role for various further tasks including tool pose estimation, tracking and control. In addition, for augmented reality, referring a segmentation mask can prevent the overlay of rendered tissue from occluding instruments.

© Springer Nature Switzerland AG 2019
D. Shen et al. (Eds.): MICCAI 2019, LNCS 11768, pp. 440–448, 2019.
https://doi.org/10.1007/978-3-030-32254-0_49

However, accurate instrument segmentation from surgical videos is very challenging, due to the complicated scene, blur from instrument motion, inevitable visual occlusion by blood or smoke, and various lighting conditions. Recognizing the instrument in greater details, e.g., separating its different parts or specifying its sub-type, is even harder given the limited inter-class variance.

To meet these challenges, early methods use hand-crafted features from color and texture, with machine learning models such as random forests and Gaussian mixture model [3,13]. Later, convolutional neural network (CNN) based methods have demonstrated new state-of-the-art on instrument segmentation. The ToolNet [5] uses a holistically-nested fully convolutional network, imposing multi-scale constraint of predictions. Laina et al. [9] propose a multi-task CNN to concurrently regress the segmentation and localization. Milletari et al. [11] use residual CNN and integrate multi-scale features of a frame via LSTM. Shvets et al. [16] design a skip-connection model trained with transfer learning, winning the 2017 EndoVis Challenge [2]. The existing works treat sequential data as static image, and perform segmentation purely using visual cues in single frame.

With the sequential nature, temporal information actually can provide valuable clues for video analysis, and has demonstrated benefit in other surgical tasks, e.g., workflow recognition [7,18], instrument detection [15], and pose estimation [1]. These methods either implicitly learn spatio-temporal features in a network (generally with LSTM), or straightforwardly take the optical flow map as an extra input channel to a network. In addition, they only need to produce coarse predictions rather than pixel-level dense segmentation. How to more interpretably utilize time cues and more explicitly incorporate it into a network, are of large importance to achieve an accurate segmentation.

We propose a novel framework integrating a prior derived from motion flow into a temporal attention pyramid network (named MF-TAPNet) for automatic instrument segmentation in minimally invasive surgery video. Our method uses the inherent temporal clues from the instrument motion to boost results. Specifically, we propagate the prediction mask of the previous frame, via optical flow in an unsupervised way, and infer a reliable prior indicating the instrument's location and shape in the current frame. Next, we make explicit use of this temporal prior, by incorporating it at the bottleneck layer of a segmentation network as an initial attention map, and evolve a pyramid of attention modules. In this way, the sequential dynamics and the attention network can complement and progressively highlight discriminative features (or suppress irrelevant regions). As an exciting additional usage, our method enables semi-supervised learning at periodically unlabeled video, simply by propagating the prior in reverse direction. We evaluate our method on three different tasks of 2017 MICCAI EndoVis Challenge. Our MF-TAPNet consistently outperforms the leaderboard methods at all tasks. Our semi-supervised setting also achieves promising results only requiring labeling 50% frames, which endorses potential value in clinical practice.

2 Method

Figure 1 presents our proposed MF-TAPNet, which incorporates motion flow based temporal prior to a designed attention pyramid network for accurate surgical instrument segmentation from video. We elaborate each component in this section.

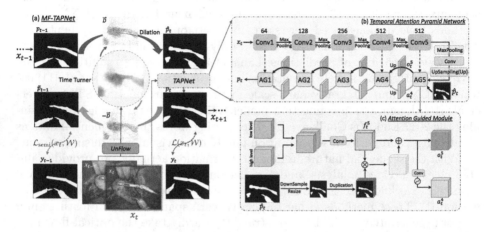

Fig. 1. Illustration of the proposed (a) MF-TAPNet for surgical instrument segmentation based on motion flow, with architecture of (b) temporal attention pyramid network and (c) attention guided module presented in detail.

2.1 Unsupervised Temporal Propagation via Motion Flow

In surgical video, instruments performed by surgeons, usually have obvious and rich motion information. Such valuable temporal inherence in the sequential data is unexplored in previous works on instrument segmentation. We propose a novel temporal prior propagation strategy, named as *time turner*, to take advantage of such domain knowledge to a large extent.

Intuitively, we argue that the motion derived from the raw images (frames in video data) also applies to their corresponding instrument masks. This generally shares the spirit with atlas-based segmentation, but here, our "deformation field" is the motion flow between sequential frames in video. In practice, we derive the apparent instrument movement using optical flow which is de-facto for motion analysis. More specifically, we use Unflow [10], a recent state-of-the-art method, to obtain a map $\vec{D}$ of displacement vector between adjacent frame pair of (x_{t-1}, x_t), showing the motion magnitude and orientation at each pixel. In the map $\vec{D}$, each displacement vector $\vec{d} = [d_a, d_b]$ directs a position from frame x_{t-1} to x_t. In our intuition, their instrument masks also follow the same location shift with such motion. Given the mask prediction p_{t-1} (output from a network given input of x_{t-1}), we can propagate it with $\vec{D}$ to infer a prediction for x_t. Formally, with denoting $\boldsymbol{u}_{t-1} = [u_a, u_b]$ as the position of one value in p_{t-1}, we infer its position in next frame as $\boldsymbol{u}_t = \boldsymbol{u}_{t-1} + \vec{\boldsymbol{d}} = [u_a + d_a, u_b + d_b]$. With operation for all positions, we obtain the inferred mask prediction for x_t, which is the referred concept of *temporal prior* in this paper. We further enhance it using morphological dilation to relieve the effects of camera zoom, The finally obtained temporal prior is denoted by $\hat{p}_t$, which is very informative and of high-quality regarding the location and shape of instrument in frame x_t. Note that in multi-class segmentation, we sum the probabilities of all positive classes and get p_{t-1} as a 2D map indicating non-background probability, therefore $\hat{p}_t$ is also a 2D map accordingly. Our prior can be obtained via propagating the prediction map by computing optical flow, no matter the instrument motion is large or mild compared with background motion. Therefore, it can be well generalizable to some unusual yet extreme conditions in surgical video, such as video clips with the large camera motion, still instruments and no instrument.

2.2 Temporal Prior Driven Attention Pyramid Network

Way of incorporating the temporal prior $\hat{p}_t$ provided by the *time turner* is crucial for taking great advantage of it. In this regard, we design a temporal attention pyramid network (TAPNet) which consists of multi-stage attention guided (AG) modules. It injects the prior at the encoder-decoder bottleneck and progressively learns attention guide-map pyramid in coarse-to-fine, see Fig. 1(b). The temporal prior serves as initialization of the series of attentions, and forms the essential focus throughout the pyramid. Some previous methods may also use multi-stage attention, however, most works implicitly learn attention maps from home-grown features within a network [4,12]. Our TAPNet is explicitly driven by the distinct temporal prior, making the model precisely focus on the instrument regions and hence the benefit of attention pyramid is maximized.

We first elaborate the operation inside an AG module in Fig. 1(c), with example of the most coarse one (AG5) where prior $\hat{p}_t$ is incorporated. In the segmentation task, we use skip connection to concatenate low/high-level features, followed by 1×1 convolution producing f_t^5. We first downsample $\hat{p}_t$, and then duplicate it to the same channels as f_t^5. Next, we conduct element-wise multiplication between f_t^5 and the processed $\hat{p}_t$, to extract features from those spatial locations recognized in temporal prior. The result is resummed with f_t^5, outputting a representation with enlarged instrument-related activation and necessary visual context. It is forwarded to a 3×3 convolution and a Sigmoid function to generate the attention map for next stage AG. Formally, for the i-th AG, output o_t^i and attention map a_t^{i-1} for its following module are obtained with:

$$o_t^i = f_t^i + a_t^i \odot f_t^i, \quad a_t^{i-1} = Sigmoid\left(\text{Conv}(o_t^i; \omega)\right). \tag{1}$$

Both o_t^i, a_t^{i-1} are upsampled by interpolation before forwarding to the next stage. Overall, we stack 5 AG modules in pyramid to gradually decode coarse features guided by attention maps, and finally obtain the dense prediction p_t for frame x_t.

With denoting the label mask of frame x_t by y_t, we adopt weighted cross-entropy loss for multi-class segmentation, computing from all pixels in frame x_t:

$$\mathcal{L}(x_t; \mathcal{W}) = \sum -\alpha \cdot \log \mathcal{P}(y_t | x_t, \hat{p}_t), \text{ where } \hat{p}_t = \vec{\boldsymbol{D}}(p_{t-1} | x_{t-1}, x_t). \quad (2)$$

Similarly, prediction p_t of frame x_t is also used to infer $\hat{p}_{t+1}$ for its future frame x_{t+1}. To the end, a beneficial circulation for the entire network training is formed, to sequentially produce accurate segmentation masks of the entire surgical video. For the very beginning frame x_0, its prior is set as zero, but this rare case cannot affect learning. The optical flow at *time turner* is precomputed, so with p_{t-1} from the network, we can compute $\hat{p}_t$ in real-time during training.

2.3   Semi-supervision via Reverse Time Turner

Annotating medical data is time-consuming and laborious, especially for surgical video with high frequency. Excitingly, our method enables semi-supervised learning with fewer annotations using *time turner*. This is achieved by leveraging the sequential consistency to transfer the prediction of unlabeled frame to that of the adjacent frame whose label is available for loss calculation.

With a video having T frames as $\boldsymbol{x} = \{x_0, x_1, \ldots, x_{T-1}\}$, we assume that $\boldsymbol{x}$ is labeled with intervals, e.g., only $\{x_0, x_2, x_4, \ldots\}$ being labeled. This is a reasonable setting in clinical practice because it is easier for surgeons to perform low hertz labeling. The whole data therefore consists of labeled subset $\mathcal{V} = \{x_k\}_{k=2n}$ and unlabeled subset $\mathcal{U} = \{x_k\}_{k=2n+1}$. If frame x_t is unlabeled, we simply execute our *time turner* in a reverse direction, to transfer its prediction p_t into $\tilde{p}_{t-1}$ which is corresponding to frame x_{t-1}. Note that a reverse flow $-\vec{\boldsymbol{D}}$ is easily obtained with element-wise negative of $\vec{\boldsymbol{D}}$, without extra computation, see green arrow in Fig. 1(a). The $\tilde{p}_{t-1}$ is expected to well overlap with label of x_{t-1}, given inherent motion consistency. Hence, we can borrow y_{t-1} to calculate semi-supervised cross entropy for x_t, as:

$$\mathcal{L}_{\text{semi}}(x_t; \mathcal{W}) = \sum -\beta \cdot (y_{t-1} \cdot \log \tilde{p}_{t-1}), \text{ where } \tilde{p}_{t-1} = -\vec{\boldsymbol{D}}(p_t | x_{t-1}, x_t). \quad (3)$$

Overall, the training uses the supervised loss in Eq. (2) if a frame x_t is labeled, otherwise it uses the semi-supervised loss in Eq. (3). By encouraging the temporal consistent predictions, the bi-directional use of *time turner* effectively benefits the network learning. Our semi-supervision enabled by motion flow is inherently general and can be applicable for other medical video analysis tasks.

3   Experiments

Dataset and Evaluation Metrics. We validate the proposed framework on the public dataset of Robotic Instrument Segmentation from the 2017 MICCAI EndoVis Challenge [2]. It consists of 10 video sequences of abdominal porcine procedures. Each video contains 300 frames obtained at sampling frequency of

Table 1. Comparison of instrument segmentation results on three tasks (mean±std).

Methods	Task1: Binary segmentation		Task2: Part segmentation		Task3: Type segmentation	
	IoU (%)	Dice (%)	IoU (%)	Dice (%)	IoU (%)	Dice (%)
U-Net [14]	75.44 ± 18.18	84.37 ± 14.58	48.41 ± 17.59	60.75 ± 18.21	15.80 ± 15.06	23.59 ± 19.87
TernausNet [16]	83.60 ± 15.83	90.01 ± 12.50	65.50 ± 17.22	75.97 ± 16.21	33.78 ± 19.16	44.95 ± 22.89
U-NetPlus [6]	83.75 ± 15.36	90.19 ± 11.77	65.75 ± 16.74	76.25 ± 15.54	34.19 ± 15.06	45.32 ± 19.86
PlainNet	81.86 ± 15.85	88.96 ± 12.98	64.73 ± 17.39	73.53 ± 16.98	34.57 ± 21.93	44.64 ± 25.16
TAPNet	84.01 ± 16.93	90.46 ± 13.56	65.84 ± 16.91	76.12 ± 16.75	34.23 ± 19.63	45.50 ± 22.55
MF-TAPNet (Ours)	**87.56 ± 16.24**	**93.37 ± 12.93**	**67.92 ± 16.50**	**77.05 ± 16.17**	**36.62 ± 22.78**	**48.01 ± 25.64**
MF-TAPNet (50%)	79.31 ± 17.13	87.18 ± 13.68	56.01 ± 15.59	68.13 ± 15.44	28.47 ± 23.41	38.39 ± 25.88
Semi-MF-TAPNet (50%)	80.03 ± 16.87	88.07 ± 13.15	56.72 ± 16.12	68.51 ± 16.11	30.04 ± 19.79	41.01 ± 23.81

2 Hz and a high resolution of 1280 × 1024. Specifically, 8 × 225-frame videos are used for training, while the remaining 8 × 75-frame videos and another 2 × 300-frame videos are used for testing; the ground-truth of test data is held-out by challenge organizer. There are three sub-tasks, i.e. binary instrument (2 classes), instrument part (4 classes), instrument type (8 classes), gradually fine-grained segmentation of an instrument. The challenge report [2] describes more details of the difficulties in the tasks. For direct and fair comparison, we follow the same evaluation manner as TernausNet [16] (challenge winner), by using 4-fold cross-validation with the same splits of 8 × 225 released training data. We also use the same evaluation metrics as [16], i.e., (1) mean intersection-over-union (IoU), which is also used in MICCAI EndoVis Challenge to evaluate participants, and (2) Dice coefficient (Dice), which is another common metric for segmentation.

Implementation Details. We reduce the resolution to 640 × 512 to save memory. We train models using an Adam optimizer [8], with learning rates initialized as 3e−5, 3e−5 and 2e−5 respectively for binary, part and type segmentation tasks. Our framework is implemented in PyTorch with 4 NVIDIA Titan Xp GPUs for training. The multiple GPUs enable the network to be trained at batch size of 8. The backbone of our network is VGG11 [17] with 5 scales of downsampling, and deeper networks did not yield much better results in experiments, so we stick to VGG11 for the sake of real-time efficiency during surgery. The code is available at https://github.com/keyuncheng/MF-TAPNet.

Comparison with State-of-the-Art Methods. We first compare our method with the state-of-the-art results in challenge on three tasks. Table 1 lists the performance of U-Net [14] (results quoted from [16]), TernausNet [16], and latest reported U-NetPlus [6] (an enhanced U-Net with batch normalized encoders and nearest neighbor interpolation). We see that MF-TAPNet consistently outperforms all other methods across all three tasks. Our IoU exceeds the challenge winner by 3.96% at binary segmentation, 2.42% at part segmentation, and 2.84% at type segmentation. Though [16] and [6] develop advanced strategies to enhance a network, our method is superior by using temporal prior to explicitly provide a reliable guidance, which helps the network learn to focus on regions of interest.

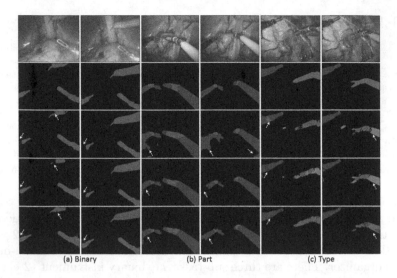

Fig. 2. Typical results for instrument (a) binary segmentation (instrument and background tissues), (b) part segmentation (shaft, wrist and jaws), (c) type segmentation (different yet looking quite similar instruments). From top to bottom, for each task, we present two continuous video frames and their corresponding ground truth, with segmentation results using PlainNet, TAPNet and our proposed MF-TAPNet.

The improvement is more obvious for binary segmentation, because our prior also aggregates probabilities from all positive classes. Under such homologous guidance, we achieve the highest Dice score 93.37%, which is useful for context-aware robot-assisted surgery. Meanwhile, there still exists a big room to boost type segmentation performance, even though we set the highest among existing methods. This reflects the natural great challenge in this task, i.e. the extremely similar appearance (shape and intensity value) in different fine-grained types. Our method is extensible for further improvement by inferring a multi-class prior, while such extension is limited for other methods. Last, as our method relies on the temporal consistency, its efficacy may degrade when unexpected motion appears, resulting in slightly higher standard deviations. This can be alleviated as advancements of more stable surgical robots.

Effectiveness of Temporal Prior and Motion Flow. We investigate effectiveness of key components in our MF-TAPNet. Table 1 also lists the results of three ablation settings: (1) a plain encoder-decoder as baseline (PlainNet); (2) our TAPNet, but directly use the previous frame's prediction p_{t-1} as temporal prior; (3) our entire framework at fully-supervised learning. The network backbone is unchanged for different settings for clear comparison. We observe that TAPNet performs better than PlainNet, especially for binary segmentation (1.50% higher Dice) and part segmentation (2.59% higher Dice). This shows that, explicitly incorporating a temporal prior can provide powerful guidance, even with the rough prediction from previous frame. Accordingly, our TAPNet can pyramidally refine the guidance and gradually concentrate on segmenting attentive objects. Here, our TAPNet can already achieve comparable results with the state-of-the-art methods. More importantly, our MF-TAPNet further largely increases performances for all tasks (averagely 2.67% IoU). It demonstrates that after involving motion dynamics derived in *time turner*, the prior presents much higher quality and can convey more accurate shape and location in current frame. Some visual results are shown in Fig. 2. MF-TAPNet can achieve complete and consistent segmentations, and largely suppress the irrelevant and incorrect regions.

Semi-supervised Variant Enabled by Time Turner. We conduct experiment with the variant of semi-supervised learning. Our setting is that the data are labeled at an interval of 2, resulting in 50% frames having labels. In Table 1, we see that our semi-supervised loss (i.e., approximating the prediction of an unlabeled frame towards a reasonable label) can better confront the performance drop at sparse annotation, compared with an ordinary training of MF-TAPNet with 50% labeled data. This is a bonus from our *time turner* with interpretable meanings, and a simply reverse execution invokes a promising potential to reduce annotation cost which is very valuable in clinical surgery.

4   Conclusion

We propose a novel framework to incorporate temporal information pyramidally in a network for automatic instrument segmentation from robot-assisted surgery. Our method consistently outperforms the state-of-the-art methods across all the three tasks on the 2017 MICCAI EndoVis Challenge dataset, by a large margin. Our temporal prior enables semi-supervised learning simply by reverse execution. The achieved outstanding results, and demonstrated potentials for extension and label efficiency, endorse a promising value of our method in clinical intervention.

Acknowledgments. The work was partially supported by HK RGC TRS project T42-409/18-R, HK RGC project CUHK14225616, and CUHK T Stone Robotics Institute, CUHK. Yueming Jin is funded by the HK Ph.D. Fellowship.

References

1. Allan, M., Ourselin, S., et al.: 3-D pose estimation of articulated instruments in robotic minimally invasive surgery. IEEE TMI **37**(5), 1204–1213 (2018)
2. Allan, M., Shvets, A., et al.: 2017 robotic instrument segmentation challenge. arXiv preprint arXiv:1902.06426 (2019)
3. Bouget, D., Benenson, R., et al.: Detecting surgical tools by modelling local appearance and global shape. IEEE TMI **34**(12), 2603–2617 (2015)

4. Chen, J., et al.: Multiview two-task recursive attention model for left atrium and atrial scars segmentation. In: Frangi, A.F., Schnabel, J.A., Davatzikos, C., Alberola-López, C., Fichtinger, G. (eds.) MICCAI 2018. LNCS, vol. 11071, pp. 455–463. Springer, Cham (2018). https://doi.org/10.1007/978-3-030-00934-2_51

5. García-Peraza-Herrera, L.C., Li, W., et al.: ToolNet: holistically-nested real-time segmentation of robotic surgical tools. In: IEEE/RSJ IROS, pp. 5717–5722 (2017)

6. Hasan, S., Linte, C.A.: U-NetPlus: a modified encoder-decoder U-Net architecture for semantic and instance segmentation of surgical instrument. arXiv preprint arXiv:1902.08994 (2019)

7. Jin, Y., Dou, Q., et al.: SV-RCNet: workflow recognition from surgical videos using recurrent convolutional network. IEEE TMI **37**(5), 1114–1126 (2018)

8. Kingma, D.P., Ba, J.: Adam: a method for stochastic optimization. arXiv preprint arXiv:1412.6980 (2014)

9. Laina, I., et al.: Concurrent segmentation and localization for tracking of surgical instruments. In: Descoteaux, M., Maier-Hein, L., Franz, A., Jannin, P., Collins, D.L., Duchesne, S. (eds.) MICCAI 2017. LNCS, vol. 10434, pp. 664–672. Springer, Cham (2017). https://doi.org/10.1007/978-3-319-66185-8_75

10. Meister, S., Hur, J., Roth, S.: UnFlow: unsupervised learning of optical flow with a bidirectional census loss. In: AAAI (2018)

11. Milletari, F., Rieke, N., Baust, M., Esposito, M., Navab, N.: CFCM: segmentation via coarse to fine context memory. In: Frangi, A.F., Schnabel, J.A., Davatzikos, C., Alberola-López, C., Fichtinger, G. (eds.) MICCAI 2018. LNCS, vol. 11073, pp. 667–674. Springer, Cham (2018). https://doi.org/10.1007/978-3-030-00937-3_76

12. Oktay, O., Schlemper, J., et al.: Attention U-Net: learning where to look for the pancreas. MIDL (2018)

13. Rieke, N., Tan, D.J., et al.: Real-time localization of articulated surgical instruments in retinal microsurgery. Med. Image Anal. **34**, 82–100 (2016)

14. Ronneberger, O., Fischer, P., Brox, T.: U-Net: convolutional networks for biomedical image segmentation. In: Navab, N., Hornegger, J., Wells, W.M., Frangi, A.F. (eds.) MICCAI 2015. LNCS, vol. 9351, pp. 234–241. Springer, Cham (2015). https://doi.org/10.1007/978-3-319-24574-4_28

15. Sarikaya, D., Corso, J.J., Guru, K.A.: Detection and localization of robotic tools in robot-assisted surgery videos using deep neural networks for region proposal and detection. IEEE TMI **36**(7), 1542–1549 (2017)

16. Shvets, A.A., Rakhlin, A., et al.: Automatic instrument segmentation in robot-assisted surgery using deep learning. In: ICMLA, pp. 624–628 (2018)

17. Simonyan, K., Zisserman, A.: Very deep convolutional networks for large-scale image recognition. arXiv preprint arXiv:1409.1556 (2014)

18. Twinanda, A.P., Shehata, S., et al.: EndoNet: a deep architecture for recognition tasks on laparoscopic videos. IEEE TMI **36**(1), 86–97 (2017)

Hard Frame Detection and Online Mapping for Surgical Phase Recognition

Fangqiu Yi and Tingting Jiang[⊠]

NELVT, Department of Computer Science, Peking University, Beijing, China
{chinayi,ttjiang}@pku.edu.cn

Abstract. Surgical phase recognition is an important topic of Computer Assisted Surgery (CAS) systems. In the complicated surgical procedures, there are lots of hard frames that have indistinguishable visual features but are assigned with different labels. Prior works try to classify hard frames along with other simple frames indiscriminately, which causes various problems. Different from previous approaches, we take hard frames as mislabeled samples and find them in the training set via data cleansing strategy. Then, we propose an Online Hard Frame Mapper (OHFM) to handle the detected hard frames separately. We evaluate our solution on the M2CAI16 Workflow Challenge dataset and the Cholec80 dataset and achieve superior results. (The code is available at https://github. com/ChinaYi/miccai19).

Keywords: Surgical phase recognition · Data cleansing · Deep learning

1 Introduction

Computer-Assisted Surgery (CAS) systems are crucial in the development of modern surgery. Surgical phase recognition is an important topic of CAS systems because it offers solutions to numerous demands of the modern operating room(OR). For instance, such recognition is an important component to develop context-aware systems to monitor surgical processes [3], schedule surgeons [1] and enhance coordination among surgical teams [10]. The surgical phase recognition can be performed online or offline. The online surgical phase recognition is more challenging than offline since we are not allowed to use the information of future frames. However, online surgical phase recognition is more suitable for practical application, since the online recognition can support decision making during the surgery, especially for junior surgeons. This paper works on the online surgical phase recognition task.

Previous online surgical phase recognition approaches can be classified into two categories. The first one is dedicated to extracting discriminative visual

Electronic supplementary material The online version of this chapter (https:// doi.org/10.1007/978-3-030-32254-0_50) contains supplementary material, which is available to authorized users.

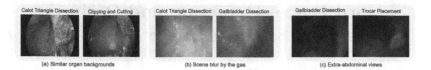

Fig. 1. Illustration of various hard frames in M2CAI16 Workflow Challenge. The text on the top of each frame indicates which phase it belongs to.

features to train a frame-wise classifier without utilizing temporal information, while the second one tries to combine temporal information in different manners. However, we observe that both approaches suffer from the existence of hard frames. As demonstrated in Fig. 1(a), (b) and (c), there are three types of hard frames. For hard frames of the same type, they have indistinguishable visual features but are assigned with different labels during the annotation. Owing to the visual similarity of hard frames, frame-wise methods perform poorly, and an example result is shown in Fig. 2(a). Combining temporal information can effectively help to classify hard frames, however, with the interference of hard frames, the captured temporal information may be heavily disturbed, resulting in additional errors, as shown in the Fig. 2(b). Moreover, the detection of spikes is not a trivial thing for online surgical workflow segmentation, resulting in severe over-segmentation problem.

One solution to address the challenge is to detect hard frames and handle them separately, which can benefit both training and testing. To be specific, for training, the negative impact of hard frames will be minimized if hard frames can be removed. For testing, the detected hard frames can be labeled as an additional class to separate from other simple frames, which can alleviate the disruption on the temporal structure. Meanwhile, the detected hard frames can be further treated by an online rectifying mechanism.

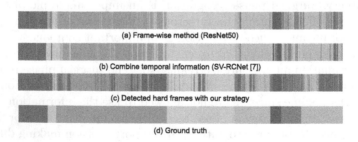

Fig. 2. Visualization of classification results on one test surgery in M2CAI16 Workflow Challenge. (a) Frame-wise method. (ResNet50 is used for illustration.) (b) Method combining temporal information. (SV-RCNet w/o post-processing [7] is used for illustration.) (c) Detected hard frames with our strategy, shown as the brown ribbon. (d) Ground truth labels.

Motivated by the above analyses, we propose a three-step approach to deal with the problems of hard frames. Since only the beginning and the end of a phase are manually annotated, hard frames that within the phase are automatically labeled. Therefore, we first take hard frames as mislabeled samples and employ a data cleansing strategy based on model predictions to find out hard frame samples in the training set. Next, these hard frames are labeled as an additional class to separate from other simple frames, and a classifier is trained to carry out both detection task for hard frames and phase recognition task for simple frames during the test, and example results are shown in Fig. 2(c). Finally, for the detected hard frames, we propose an Online Hard Frame Mapper (OHFM) to map them to corresponding phases. We extensively evaluate our solution on the M2CAI16 Workflow Challenge dataset and Cholec80 dataset. Our main contributions are summarized as follows. (1) For the first time, we explicitly raise the issues of hard frames and propose a novel solution for surgical phase recognition. (2) Our proposed solution achieves superior results on two benchmark datasets.

2   Related Work

Surgical Phase Recognition. Numerous approaches have been proposed to perform the surgical phase recognition task. Early studies use a frame-wise classifier to tackle videos frame-by-frame without using temporal information. These works focus on extracting discriminative visual features, such as various hand-crafted features [2,8] or deep CNN features [16]. The other type of approaches tries to combine temporal models in different manners. For example, a number of works utilize dynamic time warping [2,13], conditional random field [15], and variations of Hidden Markov Model (HMM) [9,12] to enforce temporal constraints to the output results. Jin et al. [7] train an end-to-end CNN-RNN model to encode both spatial and temporal information, which is referred to as SV-RCNet. However, the captured temporal information may contain noises caused by hard frames, leading to unreliable classification results. Furthermore, some works apply post-processing strategy to rectify the results, such as PKI [7], avg-smoothing [4]. However, the improvement by post-processing may highly depend on the hyper-parameters, and the generalization ability is limited.

Data Cleansing. Many methods have been proposed to cleanse training sets, with different degrees of success [5]. Some methods detect mislabeled instances with measures like the classification confidence [14] or the model complexity [6]. However, these methods are applicable to the condition where mislabeled samples are only a small part of the training set. While in surgical videos, the ratio of hard frames may be relatively large according to our experiment. Another type of methods relies on the predictions of classifiers [11]. They use a K-fold cross-validation scheme to obtain the predictions on every validation set, and then determine from the validation results whether a sample is mislabeled or not. In this paper, we adopt the second type of methods, but we take the detected samples as an additional class rather than ignoring it.

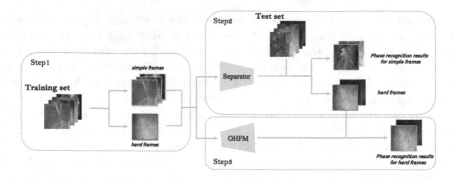

Fig. 3. The overview of our three-step solution for phase recognition task.

3   Methodology

The input of online phase recognition task is a video sequence $X = \{x_1, x_2, ..., x_m\}$ with N_p phases, the output is the corresponding phases $\{c_1, c_2, ..., c_m\}$ for each frame in the video sequence, where $c \in \{1, 2, ..., N_p\}$. Our solution consists of three main steps to tackle the phase recognition task, as illustrated in Fig. 3, and will be described in detail in following sections.

3.1   Data Cleansing for Training

Motivated by the observations that frame-wise classifiers often make mistakes on hard frames, we use a model-prediction based data cleansing strategy [5] which has two stages. The first stage consists of using a K-fold cross-validation scheme. Specifically, we randomly partition the training videos into K groups of equal size. Each time, a single group is retained for validation, and the remaining $K - 1$ groups are used to train a frame-wise classifier. In our experiment, we use *ResNet50* as our classifier, but it can be replaced with any frame-wise classification method. The second stage is to determine from the validation results whether a sample is hard or not. We simply take samples that are misclassified as hard frames.

3.2   Hard Frame Detection for Testing

We take hard frames in the training set as an additional class and train another ResNet50 classifier with $(N_p + 1)$ classes, which is referred to as "*Separator*" for further discussion. *Separator* carries out the detection task for hard frames and the recognition task for simple frames simultaneously by outputting the class label $\hat{c}$ for the input frame x, where $\hat{c} \in \{0, 1, 2, ..., N_p\}$. To be specific, $\hat{c} \in \{1, 2, ..., N_p\}$ represents the phase recognition results while $\hat{c} = 0$ stands for the detected hard frame, which will be further rectified by the Online Hard Frame Mapper (OHFM).

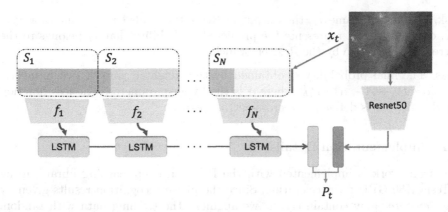

Fig. 4. Architecture of OHFM network for hard frame mapping. In LSTM branch, previous prediction sequence is split into N sub-sequences of equal length, denoted as $\{S_1, S_2, ..., S_N\}$. f_i is the extracted feature for each sub-sequence. LSTM take $\{f_i\}$ as input to obtain the prediction result for hard frame x_t. In the ResNet branch, visual features are extracted by ResNet50 to help with the mapping task.

3.3 Online Hard Frame Mapper

For a detected hard frame x_t, we proposed an Online Hard Frame Mapper (OHFM) to map it to its corresponding phase with two branches. The LSTM branch is designed for utilizing the classification sequence of previous frames while the ResNet branch tries to extract useful visual features of x_t. The architecture of OHFM is illustrated in Fig. 4.

LSTM Branch. Previous predictions are very helpful for us to map hard frame samples to its correct phase. Suppose $C_{t-1} = \{\hat{c}_1, \hat{c}_2, ..., \hat{c}_{t-1}\}$ is the previous prediction sequence given by the *Separator* which is described in Sect. 3.2. Note that hard frames are labeled as an additional class to be different from original phases. Therefore, the temporal interruption caused by the hard frames can be alleviated. We split sequence C_{t-1} into N sub-sequences of equal size, denoted as $\{S_1, S_2, ..., S_N\}$. For each sub-sequence S_i, two types of features are extracted. First, we find out the phase that appears most frequently and encode it with one-hot encoding, denoted as $M(S_i)$. Then, we calculate the proportion of each phase, denoted as $Pr(S_i)$. The change in proportion of phases in each bin is used to reflect the surgical procedure since the timestamp is not available in online surgical workflow segmentation. Both $M(S_i)$ and $Pr(S_i)$ are $(N_p + 1)$-dimension vectors, and then are concatenated to form the final feature f_i. The LSTM network takes $\{f_i\}$ as input. The output of the last LSTM cell is a N_p-dimension vector, denoted as P_{lb}, which represents the predicted probability that x_t belongs to the corresponding phases by the LSTM branch.

ResNet Branch. Visual features can be helpful in the condition where the LSTM branch is not confident about its predictions. Therefore, we construct a 50-layer ResNet and try to extract useful visual information to help with the mapping task. For a hard frame x_t, the output of ResNet50 is also a N_p-dimension vector, denoted as P_{rb}, represents the predicted probability that x_t belongs to the corresponding phase by the ResNet branch.

Loss. The final probability is obtained by the weighted sum of two branches: $P_t = \alpha * P_{lb} + (1 - \alpha) * P_{rb}$, where α is the hyper-parameter. The loss function for the mapper is defined as a cross-entropy loss.

3.4   Implementation Details

Our framework is implemented with the PyTorch deep learning library, using 8 Tesla K80 GPU for acceleration. Since the phase recognition results given by the *Separator* may contain errors, we augment the training data with random noise to effectively train our OHFM. Specifically, for the phase that appears most frequently in each sub-sequence, it will be randomly changed to any other phases with the probability of 15%. We set $N = 240$ and $\alpha = 0.95$ for our experiment. The frames before $N = 240$ are labeled as the initial phase of the surgical video.

4   Experiment

4.1   Dataset

M2CAI16 Workflow Challenge. The M2CAI16 Workflow Challenge dataset contains 41 laparoscopic videos that are acquired at 25 fps of cholecystectomy procedures, and 27 of them are used for training and 14 videos are used for testing. These videos are segmented into 8 phases by experienced surgeons.

Cholec80. The Cholec80 dataset contains 80 videos of cholecystectomy surgeries performed by 13 surgeons. The dataset is divided into training set (40 videos) and testing set (40 videos). The videos are divided into 7 phases and are captured at 25 fps.

For training data preparation, the original videos are downsampled from 25 fps to 5 fps. The resolution of the frames is resized to 256×256 to save the GPU memory. All the results are reported on the full test set.

4.2   Data Cleansing Result

We set $K = 9$ (3 videos in 1 group) for M2CAI16 Workflow Challenge and $K = 10$ (4 videos in 1 group) for Cholec80. Table 1 shows the proportion of hard frames in each phase. As shown in Table 1, almost half of the frames in the *Preparation* phase are cleaned up as hard frames. This makes sense because illumination and extra-abdominal views are more likely to occur during instrument insertion in the preparation phase. The example hard frames can be found in the supplementary material.

To verify the effectiveness of our method, a simple experiment is conducted. The ResNet50 network is respectively trained by the original training set and

Table 1. The statistics of hard frames in the traning set.

	M2CAI16	Cholec80
TrocarPlacement	0.27	-
Preparation	0.60	0.45
CalotTriangleDissection	0.22	0.16
ClippingCutting	0.33	0.31
GallbladderDissection	0.28	0.17
GallbladderPackaging	0.27	0.38
CleaningCoagulation	0.29	0.38
GallbladderRetraction	0.40	0.41
Overall	**0.30**	**0.23**

Table 2. The performance gain of ResNet50 after removing hard frames.

	M2CAI16 Workflow Challenge		Cholec80	
	Accuracy ↑	Jacc ↑	Accuracy ↑	Jacc ↑
Clean training set	**1.0%** ↑	**3.1%** ↑	**2.4%** ↑	**4.1%** ↑

the clean training set, from which the hard frames we find are removed. The experiment is repeated 3 times, and the average results are reported. Table 2 shows the performance gain after the hard frames are removed. As the result shows, the existence of hard frames will cause negative impacts to the training process, and it is feasible to mine these hard frames out via data cleansing strategy.

Table 3. Phase recognition results

	M2CAI16		Cholec80	
	Accuracy	Jacc	Accuracy	Jacc
ResNet50	76.3 ± 8.9	56.4 ± 10.4	78.3 ± 7.7	52.2 ± 15.0
PhaseNet [17]	79.5 ± 12.1	64.1 ± 10.3	78.8 ± 4.7	-
EndoNet [16]	-	-	81.7 ± 4.2	-
EndoNet-GTbin [16]	-	-	81.9 ± 4.4	-
SV-RCNet w/o PKI [7]	81.7 ± 8.1	65.4 ± 8.9	85.3 ± 7.3	
Ours[a]	$\mathbf{85.2 \pm 7.5}$	$\mathbf{68.8 \pm 10.5}$	$\mathbf{87.3 \pm 5.7}$	$\mathbf{67.0 \pm 13.3}$
Cadene et al.(nearest online)[4]	86.9 ± 11.0	71.9 ± 12.7	-	-
SV-RCNet + PKI [7]	90.7 ± 6.9	78.2 ± 11.0	92.4 ± 6.9	
Ours + PKI*	$\mathbf{91.2 \pm 5.0}$	$\mathbf{78.7 \pm 13.1}$	$\mathbf{92.4 \pm 5.6}$	$\mathbf{77.0 \pm 11.8}$

[a] We evaluate the experiment on the complete test set for 3 times, and the average results are reported.

4.3   Phase Recognition Results

Table 3 shows a comparison of our solution and others. We first compare our results with the top methods that took part in M2CAI16 Challenge without post-processing strategy. Our solution achieves better performance than the state-of-the-art SV-RCNet [7] by a significant margin, improving accuracy from 81.7% to 85.2% on M2CAI16 Workflow Challenge, and from 85.3% to 87.3% on Cholec80. Note that some methods employ a post-processing scheme for further improvement. To make a fair comparison, we simply modify the PKI [7] post-processing scheme for our solution, denoted as PKI*, which integrates the phase-transition priors. Our final results that integrate post-processing scheme (PKI*) outperform all other approaches.

4.4   Discussion

The main difference between OHFM and PKI scheme is that PKI explicitly use the human-predefined phase transition priors while OHFM learns it from the training data. Compared to PKI scheme and its variants, the OHFM is more general to the unknown surgical videos in real word scenarios and is not sensitive to the hyper parameters. However, it is hard to learn the phase transition well with small amount of training videos.

5   Conclusion and Future Work

In this paper, we focus on the problems of hard frames in surgical phase recognition task and propose a novel solution by detecting hard frames during training and testing. Different from previous works that classify all frames indiscriminately, we first classify those simple frames, and the remaining hard frames are tackled by a further rectifying mechanism. The current results are promising, we believe that there is more room for further improvement in this direction.

Acknowledgement. This work was partially supported by the National Basic Research Program of China (973 Program) under contract 2015CB351803, the Natural Science Foundation of China under contracts 61572042 and 61527804. We also acknowledge the Clinical Medicine Plus X-Young Scholars Project, and High-Performance Computing Platform of Peking University for providing computational resources.

References

1. Beenish, B., Tim, O., Yan, X., Peter, H.: Real-time identification of operating room state from video. In: Proceedings of the 19th Conference on Innovative Applications of Artificial Intelligence, vol. 2, pp. 1761–1766 (2007)
2. Blum, T., Feußner, H., Navab, N.: Modeling and segmentation of surgical workflow from laparoscopic video. In: Jiang, T., Navab, N., Pluim, J.P.W., Viergever, M.A. (eds.) MICCAI 2010. LNCS, vol. 6363, pp. 400–407. Springer, Heidelberg (2010). https://doi.org/10.1007/978-3-642-15711-0_50

3. Bricon-Souf, N., Newman, C.R.: Context awareness in health care: a review. Int. J. Med. Inform. **76**(1), 2–12 (2007)
4. Cadène, R., Robert, T., Thome, N., Cord, M.: MICCAI workflow challenge: convolutional neural networks with time smoothing and Hidden Markov Model for video frames classification. arxiv abs/1610.05541 (2016)
5. Frenay, B., Verleysen, M.: Classification in the presence of label noise: a survey. IEEE Trans. Neural Netw. Learn. Syst. **25**(5), 845–869 (2014)
6. Gamberger, D., Lavrac, N., Dzeroski, S.: Noise detection and elimination in data preprocessing: experiments in medical domains. Appl. Artif. Intell. **14**(2), 205–223 (2000)
7. Jin, Y., et al.: SV-RCNet: workflow recognition from surgical videos using recurrent convolutional network. IEEE Trans. Med. Imaging **37**(5), 1114–1126 (2018)
8. Lalys, F., Riffaud, L., Bouget, D., Jannin, P.: A framework for the recognition of high-level surgical tasks from video images for cataract surgeries. IEEE Trans. Biomed. Eng. **59**(4), 966–976 (2012)
9. Lalys, F., Riffaud, L., Morandi, X., Jannin, P.: Surgical phases detection from microscope videos by combining SVM and HMM. In: Menze, B., Langs, G., Tu, Z., Criminisi, A. (eds.) MCV 2010. LNCS, vol. 6533, pp. 54–62. Springer, Heidelberg (2011). https://doi.org/10.1007/978-3-642-18421-5_6
10. Lin, H.C., Shafran, I., Murphy, T.E., Okamura, A.M., Yuh, D.D., Hager, G.D.: Automatic detection and segmentation of robot-assisted surgical motions. In: Duncan, J.S., Gerig, G. (eds.) MICCAI 2005. LNCS, vol. 3749, pp. 802–810. Springer, Heidelberg (2005). https://doi.org/10.1007/11566465_99
11. Miranda, A.L.B., Garcia, L.P.F., Carvalho, A.C.P.L.F., Lorena, A.C.: Use of classification algorithms in noise detection and elimination. In: Corchado, E., Wu, X., Oja, E., Herrero, Á., Baruque, B. (eds.) HAIS 2009. LNCS (LNAI), vol. 5572, pp. 417–424. Springer, Heidelberg (2009). https://doi.org/10.1007/978-3-642-02319-4_50
12. Padoy, N., Blum, T., Feussner, H., Berger, M.O., Navab, N.: On-line recognition of surgical activity for monitoring in the operating room. In: Proceedings of the 20th Conference on Innovative Applications of Artificial Intelligence, vol. 3, pp. 1718–1724 (2008)
13. Padoy, N., Blum, T., Ahmadi, S.A., Feussner, H., Berger, M.O., Navab, N.: Statistical modeling and recognition of surgical workflow. Med. Image Anal. **16**(3), 632–641 (2012)
14. Sun, J., Zhao, F., Wang, C., Chen, S.: Identifying and correcting mislabeled training instances. In: Future Generation Communication and Networking (FGCN 2007), vol. 1, pp. 244–250 (2007)
15. Tao, L., Zappella, L., Hager, G.D., Vidal, R.: Surgical gesture segmentation and recognition. In: Mori, K., Sakuma, I., Sato, Y., Barillot, C., Navab, N. (eds.) MICCAI 2013. LNCS, vol. 8151, pp. 339–346. Springer, Heidelberg (2013). https://doi.org/10.1007/978-3-642-40760-4_43
16. Twinanda, A.P., Shehata, S., et al.: EndoNet: a deep architecture for recognition tasks on laparoscopic videos. IEEE Trans. Med. Imaging **36**(1), 86–97 (2017)
17. Twinanda, A.P., Mutter, D., et al.: Single- and multi-task architectures for surgical workflow challenge at M2CAI 2016. arxiv abs/1610.08844 (2016)

Automated Surgical Activity Recognition with One Labeled Sequence

Robert DiPietro[(⊠)] and Gregory D. Hager

Department of Computer Science, Johns Hopkins University, Baltimore, MD, USA
rdipietro@gmail.com

Abstract. Prior work has demonstrated the feasibility of automated activity recognition in robot-assisted surgery from motion data. However, these efforts have assumed the availability of a large number of densely-annotated sequences, which must be provided manually by experts. This process is tedious, expensive, and error-prone. In this paper, we present the first analysis under the assumption of scarce annotations, where as little as *one annotated sequence* is available for training. We demonstrate feasibility of automated recognition in this challenging setting, and we show that learning representations in an unsupervised fashion, before the recognition phase, leads to significant gains in performance. In addition, our paper poses a new challenge to the community: how much further can we push performance in this important yet relatively unexplored regime?

Keywords: Surgical activity recognition · Gesture recognition · Maneuver recognition · Semi-supervised learning

1 Introduction

The advent of robot-assisted surgery has spawned many new research areas, in large part because it allows the capture of high-quality surgical-motion data at scale. Two examples are objective performance assessment [15,16] and automated feedback for trainees [5], which have the potential to transform surgical training curricula and in turn improve patient outcomes [2]. An important prerequisite task toward these goals and others is *surgical activity recognition*, where we aim to automatically segment and label surgical-motion data according to the activities being performed by a surgeon or trainee.

Significant progress has been made in surgical activity recognition, especially within the context of simulated training [1,6,8], an important part of current training curricula [14]. Though promising, these approaches have relied on large amounts of annotated data, which, unlike the surgical-motion data itself, must be provided *manually* by experts. This process is expensive, error-prone, and often subjective, especially when carried out at scale.

Despite these difficulties, literature has largely ignored activity recognition in the context of scarce annotations. To our knowledge, the only exceptions have been in the form of preprints, and have focused on video-based recognition

© Springer Nature Switzerland AG 2019
D. Shen et al. (Eds.): MICCAI 2019, LNCS 11768, pp. 458–466, 2019.
https://doi.org/10.1007/978-3-030-32254-0_51

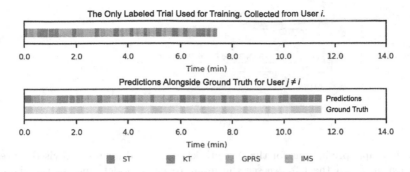

Fig. 1. Example predictions for maneuver recognition, using only a single labeled sequence for training. Here representations were learned with the RNN-Based Future Prediction model prior to recognition. It exhibits a representative error rate (19.4%) and an edit distance that is worse than average (40.7%). Results are similar for the RNN-Based Generative Model. The activities are *suture throw* (ST), *knot tying* (KT), *grasp pull run suture* (GPRS), and *intermaneuver segment* (IMS).

rather than motion-based recognition [4,17,18]. The most closely related work to this paper is [7], in which we explored unsupervised learning of surgical motion via future prediction. Two limitations of [7] are 1. considering applications to motion-based search rather than the predominant task of activity recognition and 2. considering models that assume independence over time, which lead to blurry, incoherent future prediction (see Fig. 2).

The primary contributions of this paper are 1. demonstrating the feasibility of activity recognition in annotation-scarce settings (e.g., Fig. 1); 2. showing that preceding recognition with unsupervised representation learning leads to significant gains in recognition performance for both maneuver recognition and gesture recognition (e.g., Figs. 3 and 5); 3. introducing a probabilistic generative model over surgical motion that makes no simplifying assumption of independence over time (Sect. 2); and 4. showing that this generative model is especially important when used to recognize activities that exhibit fine-grained structure over short time scales (Fig. 5).

2   Methods

We let $\mathbf{X} \equiv \{\mathbf{x}_t\}_1^T$ denote a sequence of kinematics, with each $\mathbf{x}_t \in \mathbb{R}^{n_x}$ (containing, e.g., joint velocities), and we let $\mathbf{Y} \equiv \{y_t\}_1^T$ denote a corresponding sequence of activities, where each y_t is an integer (specifying an activity). We aim to learn a mapping from $\mathbf{X}$ to $\mathbf{Y}$, which corresponds to joint segmentation and classification. This is accomplished in two phases. The first is representation learning, where we learn a transformation from $\mathbf{X}$ to $\tilde{\mathbf{X}} \equiv \{\tilde{\mathbf{x}}_t\}_1^T$ through an auxiliary task that requires no annotations. The second is recognition, in which we learn a mapping from $\tilde{\mathbf{X}}$ to $\mathbf{Y}$.

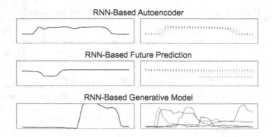

Fig. 2. Example predictions for the three tasks considered for unsupervised representation learning. On the left, we see the input to each model; and on the right, we see sampled predictions. The autoencoder reconstructs the input window; the future-prediction model predicts a window assuming independence over time steps, conditioned on a previous window; and the generative model predicts coherent futures of any length, conditioned on the entire past (5 sampled trajectories are shown).

Representation Learning Overview. We consider three models for representation learning. The first two mimic those from [7], where they were used for motion-based search. The first, the RNN-Based Autoencoder, aims to reconstruct a given window of kinematics through a bottleneck; and the second, RNN-Based Future Prediction, models a *window* of future motion conditioned on a *window* of previous motion, *assuming conditional independence over time.* The third model, which we introduce here and refer to as the RNN-Based Generative Model, is a generative model over all of $\mathbf{X}$, *without* any simplifying assumption of independence over time. Here we describe the RNN-Based Generative Model in detail, and we refer the reader to [7] for a full description of the RNN-Based Future Prediction and RNN-Based Autoencoder models.

The RNN-Based Generative Model. The RNN-Based Generative Model models the full joint distribution over $\mathbf{X}$ by making use of the chain rule,

$$p(\mathbf{x}_1, \mathbf{x}_2, \dots, \mathbf{x}_T) = p(\mathbf{x}_1)p(\mathbf{x}_2 \mid \mathbf{x}_1)p(\mathbf{x}_3 \mid \mathbf{x}_1, \mathbf{x}_2) \cdots p(\mathbf{x}_T \mid \mathbf{x}_1, \dots, \mathbf{x}_{T-1}) \quad (1)$$

This representation facilitates the use of recurrent neural networks and mixture density networks [3] to model each factor in the product sequentially: At time t, we use long short-term memory (LSTM) [12,13] to map from the previous kinematics vector $\mathbf{x}_{t-1}$ and previous hidden state $\mathbf{h}_{t-1}$ to a new hidden state (the LSTM cell $\mathbf{c}_t$ is omitted here for simplicity):

$$\mathbf{h}_t = \mathrm{LSTM}(\mathbf{x}_{t-1}, \mathbf{h}_{t-1}) \quad (2)$$

Next, we map from $\mathbf{h}_t$ to the parameters that govern the distribution $p(\mathbf{x}_t \mid \mathbf{x}_1, \dots, \mathbf{x}_{t-1})$. This can be any reasonable distribution of our choosing. Following [7] for simplicity and fair comparisons, we map from $\mathbf{h}_t$ to the parameters of a mixture of Gaussians with diagonal covariance via

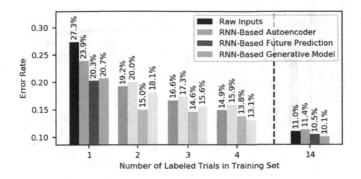

Fig. 3. MISTIC-SL maneuver recognition: error rate vs. number of labeled trials. The bottom of the y axis is set to 8.7%, the best published result using LSTM ($\sim$36 labeled trials). The non-transparent results are reported over exhaustive, deterministic splits (see Sect. 3.2) which can be compared to in future work.

$$\boldsymbol{\pi}_t = \text{softmax}(\mathbf{W}_\pi\,\mathbf{h}_t + \mathbf{b}_\pi) \tag{3}$$

$$\boldsymbol{\mu}_t^{(c)} = \mathbf{W}_\mu^{(c)}\,\mathbf{h}_t + \mathbf{b}_\mu^{(c)} \tag{4}$$

$$\mathbf{v}_t^{(c)} = \text{softplus}(\mathbf{W}_v^{(c)}\,\mathbf{h}_t + \mathbf{b}_v^{(c)}) \tag{5}$$

with the conditional distribution over $\mathbf{x}_t$ then specified as

$$p(\mathbf{x}_t \mid \mathbf{x}_1, \dots, \mathbf{x}_{t-1}) = \sum_c \pi_t^{(c)}\,\mathcal{N}\left(\mathbf{x}_t;\ \boldsymbol{\mu}_t^{(c)}, \mathbf{v}_t^{(c)}\right) \tag{6}$$

All weight matrices $\mathbf{W}$ and all biases $\mathbf{b}$, in both the LSTM and in the mapping from hidden states to distribution parameters, are learned by maximizing (the logarithm of) Eq. 1. After training, the sequence of hidden states from the LSTM, $\mathbf{H}$, is used as inputs in the recognition phase: $\tilde{\mathbf{X}} = \mathbf{H}$.

Recognition Overview. We discriminatively model $p(\mathbf{Y} \mid \tilde{\mathbf{X}})$ using the multi-layered, bidirectional LSTM architecture from [6]. First, $\tilde{\mathbf{X}}$ is transformed into a sequence of hidden states $\mathbf{H}$ (simply LSTM hidden states, distinct from $\mathbf{H}$ of the previous section), and these hidden states are then mapped in the standard fashion (through affine transformations) to the parameters that govern the categorical distributions over each $p(y_t \mid \tilde{\mathbf{X}})$. Training is carried out by maximizing conditional likelihood under this model, or equivalently by minimizing cross entropy. Please see [6] for more detail.

3 Experiments

Here we study recognition performance in the annotation-scarce setting across two datasets and four approaches: recognition from raw inputs and recognition from learned representations using the autoencoder, the future-prediction model,

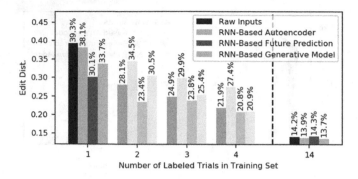

Fig. 4. MISTIC-SL maneuver recognition: edit distance vs. number of labeled trials. The bottom of the y axis is set to 12.1%, the best published result using LSTM ($\sim$36 labeled trials). The non-transparent results are reported over exhaustive, deterministic splits (see Sect. 3.2) which can be compared to in future work.

and the full generative model. For recognition, we use the state-of-the-art model from [6]. We also carry over the same hyperparameters, which were optimized in [6] for recognition using raw inputs. Thus any improvements from using learned representations are not due to tuning.

3.1   Datasets

The two datasets used are the Minimally Invasive Surgical Training and Innovation Center – Science of Learning dataset (MISTIC-SL) [9,11] and the JHU-ISI Gesture and Skill Assessment Working Set (JIGSAWS) [1,10]. Both datasets consist of two distinct components: 1. Measurements recorded automatically over time as a trainee operates the *da Vinci*, including motion data, and 2. dense activity labels over time that were provided manually by experts.

MISTIC-SL focuses on recognizing maneuvers, with each activity label being 1 of 4 different manuevers: *suture throw* (ST), *knot tying* (KT), *grasp pull run suture* (GPRS), or *intermaneuver segment* (IMS). As input, we use 14 kinematic signals: velocities along the 3 axes, angular velocities along the 3 axes, and gripper angle, all for both the left and right hands. All signals are provided at 50 Hz, which following [6,8] we downsample by a factor of 6. The data was collected in a benchtop training environment. We follow [8,11] and use 39 right-handed trials from 15 subjects, most of whom were residents.

JIGSAWS focuses on recognizing gestures – short, low-level activities such as *pushing needle through tissue* (see [1] for a full list). We follow the majority of prior work and focus on the *Suturing* task. Here each activity label is 1 of 10 different gestures. As input, we use the same 14 kinematic signals. Here, all signals are provided at 30 Hz, and following [6,8] we downsample by a factor of 6. The data was collected in a benchtop training environment and consists of 39 trials from 8 different subjects, most of whom were medical students.

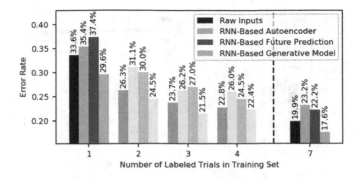

Fig. 5. JIGSAWS gesture recognition: error rate vs. number of labeled trials. The bottom of the y axis is set to 15.3%, the best published result using LSTM (~35 labeled trials). The non-transparent results are reported over exhaustive, deterministic splits (see Sect. 3.2) which can be compared to in future work.

3.2   Experimental Design

The recognition model from [6] consists of bidirectional LSTM with 3 layers, each with 64 hidden units, and is optimized using Adam and a learning rate of $10^{-2.5}$. All hyperparameters are carried over unchanged except the batch size: we use a batch size of 1 because it is the only possible option in many of our experiments. Training is carried out for 100 epochs. The metrics considered are frame-wise error rate and segment-wise edit distance (Levenshtein distance), normalized by the maximum number of segments in any one trial to aid interpretability, following prior work. In focusing on generalization across users, *any particular training set consists of exactly one labeled trial per user*, with between 1 and $u-1$ labeled trials, where u is the number of users in the dataset. In all cases, results are averaged over splits, exhaustively for 1 trial and $u-1$ trials and randomly otherwise (in this case 10 splits are randomly sampled).

During the representation-learning phase, the most important hyperparameters are the number of LSTM hidden units (n_h) and the number of components in the Gaussian mixture model (n_c). For the autoencoder and future-prediction models, these were tuned in [7] to maximize performance on a held-out set of 4 MISTIC-SL users, and here we use the same values ($n_h = 64, n_c = 16$). We followed the same process for the RNN-Based Generative Model. Tuning is carried out using the unsupervised-learning objective, not the recognition objective. This led to values of $n_h = 128, n_c = 8$. In all cases, training was carried out for 100 epochs using Adam, with a learning rate of 0.005.

3.3   Results and Discussion

Figure 2 shows examples of the gripper-angle signal from MISTIC-SL to illustrate the three unsupervised-learning tasks. Future prediction yields blurred, incoherent futures, whereas the generative model samples detailed trajectories.

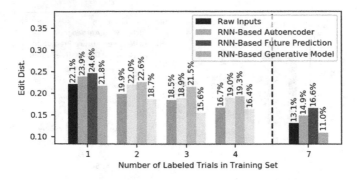

Fig. 6. JIGSAWS gesture recognition: edit distance vs. number of labeled trials. The bottom of the y axis is set to 8.4%, the best published result using LSTM (~35 labeled trials). The non-transparent results are reported over exhaustive, deterministic splits (see Sect. 3.2) which can be compared to in future work.

This suggests that the generative model's representations may be better suited for fine-grained activities; and this is confirmed below in the case of JIGSAWS.

Figure 3 shows error rate vs. the number of labeled trials for maneuver recognition (MISTIC-SL). Using only one labeled trial, raw inputs for recognition lead to an error rate of 27.3%; the autoencoder representations lead to an improvement, obtaining 23.9%; and the future-prediction and generative models lead to further improvements, obtaining 20.3% and 20.7% respectively. Figure 1 shows qualitative results using only 1 labeled trial with future prediction (results are similar for the generative model). When 14 labeled trials are used, the generative model yields the lowest error rate (10.1%). For reference, the state-of-the-art LSTM result using 36 labeled trials is 8.7% [6]. Figure 4 shows results for edit distance; the same general trends hold.

Figure 5 shows error rate vs. the number of labeled trials for gesture recognition (JIGSAWS). Using only one labeled trial, raw inputs lead to an error rate of 33.6%. Representations from the full generative model reduce the error rate to 29.6%, while the autoencoder and future-prediction based representations both degrade performance. This is not surprising: we have no reason to believe that the autoencoder's task of signal reconstruction is well aligned with the task of activity recognition; and for future prediction, we have seen above that blurry, uncoherent futures are obtained, and this is likely detrimental to recognizing fine-grained activities such as gestures. When 7 labeled trials are used for training, the generative model again yields the lowest error rate (17.6%). For reference, the state-of-the-art LSTM result using 35 labeled trials is 15.3% [6]. Figure 6 shows results for edit distance; the same general trends hold.

4   Conclusions and Future Work

Automated activity recognition in the presence of few annotations is an important problem which we believe warrants more attention. This work presented the first analysis of surgical activity recognition in this setting. We found that recognition is feasible using only one annotated sequence, and that leveraging learned representations, obtained in an unsupervised fashion, leads to performance boosts at recognition time. The RNN-based generative model introduced in this work is particularly strong for this purpose, especially when recognizing activities that occur over short time scales, as in gesture recognition. That said, a significant gap still exists in performances when fewer annotated sequences are available for training. We hope that the community will join us in seeing how much we can improve performance in this important annotation-limited regime.

Acknowledgements. This work was supported by a fellowship for modeling, simulation, and training from the Link Foundation. We also thank Anand Malpani, Madeleine Waldram, Swaroop Vedula, Gyusung I. Lee, and Mija R. Lee for procuring the MISTIC-SL dataset. The procurement of MISTIC-SL was supported by the Johns Hopkins Science of Learning Institute.

References

1. Ahmidi, N., et al.: A dataset and benchmarks for segmentation and recognition of gestures in robotic surgery. IEEE Trans. Biomed. Eng. **64**(9), 2025–2041 (2017)
2. Birkmeyer, J.D., et al.: Surgical skill and complication rates after bariatric surgery. New Engl. J. Med. **369**(15), 1434–1442 (2013)
3. Bishop, C.M.: Mixture density networks. Technical report, Aston University (1994)
4. Bodenstedt, S., et al.: Unsupervised temporal context learning using convolutional neural networks for laparoscopic workflow analysis. arXiv preprint arXiv:1702.03684 (2017)
5. Chen, Z., et al.: Virtual fixture assistance for needle passing and knot tying. In: Intelligent Robots and Systems (IROS), pp. 2343–2350 (2016)
6. DiPietro, R., et al.: Segmenting and classifying activities in robot-assisted surgery with recurrent neural networks. Int. J. Comput. Assist. Radiol. Surg. (2019)
7. DiPietro, R., Hager, G.D.: Unsupervised learning for surgical motion by learning to predict the future. In: Frangi, A.F., Schnabel, J.A., Davatzikos, C., Alberola-López, C., Fichtinger, G. (eds.) MICCAI 2018. LNCS, vol. 11073, pp. 281–288. Springer, Cham (2018). https://doi.org/10.1007/978-3-030-00937-3_33
8. DiPietro, R., et al.: Recognizing surgical activities with recurrent neural networks. In: Ourselin, S., Joskowicz, L., Sabuncu, M.R., Unal, G., Wells, W. (eds.) MICCAI 2016. LNCS, vol. 9900, pp. 551–558. Springer, Cham (2016). https://doi.org/10.1007/978-3-319-46720-7_64
9. Gao, Y., Vedula, S.S., Lee, G.I., Lee, M.R., Khudanpur, S., Hager, G.D.: Query-by-example surgical activity detection. Int. J. Comput. Assist. Radiol. Surg. **11**(6), 987–996 (2016)
10. Gao, Y., et al.: Language of surgery: a surgical gesture dataset for human motion modeling. In: Modeling and Monitoring of Computer Assisted Interventions (2014)
11. Gao, Y., Vedula, S., Lee, G.I., Lee, M.R., Khudanpur, S., Hager, G.D.: Unsupervised surgical data alignment with application to automatic activity annotation. In: 2016 IEEE International Conference on Robotics and Automation (ICRA) (2016)
12. Gers, F.A., Schmidhuber, J., Cummins, F.: Learning to forget: continual prediction with LSTM. Neural Comput. **12**(10), 2451–2471 (2000)

13. Hochreiter, S., Schmidhuber, J.: Long short-term memory. Neural Comput. **9**(8), 1735–1780 (1997)
14. Jacobs, D.M., Poenaru, D. (eds.): Surgical Educators' Handbook. Association for Surgical Education, Los Angeles (2001)
15. Reiley, C.E., Akinbiyi, T., Burschka, D., Chang, D.C., Okamura, A.M., Yuh, D.D.: Effects of visual force feedback on robot-assisted surgical task performance. J. Thorac. Cardiovasc. Surg. **135**(1), 196–202 (2008)
16. Vedula, S.S., Malpani, A., Ahmidi, N., Khudanpur, S., Hager, G., Chen, C.C.G.: Task-level vs. segment-level quantitative metrics for surgical skill assessment. J. Surg. Educ. **73**(3), 482–489 (2016)
17. Yengera, G., Mutter, D., Marescaux, J., Padoy, N.: Less is more: surgical phase recognition with less annotations through self-supervised pre-training of CNN-LSTM networks. arXiv preprint arXiv:1805.08569 (2018)
18. Yu, T., Mutter, D., Marescaux, J., Padoy, N.: Learning from a tiny dataset of manual annotations: a teacher/student approach for surgical phase recognition. arXiv preprint arXiv:1812.00033 (2018)

Using 3D Convolutional Neural Networks to Learn Spatiotemporal Features for Automatic Surgical Gesture Recognition in Video

Isabel Funke[1]([✉])[iD], Sebastian Bodenstedt[1][iD], Florian Oehme[2],
Felix von Bechtolsheim[2], Jürgen Weitz[2,3], and Stefanie Speidel[1,3]

[1] Division of Translational Surgical Oncology,
National Center for Tumor Diseases (NCT), Partner Site Dresden, Dresden, Germany
Isabel.Funke@nct-dresden.de
[2] Department for Visceral, Thoracic and Vascular Surgery,
University Hospital Carl Gustav Carus, TU Dresden, Dresden, Germany
[3] Centre for Tactile Internet with Human-in-the-Loop (CeTI),
TU Dresden, Dresden, Germany

Abstract. Automatically recognizing surgical gestures is a crucial step towards a thorough understanding of surgical skill. Possible areas of application include automatic skill assessment, intra-operative monitoring of critical surgical steps, and semi-automation of surgical tasks. Solutions that rely only on the laparoscopic video and do not require additional sensor hardware are especially attractive as they can be implemented at low cost in many scenarios. However, surgical gesture recognition based only on video is a challenging problem that requires effective means to extract both visual and temporal information from the video. Previous approaches mainly rely on frame-wise feature extractors, either handcrafted or learned, which fail to capture the dynamics in surgical video. To address this issue, we propose to use a 3D Convolutional Neural Network (CNN) to learn spatiotemporal features from consecutive video frames. We evaluate our approach on recordings of robot-assisted suturing on a bench-top model, which are taken from the publicly available JIGSAWS dataset. Our approach achieves high frame-wise surgical gesture recognition accuracies of more than 84%, outperforming comparable models that either extract only spatial features or model spatial and low-level temporal information separately. For the first time, these results demonstrate the benefit of spatiotemporal CNNs for video-based surgical gesture recognition.

Keywords: Surgical gesture · Spatiotemporal modeling · Video understanding · Action segmentation · Convolutional Neural Network

Electronic supplementary material The online version of this chapter (https:// doi.org/10.1007/978-3-030-32254-0_52) contains supplementary material, which is available to authorized users.

1   Introduction

Surgical gestures [1] are the basic elements of every surgical process. Recognizing which surgical gesture is being performed is crucial for understanding the current surgical situation and for providing meaningful computer assistance to the surgeon. Automatic surgical gesture recognition also offers new possibilities for surgical training. For example, it may enable a computer-assisted surgical training system to observe whether gestures are performed in the correct order or to identify with which gestures a trainee struggles the most.

Especially appealing is the exploitation of ubiquitous video feeds for surgical gesture recognition, such as the feed of the laparoscopic camera, which displays the surgical field in conventional and robot-assisted minimally invasive surgery. The problem of *video-based* surgical gesture recognition is formalized as follows: A video of length T is a sequence of video frames $v_t, t = 1, ..., T$. The problem is to predict the gesture $g(t) \in \mathcal{G}$ performed at time t for each $t = 1, ..., T$, where $\mathcal{G} = \{1, ..., G\}$ is the set of surgical gestures. Variations of surgical gesture recognition differ in the amount of information that is available to obtain an estimate $\hat{g}(t)$ of the current gesture, e.g., (i) only the current video frame, i.e., $\hat{g}(t) = \hat{g}(v_t)$ (*frame-wise* recognition), (ii) only frames up until the current timestep, i.e., $\hat{g}(t) = \hat{g}(v_k, ..., v_t), k \geq 1$ (*on-line* recognition), or (iii) the complete video, i.e., $\hat{g}(t) = \hat{g}(v_1, ..., v_T)$ (*off-line* recognition).

The main challenge in video-based surgical gesture recognition is the high dimensionality, high level of redundancy, and high complexity of video data. State-of-the-art methods tackle the problem by transforming video frames into feature representations, which are fed into temporal models that infer the sequence of gestures based on the input sequence. These temporal models have been continuously improved in the last years, starting with variants of Hidden Markov Models [12] and Conditional Random Fields [9,13] and evolving into deep learning-based methods such as Recurrent Neural Networks [3], Temporal Convolutional Networks (TCN) [10], and Deep Reinforcement Learning (RL) [11].

To obtain feature representations from video frames, early approaches compute bag-of-features histograms from feature descriptors extracted around space-time interest points or dense trajectories [13]. More recently, *Convolutional Neural Networks (CNNs)* became a popular tool for visual feature extraction. For example, Lea et al. train a CNN (*S-CNN*) for frame-wise gesture recognition [9] and use the latent video frame encodings as feature representations, which are further processed by a TCN for gesture recognition [10]. A TCN combines 1D convolutional filters with pooling and channel-wise normalization layers to hierarchically capture temporal relationships at low-, intermediate-, and high-level time scales.

Features extracted from individual video frames cannot represent the dynamics in surgical video, i.e., changes between adjacent frames. To alleviate this problem, Lea et al. [10] propose adding a number of difference images to the input fed to the S-CNN. For timestep t, difference images are calculated within a window of 2 s around frame v_t. Also, they suggest to use a *spatiotemporal CNN*

(ST-CNN) [9], which applies a large temporal 1D convolutional filter to the latent activations obtained by a S-CNN. In contrast, we propose to use a 3D CNN to learn spatiotemporal features from stacks of consecutive video frames, thus modeling the temporal evolution of video frames directly.

To the best of our knowledge, we are the first to design a 3D CNN for surgical gesture recognition that predicts gesture labels for consecutive frames of surgical video. An evaluation on the suturing task of the publicly available JIGSAWS [1] dataset demonstrates the superiority of our approach compared to 2D CNNs that estimate surgical gestures based on spatial features extracted from individual video frames. Averaging the dense predictions of the 3D CNN over time even achieves compelling frame-wise gesture recognition accuracies of over 84%. Source code can be accessed at https://gitlab.com/nct_tso_public/surgical_gesture_recognition.

2   Methods

In the following, we detail the architecture and training procedure of the proposed 3D CNN for video-based surgical gesture recognition.

2.1   Network Architecture

Ji et al. [6] proposed *3D CNNs* as a natural extension of well-known (2D) CNNs. While 2D CNNs apply 2D convolutions and 2D pooling kernels to extract features along the spatial dimensions of a video frame $v \in \mathbb{R}^{C \times H \times W}$, 3D CNNs apply 3D convolutions and 3D pooling kernels to extract features along the spatial and temporal dimensions of a stack of video frames $\vartheta = [v_k, v_{k+1}, ..., v_{k+L-1}] \in \mathbb{R}^{C \times L \times H \times W}$. Recently, Carreira et al. [2] suggested to create 3D CNN architectures by *inflating* established deep 2D CNN architectures along the temporal dimension. This basically means that all $N \times N$ kernels are expanded into their cubic $N \times N \times N$ counterparts.

The proposed 3D CNN for surgical gesture recognition is based on 3D ResNet-18 [4], which is created by inflating an 18-layer residual network [5]. Input to the network are stacks of 16 consecutive video frames (as proposed in [4]) with a resolution of 224×224 pixels. More precisely, to obtain an estimate $\hat{g}(t)$ of the gesture being performed at time t, we feed the video snippet $\vartheta_t = (v_{t-15}, ..., v_{t-1}, v_t)$ to the network. Because we process the video at 5 fps, the network can refer to the previous three seconds of video in order to infer $\hat{g}(t)$. At this point, we abstain from feeding future video frames to the network so that the method is applicable for online gesture recognition.

The original 3D ResNet-18 architecture is designed to predict one distinct action label per video snippet using a one-hot encoding. In contrast, surgical gesture recognition is a dense labeling problem, where each frame v_k of a video snippet has a distinct label $g(k)$. This means that one video snippet may contain frames that belong to different gestures. To account for this, we adapt our network to output dense gesture label estimates $\hat{\gamma}_t = (\hat{g}_t(t-15), ..., \hat{g}_t(t-1), \hat{g}_t(t)) \in$

Table 1. Network architecture. For each layer type, we specify kernel size, number of output feature maps, and, if applicable, stride or number of residual blocks. Square brackets indicate shortcut connections.

Layer type		Output size
conv	$7 \times 7 \times 7$, 64, stride(1, 2, 2)	$16 \times 112 \times 112$
max pool	$1 \times 3 \times 3$, 64, stride(1, 2, 2)	$16 \times 56 \times 56$
res block	$\begin{bmatrix} 3 \times 3 \times 3, 64 \\ 3 \times 3 \times 3, 64 \end{bmatrix} \times 2$	
res block	$\begin{bmatrix} 3 \times 3 \times 3, 128 \\ 3 \times 3 \times 3, 128 \end{bmatrix} \times 2$	$8 \times 28 \times 28$
res block	$\begin{bmatrix} 3 \times 3 \times 3, 256 \\ 3 \times 3 \times 3, 256 \end{bmatrix} \times 2$	$4 \times 14 \times 14$
res block	$\begin{bmatrix} 3 \times 3 \times 3, 512 \\ 3 \times 3 \times 3, 512 \end{bmatrix} \times 2$	$2 \times 7 \times 7$
avg pool	$1 \times 7 \times 7, 512$	2
conv^T	11, G stride 5	16

$\mathbb{R}^{G \times 16}$. Here, G denotes the number of distinct surgical gestures. The component $\hat{g}_t(t - i), i = 0, ..., 15$, of $\hat{\gamma}_t$ is the estimate for gesture label $g(t - i)$, obtained at time t.

Specifically, we adapt the max pooling layer of 3D ResNet-18 so that downsampling is only performed along the spatial dimensions. Thus, the feature maps after the final average pooling layer have a dimension of 512×2. This is upsampled to the output dimension $G \times 16$ using a transposed 1D convolution (conv^T) with kernel size 11 and stride 5.

An overview of the network architecture is given in Table 1. The input is downsampled in the initial convolutional and max pooling layers and then passed through a number of residual blocks. When convolutions are applied with stride 2 to downsample feature maps, the number of feature maps is doubled. For details on residual blocks, please see the original papers [4,5]. We apply batch normalization and the ReLU non-linearity after each convolutional layer. An exception is the final transposed convolution, which is normalized using a softmax layer.

2.2 Network Training

We train our 3D CNN on video snippets $\vartheta_t = (v_{t-15}, ..., v_{t-1}, v_t)$ to predict the corresponding ground truth gesture labels $\gamma_t = (g(t - 15), ..., g(t - 1), g(t))$. Therefore, we minimize the loss $\mathcal{L}(\gamma_t, \hat{\gamma}_t) = \sum_{i=0}^{15} w_i \mathcal{L}_{CE}(g(t-i), \hat{g}_t(t-i))$, where $\mathcal{L}_{CE}$ denotes the cross entropy loss. We found it to be beneficial to penalize the errors made on more current predictions harder and therefore train with weighting factors $\omega_i = \frac{(16-i)^2}{\sum_{i=0}^{15}(16-i)^2}$.

Because of their large number of parameters, 3D CNNs are difficult to train, especially on small datasets [4]. Thus, it is important to begin training from a suitable initialization of network parameters. We investigate two approaches for network initialization: (i) Initializing the network with parameters obtained by training on Kinetics [2], one of the largest human action datasets available so far. For this, a publicly available pretrained 3D ResNet-18 model[1] [4] is used. (ii) Bootstrapping network parameters from an ImageNet-pretrained 2D ResNet-18 model that was further trained on individual video frames to perform frame-wise gesture recognition. As described in [2], the 3D filters of the 3D ResNet-18 are initialized by repeating the weights of the corresponding 2D filters N times along the temporal dimension and then dividing them by N.

During training, we sample video snippets ϑ_t at random temporal positions t from the training videos. Per epoch, we sample about 3000 snippets in a class-balanced manner, which means that we ensure that each gesture $g \in \mathcal{G}$ is represented equally in the set of sampled snippets. For data augmentation, we use scale jittering and corner cropping as proposed in [14]. Here, all frames within one training snippet are augmented in the same manner. We train the 3D CNN for 250 epochs using the Adam [7] optimizer with a batch size of 32 and an initial learning rate of $2.5 \cdot 10^{-4}$. The learning rate is divided by factor 5 every 50 epochs. Our 3D CNN implementation is based on code[2] provided by [4].

3   Evaluation

We evaluate our approach on 39 videos of robot-assisted suturing tasks performed on a bench-top model, which are taken from the *JHU-ISI Gesture and Skill Assessment Working Set (JIGSAWS)* [1]. The recorded tasks were performed by eight participants with varying surgical experience. The videos were annotated with surgical gestures such as *positioning the tip of the needle* or *pushing needle through the tissue*. In total, $G = 10$ different gestures are used. We follow the leave-one-user-out (LOUO) setup for cross-validation as defined in [1]. Thus, for each experiment, we train one model per left-out user.

We report the following evaluation metrics: (i) Frame-wise accuracy, i.e., the ratio of correctly predicted gesture labels in a video. (ii) Average F_1 score, where we calculate the F_1 score, i.e., the harmonic mean of precision and recall, with respect to each gesture class and average the results over all classes. (iii) Edit score, as proposed in [9], which employs the Levenshtein distance to assess the quality of predicted gesture segments. (iv) Segmental F_1 score with threshold 10% (F_1@10), as proposed in [8]. Here, a predicted gesture segment is considered a true positive if its intersection with the corresponding ground truth segment is over 10%, and the F_1 score is calculated regarding the total number

---

[1] https://github.com/kenshohara/3D-ResNets-PyTorch#pre-trained-models.
[2] https://github.com/kenshohara/3D-ResNets-PyTorch.

Table 2. Experimental results on the suturing task of JIGSAWS. The column captioned with *look ahead* indicates how much future video a method needs to see to estimate the current gesture. Evaluation measures that were not reported in related work are denoted as –. All measures are given in %.

Method	Look ahead	Acc	Avg. F_1	Edit	F_1@10
Evaluation at 5 fps					
2D ResNet-18	0 s	79.9	73.3	41.4	55.4
3D CNN (B)	0 s	79.9	73.7	64.0	75.2
3D CNN (K)	0 s	81.8	75.8	58.7	71.1
3D CNN (B) + window	3 s	84.0	**78.4**	**80.7**	**87.2**
3D CNN (K) + window	3 s	**84.2**	**78.4**	80.0	87.1
Evaluation at 10 fps					
S-CNN [10]	1 s	74.0	–	37.7	–
S-CNN + TCN, $C = 10$, causal	1 s	76.8	71.5	57.3	69.6
S-CNN + TCN, $C = 10$	3 s	76.1	69.9	68.2	77.9
ST-CNN [10]	10 s	77.7	–	68.0	–
S-CNN + TCN, $C = 75$	22.5 s	81.4	77.6	84.9	89.6
S-CNN + TCN + Deep RL [11]	–	81.4	–	**88.0**	**92.0**
2D ResNet-18	0 s	79.5	73.1	30.6	44.2
3D CNN (B)	0 s	79.5	73.6	49.5	62.8
3D CNN (K)	0 s	81.3	75.1	46.3	60.1
3D CNN (B) + window	3 s	84.0	78.6	80.6	87.0
3D CNN (K) + window	3 s	**84.3**	**78.6**	80.0	87.0

of true positives, false positives, and false negatives. For each experiment, evaluation metrics are calculated for every video in the dataset and then averaged.

As baseline experiment, we train a 2D ResNet-18 [5], i.e., the 2D counterpart to the proposed 3D CNN, for frame-wise gesture recognition. Here, we follow the training procedure described in Sect. 2.2 except for the fact that we train on video snippets of size 1, i.e., individual video frames. The 2D ResNet-18 is initialized with ImageNet-pretrained weights.

Additionally, we perform two experiments where we train the proposed 3D CNN for surgical gesture recognition: one where we initialize the 3D CNN with Kinetics-pretrained weights *(3D CNN (K))* and one where we bootstrap weights from a pretrained 2D ResNet-18 as described in Sect. 2.2 *(3D CNN (B))*. To account for the stochastic nature of CNN optimization, we repeat the three experiments four times and report the averaged results. For the *3D CNN (B)* experiment, we initialize the models in the ith experiment repetition by bootstrapping weights from the corresponding 2D ResNet-18 models (with respect to the LOUO splits) that were trained during the ith repetition of the baseline experiment.

We evaluate the trained 3D CNN models either snippet-wise or in combination with a sliding window ($+$ $window$). For snippet-wise evaluation, the estimated gesture label $\hat{g}(t)$ at time t is simply $\hat{g}_t(t)$. With the sliding window approach, we accumulate the dense predictions of the 3D CNN over time. This yields the overall estimate $\bar{\hat{g}}(t) = \sum_{i=0}^{15} \hat{g}_{t+i}(t)$ for the gesture at time t. To obtain $\bar{\hat{g}}(t)$, information of 15 future time steps is used, which corresponds to the next three seconds of video.

To make comparisons to prior studies possible, we additionally evaluate the 2D ResNet-18 and the 3D CNN models at 10 fps. This means that we extract video snippets at 10 Hz, instead of 5 Hz, from the video. For the 3D CNNs, the individual snippets still consist of 16 frames sampled at 5 fps. To apply the sliding window approach, we temporally upsample the prediction $\hat{\gamma}_t \in \mathbb{R}^{G \times 16}$ to $\tilde{\gamma}_t \in \mathbb{R}^{G \times 32}$, where

$$\tilde{\gamma}_t[j] = \begin{cases} \hat{\gamma}_t[0], & \text{if } j = 0, \\ 0.5 \cdot \hat{\gamma}_t[\lfloor \frac{j-1}{2} \rfloor] + 0.5 \cdot \hat{\gamma}_t[\lceil \frac{j-1}{2} \rceil], & \text{if } j = 1, ..., 31. \end{cases}$$

The experimental results are listed in Table 2. For comparison, we state the results of some previous methods that were described in Sect. 1. Further experiments can be found in the supplementary document.

S-CNN $+$ TCN refers to the method where spatial features are extracted from video frames using a S-CNN and fed to a TCN that predicts surgical gestures [8,10]. Here, the results were reproduced using the ED-TCN architecture described in [8] with 2 layers and temporal filter size C. For causal evaluation, filters are applied from v_{t-C} to v_t instead of $v_{t-C/2}$ to $v_{t+C/2}$. We use source code[3] provided by the authors of [8,10]. The reported results are averaged over four LOUO cross-validation runs.

4 Discussion

As can be seen in Table 2, the proposed variant of 3D ResNet-18 for snippet-wise gesture recognition yields comparable or better frame-wise evaluation results (accuracy and average F_1) and considerably better segment-based evaluation results (edit score and $F_1@10$) compared to the 2D counterpart. This demonstrates the benefit of modeling several consecutive video frames to capture the temporal evolution of video.

Accumulating the 3D CNN predictions using a sliding window with a duration of three seconds provides a further boost to recognition performance. Not only does the sliding window approach produce better gesture segments, it also improves frame-wise accuracies. Considering future video snippets most likely helps to resolve ambiguities in individual snippets.

Minor differences can be observed between both network initialization variants, Kinetics pretraining (K) and 2D weight bootstrapping (B): while pretraining on Kinetics yields higher frame-wise accuracies, the other approach yields

---

[3] https://github.com/colincsl/TemporalConvolutionalNetworks.

better gesture segments. In combination with the sliding window the differences are marginal.

When testing at 10 fps instead of 5 fps, we observe a notable degradation of the segment-based measures for both the 2D ResNet-18 and the 3D variants. Most likely, the high evaluation frequency enhances noise in the gesture predictions, which is penalized by the edit score and the F_1@10 metric. For the 3D CNNs, this effect can be alleviated by filtering with the sliding window.

Compared to the ST-CNN, the 3D CNN yields considerably better results with regards to all evaluation metrics when being evaluated with the sliding window approach. Apparently, for the given task, modeling spatiotemporal features in video snippets achieves better results than modeling spatial and temporal information separately, as is the case for the ST-CNN.

In combination with the sliding window, the proposed 3D CNN also outperforms the state-of-the-art methods *S-CNN + TCN* and *S-CNN + TCN + Deep RL* in terms of accuracy and average F_1. These methods apply very long temporal filters while the proposed approach only processes a few seconds of video to estimate the current gesture. Thus, it is surprising that the quality of gesture segments, as measured by edit score and F_1@10, is almost equal.

Note that the proposed method operates with a delay of only 3 s and can therefore provide information, such as feedback in a surgical training scenario, in a more timely manner than methods with a longer *look ahead* time.

5   Conclusion

We present a 3D CNN to predict dense gesture labels for surgical video. The conducted experiments demonstrate the benefits of using an inherently spatiotemporal model to extract features from consecutive video frames. Future work will investigate options for combining spatiotemporal feature extractors with models that capture high-level temporal dependencies, such as LSTMs or TCNs.

Acknowledgements. The authors thank Colin Lea for sharing code and precomputed S-CNN features to reproduce results from [10] as well as the Helmholtz-Zentrum Dresden-Rossendorf (HZDR) for granting access to their GPU cluster.

References

1. Ahmidi, N., Tao, L., Sefati, S., Gao, Y., Lea, C., Haro, B.B., et al.: A dataset and benchmarks for segmentation and recognition of gestures in robotic surgery. IEEE Trans. Biomed. Eng. **64**(9), 2025–2041 (2017)
2. Carreira, J., Zisserman, A.: Quo vadis, action recognition? A new model and the Kinetics dataset. In: CVPR, pp. 4724–4733. IEEE (2017)
3. DiPietro, R., Lea, C., Malpani, A., Ahmidi, N., Vedula, S.S., Lee, G.I., et al.: Recognizing surgical activities with recurrent neural networks. In: Ourselin, S., Joskowicz, L., Sabuncu, M.R., Unal, G., Wells, W. (eds.) MICCAI 2016. LNCS, vol. 9900, pp. 551–558. Springer, Cham (2016). https://doi.org/10.1007/978-3-319-46720-7_64

4. Hara, K., Kataoka, H., Satoh, Y.: Learning spatio-temporal features with 3D residual networks for action recognition. In: ICCV-W, pp. 3154–3160. IEEE (2017)
5. He, K., Zhang, X., Ren, S., Sun, J.: Deep residual learning for image recognition. In: CVPR, pp. 770–778. IEEE (2016)
6. Ji, S., Xu, W., Yang, M., Yu, K.: 3D convolutional neural networks for human action recognition. IEEE Trans. Pattern Anal. Mach. Intell. **35**(1), 221–231 (2013)
7. Kingma, D.P., Ba, J.: Adam: a method for stochastic optimization. In: ICLR (2015)
8. Lea, C., Flynn, M.D., Vidal, R., Reiter, A., Hager, G.D.: Temporal convolutional networks for action segmentation and detection. In: CVPR, pp. 156–165. IEEE (2017)
9. Lea, C., Reiter, A., Vidal, R., Hager, G.D.: Segmental spatiotemporal CNNs for fine-grained action segmentation. In: Leibe, B., Matas, J., Sebe, N., Welling, M. (eds.) ECCV 2016. LNCS, vol. 9907, pp. 36–52. Springer, Cham (2016). https://doi.org/10.1007/978-3-319-46487-9_3
10. Lea, C., Vidal, R., Reiter, A., Hager, G.D.: Temporal convolutional networks: a unified approach to action segmentation. In: Hua, G., Jégou, H. (eds.) ECCV 2016. LNCS, vol. 9915, pp. 47–54. Springer, Cham (2016). https://doi.org/10.1007/978-3-319-49409-8_7
11. Liu, D., Jiang, T.: Deep reinforcement learning for surgical gesture segmentation and classification. In: Frangi, A.F., Schnabel, J.A., Davatzikos, C., Alberola-López, C., Fichtinger, G. (eds.) MICCAI 2018. LNCS, vol. 11073, pp. 247–255. Springer, Cham (2018). https://doi.org/10.1007/978-3-030-00937-3_29
12. Tao, L., Elhamifar, E., Khudanpur, S., Hager, G.D., Vidal, R.: Sparse hidden Markov models for surgical gesture classification and skill evaluation. In: Abolmaesumi, P., Joskowicz, L., Navab, N., Jannin, P. (eds.) IPCAI 2012. LNCS, vol. 7330, pp. 167–177. Springer, Heidelberg (2012). https://doi.org/10.1007/978-3-642-30618-1_17
13. Tao, L., Zappella, L., Hager, G.D., Vidal, R.: Surgical gesture segmentation and recognition. In: Mori, K., Sakuma, I., Sato, Y., Barillot, C., Navab, N. (eds.) MICCAI 2013. LNCS, vol. 8151, pp. 339–346. Springer, Heidelberg (2013). https://doi.org/10.1007/978-3-642-40760-4_43
14. Wang, L., Xiong, Y., Wang, Z., Qiao, Y., Lin, D., Tang, X., et al.: Temporal segment networks: towards good practices for deep action recognition. In: Leibe, B., Matas, J., Sebe, N., Welling, M. (eds.) ECCV 2016. LNCS, vol. 9912, pp. 20–36. Springer, Cham (2016). https://doi.org/10.1007/978-3-319-46484-8_2

Surgical Skill Assessment on In-Vivo Clinical Data via the Clearness of Operating Field

Daochang Liu[1], Tingting Jiang[1(✉)], Yizhou Wang[1,3,4], Rulin Miao[2], Fei Shan[2], and Ziyu Li[2]

[1] NELVT, Department of Computer Science, Peking University, Beijing, China
{daochang,ttjiang}@pku.edu.cn
[2] Peking University Cancer Hospital, Beijing, China
[3] Peng Cheng Lab, Shenzhen, China
[4] Deepwise AI Lab, Beijing, China

Abstract. Surgical skill assessment is important for surgery training and quality control. Prior works on this task largely focus on basic surgical tasks such as suturing and knot tying performed in simulation settings. In contrast, surgical skill assessment is studied in this paper on a real clinical dataset, which consists of fifty-seven in-vivo laparoscopic surgeries and corresponding skill scores annotated by six surgeons. From analyses on this dataset, the clearness of operating field (COF) is identified as a good proxy for overall surgical skills, given its strong correlation with overall skills and high inter-annotator consistency. Then an objective and automated framework based on neural network is proposed to predict surgical skills through the proxy of COF. The neural network is jointly trained with a supervised regression loss and an unsupervised rank loss. In experiments, the proposed method achieves 0.55 Spearman's correlation with the ground truth of overall technical skill, which is even comparable with the human performance of junior surgeons.

Keywords: Surgical skill assessment · Clinical data · Neural networks

1 Introduction

Surgical skill assessment is crucial for the improvement of surgeons' competency during both training and practice [16]. Traditionally, surgical skills are evaluated by experts with onsite observation, which is prone to subjective biases. Although OSATS [13] can reduce such subjectivity to some extent, it requires intensive efforts from experts for manual grading. Thus computer-aided approaches, which

Electronic supplementary material The online version of this chapter (https://doi.org/10.1007/978-3-030-32254-0_53) contains supplementary material, which is available to authorized users.

provide objective and scalable skill predictions, draw increasing attention from the community. This paper works on computer-aided surgical skill assessment.

Prior works on this task [1,6–8,11,15,17–21] have been mainly set up on simulated datasets such as JIGSAWS [3], in which basic suturing/tying tasks are performed on benchtop models. Although some benchtop models can have high fidelity of human anatomy and accurate imitation of procedure steps, there is still a large gap between simulated scenarios and real-world clinical ones in terms of varying patient condition, working dynamics, stress level and so on. Only few studies [2,4,12,14] have been conducted on clinical data. As for surgery type, clinical open surgeries have been studied in [2,4] and laparoscopies in [12,14]. The modality of these clinical datasets can be surgery videos [4,12] or the data from external sources [2,14]. The limitations of the two existing clinical video datasets are that [4] only targets at short suturing/tying clips manually segmented from long surgeries and [12] annotates only four videos with skill labels. Different from previous works, we construct a new clinical laparoscopic video dataset, which consists of *fifty-seven long* procedures.

On the other hand, from the perspective of assessment method, most of the existing works are motion-based. In these works, surgical skills are determined with hand/tool/eye motions, obtained from robotic kinematics [1,8,11,17,19] or external sensors [2,7,14,20] or visual tracking/interest points [4,12,15,18,20,21]. However, acquiring motion trajectories is difficult for clinical data because that (1) robotic kinematics are restricted to only robotic surgeries (2) external sensors interrupt normal workflows and are hard to implement in operating rooms (3) visual tracking is not robust enough and often involves manual corrections. Unlike these prior works, we utilize the clearness of operating field (COF) rather than motion for skill assessment. The COF reflects the amount of bleeding and the visibility of anatomy landmarks. Prediction of the COF relies on appearance information carried in surgery videos, which is more obtainable and robust than motions in clinical settings. Statistical analyses on our clinical dataset identify that the COF is a good skill proxy, for its strong correlation with overall skills and high consistency across annotators. For a detailed review of previous studies, please refer to this survey [16].

In this paper, a new clinical dataset is collected, which includes fifty-seven videos of laparoscopic gastrectomy conducted in operating rooms (OR). Six surgeons annotate the videos with not only technical OSATS scores but also newly designed procedural scores and the COF score. Then we propose an objective video-based method to predict surgical skills via the proxy of COF. A neural network taking in color and semantic features is trained with a supervised regression loss and an unsupervised rank loss collectively. The proposed method outputs skill scores at frame-level to provide feedback. Experiments show that predicting overall skills via the proxy of COF performs better than predicting them directly without proxy. The Spearman's correlation between predicted overall technical skill and ground truth ratings is 0.55, which is promising and even comparable with the human performance of junior surgeons. In summary, our contributions are three-fold: (1) An in-vivo clinical dataset collected from real operating rooms. (2) The identification of COF as a good skill proxy. (3) A video-based method without extra equipment and intensive human efforts.

Table 1. Skill metrics

ID	General metrics	ID	Procedure-specific metrics
1	Gentleness	7	Dissection in correct planes
2	Time and motion	8	Vessel exposure and transection
3	Instrument handling	9	Venous breakpoint selection
4	Flow of operation	10	Arterial breakpoint selection
5	Tissue exposure	11	Infrapyloric artery exposure
6	Overall technical skill (OTS)	12	Care for adjacent organs
14	Clearness of operating field	13	Overall procedural skill (OPS)

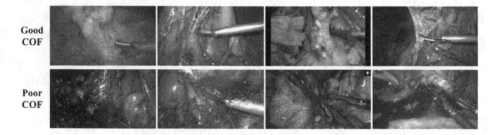

Fig. 1. Example frames from cases with good or poor COF scores.

2 Dataset

Data. The dataset includes videos of 57 in-vivo laparoscopic gastrectomy surgeries for gastric cancer. Videos are captured by the built-in camera (Karl Storz, Olympus or Sony) and are formatted to 960×540 and 25 fps. The procedures are performed by one surgeon. It is assumed that the performance of a same primary surgeon can vary across cases, due to different case complexity, fatigue condition, team members, operating time and so on. To lighten the annotation burden, the infrapyloric area [10], which is one of the four major parts of gastrectomy, is used for skill assessment in this study. The duration of infrapyloric procedure ranges from 8 to 57 min and the average is 26 min. Surgical skills are annotated by 6 surgeons on 14 metrics with the Likert scale of 1–5. The 6 surgeons include 3 senior surgeons with more than 8 years experience and 3 junior surgeons with less than 4 years experience. For each metric, the ground truth is defined as the mean score of the three seniors.

Skill Metrics. As listed in Table 1, the surgeries are evaluated on 14 metrics, including technical OSATS metrics, procedural metrics, and the COF metric. For OSATS metrics (ID 1–6), a modified version from [5] is employed. Since OSATS metrics only measure the general surgical technique and are procedure-independent, we also design 7 new procedure-specific metrics (ID 7–13) according to [10] to provide fine-grained ratings of surgeons' compliance with gastrectomy

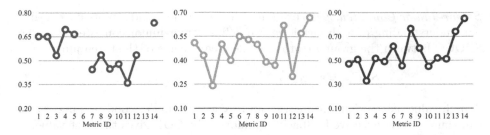

Fig. 2. Metric analyses. *Left:* Correlation with overall skills. *Middle:* Inter-senior consistency. *Right:* Senior-junior consistency. COF (ID 14) is a good skill proxy.

instructions. In addition, based on the suggestion of surgeons, the COF metric (ID 14) is proposed to represent how much the bleeding and burned tissues impact on the identification of anatomical structures. Examples are shown in Fig. 1. In cases with good COF, there is no obvious bleeding and the anatomical planes and landmarks can be recognized clearly, while in poor cases the bleeding is excessive and severely affects the recognition of planes and landmarks.

Analysis. As shown in Fig. 2, skill metrics are analyzed statistically on all 57 cases in terms of correlation with overall surgical skills and inter-annotator consistency. In the following analyses, r_{im} denotes the 57 scores from surgeon i on metric m. $\mathcal{S}$ and $\mathcal{J}$ denote the sets of seniors and juniors respectively. And srocc$(\cdot, \cdot)$ is the function of Spearman's rank correlation coefficient (SROCC).

Correlation with Overall Skills. We consider the correlations with both overall technical skill (OTS) and overall procedural skill (OPS). Concretely, the correlation with overall skills for a non-overall metric m is defined as:

$$CORR_m = \tfrac{1}{2 \times |\mathcal{S}|} \sum_{i \in \mathcal{S}} \sum_{k \in \{6,13\}} \text{srocc}(r_{im}, r_{ik}) \quad m \notin \{6,13\} \qquad (1)$$

where the SROCC between this metric and either OTS or OPS is computed, and the results from three seniors are averaged. This value is the largest when $m = 14$, indicating that COF has the best correlation with overall skills.

Inter-senior Consistency. This value reflects how seniors agree on a metric. Specifically, the inter-senior consistency for metric m is defined as the averaged SROCCs between the scores of this metric from each two seniors:

$$ISC_m = \tfrac{1}{|\mathcal{S}| \times (|\mathcal{S}|-1)} \sum_{i,j \in \mathcal{S}, i \neq j} \text{srocc}(r_{im}, r_{jm}). \qquad (2)$$

The higher this value is, the metric is less affected by subjective biases. Among the 14 metrics, the COF achieves the highest inter-senior consistency.

Senior-Junior Consistency. To examine whether juniors and seniors have a similar understanding of each metric m, we define senior-junior consistency as the SROCC between the ground truth and the mean scores of the three juniors:

$$SJC_m = \mathrm{srocc}(\tfrac{1}{|\mathcal{S}|} \textstyle\sum_{i \in \mathcal{S}} \mathbf{r}_{im}, \tfrac{1}{|\mathcal{J}|} \textstyle\sum_{j \in \mathcal{J}} \mathbf{r}_{jm}). \tag{3}$$

A high value means that this metric can be correctly understood by juniors and can thus provide effective feedback to juniors. The COF gives the best value.

In addition to the above reasons, the assessment of COF only relies on appearance information carried in video data. Hand/tool motions and extra devices are not involved. Therefore the COF is identified as a good proxy for overall skills.

3   Method

In this section, an objective video-based method is devised to regress surgical skills via the proxy of COF. The proposed approach takes a video as input and predicts its COF score, which is directly regarded as overall surgical skills.

Preprocessing. The input video is first downsampled to 1 fps to reduce data redundancy. Then extra-abdominal views are removed manually. Note that this can be efficiently done by non-professionals.

Feature Extraction. Since the COF is a measure for bleeding amount and anatomical recognition, we extract color features to describe the severity of bleeding and semantic features to provide anatomy information. For color features, color histograms in RGB space, HSV space, and Red-ratio space (R/G and R/B) are computed in every video frame. In our dataset, videos can have inconsistent color distributions due to different recording devices and patient conditions. Thus the color features are normalized using the first 30% of each video, given the observation that the first 30% is unlikely to contain heavy bleeding and should be of similar color and COF across cases. In detail, for each video, the mean color feature of the first 30% is subtracted from the color feature of each frame. As for the semantic features, the ResNet-101 [9] pretrained on ImageNet is employed in each frame. Then the two types of features are concatenated. After feature extraction, the video is transformed into a feature sequence, denoted by $X \in \mathbb{R}^{T \times D}$. T is the number of frames and D is the feature dimension.

Model. A neural network model is designed for automated skill assessment, which consists of a score branch to evaluate frame quality and a weight branch to provide frame importance. Both of the branches are frame-wise multilayer perceptrons (MLP). Given the feature of a video frame, the score branch produces a score of this frame, while the weight branch outputs a frame weight. In this way, the feature sequence X of the input video is transformed into a score sequence denoted by $A \in \mathbb{R}^{T \times 1}$ and a weight sequence represented by $U \in \mathbb{R}^{T \times 1}$. The

Table 2. Performance of COF prediction

Method	Feature	PLCC	SROCC
Baseline	Red	0.164	0.130
Baseline	Saturation.	0.233	0.178
Baseline	Duration	0.229	0.191
$\mathcal{L}_{reg}$	Color + ResNet	0.580	0.595
$\mathcal{L}_{rank}$	Color + ResNet	0.433	0.457
$\mathcal{L}_{reg} + \mathcal{L}_{rank}$	Color	0.447	0.446
$\mathcal{L}_{reg} + \mathcal{L}_{rank}$	ResNet	0.622	0.601
$\mathcal{L}_{reg} + \mathcal{L}_{rank}$	Color + ResNet	**0.641**	**0.647**
Junior surgeon	–	0.670	0.657
Senior surgeon	–	**0.880**	**0.869**

Table 3. Performance of overall skills prediction

Method	PLCC (OTS/OPS)	SROCC (OTS/OPS)
No proxy ($\mathcal{L}_{reg}$)	0.46/0.18	0.47/0.18
No proxy ($\mathcal{L}_{reg} + \mathcal{L}_{rank}$)	0.45/0.21	0.45/0.24
With proxy ($\mathcal{L}_{reg} + \mathcal{L}_{rank}$)	**0.56/0.40**	**0.55/0.41**
Junior surgeon (COF)	0.56/0.61	0.56/0.60
Junior surgeon (OTS/OPS)	0.42/0.64	0.41/0.62
Senior surgeon (COF)	0.74/0.74	0.73/0.73
Senior surgeon (OTS/OPS)	**0.82/0.84**	**0.82/0.83**

weight branch is additionally followed by a softmax function so that the weights of all frames sum to one. Then the video-level score q is obtained by the weighted sum of frame-level scores: $q = \sum_{t=1}^{T} U_t A_t$.

Loss. The loss function comprises a supervised regression loss and an unsupervised rank loss. The regression loss is a standard L1 loss: $L_{reg} = |y - q|$, where y denotes the ground truth COF score and q is the predicted score. In addition, we devise a rank loss based on the observation that the quality of COF decreases over time as the bleeding accumulates. It is assumed that the COF is better at the start of the surgery than in the end. As recommended by surgeons, we define the start section as the first 30% of the surgery and the end section as 60% to 90%. The last 10% is not used for the end section because surgeons commonly clean the operating field thoroughly when finishing. Then the rank loss is proposed to enforce the score of the start section to be higher than the end section by a margin:

$$L_{rank} = \max(0, 1 - (q_s - q_e)) \tag{4}$$

where $q_s = \sum_{t=1}^{0.3T} U_t A_t$ is the predicted score for the start section and $q_e = \sum_{t=0.6T}^{0.9T} U_t A_t$ is for the end section. This rank loss is only applied to the training cases with COF score no more than 3, since in good cases the COF quality might stay high through the whole surgery. Note that frame weights U are normalized with softmax within the defined ranges when computing q_s and q_e. Then the neural network is trained with the regression loss and the rank loss jointly.

4   Experiments

The proposed method is evaluated on the newly introduced clinical dataset. We repeat three-fold cross-validation 15 times, with 45 runs in total. In each run, 38 videos are chosen randomly for training and the rest 19 videos are for testing. We report the Spearman's rank correlation coefficient (SROCC) and the Pearson linear correlation coefficient (PLCC) between the ground truth and the prediction, which are averaged over all 45 runs. Results of COF prediction and overall skills prediction are both presented.

COF Prediction. Results of COF prediction are provided in Table 2. First, three baselines are tested, which simply depend on the mean red value, the mean saturation value, or duration of the video. Then ablation studies are performed to investigate the impact of feature and loss design. At last, human performances of senior and junior surgeons are computed by using annotations of each individual surgeon as the prediction and then averaging the results over juniors or seniors. Our full model surpasses the baselines and the ablated models, which is even comparable with junior surgeons.

Overall Skills Prediction. For overall skills, both OTS and OPS are predicted with or without the proxy of COF. When with the proxy, the predicted overall skills are set the same as the predicted COF. When without proxy, same models are trained to regress overall skills directly by setting the OTS or OPS as the learning target y in the loss. To facilitate the comparison between the proposed method and human performances, performances of surgeons are also computed with proxy (COF as overall skills) or without the proxy. As the results in Table 3, predicting overall skills via the proxy is better than directly regressing them without proxy, which further validates that COF is a good skill proxy. For OTS, the SROCC is 0.55, which is promising and comparable with the human performance of junior surgeons. For OPS, the SROCC is 0.41, which can be improved in the future by explicitly modeling the procedure steps. Note that previous works are not applicable due to different data modality and surgery setting.

Feedback. As shown in Fig. 3, the proposed method generates frame-level scores to indicate which parts are of low quality and frame-level weights to identify which parts should receive more attention. In this test example, the score drop

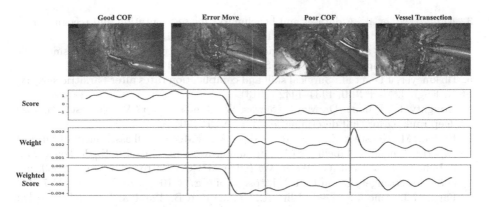

Fig. 3. Frame-level COF scores for a test surgery. The scores have been normalized.

(the 2nd image) corresponds to an error move that the surgeon needs to improve, and the increase of weight (the 4th image) corresponds to the vessel transection that the surgeon should perform with special care. Video demos are provided in the supplementary. The quantification of such feedback is left for future research.

5   Conclusion and Future Work

In this work, a clinical dataset for surgical skill assessment is compiled. Statistical analyses and empirical results both show that the clearness of operating field is a good skill proxy. A video-based objective model is proposed to predict overall skills via this proxy, which achieves promising results in experiments. The limitation of this work is that the dataset only includes gastrectomy procedures performed by a single surgeon. The generalizability to other procedures and across surgeons needs to be further validated. Future works should also focus on (1) temporal structure modeling (2) incorporating more domain knowledge (3) explicitly modeling the surgery steps and human anatomy.

Acknowledgement. This work was partially supported by National Basic Research Program of China (973 Program) under contract 2015CB351803, the Natural Science Foundation of China under contracts 61572042, 61527804 and 61625201. We also acknowledge the Clinical Medicine Plus X-Young Scholars Project and High-Performance Computing Platform of Peking University.

References

1. Ahmidi, N., et al.: String motif-based description of tool motion for detecting skill and gestures in robotic surgery. In: Mori, K., Sakuma, I., Sato, Y., Barillot, C., Navab, N. (eds.) MICCAI 2013. LNCS, vol. 8149, pp. 26–33. Springer, Heidelberg (2013). https://doi.org/10.1007/978-3-642-40811-3_4
2. Ahmidi, N., et al.: Automated objective surgical skill assessment in the operating room from unstructured tool motion in septoplasty. IJCARS **10**, 981–991 (2015)

3. Ahmidi, N., et al.: A dataset and benchmarks for segmentation and recognition of gestures in robotic surgery. IEEE TBE **64**, 2025–2041 (2017)
4. Azari, D.P., et al.: Modeling surgical technical skill using expert assessment for automated computer rating. Ann. Surg. **269**, 574–581 (2019)
5. Birkmeyer, J.D., et al.: Surgical skill and complication rates after bariatric surgery. N. Engl. J. Med. **369**, 1434–1442 (2013)
6. Doughty, H., Damen, D., Mayol-Cuevas, W.: Who's better? Who's best? Pairwise deep ranking for skill determination. In: CVPR (2018)
7. Ershad, M., Koesters, Z., Rege, R., Majewicz, A.: Meaningful assessment of surgical expertise: semantic labeling with data and crowds. In: Ourselin, S., Joskowicz, L., Sabuncu, M.R., Unal, G., Wells, W. (eds.) MICCAI 2016. LNCS, vol. 9900, pp. 508–515. Springer, Cham (2016). https://doi.org/10.1007/978-3-319-46720-7_59
8. Fard, M.J., Ameri, S., Darin Ellis, R., Chinnam, R.B., Pandya, A.K., Klein, M.D.: Automated robot-assisted surgical skill evaluation: predictive analytics approach. Int. J. Med. Robot. Comput. Assist. Surg. **14**, e1850 (2018)
9. He, K., Zhang, X., Ren, S., Sun, J.: Deep residual learning for image recognition. In: CVPR (2016)
10. Huang, C.M., Zheng, C.H.: Laparoscopic Gastrectomy for Gastric Cancer: Surgical Technique and Lymphadenectomy. Springer, Netherlands (2015). https://doi.org/10.1007/978-94-017-9873-0
11. Ismail Fawaz, H., Forestier, G., Weber, J., Idoumghar, L., Muller, P.-A.: Evaluating surgical skills from kinematic data using convolutional neural networks. In: Frangi, A.F., Schnabel, J.A., Davatzikos, C., Alberola-López, C., Fichtinger, G. (eds.) MICCAI 2018. LNCS, vol. 11073, pp. 214–221. Springer, Cham (2018). https://doi.org/10.1007/978-3-030-00937-3_25
12. Jin, A., et al.: Tool detection and operative skill assessment in surgical videos using region-based convolutional neural networks. In: WACV (2018)
13. Martin, J., et al.: Objective structured assessment of technical skill (OSATS) for surgical residents. Br. J. Surg. **84**, 273–278 (1997)
14. Richstone, L., Schwartz, M.J., Seideman, C., Cadeddu, J., Marshall, S., Kavoussi, L.R.: Eye metrics as an objective assessment of surgical skill. Ann. Surg. **252**, 177–182 (2010)
15. Sharma, Y., et al.: Automated surgical OSATS prediction from videos. In: ISBI (2014)
16. Vedula, S.S., Ishii, M., Hager, G.D.: Objective assessment of surgical technical skill and competency in the operating room. Annu. Rev. Biomed. Eng. **19**, 301–325 (2017)
17. Wang, Z., Fey, A.M.: Deep learning with convolutional neural network for objective skill evaluation in robot-assisted surgery. IJCARS **13**, 1959–1970 (2018)
18. Zhang, Q., Li, B.: Relative hidden Markov models for video-based evaluation of motion skills in surgical training. TPAMI **37**, 1206–1218 (2015)
19. Zia, A., Essa, I.: Automated surgical skill assessment in RMIS training. IJCARS **13**, 731–739 (2018)
20. Zia, A., Sharma, Y., Bettadapura, V., Sarin, E.L., Essa, I.: Video and accelerometer-based motion analysis for automated surgical skills assessment. IJCARS **13**, 443–455 (2018)
21. Zia, A., et al.: Automated video-based assessment of surgical skills for training and evaluation in medical schools. IJCARS **11**, 1623–1636 (2016)

Graph Neural Network for Interpreting Task-fMRI Biomarkers

Xiaoxiao Li[1(✉)], Nicha C. Dvornek[5], Yuan Zhou[5], Juntang Zhuang[1],
Pamela Ventola[4], and James S. Duncan[1,2,3,5]

[1] Biomedical Engineering, Yale University, New Haven, CT, USA
xiaoxiao.li@yale.edu
[2] Electrical Engineering, Yale University, New Haven, CT, USA
[3] Statistics and Data Science, Yale University, New Haven, CT, USA
[4] Child Study Center, Yale School of Medicine, New Haven, CT, USA
[5] Radiology and Biomedical Imaging, Yale School of Medicine, New Haven, CT, USA

Abstract. Finding the biomarkers associated with ASD is helpful for understanding the underlying roots of the disorder and can lead to earlier diagnosis and more targeted treatment. A promising approach to identify biomarkers is using Graph Neural Networks (GNNs), which can be used to analyze graph structured data, i.e. brain networks constructed by fMRI. One way to interpret important features is through looking at how the classification probability changes if the features are occluded or replaced. The major limitation of this approach is that replacing values may change the distribution of the data and lead to serious errors. Therefore, we develop a 2-stage pipeline to eliminate the need to replace features for reliable biomarker interpretation. Specifically, we propose an inductive GNN to embed the graphs containing different properties of task-fMRI for identifying ASD and then discover the brain regions/subgraphs used as evidence for the GNN classifier. We first show GNN can achieve high accuracy in identifying ASD. Next, we calculate the feature importance scores using GNN and compare the interpretation ability with Random Forest. Finally, we run with different atlases and parameters, proving the robustness of the proposed method. The detected biomarkers reveal their association with social behaviors and are consistent with those reported in the literature. We also show the potential of discovering new informative biomarkers. Our pipeline can be generalized to other graph feature importance interpretation problems.

Keywords: Graph Neural Network · Task-fMRI · ASD biomarker

1 Introduction

Autism spectrum disorders (ASD) affect the structure and function of the brain. To better target the underlying roots of ASD for diagnosis and treatment, efforts to identify reliable biomarkers are growing [8]. Significant progress has been made using functional magnetic resonance imaging (fMRI) to characterize the

© Springer Nature Switzerland AG 2019
D. Shen et al. (Eds.): MICCAI 2019, LNCS 11768, pp. 485–493, 2019.
https://doi.org/10.1007/978-3-030-32254-0_54

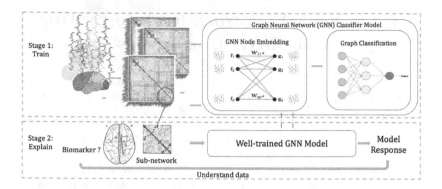

Fig. 1. Pipeline for interpreting important features from a GNN

brain remodeling in ASD [9]. Recently, emerging research on Graph Neural Networks (GNNs) has combined deep learning with graph representation and applied an integrated approach to fMRI analysis in different neuro-disorders [11]. Most existing approaches (based on Graph Convolutional Network (GCN) [10]) require all nodes in the graph to be present during training and thus lack natural generalization on unseen nodes. Also, it is necessary to interpret the important feature in the data used as evidence for the model, but currently no tool exists that can interpret and explain GNNs while recent CNN explanation algorithms cannot directly work on graph input.

Our main contributions include the following three points: (1) We develop a method to integrate all the available connectivity, geometric, anatomic information and task-fMRI (tfMRI) related parameters into graphs for deep learning. Our approach alleviates the problem of predetermining the best features and measures of functional connectivity, which is often ambiguous due to the intrinsic complex structure of task-fMRI. (2) We propose a generalizable GNN inductive learning model to more accurately classify ASD v.s. healthy controls (HC). Different from the spectral GCN [10], our GNN classifier is based on graph isomorphism, which can be applied to multigraphs with different nodes/edges (e.g. sub-graphs), and learn local graph information without binding to the whole graph structure. (3) The GNN architecture enables us to train the model on the whole graph and validate it on subgraphs. We directly evaluate the importance scores on sub-graphs and nodes (i.e. regions of interest (ROIs)) by examining model responses, without resampling value for the occluded features. The 2-stage pipeline to interpret important sub-graphs/ROIs, which are defined as biomarkers in our setting, is shown in Fig. 1.

2   Methodology

2.1   Graph Definition

We firstly parcellate the brain into N ROIs based on its T1 structural MRI. We define ROIs as graph nodes. We define an undirected multigraph $\boldsymbol{G} = (\boldsymbol{V}, \boldsymbol{E})$, where $V = (v_1, v_2, \ldots, v_N)^T \in \mathbb{R}^{N \times D}$ and $E = [e_{ij}] \in \mathbb{R}^{N \times N \times F}$, D and F are the attribute dimensions of nodes and edges respectively. For node attributes, we concatenate handcrafted features: degree of connectivity, General Linear Model (GLM) coefficients, mean, standard deviation of task-fMRI, and ROI center coordinates. We applied the Box-Cox transformation [13] to make each feature follow a normal distribution (parameters are learned from the training set and applied to the training and testing sets). The edge attribute e_{ij} of node i and j includes the Pearson correlation, partial correlation calculated using residual fMRI, and $exp(-r_{ij}/10)$ where r_{ij} is the geometric distance between the centers of the two ROIs. We thresholded the edges under the 95th percentile of partial correlation values to ensure sparsity for efficient computation and avoiding oversmoothing.

2.2 Graph Neural Network (GNN) Classifier

The architecture of our proposed GNN is shown in Fig. 2 (node, edge attribute definition, kernel sizes are denoted). The model inductively learns node representation by recursively aggregating and transforming feature vectors of its neighboring nodes. Below, we define the layers in the proposed GNN classifier.

Convolutional Layer. Following Message Passing Neural Networks (NNconv) [7], which is invariant to graph symmetries, we leverage node degree in the embedding. The embedded representation of the lth convolutional layer $v_i^{(l)} \in \mathbb{R}^{d^{(l)}}$ is

$$v_i^{(l)} = \frac{1}{|\mathcal{N}(i)| + 1} \sigma(\Theta v_i^{(l-1)} + \sum_{j \in \mathcal{N}(i)} h_\phi(e_{ij}) v_j^{(l-1)}), \qquad (1)$$

where $\sigma(\cdot)$ is a nonlinear activation function (we use `relu` here), $\mathcal{N}(i)$ is node i's 1-hop neighborhood, $\Theta \in \mathbb{R}^{d^{(l)} \times d^{(l-1)}}$ is a learnable propagation matrix, h_ϕ denotes a Multi-layer Perceptron (MLP), which maps the edge attributes e_{ij} to a $d^{(l)} \times d^{(l-1)}$ matrix, and we initialize $v_i^{(0)} = v_i$.

Pooling Aggregation Layer. To make sure that down-sampling layers behave idiomatically with respect to different graph sizes and structures, we adopt the approach in [2] for reducing graph nodes. The choice of which nodes to drop is done based on projecting the node attributes on a learnable vector $w^{(l-1)} \in$

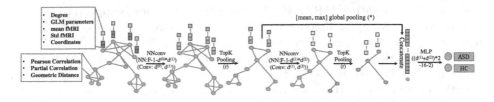

Fig. 2. The architecture of the GNN classifier

$\mathbb{R}^{d^{(l-1)}}$. The nodes receiving lower scores will experience less feature retention. Fully written out, the operation of this pooling layer (computing a pooled graph, $(\boldsymbol{V}^{(l)}, \boldsymbol{E}^{(l)})$, from an input graph, $(\boldsymbol{V}^{(l-1)}, \boldsymbol{E}^{(l-1)})$), is expressed as follows:

$$\boldsymbol{y} = \frac{\boldsymbol{V}^{(l-1)}\boldsymbol{w}^{(l-1)}}{\|\boldsymbol{w}^{(l-1)}\|} \quad \boldsymbol{i} = \text{top}k(\boldsymbol{y}, k) \quad \boldsymbol{V}^{(l)} = (\boldsymbol{V}^{(l-1)} \odot \tanh(\boldsymbol{y}))_{\boldsymbol{i},:} \quad \boldsymbol{E}^{(l)} = \boldsymbol{E}^{(l-1)}_{\boldsymbol{i},\boldsymbol{i}} . \quad (2)$$

Here $\| \cdot \|$ is the L_2 norm, top$k$ finds the indices corresponding to the largest k elements in vector $\boldsymbol{y}$, $\odot$ is (broadcasted) element-wise multiplication, and $(\cdot)_{\boldsymbol{i},\boldsymbol{j}}$ is an indexing operation which takes elements at row indices specified by $\boldsymbol{i}$ and column indices specified by $\boldsymbol{j}$ (colon denotes all indices). The pooling operation trivially retains sparsity by requiring only a projection, a point-wise multiplication and a slicing into the original feature and adjacency matrix. Different from [2], we induce constraint $\|\boldsymbol{w}^{(l)}\|_2 = 1$ implemented by adding an additional `regularization loss` $\lambda \sum_{l=1}^{L}(\|\boldsymbol{w}^{(l)}\|_2 - 1)^2$ to avoid identifiability issues.

Readout Layer. Lastly, we seek a "flattening" operation to preserve information about the input graph in a fixed-size representation. Concretely, to summarise the output graph of the lth conv-pool block, $(\boldsymbol{V}^{(l)}, \boldsymbol{E}^{(l)})$, we use

$$\boldsymbol{s}^{(l)} = (\frac{1}{N^{(l)}} \sum_{i=1}^{N^{(l)}} \boldsymbol{v}_i^{(l)}) \parallel \max(\{\boldsymbol{v}_i^{(l)} : i = 1, ..., N^{(l)}\}), \quad (3)$$

where $N^{(l)}$ is the number of graph nodes, $\boldsymbol{v}_i^{(l)}$ is the ith node's feature vector, max operates elementwise, and $\parallel$ denotes concatenation. The final summary vector is obtained as the concatenation of all those summaries (i.e. $\boldsymbol{s} = \boldsymbol{s}^{(1)} \parallel \boldsymbol{s}^{(2)} \parallel \cdots \parallel \boldsymbol{s}^{(L)}$) and submitted to a MLP for obtaining final predictions.

2.3 Explain Input Data Sensitivity

To explain input data sensitivity, we cluster the whole brain graph into subgraphs first. Then we investigate the predictive power of each sub-graph, further assign importance score to each ROI.

Network Community Clustering. From now on we add the subscript to the graph as $\boldsymbol{G}_s = (\boldsymbol{V}_s, \boldsymbol{E}_s)$ for the sth instance, $s = 1, ..., S$, where S is the number of graphs. Concatenating the sparsified non-negative partial correlation matrices $(\boldsymbol{E}_s)_{:,:,2}$ for all the graphs, we can create a 3rd-order tensor τ of dimension $N \times N \times S$. Non-negative PARAFAC [3] tensor decomposition is applied to tensor τ to discover overlapping functional brain networks. Given decomposition rank R, $\tau \approx \sum_{j=1}^{R} \boldsymbol{a}_j \otimes \boldsymbol{b}_j \otimes \boldsymbol{c}_j$, where loading vectors $\boldsymbol{a}_j \in \mathbb{R}^N$, $\boldsymbol{b}_j \in \mathbb{R}^N$, $\boldsymbol{c}_j \in \mathbb{R}^S$ and $\otimes$ denotes the vector outer product. $\boldsymbol{a}_j = \boldsymbol{b}_j$ since the connectivity matrix is symmetric. The ith element of $\boldsymbol{a}_j$, a_{ji} provides the membership of region i in the community j. Here, we consider region i belongs to community j if $a_{ji} > mean(\boldsymbol{a}_j) + std(\boldsymbol{a}_j)$ [12]. This gives us a collection of community indices indicating region membership $\{\boldsymbol{i}_j \subset \{1, ..., N\} : j = 1, ..., R\}$.

Graph Salience Mapping. After decomposing all the brain networks into community sub-graphs $\{G_{sj} = ((V_s)_{i_j,:}, (E_s)_{i_j,i_j}) : s = 1, ..., S, j = 1, ..., R\}$, we use a salience mapping method to assign each sub-graph an importance score. In our classification setting, the probability of class $c \in \{0, 1\}$ (0: HC, 1: ASD) given the original network G is estimated from the predictive score of the model: $p(c|G)$. To calculate $p(c|G_{sj})$, different from CNN or GCN, we can directly input the sub-graph into the pre-trained classifier. We denote c_s as the class label for instance s and define *Evidence for Correct Class (ECC)* for each community:

$$ECC_j = \frac{1}{S} \sum_s \tanh(\log_2(p(c = c_s|G_{sj})/(1 - p(c = c_s|G_{sj})))), \qquad (4)$$

where laplace correction $(p \leftarrow (pS + 1)/(S + 2))$ is used to avoid zero denominators. Note that log odds-ratio is commonly used in logistic regression to make p more separable. The nonlinear tanh function is used for bounding *ECC*. *ECC* can be positive or negative. A positive value provides evidence for the classifier, whereas a negative value provides evidence against the classifier. The final importance score for node k is calculated by $\sum_{j:k \in i_j} ECC_j/|i_j|$. The larger the score, the more possible the node can be used as a distinguishable marker.

3 Experiments and Results

3.1 Data Acquisition and Preprocessing

We tested our method on a group of 75 ASD children and 43 age and IQ-matched healthy controls collected at Yale Child Study Center. Each subject underwent a task fMRI scan (BOLD, TR = 2000 ms, TE = 25 ms, flip angle = 60°, voxel size $3.44 \times 3.44 \times 4 \text{ mm}^3$) acquired on a Siemens MAGNETOM Trio TIM 3T scanner. For the fMRI scans, subjects performed the "biopoint" task, viewing point light animations of coherent and scrambled biological motion in a block design [9] (24 s per block). The fMRI data was preprocessed following the pipeline in [14].

The mean time series for each node were extracted from a random 1/3 of voxels in the ROI (given an atlas) of preprocessed images by bootstrapping. We augmented the ASD data 10 times and the HC data 20 times, resulting in 750 ASD graphs and 860 HC graphs separately. We split the data into 5 folds based on subjects. Four folds were used as training data and the left out fold was used for testing. Based on the definition in Sect. 2.1, each node attribute $v_i \in \mathbb{R}^{10}$ and each edge attribute $e_{ij} \in \mathbb{R}^3$. Specifically, the GLM parameters of "biopoint task" are: β_1: coefficient of biological motion matrix; β_3: coefficient of scramble motion matrix; β_2 and β_4: coefficients of the previous two matrices' derivatives.

3.2 Step 1: Train ASD/HC Classification Model

Firstly, we tested classifier performance on the Destrieux atlas [5] (148 ROIs) using proposed GNN. Since our pipeline integrated interpretation and classification, we apply a random forest (RF) using 1000 trees as an additional "reality check", while the other existing graph classification models either cannot

Table 1. Performance of different models (mean ± std)

Model	RF(V)	RF(E)	RF(V+E)	GNN(r = 0.3)	GNN(r = 0.5)	GNN(r = 0.8)
Accuracy	0.71 ± 0.05	0.66 ± 0.06	0.68 ± 0.06	0.67 ± 0.14	**0.76 ± 0.06**	0.73 ± 0.07
F-score	0.69 ± 0.06	0.68 ± 0.06	0.63 ± 0.12	0.68 ± 0.09	**0.79 ± 0.08**	0.71 ± 0.10
Precision	0.68 ± 0.06	0.61 ± 0.06	0.69 ± 0.12	0.65 ± 0.19	**0.76 ± 0.12**	0.68 ± 0.08
Recall	0.73 ± 0.12	0.76 ± 0.10	0.77 ± 0.09	0.74 ± 0.07	**0.82 ± 0.06**	0.75 ± 0.08

achieve the performance as GNN [2,7] or do not have straightforward and reliable interpretation ability [1]. We flattened the features to $V \in \mathbb{R}^{1480}$ and $E \in \mathbb{R}^{65712}$ ($65712 = 148 \times 148 \times 3$) and used this input to the RF. In our GNN, $d^{(0)} = D = 10$, $d^{(1)} = 16, d^{(2)} = 8$, resulting in 2746 trainable parameters and we tried different pooling ratios r ($k = r \times N$) in Fig. 2, which was implemented based on [6]. We applied `softmax` after the network output and combined `cross entropy loss` and `regularization loss` with $\lambda = 0.001$ as the objective function. We used the Adam optimizer with initial learning 0.001, then decreased it by a factor of 10 every 50 epochs. We trained the network 300 epochs for all of the splits and measured the instance classification by accuracy, F-score, precision and recall (see Table 1). Our proposed model significantly outperformed the alternative method, due to its ability to embed high dimensional features based on the structural relationship. We selected the best GNN model with $r = 0.5$ in the next step: interpreting biomarkers.

3.3   Step 2: Interpret and Explain Biomarkers

We put forth the hypothesis that the more accurate the classifier, the more reliable biomarkers can be found. We used the best RF model using V as inputs (77.4% accuracy on testing set) and used the RF-based feature importance (mean Gini impurity decrease) as a form of standard method for comparison. For GNN interpretation, we also chose the best model (83.6% accuracy on testing set). Further, to be comparable with RF, all of the interpretation experiments were performed on the training set only. The interpretation results are shown in Fig. 3, where the top 30 important ROIs (averaged over node features and instances)

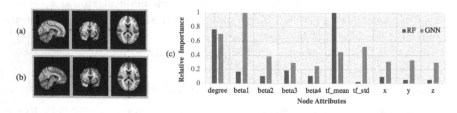

Fig. 3. (a) Top 30 important ROIs (colored in yellow) selected by RF; (b) Top 30 important ROIs selected by GNN ($R = 20$) (colored in red) laying over (a); (c) Node attributes' relative importance scores in the two methods. (Color figure online)

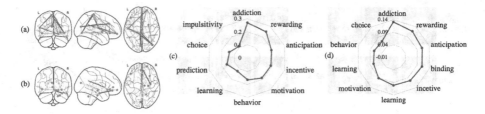

Fig. 4. (a), (c) Top scoring sub-graph and corresponding functional decoding keywords and coefficients. (b), (d) The 2nd high scoring sub-graph and corresponding functional decoding keywords and coefficients.

selected by RF are shown in yellow and the top 30 important ROIs selected by our proposed GNN in red. Nine important ROIs were selected by both methods. In addition, for node attribute importance, we averaged the importance score over ROIs and instances for RF. For GNN, we averaged *gradient explanation* over all the nodes and instances, i.e. $\mathbb{E}(\frac{1}{N}\sum_i|\frac{\partial y}{\partial v_{ij}}|)$, where $y = p(c = 1|G)$, which quantifies the sensitivity of the jth node attribute. From Fig. 3(c) we show the relative importance to the most important node attribute, our proposed method assigned more uniform importance to each node attribute, among which the biological motion parameter β_1 was the most important. In addition, similar features, mean/std of task-fMRI (tf_mean/tf_std) and coordinates (x, y, z), have similar scores, which makes more sense for human interpretation. Notice that our proposed pipeline is also able to identify sub-graph importance from Eq. (4), which is helpful for understanding the interaction between different brain regions. We selected the top 2 sub-graphs ($R = 20$) and used Neurosynth [15] to decode the functional keywords associated with the sub-graphs (shown in Fig. 4). These networks are both associated with high-level social behaviors. To illustrate the predictive power of the 2 sub-graphs, we retrained the network using the graph slicing on those 19 ROIs of the 2 sub-graphs as input. Accuracy on the testing set (in the split of the best model) was 78.9%, achieving comparable performance to using the whole graph.

3.4   Evaluation: Robustness Discussion

To examine the potential influence of different graph building strategies on the reliability of network estimates, the functional and anatomical data were registered and parcellated by the Destrieux atlas (*A1*) and the Desikan-Killiany atlas (*A2*) [4]. We also showed the robustness of the results with respect to the number of clusters for $R = 10, 20, 30$. The results are shown in Fig. 5. We ranked *ECC*s for each node and indicated the top 30 ROIs in *A1* and top 15 ROIs in *A2*. The atlas and number of clusters are indicated on the left of each sub-figure. Orbitofrontal cortex and ventromedial prefrontal cortex are selected in all the cases, which are social motivation related and have previously been shown to be associated with ASD [9]. We also validated the results by decoding the neurological functions of the important ROIs overlapped with Neurosynth.

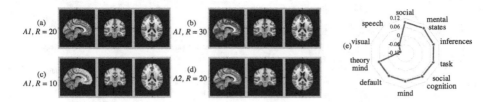

Fig. 5. (a) The biomarkers (red) interpreted on *A1* with 20 clusters; (b)–(d) The biomarkers interpreted by different *R* and atlas laying over on (a) with different colors; (e) The correlation between overlapped ROIs and functional keywords. (Color figure online)

4   Conclusion and Future Work

In this paper, we proposed a framework to discover ASD brain biomarkers from task-fMRI using GNN. It achieved improved accuracy and more interpretable features than the baseline method. We also showed our method performed robustly on different atlases and hyper-parameters. Future work will include investigating more hyper-parameters (i.e. suitable size of sub-graphs communities), testing the results on functional atlases and different graph definition methods. The pipeline can be generalized to other feature importance analysis problems, such as resting-fMRI biomarker discovery and vessel cancer detection.

Acknowledgment. This work was supported by NIH Grant R01 NS035193.

References

1. Adebayo, J., et al.: Sanity checks for saliency maps. In: Advances in Neural Information Processing Systems, pp. 9505–9515 (2018)
2. Cangea, C., et al.: Towards sparse hierarchical graph classifiers. arXiv preprint arXiv:1811.01287 (2018)
3. Carroll, J.D., Chang, J.J.: Analysis of individual differences in multidimensional scaling via an N-way generalization of "Eckart-Young" decomposition. Psychometrika **35**(3), 283–319 (1970)
4. Desikan, R.S., et al.: An automated labeling system for subdividing the human cerebral cortex on MRI scans into gyral based regions of interest. NeuroImage **31**(3), 968–980 (2006)
5. Destrieux, C., et al.: Automatic parcellation of human cortical gyri and sulci using standard anatomical nomenclature. NeuroImage **53**(1), 1–15 (2010)
6. Fey, M., Lenssen, J.E.: Fast graph representation learning with PyTorch geometric. CoRR abs/1903.02428 (2019)
7. Gilmer, J., et al.: Neural message passing for quantum chemistry. In: ICML 2017, pp. 1263–1272. JMLR.org (2017)
8. Goldani, A.A., et al.: Biomarkers in autism. Front. Psychiatry **5**, 100 (2014)
9. Kaiser, M.D., et al.: Neural signatures of autism. Proc. Nat. Acad. Sci. **107**(49), 21223–21228 (2010)

10. Kipf, T.N., Welling, M.: Semi-supervised classification with graph convolutional networks. arXiv preprint arXiv:1609.02907 (2016)
11. Ktena, S.I., et al.: Distance metric learning using graph convolutional networks: application to functional brain networks. In: Descoteaux, M., Maier-Hein, L., Franz, A., Jannin, P., Collins, D.L., Duchesne, S. (eds.) MICCAI 2017. LNCS, vol. 10433, pp. 469–477. Springer, Cham (2017). https://doi.org/10.1007/978-3-319-66182-7_54
12. Loe, C.W., Jensen, H.J.: Comparison of communities detection algorithms for multiplex. Physica A: Stat. Mech. Appl. **431**, 29–45 (2015)
13. Nishii, R.: Box-Cox Transformation. Encyclopedia of Mathematics. Springer, New York (2001)
14. Yang, D., et al.: Brain responses to biological motion predict treatment outcome in young children with autism. Transl. Psychiatry **6**(11), e948 (2016)
15. Yarkoni, T., et al.: Large-scale automated synthesis of human functional neuroimaging data. Nat. Methods **8**(8), 665 (2011)

Achieving Accurate Segmentation of Nasopharyngeal Carcinoma in MR Images Through Recurrent Attention

Jia-bin Huang[1], Enhong Zhuo[1], Haojiang Li[2], Lizhi Liu[2], Hongmin Cai[1(✉)], and Yangming Ou[3(✉)]

[1] South China University of Technology, Guangzhou 510006, China
hmcai@scut.edu.cn
[2] Guangdong Key Laboratory of Nasopharyngeal Carcinoma Diagnosis and Therapy, Collaborative Innovation Center for Cancer Medicine, Sun Yat-sen University Cancer Center, Guangzhou 510060, China
[3] Harvard Medical School, Boston, MA 02115, USA
yangming.ou@childrens.harvard.edu

Abstract. Automatic nasopharyngeal carcinoma (NPC) segmentation in magnetic resonance (MR) images remains challenging since NPC is infiltrative and typically has a small or even tiny volume, making it indiscernible from tightly connected surrounding tissues. Recent methods using deep learning models performed unsatisfactorily since the boundary between NPC and its neighbor tissues is difficult to distinguish. In this paper, a novel Convolutional Neural Network (CNN) with recurrent attention modules (RAMs) is proposed to tackle the problem. To enhance the performance of NPC segmentation, the proposed fully automatic NPC segmentation method with recurrent attention exploits the semantic features in higher layers to guide the learning of features in lower layers. Features are fed into RAMs iteratively from the higher layers to the lower ones. The lower layers are updated iteratively by the guidance of higher layers to render with discriminative capability. Our proposed method was validated in a dataset including 596 patients, experimental results demonstrate that our method outperforms state-of-the-art methods.

Keywords: Nasopharyngeal carcinoma segmentation · Recurrent attention · Convolutional neural network

1 Introduction

Nasopharyngeal carcinoma (NPC) is a malignant tumor originating in the nasopharynx, and is prevalent in South China, Northern Africa, and Alaska [1]. With high resolution for soft tissues, magnetic resonance (MR) images can be utilized to evaluate the location and shape of NPC. Reliable automatic NPC segmentation in MR images is important for treatment planning as well as follow-up

© Springer Nature Switzerland AG 2019
D. Shen et al. (Eds.): MICCAI 2019, LNCS 11768, pp. 494–502, 2019.
https://doi.org/10.1007/978-3-030-32254-0_55

evaluation [2]. However, there exists an indiscernible boundary between NPC and surrounding tissues, and intensity inhomogeneity usually happens in MR images, making automatic NPC segmentation a challenging but significant task.

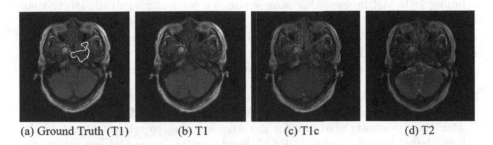

(a) Ground Truth (T1)   (b) T1   (c) T1c   (d) T2

Fig. 1. Example MR images with 3 sequences including T1-weighted (T1), enhanced contrast T1-weighted (T1c) and T2-weighted (T2). Red contour represents the indiscernible boundary between NPC and surrounding tissues. (Color figure online)

There are a few approaches proposed to tackle NPC segmentation in MR images in the last few years. Huang *et al.* [3] performed an automatic NPC segmentation in MR images with a hidden Markov random field model. Huang *et al.* [4] proposed two semi-supervised region-based NPC segmentation. Zhou *et al.* [5] introduced a two-class SVM-based NPC segmentation method by learning the distribution of MR images data with the help of kernel learning. Recently, Convolutional Neural Networks (CNNs), including fully convolutional network (FCN) [6] and U-Net [7], have been proven to be powerful for semantic segmentation. Men *et al.* [8] used a deep deconvolutional neural network to achieve NPC segmentation in planning computed tomography (CT) images. However, neither the traditional hand-engineered models nor the automatic deep learning models performed on a large number of samples. Moreover, current deep learning models perform unsatisfactorily for NPC segmentation due to a lack of refining lower layers with the guidance of contextual information from higher layers.

Different layers in deep learning models have different receptive fields and create different latent features. In lower layers of a neural network, basic image characteristics such as the edge and contour information are learned. In comparison, more contextual information but less spatial information are learned in the higher layers due to the larger receptive field and smaller feature maps. One of the major difficulties in NPC segmentation is to discriminate the boundary between the tumor and surrounding tissues, as shown in Fig. 1. Therefore spatial information is particularly important for NPC segmentation. Alternatively, the feature maps in the lower layer with more spatial information can be refined by utilizing discriminative information in the higher layers of the network. To use the feedback of higher layers to help the learning of lower layer features, we proposed two kinds of Recurrent Attention Modules (RAMs) to extract discriminative information from higher layer using Long Short-Term Memory (LSTM), which can remember the information of the previous iterations. RAMs use discriminative information of the higher layer to guide the learning of the lower layer in neural networks iteratively to focus on significant information and region relevant to NPC. This study aims to improve accuracy in a dataset of 596 NPC patients including 1804 MR images. Our sample size is a level of magnitude larger than the sample sizes in existing studies (e.g. 26 patients in [3], 40 patients in [4], 9 patients in [5] and 230 patients in [8]), allowing us to fully test the generality of the proposed method.

Our contributions and novelties are summarized as follows:

- A channel-wise RAM, called cRAM, is proposed to exploit features of the lower layers by passing through cRAM after features of the higher layers, with their semantic guidance for iterative learning to refine features of the lower layers. By channel-wise RAM, low layers in our model can selectively suppress the features with low relevance to the segmentation target since different channels mean different kinds of features;
- A region-wise RAM, called rRAM is proposed to utilize the higher layer semantic features to guide features of the lower layer to assign different levels of attention to neighbor region. Region more relevant to NPC tends to obtain a larger weight;

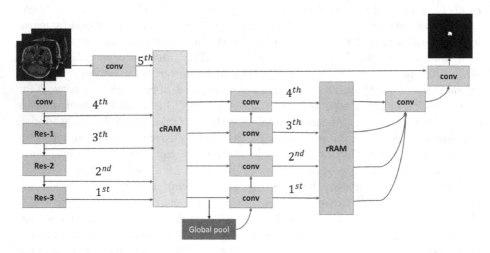

Fig. 2. Overview of our proposed model with RAMs. The black and red lines represent the downsample and upsample operations respectively, and the blue lines represent data flow without changing the resolution of the feature map. (Color figure online)

2 Methods

2.1 Method Overview

The proposed network with recurrent attention employs an "Encoder-Decoder" architecture, which is illustrated in Fig. 2. The network takes T1-weighted (T1), enhanced contrast T1-weighted (T1c) and T2-weighted (T2) MR images as input and outputs the segmentation result. We use two convolution layers to obtain feature maps with the same resolution as the input images, and utilize ResNet [9] pretrained on ImageNet [10] to extract feature maps with different resolution in the encoder phase. The obtained feature maps are fed into a cRAM from the highest layer to the lowest layer iteratively to produce attentional feature maps. Global average pooling is then performed on the highest attentional map to obtain a global contextual feature map. In the decoder phase, up-sampling results are combined with the attentional feature map in the previous layer successively in each layer. We further use an rRAM to generate region-wise attentional features iteratively. Finally, attentional feature maps from rRAM are convoluted together with the last feature map from cRAM to obtain final segmentation.

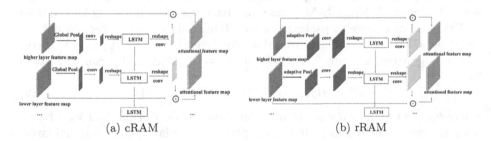

(a) cRAM   (b) rRAM

Fig. 3. Schematic illustration of RAMs. The black and red lines represent the downsample and upsample operations respectively, and the blue lines represent data flow without changing the size of the feature map. (a) cRAM. (b) rRAM. (Color figure online)

2.2 Recurrent Attention Module

Channel-Wise Recurrent Attention Module (cRAM). The cRAM inspired by Squeeze-and-Excitation (SE) networks [11] aims to make features maps focus on the channels whose features have more discriminative information for NPC. Features in lower layers are recalibrated with feedback from LSTM, which preserves contextual information from higher layers. Let $X = [X_1, X_2, \ldots, X_n]$, $X_i \in \mathbb{R}^{C \times H \times W}$ denotes the feature maps from different layers fed into the cRAM, where n is the number of layers, C, H and W denote the channel, height and width of X_i, respectively. At each iteration, feature maps

X_i passes through a global average pooling layer and a convolutional layer, and then is reshaped to a vector v_i. As presented in Fig. 3(a), the LSTM takes v_i as input and h_{i-1} as hidden state, generates $v_i' = F_{LSTM}(v_i; h_{i-1})$. h_{i-1} is the hidden state at previous iteration $i-1$, encoding contextual information from the higher layers fed into the LSTM previously. Vector v_i' is then reshaped to a tensor and passes through a convolutional layer to obtain attention weights W_i. After that, the recurrent channel-wise attention map $A_i \in \mathbb{R}^{C \times 1 \times 1}$ (gray feature maps in Fig. 3(a)) is obtained by $\sigma(W_i)$, where σ denotes the Sigmoid function. The attentional feature maps U_i can finally be achieved by

$$U_i = A_i \odot X_i, i \in \{1, 2, \ldots, n\} \tag{1}$$

where $\odot$ is the element-wise multiplication operator using array broadcasting.

We utilize the channel-wise RAM module on each layer to iteratively refine its features with the contextual guidance from higher layers. With the attention map A_i, the output feature map U_i in the cRAM tends to suppress the channels with less discriminative information.

Region-Wise Recurrent Attention Module. The rRAM aims to make the feature maps focus on the region which is important to the segmentation targets. Similar to cRAM, rRAM utilizes feedback with a semantic guidance from LSTM to refine feature maps, learning an attentional map across regions but not channels. Given feature maps from different layers $X = [X_1, X_2, \ldots, X_n]$, corresponding attention maps for each layer $A^r = [A_1^r, A_2^r, \ldots, A_n^r]$ can be learned by

$$A_i^r = \sigma(f(X_i, h_i - 1)), i \in \{1, 2, \ldots, n\} \tag{2}$$

where h_{i-1} is the hidden state at previous iteration $i-1$ of the LSTM. f represents successive operations including adaptive pooling layer, convolutional layers and the LSTM. The adaptive pooling layer firstly takes feature maps X_i as input and outputs regional statistics Z_i with size $C \times S \times S$, where S is a preset size for Z_i and $S < min(H, W)$. Then Z_i passes through a convolutional layer and is reshaped to a vector v_i. LSTM takes v_i as input and generates an attentional vector v_i' that contains contextual information from the higher layers. v_i' is then reshaped to a tensor and passes through a convolutional layer. After upsampling and normalization to [0,1] by a Sigmoid function, an attention map A_i^r is finally achieved to recalibrate features. In the end, we fuse A_i^r with X_i through element-wise multiplication to produce the final output attentional feature map, which emphasizes regions more important to the segmentation targets.

3   Experiments

3.1   Dataset

Our experiments were conducted on MR images in the axial view with three sequences including T1, T1c and T2, which were acquired from 596 patients in

Sun Yat-sen University Cancer Center. We collected 1804 image samples (thus 5512 images in total for three sequences) with ground truth manually drawn by four experienced radiologists to conduct our experiments. Each image was first resized to 384 × 384 since there were several sizes in which 384 × 384 was the smallest. We augmented (including rotation and horizontally flipping) 1400 images of 430 patients to 8400 images as the training set, while the rest 404 images from 166 patients were used as testing set.

Table 1. Metric results of different NPC segmentation methods. (The best result is highlighted in bold.)

Methods	Precision	Recall	Dice	CC
U-Net	0.7089	0.6299	0.6671	0.0018
U-Net+SE	0.7227	0.6741	0.6976	0.1329
U-Net+cRAM	0.7320	0.7058	0.7187	0.2171
U-Net+rRAM	0.7027	0.7194	0.7110	0.1870
U-Net+cRAM+rRAM	0.7027	0.7538	0.7231	0.2502
DenseNet	0.5332	0.7025	0.6063	−0.2990
DDNN	0.6985	0.7214	0.7098	0.1822
Ours	0.7554	0.7991	0.7766	0.4248
Ours (weighted loss)	**0.7824**	**0.8107**	**0.7963**	**0.4884**

3.2 Implementation Details

The boundary pixel of the NPC is important to delineate the tumor from the surrounding tissues. To exploit and strengthen the boundary information, we introduced a pixel-wise weighted cross-entropy loss function to guide penalizing the learning. Those pixels with a distance to the border of NPC smaller than $d > 1$ were penalized by a larger weight w_b, otherwise, it stays the same with a weighting coefficient of 1. Throughout our experiments, we set $d = 3$ and $w_b = 1.5$.

Stochastic gradient descent (SGD) with momentum 0.9 and weight decay $4e^{-3}$ is adopted as optimizer to train our model. We set the learning rate to 0.004 and become one-tenth in every 10 epochs, and $S = 7$ in rRAM. Our model is trained and evaluated on two NVIDIA GTX1080TI GPUs with batch size 10.

3.3 Experimental Results

We compare NPC segmentation results of our method with several state-of-the-art methods on our dataset, including U-Net [7], Fully Convolutional DenseNet [12] and a deep deconvolutional neural network (DDNN) proposed by Men et al. [8]. Some common evaluation metrics for semantic segmentation are provided for quantitative comparison, including Precision, Recall, Dice Similarity Coefficient (Dice) and Conformity Coefficient (CC). For a fair competition,

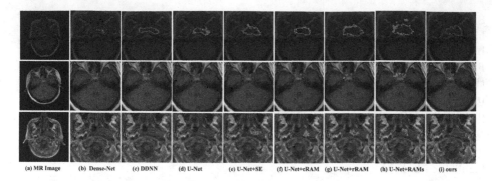

(a) MR Image   (b) Dense-Net   (c) DDNN   (d) U-Net   (e) U-Net+SE   (f) U-Net+cRAM   (g) U-Net+rRAM   (h) U-Net+RAMs   (i) ours

Fig. 4. Results comparison for NPC segmentation. Red contour represents ground truth, and other colors of contours represent segmentation results from different methods. The first column represents T1-weighted MR images, segmentation results of different methods are enlarged for visualization in the rest columns. Each row stands for segmentation results for one slice of MR images. U-Net+RAMs represents U-Net+cRAM+rRAM. (Color figure online)

all methods adopt the cross-entropy as the loss function. Metric results of different methods are listed in Table 1, our method obviously outperforms other methods on all the metrics.

Moreover, to measure the effect of RAMs, we incorporate RAMs into U-Net since the architecture of our model is similar to U-Net. RAMs improve U-Net significantly by increasing a Dice score of 5.60%. U-Net with cRAM also outperforms U-Net with SE Blocks [11] (in the same place we add cRAM) on all the metrics. In addition, we visualize NPC segmentation results of our method (using pixel-wise weighted loss function) and the compared methods in Fig. 4. DDNN obtains unsatisfactory results without a similar boundary to the ground truth, the probable reason is that their method does not take full advantage of the spatial information from the lower layers. Our method achieved segmentation results similar to the ground truth in the second row of Fig. 4, whereas other methods get unsatisfactory results with few positives in the predicted mask.

The segmentation results by other methods contain more false clusters and thus leading to an unsmoothed boundary between NPC and surrounding tissues. As is illustrated in Fig. 5, our method obtains a highly accurate segmentation with a smooth boundary.

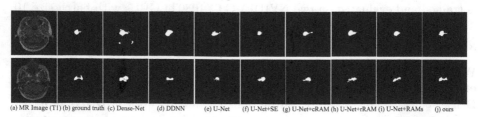

(a) MR Image (T1) (b) ground truth (c) Dense-Net   (d) DDNN   (e) U-Net   (f) U-Net+SE (g) U-Net+cRAM (h) U-Net+rRAM (i) U-Net+RAMs   (j) ours

Fig. 5. NPC segmentation results on two typical examples. Each row stands for segmentation results for one slice of MR images. U-Net+RAMs represents U-Net+cRAM+rRAM.

4   Conclusion

In this paper, a novel convolutional neural network with two kinds of RAMs is proposed for NPC segmentation in MR images. These two kinds of RAMs, cRAM and rRAM, are designed to exploit discriminative information across channels and regions, respectively. RAMs work iteratively to refine feature maps from each layer by using discriminative information remembered by LSTM. We applied the obtained feature maps from RAMs to guide NPC segmentation in MR images. Experimental results for NPC segmentation demonstrate that our method outperforms state-of-the-art semantic segmentation neural networks. The superior performance of the two RAMs when being equipped in the benchmark network proved that they are potentially valuable to address challenging segmentation tasks.

Acknowledgments. This work was supported by grants from the National Natural Science Foundation of China (no. 61771007, no. 81572652), Health & Medical Collaborative Innovation Project of Guangzhou City, China (grants 201604020003, 201803010021), Science and Technology Planning Projects of Guangdong Province (2016A010101013, 2017B020226004), and the Fundamental Research Fund for the Central Universities (2017ZD051).

References

1. Wei, W.I., Sham, J.S.: Nasopharyngeal carcinoma. Lancet **365**(9476), 2041–2054 (2005)
2. King, A.D., et al.: Neck node metastases from nasopharyngeal carcinoma: MR imaging of patterns of disease. J. Sci. Spec. Head Neck **22**(3), 275–281 (2000)
3. Huang, K.W., Zhao, Z.Y., Gong, Q., Zha, J., Chen, L., Yang, R.: Nasopharyngeal carcinoma segmentation via HMRF-EM with maximum entropy. In: 2015 37th Annual International Conference of the IEEE Engineering in Medicine and Biology Society (EMBC), pp. 2968–2972. IEEE (2015)
4. Huang, W., Chan, K.L., Zhou, J.: Region-based nasopharyngeal carcinoma lesion segmentation from MRI using clustering- and classification-based methods with learning. J. Digit. Imaging **26**(3), 472–482 (2013)
5. Zhou, J., Chan, K.L., Xu, P., Chong, V.F.: Nasopharyngeal carcinoma lesion segmentation from MR images by support vector machine. In: 3rd IEEE International Symposium on Biomedical Imaging: Nano to Macro, pp. 1364–1367. IEEE (2006)
6. Long, J., Shelhamer, E., Darrell, T.: Fully convolutional networks for semantic segmentation. In: Proceedings of the IEEE Conference on Computer Vision and Pattern Recognition, pp. 3431–3440 (2015)
7. Ronneberger, O., Fischer, P., Brox, T.: U-Net: convolutional networks for biomedical image segmentation. In: Navab, N., Hornegger, J., Wells, W.M., Frangi, A.F. (eds.) MICCAI 2015. LNCS, vol. 9351, pp. 234–241. Springer, Cham (2015). https://doi.org/10.1007/978-3-319-24574-4_28
8. Men, K., et al.: Deep deconvolutional neural network for target segmentation of nasopharyngeal cancer in planning computed tomography images. Front. Oncol. **7**, 315 (2017)

9. He, K., Zhang, X., Ren, S., Sun, J.: Deep residual learning for image recognition. In: Proceedings of the IEEE Conference on Computer Vision and Pattern Recognition, pp. 770–778 (2016)
10. Russakovsky, O., et al.: Imagenet large scale visual recognition challenge. Int. J. Comput. Vision **115**(3), 211–252 (2015)
11. Hu, J., Shen, L., Sun, G.: Squeeze-and-excitation networks. In: Proceedings of the IEEE Conference on Computer Vision and Pattern Recognition, pp. 7132–7141 (2018)
12. Jégou, S., Drozdzal, M., Vazquez, D., Romero, A., Bengio, Y.: The one hundred layers tiramisu: fully convolutional densenets for semantic segmentation. In: Proceedings of the IEEE Conference on Computer Vision and Pattern Recognition Workshops, pp. 11–19 (2017)

Brain Dynamics Through the Lens of Statistical Mechanics by Unifying Structure and Function

Igor Fortel[1], Mitchell Butler[1], Laura E. Korthauer[2,4], Liang Zhan[3], Olusola Ajilore[1], Ira Driscoll[2], Anastasios Sidiropoulos[1], Yanfu Zhang[3], Lei Guo[3], Heng Huang[3], Dan Schonfeld[1], and Alex Leow[1(✉)]

[1] University of Illinois at Chicago, Chicago, IL, USA
aleow@psch.uic.edu
[2] University of Wisconsin-Milwaukee, Milwaukee, WI, USA
[3] University of Pittsburgh, Pittsburgh, PA, USA
[4] Alpert Medical School of Brown University, Providence, RI, USA

Abstract. This paper introduces a novel method that unifies structural connectivity and functional time series to form a signed coupling inter-action network or "signed resting state structural connectome" (signed rs-SC) to describe neural excitation and inhibition. We employ an energy representation of neural activity based on the Ising model from statistical mechanics, hereby bypassing traditional BOLD correlations. The spin model is a function of a coupling interaction (traditionally positive or negative) and spin-states of paired brain regions. Observed functional time series represent brain states over time. A maximum pseudolikelihood with a constraint is used to estimate the coupling interaction. The constraint is introduced as a penalty function such that the learned interactions are scaled relative to structural connectivity; the sign of the interactions may infer inhibition or excitation over an underlying structure. We evaluate our method by comparing a group of otherwise healthy APOE-e4 carriers with a control group of non APOE-e4 subjects. Our results identify a global shift in the excitation-inhibition balance of the APOE e4 signed rs-SC compared to the control group, providing the first connectomics-based support for hyperexcitation related to APOE e4.

Keywords: Ising model · Maximum Likelihood · Brain dynamics · Functional connectivity · Structure connectome · MRI

1 Introduction

The relationship between structure and function is an open question that some researchers have investigated using the Ising model from statistical mechanics [7,11,16,17]. Communication between neurons involves the release of certain neurotransmitters that drive an excitatory or inhibitory response. At a macroscopic level, this can be interpreted as a pair of brain regions having an activating

© Springer Nature Switzerland AG 2019
D. Shen et al. (Eds.): MICCAI 2019, LNCS 11768, pp. 503–511, 2019.
https://doi.org/10.1007/978-3-030-32254-0_56

or inhibiting influence on each other. It is hypothesized that a core abnormality of early AD is "hyperexcitability" in neuronal circuits, supported by recent whole-cell recordings in animal AD models demonstrating that β-Amyloid (Aβ) induces synaptic hyperexcitation and perturbs the excitation-inhibition (E-I) balance in regions such as the entorhinal cortex and anterior cingulate via depressing inhibitory transmission [14,15]. Our main contribution is a novel approach to evaluate this hypothesis, by computationally infering the nature (excitatory vs inhibitory) of structural connectivity using statistical mechanics to yield a signed interaction network or "signed resting state structural connectome" (signed rs-SC).

2   Ising Model

A functional connectome can be represented mathematically as an undirected graph where vertices (V) correspond to regions of interest (ROIs), and edges (E) describe some measure of connectivity between pairs of vertices. In conventional descriptions of functional connectivity (FC), each edge $e_{i,j} \in E$ is associated with a weight, computed using a pairwise BOLD correlation. In this work we use the Ising model, a special case of a Markov random field model in which each ROI can exhibit two possible states $s = \pm 1$. Previous studies have shown this to accurately model neuronal activity under the assumption that connectivity between neurons can either be active (+1) or inactive (-1) [16,18].

First, we formulate the system energy as given by the Hamiltonian $H(\mathbf{s}) = -\sum_{i<j} J_{i,j} s_i s_j \ \forall \ i,j \in \{1,2,\dots,N\}$ where the spin configuration $\mathbf{s}$ is defined as the column vector $\mathbf{s} = [s_1, s_2, .., s_N]^T$, N is the number of regions, s_i and s_j are the spin states of region i and region j, and $J_{i,j}$ represents a pairwise interaction between those regions. This formulation is under the assumption that there is no external influence (i.e resting-state). Unless otherwise stated, summations in this paper are for $i < j$ to avoid double counting and exclude self-connections. The probability of observing a specific configuration is given by the Boltzmann distribution: $Pr(\mathbf{s}) = \frac{1}{Z} exp\left(-\beta H(\mathbf{s})\right)$, where β is the inverse temperature and Z is the partition function defined as $Z = \sum_\mathbf{s} exp(-\beta H(\mathbf{s}))$. Here, the summation is over all possible configurations of states. Ising model simulation is described in algorithm 1 to find an equilibrium time evolution of states for each ROI [4]. Ising model dynamics have been previously used in multiple studies to estimate functional connectivity [6,11,17].

Our method aims to solve the "inverse problem", using observed functional time series to infer coupling interactions. Similar to previous work, we use a gradient ascent scheme [17,18]. However, where previous methods estimated network structure properties, we embed the structure into the estimation. This is achieved by using a gradient ascent procedure on the log likelihood of the observed data [1]. The computation of Maximum Likelihood, in this case, requires calculations over all 2^N possible spin configurations [12]. For large sample size, the pseudolikelihood (PL) approximation converges to the maximum likelihood with lower computational cost [3]. Ezaki et al. demonstrated the viability of a pseudolikelihood-based model to estimate features on functional time series [6].

Algorithm 1. Ising Model Simulations

1: Define: J, the maximum number of simulations σ, and a range of β values
2: **procedure** MONTE CARLO SIMULATIONS FOR EACH TEMPERATURE
3:    Initialize: random configuration of spin states
4:    for each simulation: randomly fix an element from the configuration, and compute the Hamiltonian relative to that fixed element, denoted by $H(s_i)$
5:    if $H(s_i) \leq 0$ or $rand(0,1) \leq exp(\frac{H(s_i)}{\beta})$, flip the state. The command $rand(0,1)$ generates a random value between 0 and 1. Complete for all states in configuration
6:    The final configuration is used as the input to for next simulation
7:    Concatenate all simulations into an $N - by - \sigma$ matrix and compute correlation by multiplying this matrix by its transpose and dividing by σ
8: Do this for each temperature in the range

---

3   Constrained Pseudolikelihood Estimation

We begin with the observed functional time series, which are binarized to be ± 1. A threshold of 0 is used for each sample due to the data being preprocessed with global signal regression (GSR) [9], resulting in a zero-mean time series; we binarize around the mean to avoid a bias towards either state. The resulting binary sequences represent the observed spin configurations, which we define as a function of the time samples: $S_{observed} = [s(1), s(2), \ldots, s(t_{max})]$. We estimate a parameter J, a set containing all $J_{i,j}$, via the maximization of the pseudolikelihood function, defined as:

$$\max_J \mathcal{L}(J, \beta), \; where \; \mathcal{L}(J, \beta) = \prod_{t=1}^{t_{max}} \prod_{i=1}^{N} Pr\left(s_i(t) | J, \beta, s_{-i}(t)\right) \tag{1}$$

Unlike traditional Maximum Likelihood, the probability is not over all spin states, but of observing one $s_i(t)$ with all the others $s_{-i}(t)$ fixed. To ensure the magnitude of the coupling interactions are scaled relative to the structural connectome, our constraint is formulated as $|J_{i,j}| = \mu W_{i,j}$, where μ is the normalization constant and $W_{i,j}$ is the structural connectivity between ROI pairs. With appropriate scaling, we assume that $\mu = 1$. We therefore pose a penalty-based optimization approach to maximize the log-pseudolikelihood function as follows:

$$\ell(J, \beta) = \frac{1}{t_{max}} \ln \mathcal{L}(J, \beta) - \frac{1}{2}\lambda \sum_{i<j} \left(J_{i,j} - \text{sgn}\left(J_{i,j}\right) W_{i,j}\right)^2 \tag{2}$$

We first evaluate the pseudolikelihood component $\frac{1}{t_{max}} \ln \mathcal{L}(J, \beta)$, which expands to: $\frac{1}{t_{max}} \sum_{t=1}^{t_{max}} \sum_{i=1}^{N} \ln \left(\frac{\exp\left(\beta \sum_{k=1}^{N} J_{i,k} s_i(t) s_k(t)\right)}{\exp\left(\beta \sum_{k=1}^{N} J_{i,k} s_k(t)\right) + \exp\left(-\beta \sum_{k=1}^{N} J_{i,k} s_k(t)\right)} \right)$. The probability distribution here stems from the Boltzmann distribution under the pseudolikelihood conditions such that the numerator of the log is the energy of the system, while the denominator is the sum of all possible energies. Thus, only two terms are present in the denominator; one is positive and one is negative as $s_i(t)$ can only be $+1$ or -1. We can now simplify the likelihood function further by letting $C_i(t) = \beta \sum_{k=1}^{N} J_{i,k} s_k(t)$, which results in a formulation as follows:

$$\ell(\boldsymbol{J}, \beta) = \frac{1}{t_{\max}} \sum_{t=1}^{t_{\max}} \sum_{i=1}^{N} C_i(t) s_i(t) - \ln \left(\exp\left(C_i(t) \right) + \exp\left(-C_i(t) \right) \right) \tag{3}$$

$$-\frac{1}{2} \lambda \sum_{i<j} \left(J_{i,j} - \operatorname{sgn}\left(J_{i,j} \right) W_{i,j} \right)^2$$

The gradient ascent procedure can be constructed with respect to $J_{i,j}$ by computing the partial derivative of the constructed log-pseudolikelihood.

$$\frac{\partial \ell}{\partial J_{i,j}} = \frac{1}{t_{\max}} \sum_{t=1}^{t_{\max}} \beta \left\{ s_i(t) s_j(t) - s_j(t) \tanh\left(C_i(t) \right) \right\} - \lambda \left(J_{i,j} - \operatorname{sgn}\left(J_{i,j} \right) W_{i,j} \right)$$

$$\tag{4}$$

where the updating scheme follows: $J_{i,j}^{n+1} = J_{i,j}^{n} + \epsilon \left. \frac{\partial \ell}{\partial J_{i,j}} \right|_{n}$ Here, n is the iteration number and ϵ is the learning rate. The partial derivative of the penalty holds under the assumption that $J_{i,j} \neq 0$ as the sgn function is continuous and constant everywhere except 0. In practice however, if there exists a $J_{i,j} = 0$, then $sgn(0) = 0$ by convention. The penalty function ensures that the inferred pairwise interaction is scaled relative to the estimated structure of the brain. To account for the β temperature constant we employ an alternating optimization strategy whereby we first assume $\beta = 1$ and compute the first step of the gradient ascent. Using the resulting coupling interaction, we can then optimize β by simulating the Ising model to find the temperature that yields the highest correlated result with the observed functional connectome. Using this new temperature we take the next step along the gradient and continue alternating between optimizing β and $J_{i,j}$ until the algorithm converges. Through simulations, we find that the optimal β is in the neighborhood of 1 for all subjects.

4   Results and Validation

Structural and functional connectivity for 38 cognitively normal Apoe-e4 carriers aged 40–60 ($\mu = 50.8$) are compared with 38 age ($\mu = 50.9$) and sex-matched (16M/22F) non-carriers (control). Imaging included T1-weighted MRI, resting state fMRI and diffusion weighted MRI. Freesurfer cortical parcellation and subcortical segmentation was performed to derive 80 ROIs. The mean time-course was extracted from the pre-processed rs-fMRI data. Probabilistic tractography was used to create the structural connectome matrices, and normalized by the way-total of the corresponding seed ROIs. More detailed information on the imaging and processing steps can be found in Korthauer et al. [9].

We first optimize λ in our constraint by estimating the coupling interactions $J_{i,j}$ for each subject using our method for a range of λ values. The estimated $J_{i,j}$

for each λ is then used to generate a correlation function $f_c(\beta)$ by simulating the Ising Model and computing the Pearson correlation between observed and simulated functional connectomes $\forall \beta$. The function $f_1(\lambda)$ contains the $max(f_c)$ achieved. To evaluate the impact of λ on our constraint, a second function $f_2(\lambda)$ computes the Pearson correlation between $|J_{i,j}|$ and $W_{i,j}$ $\forall$ i, j.

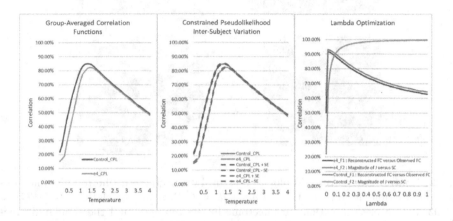

Fig. 1. Right: $f_1(\lambda)$ and $f_2(\lambda)$ curves are averaged over all 38 subjects in each group for $\lambda = (0, 0.05, ..., 1.00)$, where $\lambda = 0$ corresponds to the unconstrained case. Both groups are consistent, with optimal λ approximately 0.1. Left: f_c curve averaged over all 38 subjects in each group for $\beta = (0.05, 0.1, ..., 4.0)$ using 3 estimates for $J_{i,j}$, namely the constrained pseudolikelihood (CPL) with $\lambda = 0.1$, the unconstrained pseudolikelihood (PL), as well as simply using the structural connectome (SC) for $J_{i,j}$. Middle: f_c curve of the CPL case with standard error (SE) ribbon describing inter-subject variation

Group-averaged $f_1(\lambda)$ and $f_2(\lambda)$ are shown in Fig. 1. To determine an optimal λ, a min-max optimization is used: $D_r = arg\ \underset{\lambda}{min}(f_r(\lambda), r = (1, 2))$ and $\lambda^* = arg\ \underset{D_r}{max}(\underset{\lambda}{min}(f_r(\lambda), r = (1, 2)))$, corresponding to the intersection point between monotonically increasing and monotonically decreasing functions. We note that $f_1(\lambda)$ is not strictly monotonic due to the data point at $\lambda = 0$; however, the condition holds with that exception. We generate an f_c curve for each subject using 3 methods of determining the coupling interactions $J_{i.j}$: (1) our constrained pseudolikelihood estimation (CPL); (2) unconstrained pseudolikelihood estimation (PL); and (3) using the structural connectome as the coupling interaction (unsigned interactions). Shown in Fig. 1, f_c averaged over all subjects using the constrained model peaks at $\beta \approx 1$ and results in $r > 0.8$ at the maximum for both groups, while the other two are much lower. The improvement demonstrated by our method over the unconstrained estimate warrants further investigation into the effect coupling scale and time-series sample size may have on the result. For the control group, we show the similarity between group-averaged observed and simulated functional connectomes, and the coupling interaction and structural connectomes in Fig. 2, with correlation $r > 0.9$ for both comparisons.

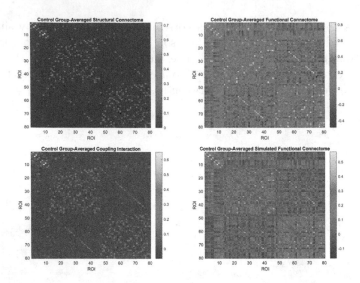

Fig. 2. Control group-averaged plots: Structural connectome in the *top left*, and coupling interaction network in the *bottom left* with Pearson correlation $r(|J|, SC) = 0.9493$, the observed functional connectome in the *top right* and the simulated functional connectome using our method (for optimal β, λ) in the *bottom right* with Pearson correlation $r = 0.9626$

One previous study using this data set computed standard graph theoretic metrics on the structural and functional networks. They found that carrier and control groups did not differ in measures of efficiency (global/local) or nodal centrality when analyzing the DTI or fMRI-derived networks separately [9]. Therefore, to investigate the significance of our estimated networks, we first compute the percent of positive and negative edges for each ROI in the signed rs-SC for each subject (control group), defined as p_c^+ and p_c^- for each ROI. For example, if an ROI has 45 positive edges and 34 negative edges, then $p_c^+ = \frac{45}{79}$ and $p_c^- = \frac{34}{79}$

ROIs with the 10 highest group-mean p_c^+ and p_c^- are shown in Fig. 3, the latter of which includes the anterior and rostral cingulate gyrus, caudate nucleus as well as the left thalamus. These are known regions with strong neural inhibitory influences on other ROIs. In particular, prefrontal cortical regions are strongly associated with cognitive control and response inhibition [2,8,10]. Sub-cortical structures including the caudate nuclei and thalamus also provide inhibitory control over motor functions through the cortico-basal ganglia-thalamo-cortical loop [13]. The correspondence between known inhibitory hubs and ROIs with higher incidence of negative interactions provides support for the insight our novel structure-function modeling may yield into the E-I balance.

We then define p_{e4}^+ similar to the control group and examine group differences between p_{e4}^+ and p_c^+ using a 2-sample T-test at the ROI-level, followed by FDR for multiple comparison correction ($q = 0.1$). This yielded 5 ROIs (shown in Fig. 3) with significant group differences. The left rostral anterior cingulate, left

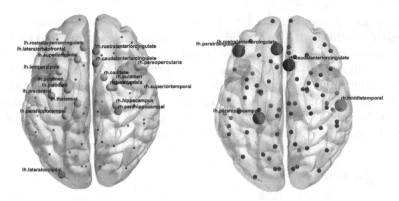

Fig. 3. Anatomical Nodes: *Left:* 10 largest group-mean p_c^+ (orange) and p_c^- (green). *Right:* ROIs with significantly higher p_{e4}^+ as compared to p_c^+ are the rostral anterior cingulate ($p = 2.598e{-}3$), parahippocampal ($p = 7.215e{-}4$), and pars triangularis ($p = 1.833e{-}3$) regions in the left hemisphere, as well as the caudal anterior cingulate ($p = 9.16e{-}4$) and middle temporal ($p = 5.359e{-}4$) regions in the right hemisphere. (Color figure online)

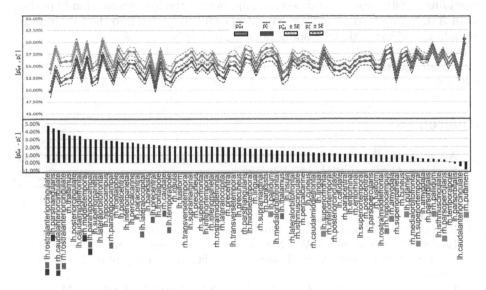

Fig. 4. Line Plots: Group-mean p_{e4}^+ and p_c^+ for each ROI, with ribbons for standard error (SE). Bar Plot: Difference between p_{e4}^+ and p_c^+. Green and Orange squares represent the 10 ROIs with the largest group-mean p_c^+ and p_c^-. Blue squares represent ROIs with significant group difference between p_{e4}^+ and p_c^+. Most ROIs in the APOE-e4 group have increased positive interactions as compared to the control group. Also, $\frac{3}{5}$ of the significant ROIs have higher p_c^- (rostral anterior cingulate, and the parahippocampal region in the left hemisphere and caudal anterior cingulate in the right hemisphere). (Color figure online)

parahippocampal, and right caudal anterior cingulate regions–are also among top p_c^-. Regions exhibiting the largest $[p_{e4}^+ - p_c^+]$ as shown in Fig. 4 tend to have fewer positive interactions in total, suggesting the presence of a shift from negative to positive interactions. Significant group differences were identified in regions of the anterior cingulate gyrus, middle temporal gyrus, inferior frontal gyrus and parahippocampal region. Moreover, white matter volume changes linked to APOE e4 [5] could also imply an increased risk for hyperexcitation, specifically in ROIs we identified after FDR correction (e.g. anterior cingulate).

5   Conclusion

We have presented here a method for estimating the positive and negative interactions between brain regions by creating a new connectome, the signed rs-SC, that embeds functional data onto a given structure. The resulting networks were validated on a sample of APOE-e4 carriers and non-carriers. When comparing the networks of the two groups, our approach identified a global shift in the E-I balance of the APOE e4 signed rs-SC as compared to the control group, thus providing the first connectomics-based support for the hyperexcitation hypothesis of AD. Future work would involve a deeper investigation into the E-I balance, including subjects with MCI and mild AD Dementia.

Acknowledgements. This study is funded in part by NIA AG056782 and NSF-IIS 1837956.

References

1. Ackley, D.H., Hinton, G.E., Sejnowski, T.J.: A learning algorithm for Boltzmann machines. Cogn. Sci. **9**(1), 147–169 (1985)
2. Badre, D., Wagner, A.D.: Selection, integration, and conflict monitoring; assessing the nature and generality of prefrontal cognitive control mechanisms. Neuron **41**, 473–487 (2004)
3. Besag, J.: Statistical analysis of non-lattice data. Statistician **24**(3), 179 (1975)
4. Binder, K., Heermann, D.W.: Monte Carlo Simulation in Statistical Physics: An Introduction. Springer, Heidelberg (2010). https://doi.org/10.1007/978-3-642-03163-2
5. Dowell, N.G., Evans, S.L., Tofts, P.S., King, S.L., Tabet, N., Rusted, J.M.: Structural and resting-state MRI detects regional brain differences in young and mid-age healthy APOE-e4 carriers compared with non-APOE-e4 carriers. NMR in Biomed. **29**(5), 614–624 (2016)
6. Ezaki, T., Watanabe, T., Ohzeki, M., Masuda, N.: Energy landscape analysis of neuroimaging data. Philos. Trans. R. Soc. A Math. Phys. Eng. Sci. **375**(2096), 20160287 (2017)
7. Fraiman, D., Balenzuela, P., Foss, J., Chialvo, D.R.: Ising-like dynamics in large-scale functional brain networks. Phys. Rev. E **79**(6), 061922 (2009)
8. Koechlin, E., Ody, C., Kouneiher, F.: The architecture of cognitive control in the human prefrontal cortex. Science **302**, 1181–1185 (2003)

9. Korthauer, L., Zhan, L., Ajilore, O., Leow, A., Driscoll, I.: Disrupted topology of the resting state structural connectome in middle-aged APOE ε4 carriers. Neuroimage **178**, 295–305 (2018)
10. MacDonald 3rd, A.W., Cohen, J.D., Stenger, V.A., Carter, C.S.: Dissociating the role of the dorsolateral prefrontal and anterior cingulate cortex in cognitive control. Science **288**, 1835–1838 (2000)
11. Marinazzo, D., Pellicoro, M., Wu, G., Angelini, L., Cortés, J.M., Stramaglia, S.: Information transfer and criticality in the ising model on the human connectome. PLoS ONE **9**(4), e93616 (2014)
12. Nguyen, H.C., Zecchina, R., Berg, J.: Inverse statistical prob-lems: from the inverse Ising problem to data science. Adv. Phys. **66**(3), 197–261 (2017)
13. Parent, A., Hazrati, L.: Functional anatomy of the basal ganglia. I. the cortico-basal ganglia-thalamo-cortical loop. Brain Res. Rev. **20**(1), 91–127 (1995)
14. Petrache, A.L.: Aberrant excitatory-inhibitory synaptic mechanisms in entorhinal cortex microcircuits during the pathogenesis of alzheimer's disease. Cereb. Cortex **29**(4), 1834–1850 (2019)
15. Ren, S., et al.: Amyloid β causes excitation/inhibition imbalance through dopamine receptor 1-dependent disruption of fast-spiking GABAergic input in anterior cingulate cortex. Sci. Rep. **8**(1), 302 (2018)
16. Schneidman, E., Berry, M.J., Segev, R., Bialek, W.: Weak pairwise correlations imply strongly correlated network states in a neural population. Nature **440**(7087), 1007–1012 (2006)
17. Watanabe, T., et al.: A pairwise maximum entropy model accurately describes resting-state human brain networks. Nat. Commun. **4**(1), 1370 (2013)
18. Yeh, F., et al.: Maximum entropy approaches to living neural networks. Entropy **12**(1), 89–106 (2010)

Synthesis and Inpainting-Based MR-CT Registration for Image-Guided Thermal Ablation of Liver Tumors

Dongming Wei[1,2,4], Sahar Ahmad[2], Jiayu Huo[1], Wen Peng[3], Yunhao Ge[4], Zhong Xue[4], Pew-Thian Yap[2], Wentao Li[5], Dinggang Shen[2(✉)], and Qian Wang[1(✉)]

[1] Institute for Medical Imaging Technology, School of Biomedical Engineering, Shanghai Jiao Tong University, Shanghai 200030, China
wang.qian@sjtu.edu.cn
[2] Department of Radiology and Biomedical Research Imaging Center (BRIC), University of North Carolina at Chapel Hill, Chapel Hill, NC 27599, USA
dgshen@med.unc.edu
[3] North China Electric Power University, Beijing, China
[4] Shanghai United Imaging Intelligence Co., Ltd., Shanghai, China
[5] Shanghai Cancer Center, Fudan University, Shanghai, China

Abstract. Thermal ablation is a minimally invasive procedure for treating small or unresectable tumors. Although CT is widely used for guiding ablation procedures, the contrast of tumors against surrounding normal tissues in CT images is often poor, aggravating the difficulty in accurate thermal ablation. In this paper, we propose a fast MR-CT image registration method to overlay a pre-procedural MR (pMR) image onto an intra-procedural CT (iCT) image for guiding the thermal ablation of liver tumors. By first using a Cycle-GAN model with mutual information constraint to generate synthesized CT (sCT) image from the corresponding pMR, pre-procedural MR-CT image registration is carried out through traditional mono-modality CT-CT image registration. At the intra-procedural stage, a partial-convolution-based network is first used to inpaint the probe and its artifacts in the iCT image. Then, an unsupervised registration network is used to efficiently align the pre-procedural CT (pCT) with the inpainted iCT (inpCT) image. The final transformation from pMR to iCT is obtained by combining the two estimated transformations, *i.e.*, (1) from the pMR image space to the pCT image space (through sCT) and (2) from the pCT image space to the iCT image space (through inpCT). Experimental results confirm that the proposed method achieves high registration accuracy with a very fast computational speed.

Keywords: Thermal ablation · Liver tumor · Image registration · Neural network

Electronic supplementary material The online version of this chapter (https://doi.org/10.1007/978-3-030-32254-0_57) contains supplementary material, which is available to authorized users.

D. Shen et al. (Eds.): MICCAI 2019, LNCS 11768, pp. 512–520, 2019.
https://doi.org/10.1007/978-3-030-32254-0_57

1   Introduction

Thermal ablation [1] elevates the temperature (55°–65° Celsius) of a focal zone in the tumor and induces irreversible cell injury and eventually tumor apoptosis and coagulative necrosis. Therefore, accurate targeting of the tumor area is critical for ablating tumor tissues only and leaving the surrounding healthy tissues intact.

CT imaging is typically used to guide the interventional procedure in thermal ablation, where pre-procedural CT (pCT) is used for planning, and intra-procedural CT (iCT) is captured during the treatment to facilitate safe placement of the ablation probe and accurate targeting of the tumor [2]. However, CT is relatively poor in tissue contrast (*e.g.*, arteries) and is susceptible to artifacts introduced by the probe during the procedure. Therefore, high-resolution pCT and pre-procedural MR (pMR) images are typically aligned during planning and then registered onto the iCT image for more precise guidance in positioning the probe to the desired region of interest (ROI) [3,4]. In liver tumor ablation, accuracy and speed of such an alignment are both important as it can compensate for deformations caused by patient positioning and respiratory motion without delay.

Most volumetric registration algorithms [5–7] are only feasible in the pre-procedural stage as they involve iterative yet time-consuming optimization. Moreover, they do not deal with the probe-induced artifacts. In order to overcome these challenges, we propose a fast image registration framework to align pMR images onto iCT images for guiding thermal ablation of the liver tumor. Meanwhile, our method also eliminates the probe artifacts so that they do not interfere during registration. The proposed registration framework consists of two stages:

1. **Pre-procedure:** Rigid and deformable registrations between pMR and pCT images. We use mutual-information (MI)-based Cycle-GAN to generate sCT from pMR images to convert the cross-modality registration into a mono-modality problem.
2. **Intra-procedure:** Fast deformable registration of the inpainted iCT (inpCT) image with the pCT image, using an unsupervised registration network (UR-Net).

Finally, the pMR image is aligned to the iCT image by composing the two transformations estimated in the above two stages.

2   Methods

In order to accurately and efficiently register pMR images onto iCT images for guiding thermal ablation of liver tumors, we propose a two-stage registration framework. First, we convert the cross-modality MR-CT image registration into mono-modality registration (CT-CT) by synthesizing sCT images from pMR images through MI-based Cycle-GAN. This mono-modality rigid and deformable registration is performed by using ANTs [8]. Then, the trained UR-Net performs

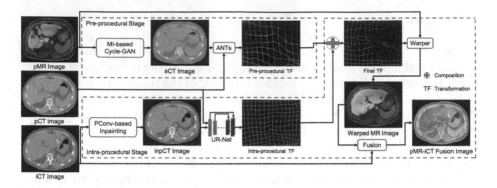

Fig. 1. The proposed image registration method consists of three deep-learning-based algorithms and the traditional ANTs algorithm.

deformable registration between pCT and inpCT, which is inpainted by a partial-convolution (PConv)-based network from the iCT image. Thus, the pMR image can be warped onto the iCT space by composing the output transformations of the two registration stages. The pipeline of our method is shown in Fig. 1.

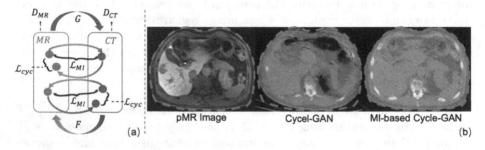

Fig. 2. Schematic illustration of MI-based Cycle-GAN. (a) The conventional Cycle-GAN algorithm, and the forward and backward synthesis steps of our method with MI as the explicit structural similarity constraint; (b) exemplar outputs of Cycle-GAN and MI-based Cycle-GAN, where the drifting of the boundaries (highlighted by red contours) can be suppressed by introducing MI-based contraint to Cycle-GAN.

2.1   Pre-procedural MR-CT Registration

MR-CT registration is challenging due to large appearance differences between the two modalities. Previous works [9] have shown that the cross-modality registration can be converted into a mono-modality registration to achieve better performance. To this end, we synthesize the sCT image from an input pMR image, which then facilitates the subsequent registration between pMR and pCT images.

The MR-to-CT synthesis is completed by using Cycle-GAN with mutual information constraint. Cycle-GAN [10], as one of the state-of-the-art image

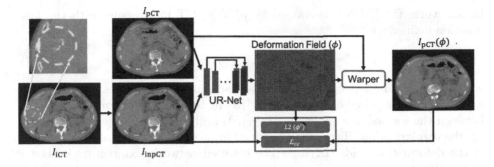

Fig. 3. Overview of unsupervised registration. The loss consists of cross-correlation between $I_{\mathrm{pCT}}(\phi)$ and I_{inpCT} and smoothness of ϕ'.

synthesis algorithms, adopts the adversarial loss given by two discriminators (D_{MR} and D_{CT}), such that the distribution of the output images of the two generators (G and F) is indistinguishable from that of the input images. It also uses the cycle-consistency (shown in Fig. 2(a)) to enforce the forward (MR-to-CT) and backward (CT-to-MR) syntheses to be bijective. However, Cycle-GAN fails to enforce structural similarity between the pMR and sCT images, which may lead to uncontrollable drifting of tissue/organ boundaries in the synthesized images (see red dashed contours in Fig. 2(b)).

Therefore, in addition to the cycle-consistency loss $\mathcal{L}_{\mathrm{cyc}}$, we propose to introduce the MI loss $\mathcal{L}_{\mathrm{MI}}$ to the generators (G and F) to directly enforce the structural similarity between the input and synthesized images (as shown in Fig. 2(a)). The MI loss is defined as:

$$\mathcal{L}_{\mathrm{MI}} = \sum\sum p(x,y)\log\frac{p(x,y)}{p(x)p(y)}, \tag{1}$$

where $p(x)$ and $p(y)$ denote the histograms of I_{MR} and $G(I_{\mathrm{MR}})$, respectively, and $p(x,y)$ refers to the joint histogram of I_{MR} and $G(I_{\mathrm{MR}})$. After synthesizing the cross-modality registration (pMR-pCT) is converted into a mono-modality registration problem (sCT-pCT). We then perform a conventional mono-modality registration using ANTs [8] to estimate the field that accounts for both rigid and deformable transformations.

2.2 Intra-procedural Registration

Due to the high computational efficiency requirement during intra-procedural stage, we propose to train a UR-Net (as shown in Fig. 3) in an unsupervised manner to perform expeditious deformable registration between pCT and inpCT images. The advantage is its fast speed by using parallel convolution on GPU during network inference. Dalca *et al.* have applied a similar unsupervised registration network to perform brain MR image registration [11], which shows comparable performance with the state-of-the-art optimization-based methods.

In our work, the UR-Net is trained by pCT-inpCT image pairs with the loss function defined as:

$$\mathcal{L} = -S(I_{\text{inpCT}}, I_{\text{pCT}}(\phi)) + \text{Reg}(\phi), \tag{2}$$

where I_{inpCT} and I_{pCT} represent the fixed and moving images, respectively. The loss function comprises of (1) similarity (S) in terms of cross-correlation ($\mathcal{L}_{\text{cc}}$) between the warped moving image ($I_{\text{pCT}}(\phi)$) and the fixed image (I_{inpCT}), and (2) the regularization (Reg) penalty defined in terms of L2-norm of the gradients of the deformation fields (L2(ϕ')). The detailed network architecture is shown in *Supplementary* file.

The probe and its artifacts, which hinder the interpretation of the underlying anatomy, may cause inaccurate registration [6]. In order to remove the probe and its streak artifacts in the iCT image, we train a PConv-based [12] 3D U-Net to obtain inpCT image (I_{inpCT}). Specifically, given a rough mask (*e.g.*, a bounding box or a polygon) covering the probe and its artifacts, the inpainting network can reconstruct the underlying tissues and update the mask layer-by-layer until the mask shrinks away. The inpainting is based on 3D convolution (Conv)-based U-Net architecture, while each convolution layer is replaced with partial convolution to ensure that the inpainted contents will not be affected by the probe and its streak artifacts in the mask. The probe and its streak artifacts exist in iCT images but not in pCT images. The mask can be manually drawn in the iCT images by clinicians during the procedure, or prepared in advance as part of the procedure planning.

3   Experiments and Results

Dataset and Pre-processing – Thirty-nine subjects undergoing liver tumor ablation were included in our experiment. Each subject was scanned with his/her own pMR, pCT and iCT images (see Table 1 for a summary of the parameters). Livers were delineated from pMR, pCT and iCT images, respectively, while tumors were delineated from pMR and pCT images but not iCT due to probe artifacts and limited contrast. We used 11 labeled subjects for testing, and the remaining 28 subjects were used for training the three networks. Before normalizing intensities into the range [0,1], the intensities of pCT and iCT images were thresholded in the range [−800, 800]. pMR images were also rigidly aligned onto pCT images. Then, all the image sizes were resampled to $256 \times 256 \times 128$ with isotropic voxel distances. If not stated otherwise, the same training/testing datasets were used.

Implementation – Three networks were trained: (1) pre-procedural stage: MI-based Cycle-GAN network for CT synthesis, and PConv-based U-Net for probe inpainting; (2) intra-procedural stage: UR-Net for deformable registration. All these networks were implemented in Keras and trained on a single NVIDIA Titan X GPU.

Table 1. The in-plane FOV, resolution and scanner used in acquisition of the pMR, pCT and iCT images.

	In-plane FOV	Resolution	Scanner
pMR image	320×260	$1.188 \times 1.188 \times 3mm^3$	Siemens 3.0T Skyra
pCT image	512×512	$0.7559 \times 0.7559 \times 3mm^3$	Philips Brilliance 64 CT
iCT image	512×512	$0.7559 \times 0.7559 \times 3mm^3$	Philips Brilliance 64 CT

Evaluation Metrics – We computed the Dice ratio over ROIs and the target registration error (TRE) over several landmarks of livers and tumors, to evaluate the registration accuracy. These two metrics are widely used for evaluation of registration performance, with higher Dice ratio (or lower TRE) characterizing better registration quality.

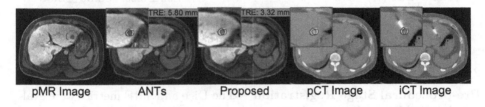

pMR Image   ANTs   Proposed   pCT Image   iCT Image

Fig. 4. Registration results by ANTs and the proposed method. The warped tumor contours by ANTs (blue), our proposed method (yellow) are visualized in zoomed-in view. The tumor contour from manually registered pCT image is used as ground-truth (red). TRE of the tumor center in this case is also reported. (Color figure online)

3.1 Registration Results for pMR and iCT

We conducted pMR-iCT image registration over the test dataset by using FSL FLIRT (rigid), ANTs (rigid and deformable) and the proposed method, respectively. As shown in Fig. 4, our proposed method achieves better accuracy against ANTs in tumor region and body alignment. Quantitative results using Dice ratio and TRE are presented in Table 2. It can be observed that our method yields better performance than ANTs. The last line of Table 2 reports the computational time in intra-procedural stage of ANTs and our proposed method, and our proposed method performed the registration in several seconds. Notice that our proposed method in the intra-procedural stage includes the iCT inpainting and the pCT-iCT image registration steps, which were computed on GPU.

Table 2. Results of pMR-iCT (rigid and deformable), pMR-pCT (rigid and deformable), and pCT-iCT (deformable only) registration.

		Rigid		Deformable	
		FLIRT	ANTs	ANTs	Proposed
pMR-iCT					
Liver	Dice (%)	48.44 ± 40.40	85.52 ± 2.92	86.59 ± 3.30	$\mathbf{86.96 \pm 3.00}$
	TRE (mm)	-	52.56 ± 9.85	5.18 ± 2.43	$\mathbf{4.93 \pm 2.72}$
pMR-pCT					
Liver	Dice (%)	48.07 ± 40.40	87.03 ± 2.60	89.55 ± 2.04	$\mathbf{90.59 \pm 1.73}$
	TRE (mm)	-	6.63 ± 2.73	5.59 ± 2.01	$\mathbf{4.67 \pm 2.00}$
Tumor	Dice (%)	12.88 ± 25.76	51.10 ± 17.13	55.34 ± 5.70	$\mathbf{62.45 \pm 4.66}$
	TRE (mm)	-	6.71 ± 2.27	6.08 ± 1.40	$\mathbf{3.89 \pm 0.99}$
pCT-iCT					
Liver	Dice (%)	-	-	87.90 ± 5.25	$\mathbf{88.63 \pm 5.53}$
	TRE (mm)	-	-	5.06 ± 3.29	$\mathbf{4.37 \pm 3.30}$

3.2 Pre-procedural Stage

Pre-procedural Stage Registration – The Dice and TRE metrics were evaluated over pMR-pCT pairs and their corresponding sCT-pCT pairs of the testing dataset. As shown in Table 2, the registration performance of our algorithm is improved over sCT-pCT pair, especially on the target tumor region (more than 7% Dice and 1.1 mm TRE improvement), which proves that our proposed synthesis algorithm can facilitate the cross-modality registration.

MR-to-CT Synthesis – We extracted 2240 slices from the transverse planes of 28 unpaired pMR and pCT images and used them as the training dataset. pMR and pCT images of each subject were linearly registered. For testing, we applied the MR-to-CT generator to synthesize CT images from pMR images slice-by-slice and then concatenated the synthesized slices into 3D volumes. As shown in Fig. 2(b), our method predicted better CT-like images from pMR images.

3.3 Intra-procedural Stage

Intra-procedural Stage Registration – UR-Net was trained by 28 rigidly registered pCT-inpCT image pairs in an unsupervised manner, where inpCT images were generated by the trained PConv-base inpainting network. We compared the UR-Net registration performance with ANTs over pCT-inpCT image pairs. The Dice and TRE metrics of liver and the intra-procedural computation time were evaluated (see Table 2). It can be seen that the UR-Net yielded better performance and was more efficient. The UR-Net method predicted a deformation field in around 3 secs for a $256 \times 256 \times 128$ image pair.

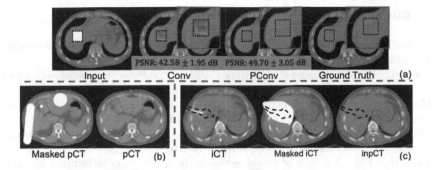

Fig. 5. (a) Qualitative and quantitative (mean ± std PSNR over test subjects) comparison results of Conv-based and PConv-based inpainting network on iCT images; (b) A training pair exemplar; (c) Results of inpainting network in clinical practice.

Inpainting – pCT images were used for training the inpainting network. Each image was augmented 500 times using 2 or 3 random 3D shapes (*i.e.*, 3D balls and bars) with random locations and sizes to imitate manual mask (cf. Fig. 5(b)). In the testing stage, we compared the inpainting results quantitatively and qualitatively on the iCT images. The results in Fig. 5(a) shows that PConv-based network obtained around 7 dB PSNR improvement in the masked region than Conv-based network. Particularly, each iCT image was combined with a cubic mask ($40 \times 40 \times 20$) in healthy tissue region and input into PConv and Conv-based networks, respectively. The PSNR is computed over the reconstructed region with the ground-truth. For clinical cases, the results are shown in Fig. 5(c). The mask was drawn in the pre-procedural images by physicians to cover the tumor and the planned puncture pathway in the tumor-centered transverse plane. Then, an appropriate height was chosen in the intra-procedural stage to ensure that the closed 3D contour can cover the probe and its artifacts. The inference time was around 2 secs for a $256 \times 256 \times 128$ subject. Note that we will further quantitatively evaluate the improvement of tumor registration, and investigate the possibility of reconstructing the tumor directly by the PConv-based inpainting network.

4   Conclusion

A learning-based registration framework is proposed to align pre-procedural MR and intra-procedural CT images for image-guided thermal ablation of liver tumor. Experimental results showed that our method can efficiently and effectively overlay pMR onto iCT during ablation with high registration accuracy, compared to the state-of-the-art ANTs algorithm. We also showed that MI-based Cycle-GAN synthesis and unsupervised registration improves the overall performance.

Acknowledgement. This work was partially supported by the National Key Research and Development Program of China (2018YFC0116400) and STCSM (19QC1400600).

References

1. Ahmed, M., Brace, C.L., Lee, F.T., Goldberg, S.N.: Principles of and advances in percutaneous ablation. Radiology **258**(2), 351–369 (2011)
2. Ahmed, M., et al.: Image-guided tumor ablation: standardization of terminology and reporting criteria-a 10-year update. Radiology **273**(1), 241–260 (2014)
3. Chu, K.F., Dupuy, D.E.: Thermal ablation of tumours: biological mechanisms and advances in therapy. Nat. Rev. Cancer **14**(3), 199–208 (2014)
4. Maybody, M.: An overview of image-guided percutaneous ablation of renal tumors. Semin. Intervent. Radiol. **27**(03), 261–267 (2010)
5. Liao, R., et al.: A review of recent advances in registration techniques applied to minimally invasive therapy. IEEE Trans. Multimed. **15**(5), 983–1000 (2013)
6. Fei, B., Lee, Z., Boll, D.T., Duerk, J.L., Lewin, J.S., Wilson, D.L.: Image registration and fusion for interventional MRI guided thermal ablation of the prostate cancer. In: Ellis, R.E., Peters, T.M. (eds.) MICCAI 2003. LNCS, vol. 2879, pp. 364–372. Springer, Heidelberg (2003). https://doi.org/10.1007/978-3-540-39903-2_45
7. Elhawary, H., et al.: Multimodality non-rigid image registration for planning, targeting and monitoring during CT-guided percutaneous liver tumor cryoablation. Acad. Radiol. **17**(11), 1334–1344 (2010)
8. Avants, B.B., Tustison, N., Song, G.: Advanced normalization tools (ANTS). Insight j. **2**, 1–35 (2011)
9. Cao, X., et al.: Dual-core steered non-rigid registration for multi-modal images via bi-directional image synthesis. Med. Image Anal. **41**, 18–31 (2017)
10. Zhu, J.Y., Park, T., Isola, P., Efros, A.A.: Unpaired image-to-image translation using cycle-consistent adversarial networks. In: CVPR, pp. 2223–2232 (2017)
11. Balakrishnan, G., et al.: An unsupervised learning model for deformable medical image registration. In: CVPR, pp. 9252–9260 (2018)
12. Liu, G., Reda, F.A., Shih, K.J., Wang, T.-C., Tao, A., Catanzaro, B.: Image inpainting for irregular holes using partial convolutions. In: Ferrari, V., Hebert, M., Sminchisescu, C., Weiss, Y. (eds.) ECCV 2018. LNCS, vol. 11215, pp. 89–105. Springer, Cham (2018). https://doi.org/10.1007/978-3-030-01252-6_6

CFEA: Collaborative Feature Ensembling Adaptation for Domain Adaptation in Unsupervised Optic Disc and Cup Segmentation

Peng Liu[1], Bin Kong[2], Zhongyu Li[3], Shaoting Zhang[4], and Ruogu Fang[1(✉)]

[1] J. Crayton Pruitt Family Department of Biomedical Engineering,
University of Florida, Gainesville, FL, USA
`ruogu.fang@bme.ufl.edu`
[2] Department of Computer Science, UNC Charlotte, Charlotte, NC, USA
[3] School of Software Engineering, Xi'an Jiaotong University, Xi'an, China
[4] Sensetime Research, Shanghai, China

Abstract. Recently, deep neural networks have demonstrated comparable and even better performance with board-certified ophthalmologists in well-annotated datasets. However, the diversity of retinal imaging devices poses a significant challenge: domain shift, which leads to performance degradation when applying the deep learning models to new testing domains. In this paper, we propose a novel unsupervised domain adaptation framework, called Collaborative Feature Ensembling Adaptation (CFEA), to effectively overcome this challenge. Our proposed CFEA is an interactive paradigm which presents an exquisite of collaborative adaptation through both adversarial learning and ensembling weights. In particular, we simultaneously achieve domain-invariance and maintain an exponential moving average of the historical predictions, which achieves a better prediction for the unlabeled data, via ensembling weights during training. Without annotating any sample from the target domain, multiple adversarial losses in encoder and decoder layers guide the extraction of domain-invariant features to confuse the domain classifier and meanwhile benefit the ensembling of smoothing weights. Comprehensive experimental results demonstrate that our CFEA model can overcome performance degradation and outperform the state-of-the-art methods in segmenting retinal optic disc and cup from fundus images.

Keywords: Domain adaptation · Adversarial learning · Ensembling · Segmentation · Retinal fundus images

1 Introduction

Many eye diseases can be revealed by the morphology of optic disc (OD) and optic cup (OC). For instance, glaucoma is usually characterized by the large cup

---

P. Liu and B. Kong—Equal contribution.

© Springer Nature Switzerland AG 2019
D. Shen et al. (Eds.): MICCAI 2019, LNCS 11768, pp. 521–529, 2019.
https://doi.org/10.1007/978-3-030-32254-0_58

to disc ratio (CDR), the ratio of the vertical diameter of the cup to the vertical diameter of the disc. Currently, determining CDR is mainly performed by pathology specialists. However, it is extremely expensive to accurately calculate CDR by human experts. Furthermore, manual delineation of these lesions also introduces subjectivity, intra- and inter-variability. Therefore, it is essential to automate the process of calculating CDR. OD and OC segmentation are commonly adopted to automatically calculate the CDR. Nevertheless, both OD and OC segmentation is challenging due to the pathological lesions on the boundaries or some regions overlapping with blood vessels.

Recently, deep learning based methods have been proposed to overcome these challenges and some of them, e.g., M-Net [2], have demonstrated impressive results. Although these methods tend to perform well when being applied to well-annotated datasets, the segmentation performance of a trained network may degrade severely on datasets with different distributions, particularly for the retinal fundus images captured with different imaging devices (e.g., different cameras,

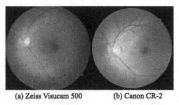

(a) Zeiss Visucam 500   (b) Canon CR-2

Fig. 1. Retinal fundus images collected by different fundus cameras.

as illustrated in Fig. 1). The variance among the diverse data domains limits deep learning's deployment in reality and impedes us from building a robust application for retinal fundus image parsing.

To tackle this challenge, existing works have mainly focused on minimizing the distance between the source and target domains to align the latent feature distributions of the different domains [7]. However, adversarial discriminative learning usually suffers the instability of its training. Numerous methods have been studied to tackle this challenge. Self-ensembling [3] is one of them recently applied to visual domain adaptation [1]. In particular, gradient descent is used to train the student network, and the exponential moving average of the weights of the student network is transferred to the teacher network after applying each training sample. The mean square difference between the outputs of the student and the teacher is used as the unsupervised loss to train the student network.

In this paper, we propose a novel unsupervised domain adaptation framework, called Collaborative Feature Ensembling Adaptation (CFEA), to further overcome the challenges underlining in domain shift. In particular, we take the advantage of the self-ensembling, which is the time-dependent weighting to the unsupervised loss for each unlabeled sample, to stabilize the adversarial discriminative learning. Most importantly, we apply the unsupervised loss by adversarial learning not only to the output space but also to the input space or the intermediate representations of the network. Thus, from a complementary perspective, adversarial learning can consistently provide various model space and time-dependent weights to self-ensembling to accelerate the learning of the domain invariant features and further enhance the stabilization of adversarial learning, forming a benign collaborative circulation and unified framework.

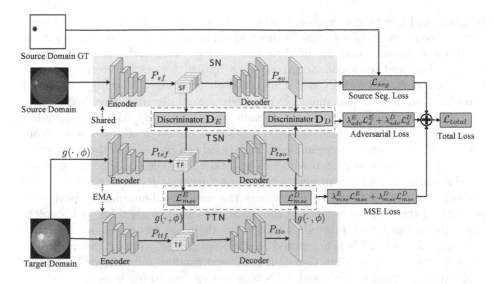

Fig. 2. Overview of the proposed model architecture.

The significant contributions of this paper are: (a) We propose the CFEA, a novel unsupervised domain adaptation framework, that exploits collaborative adversarial learning and self-ensembling for feature adaptation to tackle domain shift in a mutual benefit and complementary manner, thus leading to a robust and accurate model. (b) We intensify feature adaptation by applying adversarial discriminative learning in two phases of the network, i.e., intermediate representation space and output space. (c) We evaluate the effectiveness of our CFEA on the challenging task of the unsupervised joint segmentation of retinal OD and OC. Our CFEA model can overcome performance degradation to domain shift and outperform the state-of-the-art methods.

2   Collaborative Feature Ensembling Adaptation

2.1   Problem Formulation

Unsupervised domain adaptation typically refers to the scenario: given a labeled source domain dataset with distribution $P(X_s)$ and the corresponding label Y_s with distribution $P(Y_s|X_s)$, as well as a target dataset with distribution $P(X_t)$ and unknown label with distribution $P(Y_t|X_t)$, where $P(X_s) \neq P(X_t)$, the goal is to train a model from both labeled data X_s and unlabeled data X_t, with which the expected model distribution $P(\hat{Y}_t|X_t)$ is close to $P(Y_t|X_t)$.

2.2   Overview of the Proposed Method

As illustrated in Fig. 2, our framework mainly includes three networks, i.e., the source domain network (SN, in blue), the target domain student network (TSN, in gray) and the target domain teacher network (TTN, in orange). Although each of the networks plays a distinctive role in guiding networks to learn domain invariant representations, all of them can interact with each other, benefit to one another, and work collaboratively as a unified framework during an end-to-end training process. SN and TSN focus on supervised learning for labeled samples from the source domain (X_s) and adversarial discriminative learning for unlabeled samples from the target domain (X_t), separately. More importantly, we allow SN and TSN to share the weights that are sequentially learned from both labeled and unlabeled samples. The labeled samples enable the network to learn accurate segmentation predictions while the unlabeled ones bring unsupervised learning and further present a type of perturbation to regularize the model training [5]. Furthermore, TTN conducts the weight self-ensembling part with replicating the average weights of the TSN instead of predictions. TTN solely takes unlabeled target images as input and then the mean square difference between TSN and TTN is computed for the same target sample. Different data augmentations (e.g., adding Gaussian noise and random intensity or brightness scaling) are applied to TSN and TTN to avoid loss vanishing issue.

Basically, the U-Net [4] with encoder-decoder structure is employed as the backbone of each network. Since U-Net is one of the most successful segmentation frameworks in medical imaging, we expect that the results can easily generalize to other medical image analysis tasks.

2.3 Adversarial Discriminative Learning

We apply two discriminators at the encoder and decoder of the networks, separately, to achieve adversarial discriminative learning. Two adversarial loss functions are calculated between SN and TSN. Each of the loss calculations is performed by two steps in each training iteration: (1) train the target domain segmentation network to maximize the adversarial loss $\mathcal{L}_{adv}$, thereby fooling the domain discriminator $\mathbf{D}$ to maximize the probability of the source domain feature P_s being classified as target features:

$$\mathcal{L}_{adv}(X_s) = \mathbb{E}_{x_s \sim X_s} \log(1 - \mathbf{D}(P_s)),\tag{1}$$

and (2) minimize the discrininator loss $\mathcal{L}_D$:

$$\mathcal{L}_d(X_s, X_t) = \mathbb{E}_{x_t \sim X_t} \log(\mathbf{D}(P_t)) + \mathbb{E}_{x_s \sim X_s} \log(1 - \mathbf{D}(P_s)),\tag{2}$$

where P_t is the target domain feature.

2.4 Self-ensembling

In self-ensembling for domain adaptation, the training of the student model is iteratively improved by the task-specific loss, a moving average (EMA) model (teacher) of the student model, which can be illustrated as:

$$\Phi'_t = \alpha \Phi'_{t-1} + (1 - \alpha)\Phi_t\tag{3}$$

where Φ_t and Φ'_t denote the paramters of the student network and the teacher network, respectively.

More specifically, at each iteration, a mini-batch of labeled source domain and unlabeled target samples are drawn from the target domain T. Then, the EMA predictions and the base predictions are generated by the teacher model and the student model respectively with different augmentation applied to the target samples. Afterward, a mean-squared error (MSE) loss between the EMA and target predictions is calculated. Finally, the MSE loss together with the task-specific loss on the labeled source domain data is minimized to update the parameters of the student network. Since the teacher model is an improved model at each iteration, the MSE loss helps the student model to learn from the unlabeled target domain images. Therefore, the student model and teacher model can work collaboratively to achieve robust and accurate predictions.

2.5   CFEA Unsupervised Domain Adaptation

Unlike existing methods, our method appropriately integrates adversarial domain confusion and self-ensembling with an encoder-decoder architecture.

Adversarial Feature Adaptation: Adversarial domain confusion is applied to both the encoded features and decoded predictions between source domain network (SN) and target domain student network (TSN) to reduce the distribution differences. According to Eqs. 1 and 2, this corresponds to the adversarial loss function $\mathcal{L}^E_{adv}$ for the encoder output of SN and TSN, and the adversarial loss function $\mathcal{L}^D_{adv}$ for the decoder output of SN and TSN:

$$\mathcal{L}^E_{adv}(X_s) = \mathbb{E}_{x_s \sim X_s} \log(1 - \mathbf{D}_E(P_{sf})), \tag{4}$$

$$\mathcal{L}^D_{adv}(X_s) = \mathbb{E}_{x_s \sim X_s} \log(1 - \mathbf{D}_D(P_{so})), \tag{5}$$

where $P_{sf} \in \mathbb{R}^{W_e \times H_e \times C_e}$ and $P_{so} \in \mathbb{R}^{W_d \times H_d \times C_d}$ are the encoder and decoder outputs, respectively. H_d and W_d are the width and height of the decoders' output; C_d refers to pixel categories of the segmentation result, which is three in our cases. H_e, W_e, and C_e are the width, height, channel of the encoders' output. $\mathbf{D}_E$ and $\mathbf{D}_D$ are the discriminator networks for the encoder and decoder outputs, respectively.

The discriminator loss $\mathcal{L}^E_d$ for the encoder feature and the discriminator loss $\mathcal{L}^D_d$ for decoder feature are as follows:

$$\mathcal{L}^E_d(X_s, X_t) = \mathbb{E}_{x_t \sim X_t} \log(\mathbf{D}_E(P_{tsf})) + \mathbb{E}_{x_s \sim X_s} \log(1 - \mathbf{D}_E(P_{sf})), \tag{6}$$

$$\mathcal{L}^D_d(X_s, X_t) = \mathbb{E}_{x_t \sim X_t} \log(\mathbf{D}_D(P_{tso})) + \mathbb{E}_{x_s \sim X_s} \log(1 - \mathbf{D}_D(P_{so})), \tag{7}$$

where $P_{tsf} \in \mathbb{R}^{W_e \times H_e \times C_e}$ is the encoder output and $P_{tso} \in \mathbb{R}^{W_d \times H_d \times C_d}$ is the decoder output of TSN.

Collaborative Adaptation with Self-ensembling: Self-ensembling is also applied to both the encoded features and decoded predictions between TSN and target domain teacher network (TTN). In this work, MSE is used for the self-ensembling. The MSE loss $\mathcal{L}_{mse}^E$ between encoder outputs of TSN and TTN, and the MSE loss $\mathcal{L}_{mse}^D$ between decoder outputs of TSN and TTN are as follows:

$$\mathcal{L}_{mse}^E(X_t) = \mathbb{E}_{x_t \sim X_t}[\frac{1}{M}\sum_{i=1}^{M}(p_i^{tsf} - p_i^{ttf})^2], \qquad (8)$$

$$\mathcal{L}_{mse}^D(X_t) = \mathbb{E}_{x_t \sim X_t}[\frac{1}{N}\sum_{i=1}^{N}(p_i^{tso} - p_i^{tto})^2]. \qquad (9)$$

where p_i^{tsf}, p_i^{ttf}, p_i^{tso}, and p_i^{tto} denote the ith element of the flattened predictions $(P_{tsf}, P_{ttf}, P_{tso},$ and $P_{tto})$ of the student encoder, student decoder, teacher encoder, teacher decoder, respectively. M and N are the number of elements in the encoder feature and decoder output, respectively.

The same spatial-challenging augmentation $g(x, \phi)$ is used for both the teacher and student at each iteration with $g(x, \phi)$ applied to the training sample of the student and $g(x, \phi)$ applied to the predictions of the teacher, where ϕ is the transformation parameter.

Total Objective Function: Finally, we use the dice loss as the segmentation loss for labeled images from the source domain. Combing Eqs. 4, 5, 6, 7, 8, and 9, the total loss is obtained, which can be formulated as below.

$$\begin{aligned}\mathcal{L}_{total}(X_s, X_t) = \mathcal{L}_{seg}(X_s) + \lambda_{adv}^E \mathcal{L}_d^E(X_s, X_t) + \lambda_{adv}^D \mathcal{L}_d^D(X_s, X_t) \\ + \lambda_{mse}^E \mathcal{L}_{mse}^E(X_t) + \lambda_{mse}^D \mathcal{L}_{mse}^D(X_t),\end{aligned} \qquad (10)$$

where λ_{adv}^E, λ_{adv}^D, λ_{mse}^E, and λ_{mse}^D balance the weights of the losses. They are cross-validated in our experiments. $\mathcal{L}_{seg}(X_s)$ is the dice segmentation loss. Based on Eq. 10, we optimize the following min-max problem:

$$\min_{f_\phi, f_{\tilde{\phi}}} \max_{\mathbf{D}_E, \mathbf{D}_D} \mathcal{L}_{total}(X_s, X_t), \qquad (11)$$

where $f_{\tilde{\phi}}$ and f_ϕ are the source domain network with trainable weight $\tilde{\phi}$ and target domain network with trainable weight ϕ.

3   Experiments and Results

Data: Extensive experiments are conducted on the REFUGE[1] dataset to validate the effectiveness of the proposed method. The dataset includes 400 source domain retinal fundus images (supervised training dataset) with size 2124×2056, acquired by a Zeiss Visucam 500 camera, 400 labeled (testing dataset) and 400 additional unlabeled (unsupervised training dataset) target

---

[1] https://refuge.grand-challenge.org/Home/.

domain retinal fundus images with size 1634 × 1634 collected by a Canon CR-2 camera. As different cameras are used, the source and target domain images have totally distinct appearances (e.g., color and texture). The optic disc and optical cup regions were carefully delineated by the experts. All of the methods in this section are supervised by the annotations of the source domain and evaluated by the disc and cup dice indices (DI), and the cup-to-disc ratio (CDR) on the target domain.

Data Preprocessing: Firstly, we detect the center of optic disc by pre-trained disc-aware ensemble network [2], and then center and crop optic disc regions with a size of 600 × 600 for supervised training dataset and 500 × 500 for unsupervised training dataset and test dataset. This is due to the different sizes of images acquired by the two cameras. During training, all images are resized to a small size of 128 × 128 in order to adapt the network's receptive field.

Training: The U-Net is used for both student and teacher network. All experiments are processed on Python v2.7, and PyTorch with GEFORCE GTX TITAN GPUs.

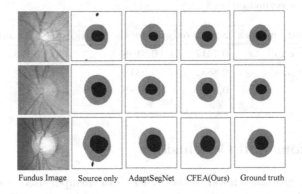

Fundus Image   Source only   AdaptSegNet   CFEA(Ours)   Ground truth

Fig. 3. The visual examples of optic disc and cup segmentation, where the black and gray region denote the cup and disc segmentations, respectively. From the left to right: fundus image, the model trained on source data only, baseline (AdaptSegNet [6]), the model trained with our domain adaptation framework, and ground truth.

Adaptation to Different Fundus Cameras: We trained our CFEA on the source domain data acquired by Zeiss Visucam 500 camera in a supervised manner and on the target domain data acquired by Canon CR-2 camera in an unsupervised manner, simultaneously. We then evaluated our fully trained segmentation network on the test dataset, which includes 400 retinal fundus images acquired by Canon CR-2 camera. To demonstrate our method's effectiveness, we trained the segmentation network on source domain data only in a supervised manner and then tested it on the test data. In addition, we also trained the baseline-AdaptSegNet [6] in the same way of training our method. Adapt-SegNet [6] represents one of the state-of-the-art unsupervised domain adaptation methods for image segmentation, which also spplies adversarial learning for domain adaptation. The main result is shown in Table 1. The model trained on source data completely fails for target data. The baseline can have satisfied results on target data. By comparing our model with the baseline, as one can see, our model outperforms the state-of-the-art method consistently for OD, OC, and CDR. These results indicate the proposed framework has a capability of overcoming domain shifts, thus allowing us to build a robust and accurate model.

Table 1. Results of adapting source to target. We evaluate our method on 400 test images. We use three metrics to evaluate our model performance, the mean Dice coefficient for the optic cups, the mean Dice coefficient for the optic disc, and the mean absolute error for the vertical cup to disc ratio (CDR). The larger value for OD and OC means better segmentation results; for CDR, the smaller value represents better results. "Source only" means the model only trained on source domain in a supervised manner. AdaptSegNet [6] is one of the state-of-the-art unsupervised domain adaptation methods for image segmentation.

Evaluation-index	Source only	AdaptSegNet [6]	CFEA (ours)
Optic cup	0.7317	0.8198	**0.8627**
Optic disk	0.8532	0.9315	**0.9416**
CDR	0.0676	0.0588	**0.0481**

4   Discussions and Conclusions

In this work, we propose a novel method CFEA for unsupervised domain adaptation of cross a diversity of retinal fundus imaging cameras. Our CFEA framework collaboratively combines adversarial discriminative learning and self-ensembling to obtain domain-invariant feature. Self-ensembling can stabilize the adversarial learning and prevent the network from getting stuck in a sub-optimal solution. From a complementary perspective, adversarial learning can consistently provide various model space and time-dependent weights to self-ensembling to accelerate the learning of the domain invariant features and further enhance the stabilization of adversarial learning, forming a benign collaborative circulation and unified framework. The collaborative mutual benefits from both adversarial feature learning and ensembling weights during an end-to-end learning process lead to a robust and accurate model. Experimental results demonstrate the superiority of our network over the state-of-the-art method. Our framework needs relatively higher computational costs during the training stage to help the segmentation network to adapt to the target domain. However, in the testing stage, the computational costs will be the same as a normal U-Net network, as the images only need to go through the TTN network. Our approach is general and can be easily extended to other unsupervised domain adaptation problems. For the future work, we will conduct the extensive ablation study of the student and teacher network and the verification study of weight sharing between the SN and TSN networks.

Acknowledgments. Research reported in this publication is partially supported by the National Science Foundation under Grant No. IIS-1564892 and IIS-1908299, the University of Florida Informatics Institute Junior SEED Program (00129436), the University of Florida Informatics Institute SEED Funds, and the UF Clinical and Translational Science Institute, which is supported in part by the NIH National Center for Advancing Translational Sciences under award number UL1 TR001427. The content is solely the responsibility of the authors and does not necessarily represent the official views of the National Institutes of Health and the National Science Foundation.

References

1. French, G., Mackiewicz, M., Fisher, M.: Self-ensembling for visual domain adaptation. arXiv preprint arXiv:1706.05208 (2017)
2. Fu, H., Cheng, J., Xu, Y., Wong, D.W.K., Liu, J., Cao, X.: Joint optic disc and cup segmentation based on multi-label deep network and polar transformation. IEEE Trans. Med. Imaging (TMI) **37**, 1597–1605 (2018)
3. Laine, S., Aila, T.: Temporal ensembling for semi-supervised learning. arXiv preprint arXiv:1610.02242 (2016)
4. Ronneberger, O., Fischer, P., Brox, T.: U-Net: convolutional networks for biomedical image segmentation. In: Navab, N., Hornegger, J., Wells, W.M., Frangi, A.F. (eds.) MICCAI 2015. LNCS, vol. 9351, pp. 234–241. Springer, Cham (2015). https://doi.org/10.1007/978-3-319-24574-4_28
5. Tarvainen, A., Valpola, H.: Mean teachers are better role models: weight-averaged consistency targets improve semi-supervised deep learning results. In: Advances in Neural Information Processing Systems, pp. 1195–1204 (2017)
6. Tsai, Y.H., Hung, W.C., Schulter, S., Sohn, K., Yang, M.H., Chandraker, M.: Learning to adapt structured output space for semantic segmentation. In: Proceedings of the IEEE Conference on Computer Vision and Pattern Recognition, pp. 7472–7481 (2018)
7. Tzeng, E., Hoffman, J., Saenko, K., Darrell, T.: Adversarial discriminative domain adaptation. In: Proceedings of the IEEE International Conference on Computer Vision (CVPR), vol. 1, p. 4 (2017)

Gastric Cancer Detection from Endoscopic Images Using Synthesis by GAN

Teppei Kanayama[1(✉)], Yusuke Kurose[1], Kiyohito Tanaka[2], Kento Aida[3], Shin'ichi Satoh[3], Masaru Kitsuregawa[4,5], and Tatsuya Harada[1,3]

[1] Graduate School of Information Science and Technology,
The University of Tokyo, Tokyo, Japan
{kanayama,kurose,harada}@mi.t.u-tokyo.ac.jp
[2] Kyoto Second Red Cross Hospital, Kyoto, Japan
kitanaka@kyoto2.jrc.or.jp
[3] Research Center for Medical Bigdata, National Institute of Informatics,
Tokyo, Japan
{aida,satoh}@nii.ac.jp
[4] Institute of Industrial Science, The University of Tokyo, Tokyo, Japan
kitsure@tkl.iis.u-tokyo.ac.jp
[5] National Institute of Informatics, Tokyo, Japan

Abstract. Datasets for training gastric cancer detection models are usually imbalanced, because the number of available images showing lesions is limited. This imbalance can be a serious obstacle to realizing a high-performance automatic gastric cancer detection system. In this paper, we propose a method that lessens this dataset bias by generating new images using a generative model. The generative model synthesizes an image from two images in a dataset. The synthesis network can produce realistic images, even if the dataset of lesion images is small. In our experiment, we trained gastric cancer detection models using the synthesized images. The results show that the performance of the system was improved.

Keywords: Endoscopy image · Generative adversarial networks · Gastric cancer detection · Dataset bias

1 Introduction

The performance of computer vision systems has been dramatically improved because of the recent development of deep learning techniques. The automatic detection of gastric cancer in endoscopic images is one of the most important

Electronic supplementary material The online version of this chapter (https://doi.org/10.1007/978-3-030-32254-0_59) contains supplementary material, which is available to authorized users.

© Springer Nature Switzerland AG 2019
D. Shen et al. (Eds.): MICCAI 2019, LNCS 11768, pp. 530–538, 2019.
https://doi.org/10.1007/978-3-030-32254-0_59

applications of these techniques. This detection task consists of detecting a cancerous tumor, regardless of its size. The automatic detection in images of the cancer's location is expected to decrease the diagnostic burden on doctors.

However, datasets for training the detection models are usually imbalanced, because the number of images showing lesions is limited. This is because the number of patients who have lesions is small and the cost of annotation for indicating the location of lesions in the images is high. This dataset imbalance can be a serious obstacle to realizing a high-performance automatic gastric cancer detection system.

In this paper, we propose a method that lessens the bias by using generative models and thus improves the performance of gastric cancer detection models, even when the dataset includes bias.

2 Related Work

The detection of objects in general images has been widely explored in recent years [12,13]. Research has also been conducted on object detection in medical images. For example, in [6] the detection of tumors from endoscopic images using the Singe Shot Detector (SSD) was described [9]. In [10], a system for glomerulus detection in light microscopic images using a faster region-based convolutional neural network (Faster R-CNN) was presented [13]. The task of detecting anomalies in images is similar to object detection tasks. In this task, an entire image is divided into regions using a grid, and the model recognizes whether the region contains anomalies. This method is advantageous in situations where the target image has stepwise anomalies. Xiao et al., for example, proposed a high performance unsupervised lesion detection system that uses a spatio-temporal pyramid that utilizes not only local but also global features [16,17]. Studies have also been conducted on detecting anomalies, i.e., lesions, in medical images. As for general images, methods that improve the performance of the system for medical images by utilizing global context information have been proposed [5,8,14]. Hayakawa et al., for example, detected lesions in endoscopic images by extracting multi-scale features using two types of convolutional neural network (CNN) [5].

A main problem that arises in the case of medical images in particular is that the number of available images is limited. To address this problem, methods for expanding datasets using generative adversarial networks (GANs) [4] have been widely explored [1–3,18]. In the study in [3], for example, computed tomography (CT) images of livers were generated by using deep convolutional GANs (DCGANs) [11]. The study's results showed that the image classification performance was improved by using the generated images. In [1], a network that can generate high resolution images using a limited dataset was proposed, and experiments on skin images were described. On the other hand, in the context of general image synthesis, GANs which use both local and global information are proposed in [15] and [19]. In [15], the authors proposed the method to synthesize images guided by sketch, color, and texture. In [19], the authors dealt with the task of generating photographic images which were conditioned on image

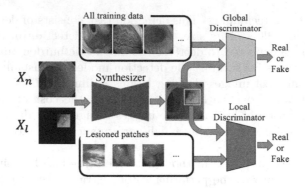

Fig. 1. Overview of gastric cancer image synthesizing system.

description expressed in natural language. Both methods require relatively large datasets compared with medical image settings.

As described above, in research studies GANs have been applied to augment datasets for image classification tasks involving medical images. These studies, however, were focused on generating entire images, and thus did not consider the lesion detection task. Therefore, images generated using these methods cannot be used for supervised lesion detection tasks, because they do not indicate the location of lesions. The studies were, furthermore, focused on reproducing the distribution in the original dataset, which cannot lessen the dataset bias mentioned in the previous section. When these generated data are used to train lesion detection models, the models detect only bright regions. In this research study, we focused on the gastric lesion detection task in endoscopic images. We propose a data augmentation method that improves the performance of the models by using generative models to produce additional images and thus lessen the dataset bias.

3   Method

Figure 1 shows an overview of the gastric cancer image synthesizing system using GAN. The system consists of three networks: a synthesizer and global and local discriminators. A normal image, i.e., an image with no lesions, and an image showing a lesion are input into the synthesizer, which outputs a new image in which the two input images are synthesized smoothly. The global discriminator determines whether the synthesized image is consistent. The local discriminator, however, has two roles. The first is to determine whether the lesion part in the generated image is realistic, and the second is to determine whether the lesion part and the normal part are connected smoothly. When designing this architecture, we used the architecture proposed in [7] as a reference.

The input into the synthesizer is a normal image and a padded patch showing a lesion. To obtain a padded lesion patch, first the patch is cropped from the part of the image that shows the lesion and then it is zero-padded such that it

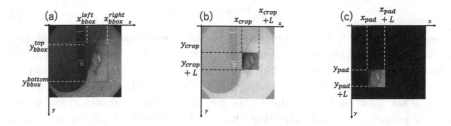

Fig. 2. Padding a lesion image. (a) Lesion image with bounding box; (b) lesion patch cropped from the lesion part of the image; (c) padded lesion patch.

is the same size as the normal image (Fig. 2). The position of the lesion patch relative to the normal image is represented by changing the position of the zero padding. The position of the padding is determined randomly. In other words, both X_n and X_l, where X_n is a normal image and X_l is a padded lesion patch, are three-dimensional tensors, which have the same shape. The normal image X_n is resized to the prescribed size in advance.

When the normal image X_n and the padded lesion patch X_l have been concatenated in the channel axis, the image is input into the synthesizer. The output of the synthesizer is a new image, in which the two images are synthesized smoothly. At this point, the position of the lesion in the synthesized image corresponds to the position of the input lesion patch (x_{pad}, y_{pad}).

The input into the global discriminator, however, is a lesion image that is either taken from the dataset or synthesized. Each image in the dataset is resized to a prescribed size in advance. The output of the global discriminator is a scalar within $[0, 1]$, which indicates the probability that the input image belongs to the dataset. The local discriminator receives as input either a lesion patch from the dataset or the lesion part of the synthesized image. Here, the synthesized image is cropped from a region slightly larger than the padded region of the input image. The purpose is to ensure that lesion patch is synthesized to the same location as the padded position in the input lesion image, and furthermore, that the boundary of the normal part and the lesion part is smooth. The output, like that of the global discriminator, is a scalar within $[0, 1]$.

Two types of loss functions are used to optimize the three networks: reconstruction and adversarial loss. The main importance of these loss functions is that the reconstruction loss function ensures the synthesized image is successfully reconstructed using the original input images and the adversarial loss function allows the boundary region between a normal image and a lesion patch to be generated flexibly. These two loss functions realize smoothly synthesized images, even when the size of the lesion image dataset is small.

The reconstruction loss is represented as

$$L_{rc}^{global} = \text{Mean}(\{X_n - G(X_n, X_l)\}^2 \odot F_1) \tag{1}$$

$$L_{rc}^{local} = \text{Mean}(\{X_l - G(X_n, X_l)\}^2 \odot F_2) \tag{2}$$

$$L_{rc} = L_{rc}^{global} + \alpha L_{rc}^{local} \tag{3}$$

where L_{rc}^{global} and L_{rc}^{local} are the reconstruction losses in the global and local discriminator, respectively, L_{rc} is the final reconstruction loss, X_n and X_a are the images from the normal and the lesion image dataset, respectively, and $G()$ is the output of the synthesizer. The squared values are the Hadamard product. Mean() is the function for calculating the mean of all the elements in the tensor. α is a hyperparameter for adjusting the weight of both the local and global reconstruction loss. F_1 and F_2 are tensors for weighting, the shape of which is the same as that of X_n. The adoption of a smoothing function such as the two-dimensional Gauss function as F_1 and F_2 makes the boundary between the normal and the lesion part become smooth.

Adversarial loss is related to the classification of the discriminator. The loss of the generator and the discriminator are respectively defined as

$$L_{adv}^{gen} = \text{Softplus}(-P_{fake}^{global}) + \text{Softplus}(-P_{fake}^{local}) \tag{4}$$

$$\begin{aligned} L_{adv}^{dis} &= \text{Softplus}(-P_{real}^{global}) + \text{Softplus}(P_{fake}^{global}) \\ &+ \beta(\text{Softplus}(-P_{real}^{local}) + \text{Softplus}(P_{fake}^{local})) \end{aligned} \tag{5}$$

where L_{adv}^{gen} and L_{adv}^{dis} are the adversarial losses of the generator and discriminator, respectively, β is a hyperparameter for adjusting the weight between the global and local adversarial loss, and Softplus is a standard softplus function. P_{real}^{global}, P_{fake}^{global}, P_{real}^{local}, and P_{fake}^{local} are respectively defined as

$$P_{real}^{global} = D_{global}(X_*') \tag{6}$$

$$P_{fake}^{global} = D_{global}(G(X_n, X_l)) \tag{7}$$

$$P_{real}^{local} = D_{local}(\lfloor X_a' \rfloor) \tag{8}$$

$$P_{fake}^{local} = D_{local}(\lfloor G(X_n, X_l) \rfloor) \tag{9}$$

where $D_{global}()$ and $D_{local}()$ are the output of the global and local discriminator, respectively. $\lfloor$ and $\rfloor$ denote the cropping lesion part. Both X and X' are images in the training data set, which in general are different. X_* indicates whether the image is from the normal or the lesion image dataset.

Based on the reconstruction and adversarial loss above, the synthesizer minimizes $L_{rc} + \gamma L_{adv}^{gen}$, and both discriminators minimize L_{adv}^{dis}, where γ is a hyperparameter for adjusting the weight between the reconstruction and adversarial loss. These optimizations are conducted simultaneously. After generating images, we replace the normal part with the original input image stepwise. The weight of the stepwise replacement is F_1 in Formula 1. This is effective, because the newly generated part is mainly around the lesion patch, and the original normal image can be reused in a part at a distance from the lesion part.

4   Experiments

Condition. In this study, we used our original endoscopic image dataset, which was extracted from an electric medical record system. Each image was annotated by the patient's attending doctor and the images showing lesions have bounding boxes on the lesion parts. This dataset contains 129,692 normal and 1,315 lesion images. The numbers of lesions by type are 1,309 tumors and 6 ulcers. The average height of the dataset is 458, and the average width is 405.

First, we divided the dataset as follows. The normal images were divided into 129,518 training images, 44 validation images, and 130 test images, and the lesion images were divided into 1,142 training images, 45 validation images, and 128 test images. Note that an individual patient's image was assigned to a unique set (training, validation, and test).

We conducted two experiments. In the first experiment, we visualized and compared the images synthesized by our method with images generated by DCGANs [11] to ensure that our method can generate clear images when the number of lesion images is small. The optimizer used was Adam ($\alpha = 0.0002, \beta = 0.5$), and the ratio of weight decay was 0.0001. The size of a minibatch was 64, and the number of training iterations was 150,000. The values of the hyperparameters alpha, beta, and gamma were 7.0, 1.0, and 0.002, respectively. For the DCGANs, the optimizer and the ratio of weight decay was the same as above. The model was trained from scratch. The size of a minibatch was 16 and the number of training iterations was 80,000.

In the second experiment, we trained the gastric cancer detection model using the synthesized lesion images and compared the performance with that when only lesion images in the dataset were used for training. As the gastric cancer detection model, the model proposed by [5] was used. For this detection model, the optimizer used was MomentumSGD (momentum: 0.9) and the learning rate was 0.01. The ratio of weight decay was 0.0005. The model was trained from scratch. The size of a minibatch was 64, and the number of training iterations was 15,000. For data augmentation, we applied the flipping, rotation by 90 degrees, grayscale, and channel shuffle techniques. In the training phase, we cropped the classification target in normal images randomly. In the case of the lesion images, however, we cropped randomly from the entire image with 50% probability and from inside the annotated bounding box with 50% probability. When determining whether the cropped part contained lesions, we considered the part to contain a lesion when the intersection-over-union (IoU) value between the cropped part and the annotated bounding box was greater than 0.4. In order to lessen the imbalance between the number of images with and without lesions, we applied oversampling to lesion images. In other words, we adjusted the parameter k to ensure that

$$N_a \times k + N_g \simeq N_n \tag{10}$$

where k is the oversampling ratio and N_a, N_g, and N_n are the numbers of lesion images, synthesized images, and normal images, respectively. In this experiment, we applied multiple numbers of synthesized images.

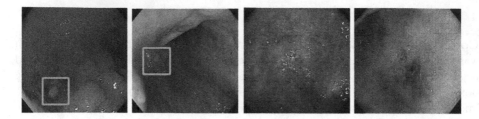

Fig. 3. Left: two images synthesized by our method with bounding boxes on the synthesized lesion patch. Right: images generated by deep convolutional generative adversarial network.

In the second experiment, the average precision (AP) metric was applied to evaluate the performance of the trained models. First, we divided each 258 images in the test dataset into 100 (10×10) grids. Then, the probability that the part contained lesions was calculated by the trained model for 64 (8×8, other than the edge) regions. Finally, we calculated the AP score according to 16,512 (258×64) predictions and annotated labels. The AP score was considered the model's score. We assigned labels as in the training phase. In the experiment, we trained the models from four different initial values and considered the mean AP values as the final score of the model.

5   Results

Figure 3 shows the results of the first experiment. Because the size of the lesion image dataset was small, mode collapse occurred in the conventional method and the resolution of the image is not very high. In contrast, our method can generate clear and various images as compared with the conventional method, because our method uses the original normal and lesion images effectively.

Table 1. Quantitative evaluation of the gastric cancer detection models. "The ratio of gen images" column shows the percentage of synthesized lesion images of all the lesion images after augmentation.

No. of gen images	No. of real images after augmentation	No. of lesion images (gen+real images)	The ratio of gen images (%)	AP
0	131330	131330	0	0.596 ± 0.029
5000	125620	130620	3.83	0.607 ± 0.032
10000	121052	131052	7.63	0.619 ± 0.013
20000	110774	130774	15.29	0.632 ± 0.013
30000	100496	130496	22.98	0.591 ± 0.030
64759	66236	130995	49.44	0.571 ± 0.007
128387	1131	129518	99.13	0.311 ± 0.030

Table 1 shows the results of the second experiment. The use of images synthesized by our proposed method improved the scores of the gastric cancer detection models. This indicates that the dataset bias was lessened, because the method allows lesion patches to be attached to various parts in normal images. When we changed the number of synthesized images input to the training dataset, we observed that the model achieved the highest AP score when 20,000 synthesized images were added, and that the performance of the model was lowered when we added a larger number of images. This indicates that the synthesized images have biases and this causes poor effects when an excessive number of synthesized images is added.

6 Summary

In this study, we focused on the imbalanced data problem for gastric cancer detection systems. To lessen the bias, we proposed a method to synthesize new lesion images by using GANs. Furthermore, we showed that the performance of a gastric cancer detection model was improved when the synthesized images were added to the training dataset.

Acknowledgements. This work was supported by a Grant for ICT infrastructure establishment and implementation of artificial intelligence for clinical and medical research from the Japan Agency of Medical Research and Development AMED (JP18lk1010028).

References

1. Baur, C., Albarqouni, S., Navab, N.: MelanoGANs: high resolution skin lesion synthesis with GANs. arXiv:1804.04338 (2018)
2. Beers, A., et al.: High-resolution medical image synthesis using progressively grown generative adversarial networks. arXiv:1805.03144 (2018)
3. Frid-Adar, M., Diamant, I., Klang, E., Amitai, M., Goldberger, J., Greenspan, H.: GAN-based synthetic medical image augmentation for increased CNN performance in liver lesion classification. Neurocomputing (2018). http://www.sciencedirect.com/science/article/pii/S0925231218310749
4. Goodfellow, I., et al.: Generative adversarial nets. In: NIPS (2014). http://papers.nips.cc/paper/5423-generative-adversarial-nets.pdf
5. Hayakawa, A., et al.: Gastric cancer detection for gastroenterological endoscopy with local and multi-scale global information. In: CARS (2019)
6. Hirasawa, T., et al.: Application of artificial intelligence using a convolutional neural network for detecting gastric cancer in endoscopic images. Gastric Cancer **21**, 653–660 (2018)
7. Iizuka, S., Simo-Serra, E., Ishikawa, H.: Globally and locally consistent image completion. ACM Trans. Graph. **36**, 107 (2017)
8. Kawahara, J., Hamarneh, G.: Multi-resolution-tract CNN with hybrid pretrained and skin-lesion trained layers. In: MICCAI (2016)
9. Liu, W., et al.: SSD: single shot MultiBox detector. In: Leibe, B., Matas, J., Sebe, N., Welling, M. (eds.) ECCV 2016. LNCS, vol. 9905, pp. 21–37. Springer, Cham (2016). https://doi.org/10.1007/978-3-319-46448-0_2

10. Lo, Y.C., et al.: Glomerulus detection on light microscopic images of renal pathology with the faster R-CNN. In: Cheng, L., Leung, A.C.S., Ozawa, S. (eds.) Neural Information Processing (2018)
11. Radford, A., Metz, L., Chintala, S.: Unsupervised representation learning with deep convolutional generative adversarial networks. In: ICLR (2016)
12. Redmon, J., Farhadi, A.: YOLOv3: an incremental improvement. arXiv:1804.02767 (2018)
13. Ren, S., He, K., Girshick, R., Sun, J.: Faster R-CNN: towards real-time object detection with region proposal networks. In: NIPS (2015)
14. Shen, W., Zhou, M., Yang, F., Yang, C., Tian, J.: Multi-scale convolutional neural networks for lung nodule classification. In: IPMI (2015)
15. Xian, W., et al.: TextureGAN: controlling deep image synthesis with texture patches. In: CVPR (2018)
16. Xiao, T., Zhang, C., Zha, H.: Learning to detect anomalies in surveillance video. IEEE Signal Process. Lett. **22**, 1477–1481 (2015)
17. Xiao T., Zhang C., Z.H.W.F.: Factorization and spatio-temporal pyramid. In: ACCV (2014)
18. Yi, X., Walia, E., Babyn, P.: Generative adversarial network in medical imaging: a review. Med. Syst. (2018)
19. Zhang, Z., Xie, Y., Yang, L.: Photographic text-to-image synthesis with a hierarchically-nested adversarial network. In: CVPR (2018)

Deep Local-Global Refinement Network for Stent Analysis in IVOCT Images

Yuyu Guo[1], Lei Bi[2], Ashnil Kumar[2], Yue Gao[3], Ruiyan Zhang[3], Dagan Feng[2], Qian Wang[1(✉)], and Jinman Kim[2]

[1] Institute for Medical Imaging Technology, School of Biomedical Engineering, Shanghai Jiao Tong University, Shanghai, China
wang.qian@sjtu.edu.cn
[2] School of Computer Science, University of Sydney, Sydney, Australia
jinman.kim@sydney.edu.au
[3] Ruijin Hospital, Shanghai Jiaotong University School of Medicine, Shanghai, China

Abstract. Implantation of stents into coronary arteries is a common treatment option for patients with cardiovascular disease. Assessment of safety and efficacy of the stent implantation occurs via manual visual inspection of the neointimal coverage from intravascular optical coherence tomography (IVOCT) images. However, such manual assessment requires the detection of thousands of strut points within the stent. This is a challenging, tedious, and time-consuming task because the strut points usually appear as small, irregular shaped objects with inhomogeneous textures, and are often occluded by shadows, artifacts, and vessel walls. Conventional methods based on textures, edge detection, or simple classifiers for automated detection of strut points in IVOCT images have low recall and precision as they are, unable to adequately represent the visual features of the strut point for detection. In this study, we propose a local-global refinement network to integrate local-patch content with global content for strut points detection from IVOCT images. Our method densely detects the potential strut points in local image patches and then refines them according to global appearance constraints to reduce false positives. Our experimental results on a clinical dataset of 7,000 IVOCT images demonstrated that our method outperformed the state-of-the-art methods with a recall of 0.92 and precision of 0.91 for strut points detection.

Keywords: Convolutional neural network (CNN) · Intravascular optical coherence tomography (IVOCT) · Stent analysis

1 Introduction

Accurate assessment of neointimal coverage after stent implantation in intravascular optical coherence tomography (IVOCT) images is important to ensure the safety and efficacy of the Percutaneous Coronary Intervention procedure [8]. Unfortunately, manual assessment requires the detection and analysis of

© Springer Nature Switzerland AG 2019
D. Shen et al. (Eds.): MICCAI 2019, LNCS 11768, pp. 539–546, 2019.
https://doi.org/10.1007/978-3-030-32254-0_60

thousands of struts within the stent, which is a challenging, tedious and time-consuming task. As shown in Fig. 1, the stent struts are small, and the visual characteristics of the region covering the thick intima (innermost layer of the artery) may make the struts inconspicuous.

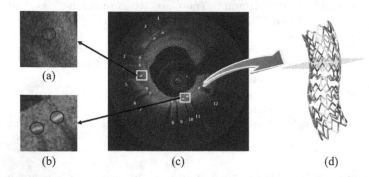

Fig. 1. Common vascular features in IVOCT images. The middle image (c) shows the manually labeled stent struts (12 in total), with two green bounding boxes of struts (a) and (b). (Color figure online)

Motivated by these challenges, a number of automated detection methods have been proposed. Existing methods typically use handcrafted features to encode the candidate strut points and then apply supervised classification to identify the struts. Commonly used handcrafted features and supervised approaches include shadow feature [11,12], decision trees [5] and wavelet based detection [3]. Besides, some studies used lumen segmentation [7,14] and stent shape models [1] to constrain the search space for the potential struts candidates. However, all these methods rely on effective pre-processing steps, such as denoising, illumination corrections and detecting lumen boundaries for producing accurate results, which thereby restricting its generalizability.

An alternative is to derive features using convolutional neural networks (CNNs) which have achieved great success in medical imaging analysis [4]. The results from the use of CNN architectures including U-Net [10] and FCN [2] demonstrate their performances in accurate detection and segmentation for large sized objects. However, because of the downsampling of the image to enlarge the receptive field and to encode the global information, the application of these CNNs to strut detection has not been validated.

We propose an automated method for stent detection in IVOCT images that overcomes the limitations above mentioned. We leverage CNNs for their ability to combine low-level appearance information with high-level semantic information in a hierarchical manner. A local network to densely detect potentially similar-struts in the image patches, and a global network that uses image appearance information to iteratively refines/removes the false predictions that are less likely to be struts. We have named our method the deep local-global refinement network (LGRN). We contribute the following to the state-of-the-art:

- To the best of our knowledge, this is the first deep learning method for strut points detection. Our method removes the reliance on pre-processing steps such as denoising and illumination corrections.
- Our coupling of a local network that has high recall with a global network that provides image level refinement, enables false positive reductions while maintaining high sensitivity and efficiency to strut point detection.
- Our global network uses an appearance constrained attention module for false positive reduction, which preserves the detected struts that fit the overall appearance of the image.

2 Method

2.1 Materials

Our dataset consists of 57 patients with stent implanted for more than 1 year. Each patient has an average of about 127 IVOCT images with stent. All the IVOCT images were acquired using a C7-XR OCT system (St. Jude Medical, St. Paul, MN, USA) with a 2.7f Dragonfly imaging catheter. Each IVOCT image has a resolution of 714×714 pixels. A cardiologist performed manual annotation of the struts and lumen on all the IVOCT images. And we follow the same protocol as in [6] to design a morphological filter applied to the annotated struts to enlarge the size, which was then used as the ground truth for evaluation.

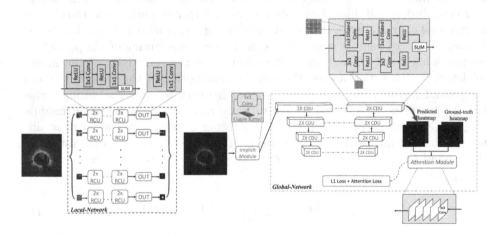

Fig. 2. Overall structure of the LGRN.

2.2 Deep Local-Global Refinement Network

Figure 2 shows the overview of the proposed local-global refinement network. Initially, Local-Network is applied to the input IVOCT image to detect all the potential struts via small input patches. After that, the detected struts together with the original IVOCT image are used as the input to Global-Network for refinement, where an appearance constrained attention module is applied to guide the overall spatial distribution of all the struts and to remove all falsely detected struts.

Local-Network: A patch-based deep CNN is used as the Local-Network for detecting all the strut points. It consists of 9 zero-padded convolutional layers with kernel size of 3 and stride of 1. Residual block is used to connect each adjacent layer. At the end of the Local-Network we use a linear 1×1 convolution layer and a Gaussian convolution kernel, where the 1×1 convolution is used to compensate for batch normalization, and the Gaussian convolution kernel is used to smooth the output, e.g., suppressing the path artifacts of the Local-Network. The patch size is set to 64×64 for the Local-Network. The network is trained with $L1$ Loss.

Global-Network: The purpose of the Global-Network is to extract high-level semantic information that can be used to guide the refinement of all the detected struts. The Global-Network uses a modified U-net [10] architecture. There are 4 downsampling layers, each with a 2×2 max-pooling operator, and 4 upsampling layers. At each down/up-sampling layer, we repeat the following parallel architecture module: one sub-branch with 3×3 convolutional kernel, and another sub-branch with 3×3 dilated convolution and 2 dilations. The outputs of these two sub-branches are added at the end of this module. This combination of regular convolution and dilated convolution has a larger receptive field thus it can learn visual characteristics that assist in inferring struts with less visual features. Therefore, global context constraints can ensure the accuracy of the prediction results, while local context learning can improve the sensitivity of the model to detect the object. However, the uneven distribution of the background and foreground makes it difficult for the global network to converge during training. To overcome this, we added an appearance constrained attention module to guide its convergence, where we used another 5 layers CNN network to different whether the predicted detection results have the similar appearance to the ground truth. To facilitate the learning process, we used two loss functions ($\ell_{similar}$ and $\ell_{attention}$) as:

$$\ell_{similar} = \ell_{L1}\Big(\lceil M \rceil * P, M\Big) + \ell_{L1}\Big(\big(1 - \lceil M \rceil\big) * P, 0\Big) \tag{1}$$

where $\lceil M \rceil$ is the ground truth annotation. P indicates the predicted results. It's used to balance the uneven distribution of foreground and background. We also add an attention loss to constrain the overall appearance of the predicted struts and this can be defined as:

$$\ell_{attention} = log\Big(A(M, I)\Big) + log\Big(1 - A(P, I)\Big) \tag{2}$$

where $A(\cdot)$ indicates the attention module that discriminates whether P is similar appearance to the ground truth.

Table 1. Detection results compared to the state-of-the-art methods

Method	Recall	Precision
Hyeong et al. [7]	0.894	0.818
Hong et al. [5]	0.804	0.826
Ancong et al. [13]	0.910	0.840
Faster-RCNN [9]	0.913	0.856
Local-network	0.914	0.833
Global-network	0.903	0.876
Ours	**0.925**	**0.903**

2.3 Implementation Details

We pre-processed the dataset with maximum normalization and cropped all images to 512 × 512. Both Local-Net and Global-Network were trained for 80 epochs with an Adam optimizer at an initial learning rate of 0.001 and batch size of 1. It took an average of 15 h to train on an 11 GB Nvidia 1080Ti GPU.

3 Results and Discussions

3.1 Experimental Setup

We randomly divided the dataset into a training set (30 patients, 3873 images) and a test set (27 patients, 3352 images) for evaluation. We performed the following experiments on the dataset: (a) comparison of the performance of our method with the state-of-the-art methods; and (b) analysis of the performance of each component in our method. The state-of-the-art methods include: (i) Wang et al. [13] - Bayesian network based detection method; (ii) Faster-RCNN [9] - Region Proposal Network (RPN) that is trained end-to-end to generate high-quality region proposals for detection. (iii) Lu et al. [5] - Bagged decision trees classifier for classifying candidate struts using structure features, and (iv) Nam et al. [7] - Neural network classifier to classify the features from gradient images. For [13], due to the unavailability of the algorithm source code, we refer to the published result as a reference acknowledging that the dataset is different. We use recall and precision for the evaluation (we followed [13] to define the true positive detection if they are within 5 pixels of the ground-truth).

3.2 State-of-the-Art Methods Comparison

Table 1 shows the detection results of our method compared to the state-of-the-art methods, where it increases recall by 1.2% and precision by 4.7%, relative to the second best results from Faster-RCNN, as shown in Fig. 3(a).

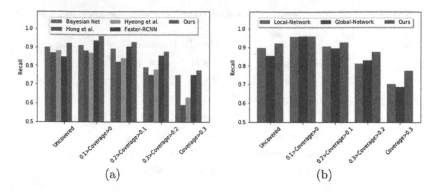

Fig. 3. Strut detection results: (a) comparison of our method to the existing methods, (b) component analysis of our method.

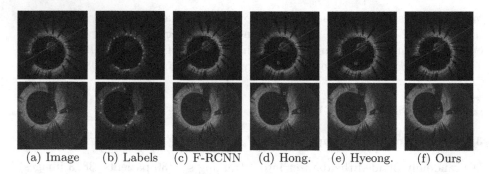

(a) Image   (b) Labels   (c) F-RCNN   (d) Hong.   (e) Hyeong.   (f) Ours

Fig. 4. Comparison of our detection results with existing comparison methods

3.3   Component Analysis

Table 1 and Fig. 3(b) show the detection results of our method at individual stages. Figure 5(a) shows the two example detection results with various thickness coverage. The Local-Network shows the higher recall while Global-Network achieved better precision results (as shown in Fig. 5(c) and (d)). As exemplified in Fig. 5(e), the proposed method integrated both Local Network and Global-Network and achieved a better consistent performance in recall and precision.

3.4   Discussion

Table 1 and Fig. 3(a) illustrate our method achieved the overall best performance when compared to the existing methods for strut detection. The traditional methods (Hyeong et al. [7], Hong et al. [5] and Ancong et al. [13]) using hand-crafted features with conventional classifiers achieved competitive performance when compared with Faster-RCNN method. Figure 4(d) and (e) show two example results where both Hyeong et al. and Hong et al. methods fail to detect strut points where there is low-contrast to the background. In contrast, Faster-RCNN

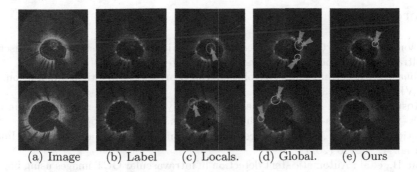

| (a) Image | (b) Label | (c) Locals. | (d) Global. | (e) Ours |

Fig. 5. Example results of struts detection. Red arrows indicate the detection errors. (Color figure online)

has the ability to combine deep semantic information and shallow appearance information in a hierarchical manner that enables it to encode image-wide location information and semantic characteristics. However, Faster-RCNN lacks constrain of the overall appearance of all the struts. Consequently, Faster-RCNN generates poor detection results for small struts (as shown in Fig. 4(c)).

Table 1, Figs. 3(b) and 5 compared the main components of our method individually to quantify their contributions to the final detection results. These results demonstrate that Local-Network has higher recall and we attribute this to the usage of patch-based network to detect all the potential strut candidates. In contrast, Global-Network achieved higher precision for its ability by adding global context, e.g., appearance information, as part of the learning process, which ensures all the detected struts are consistent with the shape of the stent. Table 1, Figs. 3(b) and 5 also show the advantages from our combination which integrates complementary detection results produced at individual components.

4   Conclusion

We propose a deep learning-based method for stent struts detection for IVOCT images. We achieved state-of-the-art struts detection performance via a local-global refinement network, where we detected potential struts which were then refined according to global appearance constraints to reduce false positives. Our experimental results demonstrate that our method achieved higher accuracy when compared to the existing state-of-the-art methods on a large clinical dataset.

Acknowledgement. This work was supported in part by Australia Research Council (ARC) grants (LP140100686 and IC170100022), the University of Sydney – Shanghai Jiao Tong University Joint Research Alliance (USYD-SJTU JRA) grants and STCSM grant (17411953300).

References

1. Ciompi, F., et al.: Computer-aided detection of intracoronary stent in intravascular ultrasound sequences. Med. Phys. **43**(10), 5616–5625 (2016)
2. Jonathan, L., et al.: Fully convolutional networks for semantic segmentation. In: CVPR, pp. 3431–3440 (2015)
3. Kostas, M., et al.: Automatic quantitative analysis of in-stent restenosis using FD-OCT in vivo intra-arterial imaging. Med. Phys. **40**(6PartI), 063101 (2013)
4. Litjens, G., et al.: A survey on deep learning in medical image analysis. Med. Image Anal. **42**, 60–88 (2017)
5. Lu, H., et al.: Automatic stent detection in intravascular OCT images using bagged decision trees. Biomed. Opt. Express **3**(11), 2809–2824 (2012)
6. Merget, D., et al.: Robust facial landmark detection via a fully-convolutional local-global context network. In: CVPR, pp. 781–790 (2018)
7. Nam, H.S., et al.: Automated detection of vessel lumen and stent struts in intravascular optical coherence tomography to evaluate stent apposition and neointimal coverage. Med. Phys. **43**(4), 1662–1675 (2016)
8. Otsuka, F., et al.: Neoatherosclerosis: overview of histopathologic findings and implications for intravascular imaging assessment. Eur. Hear. J. **36**(32), 2147–2159 (2015)
9. Ren, S., et al.: Faster R-CNN: towards real-time object detection with region proposal networks. In: NIPS, pp. 91–99 (2015)
10. Ronneberger, O., Fischer, P., Brox, T.: U-Net: convolutional networks for biomedical image segmentation. In: Navab, N., Hornegger, J., Wells, W.M., Frangi, A.F. (eds.) MICCAI 2015. LNCS, vol. 9351, pp. 234–241. Springer, Cham (2015). https://doi.org/10.1007/978-3-319-24574-4_28
11. Ughi, G.J., et al.: Automatic segmentation of in-vivo intra-coronary optical coherence tomography images to assess stent strut apposition and coverage. Int. J. Cardiovasc. Imagin **28**(2), 229–241 (2012)
12. Wang, A., et al.: Automatic stent strut detection in intravascular optical coherence tomographic pullback runs. Int. J. Cardiovasc. Imaging **29**(1), 29–38 (2013)
13. Wang, A., et al.: 3-D stent detection in intravascular OCT using a Bayesian network and graph search. IEEE Trans. Med. Imaging **34**(7), 1549–1561 (2015)
14. Yong, Y.L., et al.: Linear-regression convolutional neural network for fully automated coronary lumen segmentation in intravascular optical coherence tomography. J. Biomed. Opt. **22**(12), 126005 (2017)

Generalized Non-rigid Point Set Registration with Hybrid Mixture Models Considering Anisotropic Positional Uncertainties

Zhe Min[1(✉)], Li Liu[1], and Max Q.-H. Meng[1,2]

[1] Robotics, Perception, and Artificial Intelligence Lab,
The Chinese University of Hong Kong, Shatin, NT, Hong Kong, China
{zmin,max}@ee.cuhk.edu.hk
[2] Shenzhen Research Institute,
The Chinese University of Hong Kong, Shenzhen, China
liliu@cuhk.edu.hk

Abstract. Image-to-patient or pre-operative to intra-operative registration is an essential problem in computer-assisted surgery (CAS). Non-rigid or deformable registration is still a challenging problem with partial overlapping between point sets due to limited camera view, missing data due to tumor resection and the surface reconstruction error intra-operatively. In this paper, we propose and validate a normal-vector assisted non-rigid registration framework for accurately registering soft tissues in CAS. Two stages including rigid and non-rigid registrations are involved in the framework. In the stage of the rigid registration that does the initial alignment, the normal vectors extracted from the point sets are used while the position uncertainty is assumed to be anisotropic. With the normal vectors incorporated, the algorithm can better recover the point correspondences and is more robust to intra-operative partial data which is often the case in a typical laparoscopic surgery. In the stage of the non-rigid registration, the anisotropic coherent point drift (CPD) method is formulated, where the isotropic error assumption is generalized to anisotropic cases. Extensive experiments on the human liver data demonstrate our proposed algorithm's several great advantages over the existing state-of-the-art ones. First, the rigid transformation matrix is recovered more accurately. Second, the proposed registration framework is much more robust to partial scan. Besides, the anisotropic CPD outperforms the original CPD significantly in terms of robustness to noise.

1 Introduction

Registration is an essential problem in both medical imaging (MI) and computer assisted surgery (CAS) or image-guided surgery (IGS). Registration problems

Electronic supplementary material The online version of this chapter (https://doi.org/10.1007/978-3-030-32254-0_61) contains supplementary material, which is available to authorized users.

© Springer Nature Switzerland AG 2019
D. Shen et al. (Eds.): MICCAI 2019, LNCS 11768, pp. 547–555, 2019.
https://doi.org/10.1007/978-3-030-32254-0_61

can be coarsely divided into rigid registrations and non-rigid registrations. In a rigid registration, the transformation is rigid, which typically includes a rotation matrix, a translation vector. In a non-rigid registration, the transformation between PSs is usually unknown and nonlinear. Compared with the rigid one, the non-rigid registration is a much more challenging problem [4,14,15].

In IGS, the pre-operative CT or MRI model has to be accurately registered with the intra-operative scan data (or so-called image-to-patient registration). This vital task especially the non-rigid registration is still challenging because of the initial pose between the two point sets (PSs), partial overlapping because of the partial visible surface during surgery, and the noisy sensor data (both pre-operatively and intra-operatively). More specifically, the camera attached to the surgical instrument only has access to a restricted region of the abdomen in a typical laparoscopic surgery [14] and the surface data from the stereo reconstruction intra-operatively is very noisy [14]. The rigid PS registration is utilized to recover the initial gross misalignment between the pre-operative and intra-operative spaces [13,14]. In terms of non-rigid registration, brain shift usually exists in the neuro-surgical procedures such as tumor resection [1]. In image-guided liver surgery (IGLS), the deformation of the liver intra-operatively comes from organ shape changes, respiration, liver mobilization, and resection [3].

Recently, Ravikumar et al. generalized the coherent point drift (CPD) method to high-dimensional points for the group-wise registration problem [12,13]. Bayer et al. adopts and reformulates the method in [13] to compensate the brain shift in a neuro-surgical procedure such as tumor resection [1]. In both stages of rigid registration and non-rigid registrations in [1,12,13], the isotropic localization error assumption is shared. However, this ideal and simple assumption actually does not fit the real scenarios in surgical navigation. For example, in a stereo camera system (such as an endoscopy or laparoscopy), the standard deviation of the point localization error in the viewing direction is three or five times than those in the other two directions [5,10]. Very recently, Min et al. considered the anisotropic positional uncertainty in the pair-wise rigid registration [10], and later for the multiple point set registration problems [6].

In this paper, we present a novel non-rigid registration framework based on the use of normal vectors and the anisotropic assumption of positional uncertainty. On one hand, the normal vectors are used to enhance the registration performance, which brings several benefits. First, the posterior probabilities representing the point correspondences can be computed more accurately. Second, the rotation matrix that aligns two point sets can be recovered more accurately. On the other hand, the anisotropic uncertainty is considered in both rigid and non-rigid registrations. The main contributions of our work are: (1) the normal-vector assisted rigid registration algorithm considering the anisotropic positional uncertainty is formally introduced in the proposed non-rigid registration framework; (2) to the best of our knowledge, the anisotropic non-rigid CPD is formulated and validated for the first time; (3) extensive simulated experiments on the human liver data sets are conducted to validate the proposed algorithms.

2   Methods

One surface represented by point sets (PSs) $\mathbf{X} = [\mathbf{x}_1, ...\mathbf{x}_n..., \mathbf{x}_N] \in \mathbb{R}^{3 \times N}$ that has been deformed is registered with the initial one $\mathbf{Y} = [\mathbf{y}_1, ...\mathbf{y}_m..., \mathbf{y}_M] \in \mathbb{R}^{3 \times M}$. The transformation between $\mathbf{X}$ and $\mathbf{Y}$ could possibly include a rigid transformation. Our proposed registration framework is overall divided into two stages: rigid and non-rigid registrations. In both stages, the registrations are formulated as maximum likelihood (ML) problems with the hidden variables being the point correspondences, and are solved under the expectation maximization (EM) framework. At the beginning of the first stage, the unit normal vector sets $\widehat{\mathbf{X}} = [\widehat{\mathbf{x}}_1, ...\widehat{\mathbf{x}}_n..., \widehat{\mathbf{x}}_N]$ and $\widehat{\mathbf{Y}} = [\widehat{\mathbf{y}}_1, ...\widehat{\mathbf{y}}_m..., \widehat{\mathbf{y}}_M]$ are extracted from $\mathbf{X}$ and $\mathbf{Y}$, where $\widehat{\mathbf{x}}_n \in \mathcal{S}^2$ and $\widehat{\mathbf{y}}_m \in \mathcal{S}^2$. Two generalized PSs are then constructed as $\mathbf{D}_x = [\mathbf{d}_1^x, ...\mathbf{d}_n^x..., \mathbf{d}_N^x]$ and $\mathbf{D}_y = [\mathbf{d}_1^y, ...\mathbf{d}_n^y..., \mathbf{d}_N^y]$, where $\mathbf{d}_n^x = (\mathbf{x}_n, \widehat{\mathbf{x}}_n)^\mathsf{T}$ and $\mathbf{d}_m^y = (\mathbf{y}_m, \widehat{\mathbf{y}}_m)^\mathsf{T}$ are both six-dimensional vectors. After the first stage, the rigid transformation including the rotation matrix $\mathbf{R} \in SO(3)$ and translation vector $\mathbf{t} \in \mathbb{R}^3$, the updated posterior probabilities and covariance matrix $\mathbf{\Sigma} \in \mathbb{S}^3$ are acquired and used in the following non-rigid stage. The model parameters in the stages of rigid and non-rigid registrations are defined as $\mathbf{\Theta} = \{\mathbf{R}, \mathbf{t}, \mathbf{\Sigma}\}$ and $\mathbf{\Theta}_p = \{v, \mathbf{\Sigma}\}$ respectively. Those parameters will be illustrated in the following.

2.1   Generalized Rigid Point Set Registration Considering Anisotropic Positional Uncertainty (HMM (Anisotropic))

Multi-Variate Gaussian and Von-Mises Fisher (VMF) distributions are used to model the positional and normal error vectors respectively [10]. By assuming that the positional and normal vectors are independent, the probability density function (PDF) of a generalized data point $\mathbf{d}_n^x$ given the current correspondence $z_n = m$ is defined in (1), where $\mathbf{z}_{mn} = \mathbf{x}_n - \mathbf{R}\mathbf{y}_m - \mathbf{t} \in \mathbb{R}^3$, $| \bullet |$ denotes the determinant of a matrix, the concentration parameter κ controls how $\widehat{\mathbf{x}}_n$ distribute about the central one $\mathbf{R}\widehat{\mathbf{y}}_m$. More specifically, the larger the value of κ is the more concentrated the sampled normal vectors are. The hybrid mixture models (HMMs) defined as $p(\mathbf{d}_n^x|\mathbf{D}_y, \mathbf{\Theta}) = w\frac{1}{N} + (1-w)\sum_{m=1}^{M} \frac{1}{M}p(\mathbf{d}_n^x|z_n = m)$ are the sum of an additional uniform distribution to account for noise or outliers and the PDF in (1). The weighting factor $w \in \mathbb{R}$ denotes the weight of the uniform distribution, and the prior probability of all the mixture components is $\frac{1}{M}$. By assuming that the data points in $\mathbf{D}_x$ are independent, the data likelihood defined as $\mathcal{L}(\mathbf{\Theta}) = \prod_{i=1}^{n} p(\mathbf{d}_n^x|\mathbf{D}_y, \mathbf{\Theta})$ is the product of the data points' PDFs. Instead of maximizing $L(\mathbf{\Theta})$, to estimate $\mathbf{\Theta}$, the expected negative log likelihood function (llh) is often minimized, which is $Q(\mathbf{\Theta})$ in (2) by ignoring the constants independent of $\mathbf{\Theta}$. In (2), $N_\mathbf{P} = \sum_{n=1}^{N} \sum_{m=1}^{M} p_{mn}$, where $p_{mn} \in \mathbb{R}$ is the posterior probability and is updated using the Bayes' rule as $p_{mn} = \frac{\frac{1}{M}p(\mathbf{d}_n^x|z_n=m)}{p(\mathbf{d}_n^x|\mathbf{D}_y, \mathbf{\Theta})}$ (E-step). The updated $\mathbf{\Sigma}$ is computed by solving $\frac{\partial Q(\mathbf{\Theta})}{\partial \mathbf{\Sigma}} = \mathbf{0}$ in (2) (M-step). The updated κ is computed by solving $\frac{\partial Q(\mathbf{\Theta})}{\partial \kappa} = 0$ $(-\frac{1}{\kappa} + \frac{e^\kappa + e^{-\kappa}}{e^\kappa - e^{-\kappa}} = \frac{1}{N_\mathbf{P}} \sum_{m=1}^{M} \sum_{n=1}^{N} p_{mn}(\mathbf{R}\widehat{\mathbf{y}}_m)^\mathsf{T}\widehat{\mathbf{x}}_n)$, which is solved using the fixed point approach (M-step). E and M steps will iterate until convergence. In the end, the transformed model PS is $\mathbf{T}(\mathbf{Y}) = [\mathbf{R}\mathbf{y}_1 + \mathbf{t}, ...\mathbf{R}\mathbf{y}_m + \mathbf{t}..., \mathbf{R}\mathbf{y}_M + \mathbf{t}] \in \mathbb{R}^{3 \times M}$.

$$
p(\mathbf{d}_n^x | z_n = m, \boldsymbol{\Theta}) = \underbrace{\frac{1}{(2\pi)^{\frac{3}{2}}|\boldsymbol{\Sigma}|^{\frac{1}{2}}} e^{-\frac{1}{2}(\mathbf{z}_{mn}))^{\mathsf{T}}\boldsymbol{\Sigma}^{-1}(\mathbf{z}_{mn})}}_{\text{Position Vectors}} \cdot \underbrace{\frac{\kappa}{2\pi(e^{\kappa} - e^{-\kappa})} e^{\kappa(\mathbf{R}\hat{\mathbf{y}}_m)^{\mathsf{T}}\hat{\mathbf{x}}_n}}_{\text{Normal Vectors}} ,
$$

(1)

$$
Q(\boldsymbol{\Theta}) = \sum_{n=1}^{N} \sum_{m=1}^{M} p_{mn} \left(\frac{1}{2}(\mathbf{x}_n - \mathbf{R}\mathbf{y}_m - \mathbf{t})^{\mathsf{T}}\boldsymbol{\Sigma}^{-1}(\mathbf{x}_n - \mathbf{R}\mathbf{y}_m - \mathbf{t}) - \kappa(\mathbf{R}\hat{\mathbf{y}}_m)^{\mathsf{T}}\hat{\mathbf{x}}_n \right)
$$
$$
+ \frac{1}{2}N_{\mathbf{P}} \log |\boldsymbol{\Sigma}| + N_{\mathbf{P}} \log (e^{\kappa} - e^{-\kappa}) - N_{\mathbf{P}} \log \kappa.
$$

(2)

2.2 Non-rigid Point Set Registration Considering Anisotropic Positional Uncertainty (Anisotropic CPD)

The rigidly aligned model $\mathbf{T}(\mathbf{Y})$ is used as an input in this stage, but is still denoted as $\mathbf{Y}$ for simplicity. The non-rigid transformation is assumed to be the initial position plus some displacement function v (i.e the warped model PS $\mathbf{T}(\mathbf{Y}) = \mathbf{Y} + v(\mathbf{Y}) \in \mathbb{R}^{3 \times M}$). The non-rigid transformation is further regularized using Tikhonov regularization, and expressed in the Reproducing Kernel Hilbert Space(RKHS)[11]. Considering the anisotropic positional uncertainty, the PDF of one data point $\mathbf{x}_n$ given the current correspondence (i.e. $z_n = m$) is defined as (3). Similar to Sect. 2.1, the mixture model is expressed as $p(\mathbf{x}_n|\mathbf{Y}, \boldsymbol{\Theta}_p) = w\frac{1}{N} + (1 - w)\sum_{m=1}^{M} \frac{1}{M}p(\mathbf{x}_n|z_n = m)$. Assuming that points in $\mathbf{X}$ are independent, the data likelihood $\mathcal{L}(\boldsymbol{\Theta}_p)$ is the product of the PDFs associated with $\mathbf{x}_n$: $\mathcal{L}(\boldsymbol{\Theta}_p) = \prod_{i=1}^{n} p(\mathbf{x}_n|\mathbf{Y}, \boldsymbol{\Theta}_p)$. The expected negative log-likelihood $Q(\boldsymbol{\Theta}_p)$ defined in (4) is minimized to seek $\boldsymbol{\Theta}_p$. In (4), $\mathbf{z}_{mn}^{\text{deform}}(\mathbf{x}_n - \mathbf{y}_m - v(\mathbf{y}_m)) \in \mathbb{R}^3$, $\lambda \in \mathbb{R}$ denotes the weight of the regularization term, and the operator P "extracted" the high frequency content part of v. As proved in [11], the function v that minimizes $Q(\boldsymbol{\Theta}_p)$ is a linear combination of radial basis functions (RBFs). To significantly facilitate the computation, the matrix form of $Q(\mathbf{W})$ is presented in (5), where $\text{tr}(\bullet)$ denotes the trace of a matrix and $\mathbf{P} \in \mathbb{R}^{M \times N}$ stores the posteriors with $p_{mn} = \frac{\frac{1}{M}p(\mathbf{x}_n|z_n = m, \boldsymbol{\Theta}_p)}{p(\mathbf{x}_n|\mathbf{Y}, \boldsymbol{\Theta}_p)}$ (E-step). In (5), $\mathbf{W} \in \mathbb{R}^{M \times 3}$ is the matrix of coefficients associated with RBFs while $\mathbf{G} \in \mathbb{S}^{M \times M}$ is a kernel matrix with elements $g_{ij} = G(\mathbf{y}_i, \mathbf{y}_j) = e^{-\frac{1}{2}||\frac{\mathbf{y}_i - \mathbf{y}_j}{\beta}||^2}$, where $\beta \in \mathbb{R}$ is the kernel bandwidth controlling PSs' local structure. By computing $\frac{\partial Q(\mathbf{W})}{\partial \mathbf{W}} = 0$ in (5) and with some matrix manipulations, we can get $\underbrace{\text{diag}(\mathbf{P1})\mathbf{G}}_{A}\underbrace{\mathbf{W}}_{X} + \underbrace{\mathbf{W}}_{X}\underbrace{\lambda\boldsymbol{\Sigma}}_{B} = \underbrace{\mathbf{PX}^{\mathsf{T}} - \text{diag}(\mathbf{P1})\mathbf{Y}^{\mathsf{T}}}_{C}$ about $\mathbf{W}$, which is solved by solving $\mathbf{AX} + \mathbf{XB} = \mathbf{C}$ in MATLAB (M-step). E and M steps will iterate until convergence. Finally we get $\mathbf{T}(\mathbf{Y}) = \mathbf{Y} + \mathbf{W}^{\mathsf{T}}\mathbf{G}^{\mathsf{T}}$.

$$
p(\mathbf{x}_n|z_n = m, \boldsymbol{\Theta}_p) = \frac{1}{(2\pi)^{\frac{3}{2}}|\boldsymbol{\Sigma}|^{\frac{1}{2}}} e^{-\frac{1}{2}(\mathbf{x}_n - \mathbf{y}_m - v(\mathbf{y}_m))^{\mathsf{T}}\boldsymbol{\Sigma}^{-1}(\mathbf{x}_n - \mathbf{y}_m - v(\mathbf{y}_m))}, \quad (3)
$$

$$Q(\Theta_p) = \frac{1}{2} \sum_{n=1}^{N} \sum_{m=1}^{M} p_{mn} \left(\mathbf{z}_{mn}^{\text{deform}}\right)^{\mathsf{T}} \mathbf{\Sigma}^{-1} \mathbf{z}_{mn}^{\text{deform}} + \frac{1}{2} N_{\mathbf{P}} \log|\mathbf{\Sigma}| + \frac{\lambda}{2} \|Pv\|^2, \quad (4)$$

$$Q(\mathbf{W}) = -\text{tr}\left(\mathbf{W}^{\mathsf{T}} \mathbf{G}^{\mathsf{T}} \mathbf{P} \mathbf{X}^{\mathsf{T}} \mathbf{\Sigma}^{-1}\right) + \text{tr}\left(\mathbf{W}^{\mathsf{T}} \mathbf{G}^{\mathsf{T}} \text{diag}(\mathbf{P1}) \mathbf{Y}^{\mathsf{T}} \mathbf{\Sigma}^{-1}\right)$$
$$+ \text{tr}\left(\mathbf{W}^{\mathsf{T}} \mathbf{G}^{\mathsf{T}} \text{diag}(\mathbf{P1}) \mathbf{G} \mathbf{W} \mathbf{\Sigma}^{-1}\right) + \frac{\lambda}{2} \text{tr}(\mathbf{W}^{\mathsf{T}} \mathbf{G} \mathbf{W}). \tag{5}$$

3 Experiments and Results

In the following series of studies, in silico liver data set in OpenCAS[1] is used [16] which contains three liver models that have been deformed by means of a non-linear biomechanical model. For each model, we note that the deformed surface points $\mathbf{X}$ (partial or full) represents the intra-operative data PS while the initial volume points $\mathbf{Y}$ (full) represents the pre-operative model PS. The normal vectors $\widehat{\mathbf{X}}$ and $\widehat{\mathbf{Y}}$ associated with $\mathbf{X}$ and $\mathbf{Y}$ are computed in MeshLab [2] with the number of neighbouring points being 10 (the default value), and afterwards $\mathbf{D}_x$ and $\mathbf{D}_y$ can be acquired afterwards. Note that the directions of the normal vectors are automatically pointing outwards the surfaces using MeshLab.

Rigid Registration Performance. In this section, $\mathbf{Y}$ (or $\mathbf{D}_y$) is rotated using a random rotation matrix $\mathbf{R}^g$ (that corresponds to an angle $\theta = 20°$). For computing efficiency, both $\mathbf{D}_x$ and rotated $\mathbf{Y}$ (or $\mathbf{D}_y$) are downsampled to own $N_{test} = 1000$ points since we have found that down sampling the PSs will not worsen the performance significantly using all registration methods. The inputs to CPD [11] are $\mathbf{X}$ and rotated $\mathbf{Y}$ while the inputs to HMM(isotropic) [7,9] and HMM(anisotropic) introduced in Sect. 2.1 are $\mathbf{D}_x$ and rotated $\mathbf{D}_y$. The rotational error values in degree are computed[2]. The above process is repeated for $N_{\text{repeat}} = 1000$ times, and afterwards the mean and standard deviation (std) of the error values are computed. Table 1 shows the results. In Table 1, the error values with the deformed partial scan (i.e. $\mathbf{X}$) are included in the second to fourth columns while those with the deformed full scan are shown in the last three columns. Because of the deformation in $\mathbf{X}$, all methods cannot recover the rigid transformation very accurately. We should notice that the error values shown in Table 1 can be further reduced (if not significantly) by first conducting a coarse registration through incorporating reliably identifiable, salient anatomical features. Two conclusions are drawn by carefully looking into Table 1: (1) HMM(anisotropic) and HMM (isotropic) outperform the rigid CPD method significantly when only partial scan of the whole liver is available intra-operatively, which is the case in laparoscopic surgery [14]; (2) The rigid registration error values with full liver scans are significantly smaller than those with partial scans using all methods.

---

[1] http://opencas.webarchiv.kit.edu/.

[2] $\theta_{deg} = \arccos\left[\frac{\text{tr}(\mathbf{R}^g \mathbf{R}^{\mathsf{T}})-1}{2}\right]/\pi \times 180$, where $\mathbf{R}^g$ and $\mathbf{R}$ denote the ground-truth and the computed rotation matrix using one specific test method, respectively.

Table 1. The mean and standard deviation of the rotational error values when the three liver models are computed and shown. All the presented results are in the degree unit. The CPD [11] and the HMM (isotropic) methods [7] are compared.

	Liver 1 (Partial)	Liver 2 (Partial)	Liver 3 (Partial)	Liver 1 (Full)	Liver 2 (Full)	Liver 3 (Full)
CPD	38.66 ± 4.65	33.08 ± 2.98	49.17 ± 7.58	9.08 ± 0.65	10.46 ± 0.81	9.22 ± 0.97
HMM	8.40 ± 0.43	$\mathbf{6.18 \pm 0.49}$	14.50 ± 0.86	$\mathbf{8.74 \pm 0.18}$	7.68 ± 0.44	$\mathbf{5.67 \pm 0.31}$
Ours	$\mathbf{8.22 \pm 0.37}$	6.81 ± 0.66	$\mathbf{13.79 \pm 0.92}$	8.79 ± 0.21	$\mathbf{7.39 \pm 0.51}$	6.23 ± 0.38

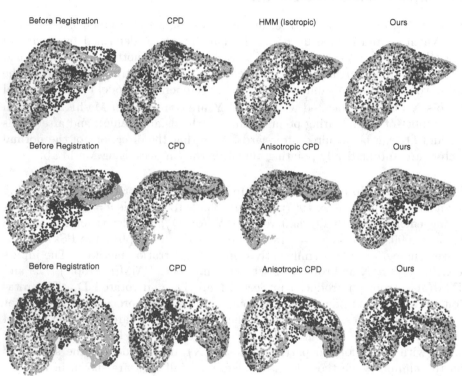

Fig. 1. The registration performances on the three liver models are shown in the three rows respectively. The two point sets before and after registration are shown in the first and in the last three columns respectively. In all sub-figures, the model and data points are represented with red and green dots respectively. The rigid HMM (anisotropic) together with the anisotropic non-rigid CPD is "ours". (Best viewed in color.)

Non-rigid Registration Performance. Since we have noticed in Table 1 that both CPD and HMM (isotropic) cannot well recover the rigid transformation, to have a fair comparison of the non-rigid registration, no gross misalignment between $\mathbf{X}$ ($\mathbf{D}_x$) and $\mathbf{Y}$ ($\mathbf{D}_y$) exists in this section. Besides, all the deformed scans (i.e. $\mathbf{X}$) are partial. To begin with, $\mathbf{X}$ ($\mathbf{D}_x$) and $\mathbf{Y}$ ($\mathbf{D}_y$) are downsampled to $N_{test} = 2000$ points. With all three liver models, the inputs into non-rigid

CPD [11] include the sampled **X** and **Y**. With all three liver models, the inputs into anisotropic CPD (introduced in Sect. 2.2) are the sampled **X** and **Y**. With all three liver models, the sampled $\mathbf{D}_x$ and $\mathbf{D}_y$ are first fed into both HMM (isotropic) [7] or HMM (anisotropic) (i.e denoted as ours), afterwards **X** and the rigidly aligned **Y** are fed into anisotropic CPD. With Liver 1, we do not show the results using anisotropic CPD since the results with anisotropic CPD are very similar with those using the CPD method. With Liver 2 and Liver 3, we do not show the results with HMM(isotropic) method, since the results with HMM(isotropic) are very similar with those using HMM (anisotropic). The qualitative results are shown in Fig. 1, where the data and model PSs **X** and **Y** are represented with green and red dots respectively. Comparing the last three sub-figures in the first row in Fig. 1, we find that (a) HMM (anisotropic) performs similarly as HMM (isotropic) [7] does, which can be explained by the fact that there exists no noise in **X**; (b) with CPD all the points in **Y** (red) are warped to all the points in **X** (green) in the end, which reflects the CPD's vulnerability to partial scan. In the second row, CPD alone or anisotropic CPD alone finds the wrong correspondences. In contrast, with our framework, the points in **X** (green) are computed to correspond to the correct corresponding partial region in **Y** (red). By carefully observing the figures (especially the edges) in the third row, we can find that ours can best register the two PSs. To briefly conclude, our proposed framework can find the correct correspondences with all three partial liver models and do the registration successfully.

Anisotropic CPD's Robustness to Positional Noise. As we have found in the last section, either only non-rigid CPD or only anisotropic non-rigid CPD without the assistance of normal vectors will fail to find correct correspondences with partial intra-operative data. Thus, to have an effective comparison, CPD only and anisotropic CPD only are compared on the liver data with full intra-operative (or deformed) scan. Different levels of noise vectors are injected into **X**, and afterwards **X** and **Y** are normalized to zero mean and unit variance to make the comparisons fair. The noise vectors are sampled from a specific covariance matrix $\mathbf{\Sigma}_{\text{test}} = a \times \text{diag}[0.01, 0.01, 9 \times 0.01]$. Notice that in $\mathbf{\Sigma}_{\text{test}}$ the standard deviation in the z direction is set to be three times of those in x and y directions to mimic the real surgical scenarios (e.g. stereo reconstruction in the laparoscopic liver surgery). The values of $a \in \mathbb{R}$ are set to increase from one to five to test the methods' robustness to noise levels. The mean surface distance (MSD) of registration is defined as the distance between computed $\mathbf{T}(\mathbf{Y})$ using CPD or anisotropic CPD and the ground-truth corresponding points' positions in the ground-truth deformed **Y**[14]. The above process is repeated for $N_{\text{repeat}} = 1000$ times, and the mean and std of MSD values can be computed. Figure 2 summarizes the corresponding results. As it is shown in Fig. 2, anisotropic CPD achieves smaller MSD values in all test cases than CPD does. In addition, our method is much more robust to the noise levels than the CPD method is with all three liver data sets. All results have passed the statistical tests (paired t-tests with the significance level $\alpha = 0.05$).

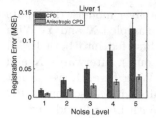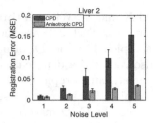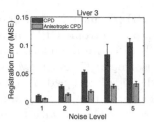

Fig. 2. From left to right, the mean and standard deviation of the registration error values (MSE) are plotted for Liver 1, Liver 2, and Liver 3.

4   Conclusions

We first show that HMM (anisotropic) can recover the rigid transformation matrix than both HMM (isotropic) and CPD more accurately (or at least comparable). This is attributed to the use of more descriptive features (i.e. normal vectors) and the anisotropic positional noise assumption. Another advantage of the proposed method is its great robustness to partial overlapping of pre-operative and intra-operative scans, which is the case in laparoscopic surgery. Finally, we demonstrate that the anisotropic CPD is much more robust to positional noise than CPD due to the generalized anisotropic noise assumption. A limitation of this paper is that we only test our methods on the liver models. In the future, we will apply our algorithm to cardiac surgery and neurosurgery that involve deformation. Another future work is to utilize the joint registration method of multiple point sets [8] in the rigid step of our non-rigid registration framework.

Acknowledgement. This project is partially supported by the Hong Kong RGC GRF grants 14210117, RGC NSFC RGC Joint Research Scheme N_CUHK448/17 and the shenzhen Science and Technology Innovation projects JCYJ20170413161616163 awarded to Max Q.-H. Meng.

References

1. Bayer, S., et al.: Intraoperative brain shift compensation using a hybrid mixture model. In: Frangi, A.F., Schnabel, J.A., Davatzikos, C., Alberola-López, C., Fichtinger, G. (eds.) MICCAI 2018. LNCS, vol. 11073, pp. 116–124. Springer, Cham (2018). https://doi.org/10.1007/978-3-030-00937-3_14
2. Cignoni, P., Callieri, M., Corsini, M., Dellepiane, M., Ganovelli, F., Ranzuglia, G.: MeshLAB: an open-source mesh processing tool. In: Eurographics Italian Chapter Conference, pp. 129–136 (2008)
3. Collins, J.A., et al.: Improving registration robustness for image-guided liver surgery in a novel human-to-phantom data framework. IEEE TMI **36**(7), 1502–1510 (2017)
4. Luo, J., et al.: Using the variogram for vector outlier screening: application to feature-based image registration. IJCARS **13**(12), 1871–1880 (2018)

5. Min, Z., Ren, H., Meng, M.Q.H.: Statistical model of total target registration error in image-guided surgery. IEEE TASE (2019). https://doi.org/10.1109/TASE.2019.2909646
6. Min, Z., Wang, J., Meng, M.Q.-H.: Joint registration of multiple generalized point sets. In: Reuter, M., Wachinger, C., Lombaert, H., Paniagua, B., Lüthi, M., Egger, B. (eds.) ShapeMI 2018. LNCS, vol. 11167, pp. 169–177. Springer, Cham (2018). https://doi.org/10.1007/978-3-030-04747-4_16
7. Min, Z., Wang, J., Meng, M.Q.H.: Robust generalized point cloud registration using hybrid mixture model. In: ICRA 2018, pp. 4812–4818. IEEE (2018)
8. Min, Z., Wang, J., Meng, M.Q.H.: Joint rigid registration of multiple generalized point sets with hybrid mixture models. IEEE TASE (2019). https://doi.org/10.1109/TASE.2019.2906391
9. Min, Z., Wang, J., Meng, M.Q.H.: Robust generalized point cloud registration with orientational data based on expectation maximization. IEEE TASE (2019). https://doi.org/10.1109/TASE.2019.2914306
10. Min, Z., Wang, J., Song, S., Meng, M.Q.H.: Robust generalized point cloud registration with expectation maximization considering anisotropic positional uncertainties. In: IROS 2018, pp. 1290–1297. IEEE (2018)
11. Myronenko, A., Song, X.: Point set registration: coherent point drift. IEEE Trans. Pattern Anal. Mach. Intell. **32**(12), 2262–2275 (2010)
12. Ravikumar, N., Gooya, A., Beltrachini, L., Frangi, A.F., Taylor, Z.A.: Generalised coherent point drift for group-wise multi-dimensional analysis of diffusion brain MRI data. Med. Image Anal. **53**, 47–63 (2019)
13. Ravikumar, N., Gooya, A., Frangi, A.F., Taylor, Z.A.: Generalised coherent point drift for group-wise registration of multi-dimensional point sets. In: Descoteaux, M., Maier-Hein, L., Franz, A., Jannin, P., Collins, D.L., Duchesne, S. (eds.) MICCAI 2017. LNCS, vol. 10433, pp. 309–316. Springer, Cham (2017). https://doi.org/10.1007/978-3-319-66182-7_36
14. Robu, M.R., et al.: Global rigid registration of ct to video in laparoscopic liver surgery. Int. J. Comput. Assist. Radiol. Surg. **13**(6), 947–956 (2018)
15. Sinha, A., Liu, X., Reiter, A., Ishii, M., Hager, G.D., Taylor, R.H.: Endoscopic navigation in the absence of CT imaging. In: Frangi, A.F., Schnabel, J.A., Davatzikos, C., Alberola-López, C., Fichtinger, G. (eds.) MICCAI 2018. LNCS, vol. 11073, pp. 64–71. Springer, Cham (2018). https://doi.org/10.1007/978-3-030-00937-3_8
16. Suwelack, S., et al.: Physics-based shape matching for intraoperative image guidance. Med. Phys. **41**(11), 111901 (2014)

A Mixed-Supervision Multilevel GAN Framework for Image Quality Enhancement

Uddeshya Upadhyay and Suyash P. Awate[✉]

Computer Science and Engineering, Indian Institute of Tehnology, Bombay, India
suyash@cse.iitb.ac.in

Abstract. Deep neural networks for image quality enhancement typically need large quantities of highly-curated training data comprising pairs of low-quality images and their corresponding high-quality images. While high-quality image acquisition is typically expensive and time-consuming, medium-quality images are faster to acquire, at lower equipment costs, and available in larger quantities. Thus, we propose a *novel generative adversarial network* (GAN) that can leverage *training data at multiple levels of quality* (e.g., high and medium quality) to improve performance while *limiting costs of data curation*. We apply our *mixed-supervision* GAN to (i) super-resolve histopathology images and (ii) enhance laparoscopy images by combining super-resolution and surgical smoke removal. Results on large clinical and pre-clinical datasets show the benefits of our mixed-supervision GAN over the state of the art.

Keywords: Image quality enhancement · Generative adversarial network (GAN) · Mixed-supervision · Super-resolution · Surgical smoke removal

1 Introduction and Related Work

Image quality enhancement using deep neural networks (DNNs) typically needs large quantities of highly-curated training data comprising corresponding pairs of low-quality and high-quality images. In this paper, "low-quality" images refer to images that have low spatial resolution and exhibit other degradations; "high-quality" images refer to high-resolution uncorrupted images. While high-quality image acquisition is typically expensive and time-consuming, medium-quality images are faster to acquire, at lower equipment costs, and available in larger quantities. Thus, we propose a novel generative adversarial network (GAN) that can leverage *training data at multiple levels of quality* (e.g., high and medium quality) to improve performance while *limiting costs of data curation*.

We thank support from Aira Matrix and the Infrastructure Facility for Advanced Research and Education in Diagnostics grant funded by Department of Biotechnology, Government of India (RD/0117-DBT0000-002).

© Springer Nature Switzerland AG 2019
D. Shen et al. (Eds.): MICCAI 2019, LNCS 11768, pp. 556–564, 2019.
https://doi.org/10.1007/978-3-030-32254-0_62

In pre-clinical and clinical digital histopathology, acquisition times increase quadratically with decreasing pixel width [3,8]. Furthermore, higher-resolution digital scanners are more expensive. Super-resolution algorithms can enable faster scanning at lower resolutions by filling-in the fine detail in a post-processing step. *Mixed-supervision* can reduce the need for data at the highest resolution and/or improve performance using medium-resolution training data; our earlier works [15,16] propose mixed-supervision for image segmentation. A class of methods for super-resolution rely on neighbor embeddings [5], sparse representation [13,22], and random forests [14]. DNNs have been successful at super-resolution with their ability to optimize features and the regression mapping jointly [4,7,10]. The class of DNNs giving among the best performances for super-resolution involve GANs [11]. Our earlier work [18] on image super-resolution proposed loss functions for robust learning in the presence of corrupted training data. Some methods [19] use a sequence of GANs for image enhancement (without super-resolution), but, unlike our approach, train each GAN independently, without defining a unified loss function. However, none of these methods leverage training data of multiple qualities for (learning) super-resolution.

In *laparoscopy*, higher-resolution imaging can offer the surgeon wider views and fine details, both, in the same frame, without needing to move the endoscope back (to get a larger field of view) and forth (to get the fine details) [21]. While some state-of-the-art laparoscopic imaging offers 8K ultra-high-definition (UHD) images, typical and affordable equipment offers lower resolution (less than 2K) images. Laparoscopic images also suffer from degradation because of surgical smoke. Super-resolution algorithms can enable low-cost equipment to produce high-resolution images. Smoke-removal algorithms, as well as super-resolution algorithms, can enhance the performance of subsequent processing involving tracking, segmentation, depth analysis, stereo vision, and augmented reality, in addition to improving the surgeon's visibility. Mixed-supervision learning can reduce the need for UHD training sets. Most methods for image desmoking [2,12,17] model the degradation analytically and propose algorithms to undo the degradation. On the other hand, a very recent approach [6] relies on learning using a DNN. In contrast, we propose a novel mixed-supervision GAN framework to leverage training data of varying image qualities to improve performance in *super-resolution coupled with image restoration*.

We propose a novel mixed-supervision GAN framework for image quality enhancement that can leverage *training data at multiple levels of quality*, e.g., high and medium quality, to improve performance while limiting costs of data curation. To the best of our knowledge, our framework is the first to propose image quality enhancement using data at multiple quality levels simultaneously. We apply our framework for (i) *super-resolution in histopathology* images and (ii) image quality enhancement in *laparoscopy images* by combining *super-resolution and surgical smoke removal*. Results on large clinical and pre-clinical datasets show the benefits of our mixed-supervision GAN over the state of the art.

2 Methods

We describe our framework's architecture, loss functions, and the training scheme.

Our Mixed-Supervision Multilevel GAN Architecture. While our framework is *not* specific to a DNN architecture, we choose to use the generator and the discriminator designs used in SRGAN [11] (Fig. 1(a)). However, our architecture (Fig. 1(b)) incorporates a sequence of generators and discriminators, with each level dealing with increasingly higher quality training data, compared to the low-quality input data. We refer to a SRGAN-like framework, equivalent to one level in our sequence, as *quality-enhancement GAN (QEGAN)*. We call our framework as *multilevel QEGAN (MLQEGAN)* (Fig. 1).

For *QEGAN*, let the generator $\mathcal{G}(\cdot; \theta)$, parametrized by set θ, take low-resolution and degraded (i.e., low-quality) input X^{LQ} and produce super-resolved and restored (i.e., high-quality) output $X^{\mathrm{HQ}} := \mathcal{G}(X^{\mathrm{LQ}}; \theta)$ to match the observed high-quality true image X^{T}. Following the GAN learning principle, let the discriminator $\mathcal{D}(\cdot; \phi)$, parametrized by set ϕ, learn to discriminate between the probability density function (PDF) of super-resolved and restored generator outputs $P(X^{\mathrm{HQ}})$ and the PDF of observed high-quality true images $P(X^{\mathrm{T}})$.

For our *MLQEGAN*, let there be L levels starting from level 1 to level L. Let level l have generator $\mathcal{G}_l(\cdot; \theta_l)$ and discriminator $\mathcal{D}_l(\cdot; \phi_l)$. Let the training data be in the form of random-vector image pairs $(Y^{\mathrm{LQ}}, Y_j^{\mathrm{T}})$, where (i) Y^{LQ} is the lowest-quality image and (ii) Y_j^{T} is the higher-quality image at quality level j with $j \in [2, L+1]$. In this paper, the levels in our MLQEGAN framework correspond to different resolutions/pixel sizes. Typical applications lead to training data in large quantities at medium quality as compared to data at higher quality. Thus, our architecture has progressively fewer parameters to optimize at higher levels, consistent with low sample sizes for higher quality training data.

Training Set. For training MLQEGAN, a higher-quality training image Y_j^{T} at level j can inform the training of generators and discriminators at all levels $i < j$. Thus, from every pair of the form $(Y^{\mathrm{LQ}}, Y_j^{\mathrm{T}})$, we create *multiple* training instances $(X^{\mathrm{LQ}}, X_m^{\mathrm{T}})$ for all levels $m \leq j$, where (i) $X^{\mathrm{LQ}} := Y^{\mathrm{LQ}}$ and (ii) X_m^{T} is the lower-resolution (corresponding to the pixel size at level m) version of Y_j^{T}; for $j = m$ we have $X_m^{\mathrm{T}} = Y_m^{\mathrm{T}}$. Thus, for training MLQEGAN, we use an *effective training set* of the form $\{(X^{\mathrm{LQ}}, X_m^{\mathrm{T}})\}$ for all $m \in [2, L+1]$. Let the set of parameters to be optimized be $\theta := \{\theta_l\}_{l=1}^L$ and $\phi := \{\phi_l\}_{l=1}^L$. Let the union of the generator parameters at levels from 1 to l be $\theta_1^l := \{\theta_k\}_{k=1}^l$.

Loss Functions. We design a loss function $\mathcal{L}(\theta, \phi)$ as the sum of loss functions corresponding to each level $l \in [1, L]$. The loss function at level l comprises a fidelity loss $\mathcal{L}_l^F(\theta_1^l)$ and an adversarial loss $\mathcal{L}_l^A(\theta_l, \phi_l)$. The generator $\mathcal{G}_1(\cdot; \theta_1)$ at level 1 takes the lowest-quality input image X^{LQ} and maps it to $X_2^{\mathrm{HQ}} := \mathcal{G}_1(X^{\mathrm{LQ}}; \theta_1)$. Let $\mathcal{G}_1^j := \mathcal{G}_j \circ \mathcal{G}_{j-1} \circ \cdots \circ \mathcal{G}_1$ be the composition of the sequence of generators from level 1 to level $j \in [2, L]$. The generator $\mathcal{G}_l(\cdot; \theta_l)$ at level l takes the lower-quality input image $\mathcal{G}_1^{l-1}(X^{\mathrm{LQ}}; \theta_1^{l-1})$ and maps it to $X_{l+1}^{\mathrm{HQ}} :=$

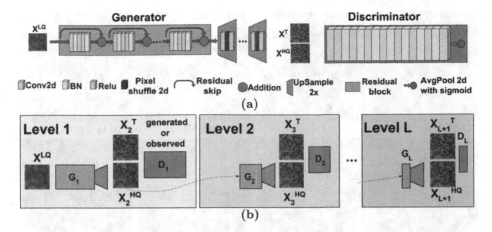

Fig. 1. Our Mixed-Supervision Multilevel GAN Framework for Quality Enhancement: MLQEGAN. (a) Architecture for generator and discriminator, used at each level, in **(b)** our multilevel architecture with mixed supervision.

$\mathcal{G}_l(\mathcal{G}_1^{l-1}(X^{\text{LQ}}; \theta_1^{l-1}); \theta_l) = \mathcal{G}_1^l(X^{\text{LQ}}); \theta_1^l)$. We propose a *fidelity loss* between the generator output X_{l+1}^{HQ} and the higher-quality image X_{l+1}^{T} as

$$\mathcal{L}_l^F(\theta_1^l) := E_{P(X^{\text{LQ}}, X_{l+1}^{\text{T}})}[F(\mathcal{G}_1^l(X^{\text{LQ}}; \theta_1^l), X_{l+1}^{\text{T}})],$$

where $F(A, B)$ measures the dissimilarity between images A and B; in this paper, $F(A, B)$ is the mean squared error (MSE). The adversarial loss is the Kullback-Leibler divergence between (i) the one-hot probability vectors (distributions) for the generated ("fake") image X_{l+1}^{HQ} and true ("real") image X_{l+1}^{T}, i.e., $[0, 1]$ or $[1, 0]$, and (ii) the probability vectors (distributions) for the generator-output image X_{l+1}^{HQ} and the higher-quality image X_{l+1}^{T}, i.e., $[\mathcal{D}_l(X_{l+1}^{\text{HQ}}; \phi_l), 1 - \mathcal{D}_l(X_{l+1}^{\text{HQ}}; \phi_l)]$ or $[\mathcal{D}_l(X_{l+1}^{\text{T}}; \phi_l), 1 - \mathcal{D}_l(X_{l+1}^{\text{T}}; \phi_l)]$, respectively. We propose the *adversarial loss*

$$\mathcal{L}_l^A(\theta_1^l, \phi_l) := E_{P(X^{\text{LQ}}, X_{l+1}^{\text{T}})}[\log(1 - \mathcal{D}_l(\mathcal{G}_1^l(X^{\text{LQ}}; \theta_1^l); \phi_l)) + \log(\mathcal{D}_l(X_{l+1}^{\text{T}}; \phi_l))].$$

We propose the overall loss $L(\theta, \phi) := \sum_{l=1}^{L} \lambda_l(\mathcal{L}_l^F(\theta_l^l) + \alpha_l \mathcal{L}_l^A(\theta_1^l, \phi_l))$, where we fix $\lambda_1 := 1$ and tune the free parameters $\{\lambda_l\}_{l=2}^L \cup \{\alpha_l\}_{l=1}^L$ using cross validation.

Training Scheme. We initialize the parameters $\theta \cup \phi$ sequentially, as follows. We first initialize $\theta_1 \cup \phi_1$ using the training subset with image pairs of the form $(X^{\text{LQ}}, X_2^{\text{T}})$ to minimize the loss function $\mathcal{L}_1^F(\theta_1) + \alpha_1 \mathcal{L}_1^A(\theta_1, \phi_1)$. Then, for increasing levels l from 2 to L, we initialize $\theta_l \cup \phi_l$ using the training subset $(X^{\text{LQ}}, X_l^{\text{T}})$ to minimize the loss function $\mathcal{L}_l^F(\theta_l^l) + \alpha_l \mathcal{L}_l^A(\theta_1^l, \phi_l)$, but fixing all previous-level generator parameters θ_1^{l-1}. After initialization, we train all GANs in a joint optimization framework using Adam [9], with internal parameters $\beta_1 := 0.9, \beta_2 := 0.999$, initial learning rate 0.002 that decays based on cosine annealing, batch size 8, and number of epochs 500.

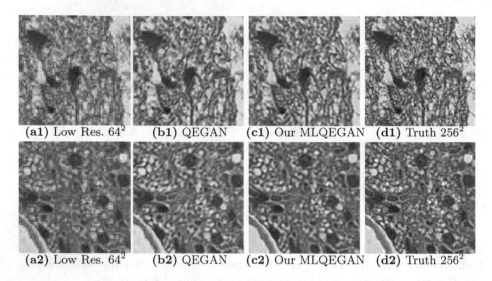

(a1) Low Res. 64^2 **(b1)** QEGAN   **(c1)** Our MLQEGAN   **(d1)** Truth 256^2

(a2) Low Res. 64^2 **(b2)** QEGAN   **(c2)** Our MLQEGAN   **(d2)** Truth 256^2

Fig. 2. Results on Histopathology Images. (a1)–(a2) Low-resolution 64^2 (from $10\times$ magnification). (RRMSE, msSSIM, QILV) for: **(b1)–(b2)** QEGAN $4\times$ super-resolution (256^2): (0.131, 0.868, 0.830), (0.117, 0.837, 0.919). **(c1)–(c2) Our MLQE-GAN** $4\times$ super-resolution (256^2): (0.117, 0.910, 0.90), (0.091, 0.922, 0.942). **(d1)–(d2)** Truth 256^2 (from $40\times$ magnification).

3   Results and Discussion

We evaluate our mixed-supervision MLQEGAN to (i) super-resolve histopathology images and (ii) enhance laparoscopy images by combining super-resolution and surgical smoke removal. We compare against a SRGAN-like architecture that is the among the state of the art for super-resolution, which we leverage additionally for quality enhancement, i.e., QEGAN. To quantitate performance, we use three complementary measures: (i) relative root MSE (RRMSE) between the DNN output, say, A^{HQ} and the corresponding true image, say, A^{T}, as $\|A^{\mathrm{HQ}} - A^{\mathrm{T}}\|_2 / \|A^{\mathrm{T}}\|_2$, (ii) multiscale structural similarity index (msSSIM) [20], and (iii) quality index based on local variance (QILV) [1]. While msSSIM is more sensitive to image noise than blur, QILV is more sensitive to image blur instead. In this paper, the cross-validation tuned free-parameter values are: $\forall l, \alpha_l = 3\mathrm{e}{-}5$; when $L = 2$, $\lambda_1 = 1\mathrm{e}{-}4$, $\lambda_2 = 1$; when $L = 3$, $\lambda_1 = 1\mathrm{e}{-}4$, $\lambda_2 = 1\mathrm{e}{-}4$, $\lambda_3 = 1$.

Results on Histopathology Images. We take 8 whole-slide histopathology images from pre-clinical Wistar rat biopsies at $40\times$ magnification from a Hamamatsu scanner, which includes images at multiple magnification levels, including $10\times$ and $20\times$. The task is to map the low-quality input data X^{LQ} at $10\times$ to the high-quality data X^{T} at $40\times$. MLQEGAN uses $L = 2$ levels.

The *training set* comprises image-pair instances of $(Y^{\mathrm{LQ}}, Y_2^{\mathrm{T}})$ and $(Y^{\mathrm{LQ}}, Y_3^{\mathrm{T}})$. We create instances of $(Y^{\mathrm{LQ}}, Y_2^{\mathrm{T}})$ by (i) randomly selecting 5000 non-overlapping patches at $20\times$ (128^2 pixels) to give Y_2^{T}; (ii) selecting the corresponding patches

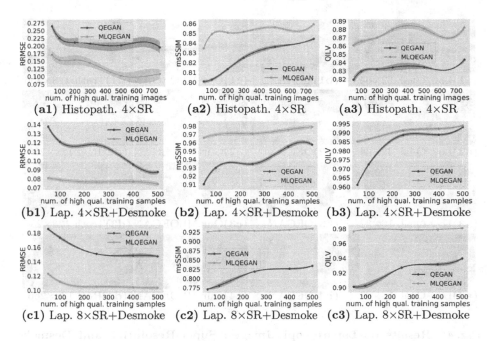

Fig. 3. Results on Histopathology and Laparoscopy Images: Quantitative Analysis. RRMSE, msSSIM, QILV for images in: **(a1)–(a3)** histopathology: 4× super-resolution; **(b1)–(b3)** laparoscopy: 4× super-resolution + desmoking; **(c1)–(c3)** laparoscopy: 8× super-resolution + desmoking. The error bars indicate the variability from randomness in data sampling and Adam [9].

at 10× (64^2 pixels) to give Y^{LQ}. We create instances of (Y^{LQ}, Y_3^T) by (i) randomly selecting non-overlapping patches at 40× (256^2 pixels) to give Y_3^T; (ii) selecting the corresponding patches at 10× (64^2 pixels) to give Y^{LQ}. We vary the number of the highest-quality image-pair instances of (Y^{LQ}, Y_3^T) from 50 to 750.

We create the *validation set* of image-pair instances of (V^{LQ}, V_3^T) by randomly choosing 100 images at 40× to give V_3^T, and their corresponding patches at 10× to give V^{LQ}. We similarly create the *test set* of 1000 instances of (Z^{LQ}, Z_3^T).

While QEGAN can leverage only a small subset of available training data comprising instances of the form (Y^{LQ}, Y_3^T), our MLQEGAN is able to leverage the entire training set including instances of the forms (Y^{LQ}, Y_3^T) and (Y^{LQ}, Y_2^T). Our MLQEGAN outputs (Fig. 2(c1)–(c2)) are much closer to the ground truth (Fig. 2(d1)–(d2)), compared to QEGAN outputs (Fig. 2(b1)–(b2)). Unlike QEGAN, MLQEGAN is able to extract useful information in the medium-quality images Y_2^T available in significantly larger quantities, compared to the highest-quality images Y_3^T. In this way, MLQEGAN clearly outperforms QEGAN in reproducing the true textural appearances (colors and features) and cell shapes. Quantitatively (Fig. 3(a1)–(a3)), while QEGAN's performance

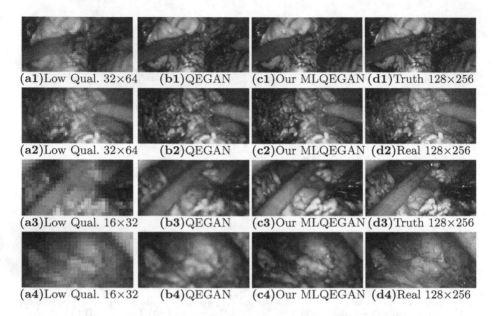

Fig. 4. Results on Laparoscopic Images: Super-Resolution and Desmoking. (RRMSE, msSSIM, QILV) are in parentheses. **(a1)** *Input with* 4× *lower-resolution, simulated smoke*; **(b1)** QEGAN: (0.112, 0.897, 0.963); **(c1) Our MLQE-GAN**: (0.065, 0.971, 0.993); **(d1)** Truth. **(a2)** *Input with* 4× *lower-resolution, real smoke*; **(b2)** QEGAN; **(c2) Our MLQEGAN**; **(d2)** Real smoky high-resolution image. **(a3)** *Input with* 8× *lower-resolution, simulated smoke*; **(b3)** QEGAN: (0.151,0.825,0.926); **(c3) Our MLQEGAN**: (0.098, 0.925, 0.988); **(d3)** Truth. **(a4)** *Input with* 8× *lower-resolution, real smoke*; **(b4)** QEGAN; **(c4) Our MLQE-GAN**; **(d4)** Real smoky high-resolution image.

reduces steadily with the reduction in the number of training-set images at the highest-quality level, our MLQEGAN's performance remains much more stable. Moreover, our MLQEGAN's performance consistently stays significantly better than QEGAN's performance, for all training-set sizes.

Results on Laparoscopic Images. We use the da Vinci dataset [23]. Our task involves smoke removal and 4× super-resolution. MLQEGAN uses $L = 2$.

The *training set* comprises image-pair instances of (Y^{LQ}, Y_2^T) and (Y^{LQ}, Y_3^T). We create instances of (Y^{LQ}, Y_2^T) by (i) randomly selecting 5000 smokeless full-resolution images and 2× downsampling them to give Y_2^T; (ii) degrading the same selected image set with smoke, and then 4× downsampling (we smooth a bit using Gaussian convolution before downsampling to prevent aliasing) to create the low-quality training set Y^{LQ}. We create instances of (Y^{LQ}, Y_3^T) by (i) randomly selecting full-resolution smokeless images to give Y_3^T; (ii) degrading and downsampling the same selected image set to give Y^{LQ}. We vary the number of the highest-quality image pairs (Y^{LQ}, Y_3^T) from 50 to 500.

We create the *validation set* of image-pair instances of (V^{LQ}, V_3^T) by randomly choosing 100 images V_3^T and creating V^{LQ} by degrading and downsampling as before. We similarly create the *test set* of 1000 instances of (Z^{LQ}, Z_3^T).

While QEGAN learning is unable to use medium-quality images, our MLQEGAN uses them to improve performance significantly. With simulated smoke, results from our MLQEGAN (Fig. 4(c1)) appear sharper than those from QEGAN (Fig. 4(b1)). We also evaluate the trained models for QEGAN and MLQEGAN on real-world smoke by selecting *smoky frames* (Fig. 4(d2)) and downsampling them by 4× to create the low-quality input (Fig. 4(a2)). The results from MLQEGAN (Fig. 4(c2)) show sharper and more realistic textures. Analogous to the aforementioned experiments, we tested all methods in a very challenging scenario with *8× downsampling*, where MLQEGAN uses $L = 3$ levels. Here as well, MLQEGAN performs better than QEGAN (Fig. 4(a3)–(d4)).

Quantitatively, with simulated smoke, for 4× and 8× downsampling (Fig. 3(b1)–(c3)) shows that MLQEGAN outperforms QEGAN in all measures.

Time Requirements. Our MLQEGAN has fewer layers and fewer parameters (by roughly 20%) than SRGAN (or QEGAN). Training time can depend on many factors, e.g., network architecture, training set sizes, and epochs needed to converge. Our MLQEGAN uses more training images at lower quality, but with smaller sizes. In general, our training time is a bit larger than that of QEGAN. For test data, our MLQEGAN produces the output a bit faster than SRGAN (or QEGAN) because we have fewer parameters and layers.

Conclusion. We proposed a novel *mixed-supervision* GAN that leverages training data at multiple levels of quality to improve performance while limiting costs of data curation. We propose a novel *multilevel* architecture with a sequence of GANs with (i) progressively decreasing complexity and (ii) loss functions using coupled generator sequences. We apply our mixed-supervision GAN to (i) *super-resolve histopathology* images and (ii) enhance *laparoscopy* images by combining *super-resolution and surgical smoke removal*. Results on large datasets show the benefits of our mixed-supervision GAN over the state of the art.

References

1. Aja-Fernandez, S., Estepar, R.J., Alberola-Lopez, C., Westin, C.: Image quality assessment based on local variance. In: IEEE EMBS Annual International Conference, p. 4815 (2006)
2. Baid, A., Kotwal, A., Bhalodia, R., Merchant, S., Awate, S.: Joint desmoking, specularity removal, and denoising of laparoscopy images via graphical models and Bayesian inference. In: IEEE International Symposium on Biomedical Imaging, pp. 732–736 (2017)
3. Bertram, C., Klopfleisch, R.: The pathologist 2.0: an update on digital pathology in veterinary medicine. Vet. Pathol. **54**(5), 756–766 (2017)
4. Bruna, J., Sprechmann, P., LeCun, Y.: Super-resolution with deep convolutional sufficient statistics. In: International Conference on Learning Representations, pp. 1–17 (2016)

5. Chang, H., Yeung, D.Y., Xiong, Y.: Super-resolution through neighbor embedding. In: IEEE Conference on Computer Vision and Pattern Recognition, pp. 275–282 (2004)
6. Chen, L., Tang, W., John, N.: Unsupervised adversarial training of surgical smoke removal. In: Medical Imaging with Deep Learning, pp. 1–3 (2018)
7. Dong, C., Loy, C.C., He, K., Tang, X.: Learning a deep convolutional network for image super-resolution. In: Fleet, D., Pajdla, T., Schiele, B., Tuytelaars, T. (eds.) ECCV 2014. LNCS, vol. 8692, pp. 184–199. Springer, Cham (2014). https://doi.org/10.1007/978-3-319-10593-2_13
8. Huisman, A., Looijen, A., van den Brink, S., van Diest, P.: Creation of a fully digital pathology slide archive by high-volume tissue slide scanning. Hum. Pathol. **41**(5), 751–757 (2010)
9. Kingma, D.P., Ba, J.: Adam: a method for stochastic optimization. In: International Conference on Learning Representations (2015)
10. Lai, W.S., Huang, J.B., Ahuja, N., Yang, M.H.: Deep Laplacian pyramid networks for fast and accurate superresolution. In: IEEE Conference on Computer Vision Pattern Recognition, pp. 5835–5843 (2017)
11. Ledig, C., et al.: Photo-realistic single image super-resolution using a generative adversarial network. In: IEEE Conference on Computer Vision and Pattern Recognition, pp. 105–114 (2017)
12. Luo, X., McLeod, A., Pautler, S., Schlachta, C., Peters, T.: Vision-based surgical field defogging. IEEE Trans. Med. Imag. **36**(10), 2021–2030 (2017)
13. Mousavi, H., Monga, V.: Sparsity-based color image super resolution via exploiting cross channel constraints. IEEE Trans. Image Process. **26**(11), 5094–5106 (2017)
14. Schulter, S., Leistner, C., Bischof, H.: Fast and accurate image upscaling with super-resolution forests. In: IEEE Conference on Computer Vision and Pattern Recognition (2015)
15. Shah, M., Bhalgat, Y., Awate, S.P.: Annotation-cost minimization for medical image segmentation using suggestive mixed supervision fully convolutional networks. In: Medical Image Meets Neural Information Processing System, pp. 1–4 (2019)
16. Shah, M., Merchant, S.N., Awate, S.P.: MS-Net: mixed-supervision fully-convolutional networks for full-resolution segmentation. In: Medical Image Computing and Computer-Assisted Intervention, pp. 379–387 (2018)
17. Tchaka, K., Pawar, V., Stoyanov, D.: Chromaticity based smoke removal in endoscopic images. In: Proceedings of SPIE, p. 101331M (2018)
18. Upadhyay, U., Awate, S.P.: Robust super-resolution GAN, with manifold-based and perception loss. In: IEEE International Symposium on Biomedical Imaging (ISBI) (2019)
19. Wang, Y., et al.: 3D conditional generative adversarial networks for high-quality PET image estimation at low dose. NeuroImage **1**(274), 550–562 (2018)
20. Wang, Z., Bovik, A., Sheikh, H., Simoncelli, E.: Image quality assessment: from error visibility to structural similarity. IEEE Trans. Image Process. **13**(4), 600–612 (2004)
21. Yamashita, H., Aoki, H., Tanioka, K., Mori, T., Chiba, T.: Ultra-high definition (8K UHD) endoscope: our first clinical success. SpringerPlus **5**(1), 1445 (2016)
22. Yang, J., Wright, J., Huang, T., Ma, Y.: Image super-resolution via sparse representation. IEEE Trans. Image Process. **19**(11), 2861–2873 (2010)
23. Ye, M., Johns, E., Handa, A., Zhang, L., Pratt, P., Yang, G.Z.: Self-supervised siamese learning on stereo image pairs for depth estimation in robotic surgery. In: Hamlyn Symposium on Medical Robotics (2017)

Combined Learning for Similar Tasks with Domain-Switching Networks

Daniel Bug[1]([✉]), Dennis Eschweiler[1], Qianyu Liu[1], Justus Schock[1],
Leon Weninger[1], Friedrich Feuerhake[2], Julia Schüler[3], Johannes Stegmaier[1],
and Dorit Merhof[1]

[1] Institute of Imaging and Computer Vision, RWTH Aachen University,
Aachen, Germany
`daniel.bug@lfb.rwth-aachen.de`
[2] Institute for Pathology, Hannover Medical School, Hannover, Germany
[3] Charles River Discovery, Research Services Germany GmbH, Freiburg, Germany

Abstract. We introduce a domain switch for deep neural networks that enables to re-weight convolutional kernels for an input of a known domain. This technique is designed to address re-occurring tasks across multiple domains that are known at runtime and to incorporate them into a single, domain-spanning network. We evaluate this approach in three distinct tasks, namely combined cell nuclei analysis across different stains and fluorescence images, facial landmark detection in grayscale and thermal infrared images, and the BraTS challenge where we treat different recording institutions as domains. We found that conventional U-nets trained on multiple domains perform similar to domain-specific U-nets. Our method improves the results in facial landmark detection significantly, but no change is measured in the other two experiments compared to multi-domain U-nets.

Keywords: Deep learning · Multi-modality · Multi-domain

1 Introduction

Without doubt, digital image analysis through machine learning based algorithms has influenced many biomedical fields. Public challenges [1,6–8,14] have been set up to provide a broader performance comparison on the dataset level. Therefore, specific solutions and evaluations targeting a single dataset or modality are very common. However, for several problems, e.g. cell nuclei analysis, facial landmark detection and brain tumor segmentation, it is possible to identify a common task across different imaging modalities. For example, in cell nuclei analysis, we are interested in counting, localizing or segmenting cell nuclei independently from the used stains or recording modalities. Typical cases are Hematoxylin and Eosin (HE) stained whole-slide images (WSI), immunohistochemically (IHC) stained WSIs or fluorescence microscopy (FLM) images. However, despite the variation in appearance, the overall task remains an analysis

© Springer Nature Switzerland AG 2019
D. Shen et al. (Eds.): MICCAI 2019, LNCS 11768, pp. 565–572, 2019.
https://doi.org/10.1007/978-3-030-32254-0_63

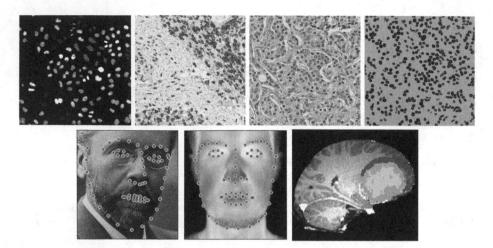

Fig. 1. Examples from the different experiments. Upper row: cell nuclei detection with FLM, IHC, HE domain and ground-truth example corresponding to the HE image. Lower row: facial landmark examples in grayscale and thermal infrared domain and brain tumor segmentation example (T1Ce image with segmentation overlay). (Color figure online)

comprising detection, localization and optionally instance segmentation. Oversimplified, the problem across all modalities is a blob-detection in various colors: violet on pink (HE), blue or brown on white (IHC) or white on black (FLM). Examples are shown in Fig. 1 (upper row). Therefore, we hypothesize that a neural network has to learn similar convolutional kernels in any of these tasks.

Our second example is facial landmark recognition in grayscale and thermal infrared images, see Fig. 1 (bottom left and middle). Thermal infrared images have been explored as an option for emotion detection, particularly stress, under medical conditions [4]. In the scope of this work, it is necessary to point out that while the appearance of faces in the infrared domain is different from conventional grayscale images, the shapes of faces and landmarks do not change with respect to edge and contour locations. Our hypothesis of related convolutional kernel features therefore also holds for the grayscale and infrared domain.

Our third and final example is the BraTS challenge [1,8], in which we predict tumor areas in MRI scans of the human brain, see Fig. 1 (bottom right). As the data was collected from multiple institutions, the task requires an implicit harmonization between the MRI scanners. Thus, we consider the recording institute as a domain in the context of this work.

All these examples have in common that the subproblems they solve are closely related and the domain that is analyzed is typically known at runtime. We hypothesize that learning from multiple domains at once improves the performance and has the potential to adapt more general features than a specialized algorithm. We propose to make the domain directly known to the neural network in the form of a switching mechanism. While past approaches use different network paths for each input domain, or implement a domain-adaptation prior to the task [3], we instead re-weight the convolutional kernels for each domain, which is highly parameter efficient.

Contribution: We implement a domain switch that adapts the network convolutions to a known target domain and enables a training with multiple datasets at once. A corresponding loss function is defined that handles varying or missing annotations between different datasets. The approach is evaluated in three different applications: cell nuclei analysis, facial landmark detection and MRI tumor segmentation in the human brain.

2   Domain Switch Implementation

The key idea is to apply a learnable weight to each convolutional kernel based on the input domain. This enables the network to re-weight features in order to distinguish common features that are required in all domains from domain-specific features.

For a task with D domains, we extend a convolutional layer with C channels with an additional weight matrix $\mathbf{M}$ of dimension $C \times D$. The layer obtains an additional input that expects a one-hot encoded vector for the domain d. Selecting the weights h for a specific domain is then achieved by a simple matrix multiplication $h = \mathbf{M} \cdot d$.

These domain-specific weights are finally multiplied to the convolutional kernels $\mathbf{W}$ and bias weights b.

$$\hat{\mathbf{W}} = \mathbf{W}_c \circ h_c$$

$$\hat{b} = \mathbf{b}_c \circ h_c$$

Herein, the domain-weight of channel c is broadcast to all other dimensions of the convolutional weights $\mathbf{W}$. Thus, we perform an element-wise multiplication similar to the Hadamard-product for matrices. The actual convolution is carried out with the re-weighted parameters $\hat{\mathbf{W}}$ and $\hat{b}$. Note that in batch-processing, an iteration over the batch will be required, since a batch usually comprises multiple domains at random. Furthermore, this implementation is independent of the dimensionality of the convolution and will apply to 1D time series, 2D images or higher dimensional ND problems. Figure 2a visualizes the proposed layer as a flowchart.

So far we have defined the domain switch, but not its role in a neural network architecture. Depending on the perspective we take on the multi-modal problem, two main architectures can be derived. If the variation between domains is abstract and unknown, the network can be given the maximum capacity of switches, i.e. replacing all convolutions by switches. However, this can lead to a very slow training given the necessary iteration over the batch. As many architectures employ subsequent convolutions in a block structure, a switch can be installed in every block, as a compromise. This is shown in Fig. 2c. Alternatively, for domains that can be expected to have very closely related features,

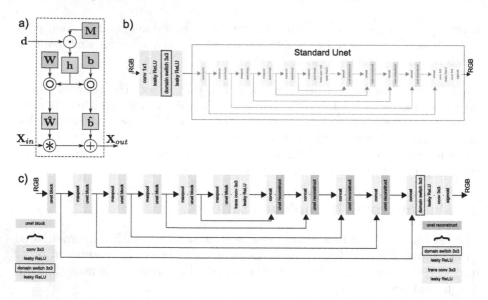

Fig. 2. Implementation of the domain switch (a) and usage together with the U-net architecture as preprocessing element (b) or in each functional block (c) (best viewed digital).

the domain switch could be incorporated in only the first layers of the network to learn a domain-specific preprocessing, seen in Fig. 2b.

Due to the multiplication in the domain switch, we have to avoid values close to zero for initializing the domain-weights $\mathbf{M}$, as they would diminish the gradients right from the beginning of the training. Hence, an initialization with a low-variance Gaussian distribution centered around one is more appropriate. For training, there are two strategies: (1) train all parameters together, or (2) *pretrain* by keeping $\mathbf{M}$ constant and *finetune* in a follow-up phase.

To combine datasets that do not feature the same set of labels, we propose a novel loss function that accumulates the provided annotations:

$$L_{\mathrm{acc}} = \frac{\sum_b \sum_c \mathrm{I}(b,c) \cdot w_c f(P,T)}{\sum_b \sum_c \mathrm{I}(b,c)} + \lambda \bar{\mu}_P,$$

where $b \in \{0, \dots B-1\}$ and $c \in \{0, \dots C-1\}$ iterate over the batch of size B and the classes C, respectively, $\mathrm{I}(b,c)$ is the indicator-function that keeps track if a class label is provided for the sample and $f(P,T)$ is a regular loss function between prediction P and target T, e.g. a binary cross entropy loss function in case of a multi-label classification problem. Note that the computation of f can be skipped, if $\mathrm{I}(b,c)$ indicates zero, i.e. label absence. The class weight w_c is used to balance the influence of rare labels. Additionally, we observed that it is beneficial to add a general cost across all predictions $\bar{\mu}_P$, i.e. the mean of the network output, with a small weight of $\lambda (=10^{-5})$, in order to draw the predictions towards zero. This has the effect of reducing artifacts as the network learns to predict only what the ground-truth demands.

3   Experiments

We continue with a description of the experiments. The results of all experiments are shown in Table 1.

3.1   Cell Nuclei Analysis

For the analysis of cell nuclei we compose a dataset from three subsets: HE [6], IHC [2] and FLM [7,14]. As the subsets have different sizes, we sample from each set with equal probability and define a training epoch by a fixed number of samples ($N = 6400$). Our baseline in this experiment are U-nets [10] trained on the individual (single) domain as well as a single U-net trained on all domains at once (without domain switching). We compare the performances to two domain switching networks that use switches along the depth of the architecture (DSnet, Fig. 2c) and as preprocessing (PPnet, Fig. 2b), All networks are trained with Adam (lr = 0.0005, weight-decay = 10^{-6}) for 70 epochs using the proposed accumulated loss L_{acc}. We predict (a) fore- and background, (b) cell nuclei boundaries, (c) cell nuclei centroids and, in case of the IHC data, (d) the presence of an immune-cell. The performance in the four cases is measured by: (a) the Dice-coefficient, (b) the Dice-coefficient, but with a two pixel wide tolerance around the ground-truth and predictions, (c) and (d) the F1-score $2 \cdot \text{tp}/2 \cdot \text{tp} + \text{fp} + \text{fn}$ by counting predictions as *true positive (tp)* if they fall within a distance of 12px (empirical) of a ground-truth nucleus, while additional predictions in the same radius count as *false positive (fp)* and entirely missing predictions in ground-truth distance as *false negative (fn)*. A six-fold cross-validation with randomized splits is repeated three times for statistical validity of the results.

3.2   Facial Landmark Detection

For the detection of facial landmarks we created a dataset out of two separate datasets: thermal infrared [4] and the grayscale images [11–13] composed of HELEN (training), LFPW (validation) and 300W (testing). We trained the same VGG-like network as proposed in [5] and compared the performance to the same network trained simultaneously on both domains and a similar network in which the first three convolutions were replaced by domain switching layers. For training, an extract of 2000 images from both datasets is used (referred to as *large* dataset) and a second subset comprising 400 images (*small*). All networks are trained with Adam (lr = 0.001), and on-plateaus scheduling (decay-factor = 0.1) for 200 epochs on images normalized into the range of $[0, 1]$. As performance measure we use the average Euclidean distances from predictions to the corresponding ground-truth landmarks, normalized to the bounding-box size. This experiment uses a fixed test set with 600 grayscale and 500 thermal infrared images.

Table 1. Summary of all evaluations. In the cell nuclei detection, *single domain* means one specific network was trained for HE, IHC, and FLM, each. For the facial landmark detection, the *single domains* are Grayscale and Thermal Infrared. Statistically significant best-performing configurations are highlighted.

Cell-Nuclei Detection	Foreground Dice mean±std (%)			Membranes Dice mean±std (%)			Centroids F1 mean±std (%)			Immune-Cells F1 mean±std (%)
Network\Dataset	HE	IHC	FLM	HE	IHC	FLM	HE	IHC	FLM	IHC
U-net, single-domain	91.2±3.9	94.3±4.4	99.6±0.2	79.2±7.0	85.4±8.5	98.4±0.7	80.5±6.8	73.7±18.0	87.9±8.4	60.2±25.1
U-net, multi-domain	90.4±4.3	93.9±4.4	99.6±0.2	76.0±8.0	84.4±8.3	97.8±1.3	77.8±7.1	74.1±17.9	87.5±6.5	55.8±23.7
PPnet	90.7±4.1	94.3±4.6	99.6±0.2	77.8±7.3	85.1±9.0	97.4±1.9	79.5±7.2	73.8±17.9	80.6±12.4	58.6±25.1
DSnet	90.5±4.5	94.0±4.6	99.6±0.2	76.7±7.7	84.6±8.5	97.5±2.0	78.6±6.8	73.1±17.6	84.2±12.1	57.0±24.9

Facial Landmark Detection	Grayscale Error mean±std		Thermal Infrared Error mean±std	
Network\Dataset	large	small	large	small
VGG, single-domain	**0.032±0.018**	0.053±0.029	**0.024±0.006**	0.058±0.047
VGG, multi-domain	0.038±0.019	0.060±0.032	0.026±0.007	0.046±0.033
DSnet	0.035±0.016	**0.048±0.020**	**0.024±0.005**	**0.037±0.019**

BraTS Challenge	Enhancing Tumor Dice mean±std (%)	Tumor Core Dice mean±std (%)	Whole Tumor Dice mean±std (%)
U-net, multi-domain	69.4±27.5	81.8±17.1	88.6±8.3
DSnet	69.5±27.6	81.7±17.1	88.1±9.7

3.3 Tumor Segmentation

In the tumor segmentation, we employ data from the BraTS 2018 training dataset including 285 cases (210 high- and 75 low-grade glioma). The complete BraTS data originates from 19 institutions over the globe with various MRI scanners. However, ground-truth labels with clear correspondence to institutions are only available in eight cases. The data from these eight institutions accounts for 244 cases, which are used in this experiment. We performed a five-fold cross-validation using a 3D-U-net as architecture, featuring 28 channels at the highest level. For the domain switch network, we applied the modifications as depicted in Fig. 1b. Both networks are trained with Adam (lr = 0.0001, weight-decay = 10^{-5}) optimizing a Dice-loss objective for 100 epochs of training. We schedule the learning rate according to $lr_n = lr \cdot (1 - n/N)^{0.9}$ [9], where n is the current epoch and N the total number of epochs. We choose a fixed input size of $128 \times 128 \times 128$ voxels and a batch size of two. During training, four such patches are cropped out of each MRI scan. Performance is assessed in terms of the Dice-coefficient between predicted and ground-truth segmentation mask. Since the state-of-the-art is to train networks on all available data, we omit the single-domain training from this experiment.

4 Results

Overall, out of the three experiments only the Facial Landmark Detection shows an improvement in favor of our hypothesis on the positive influence of combined learning from multiple datasets via domain switches. For the large Facial Landmark dataset, DSnet is on par with the single domain U-net in the IR domain and comes close on the grayscale domain with slightly higher mean, but less variance. On the small Facial Landmark dataset, the DSnet outperforms both single- and multi-domain U-net.

On the cell nuclei detection and BraTS challenge data, the differences in the individual tasks are not statistically significant. The exception is the single-domain U-net, which in some cases outperforms the competing networks by a small margin. While this can be expected from a specialized network, we were surprised to find that the overall difference in performance is very small. Furthermore, the multi-domain U-net performs at the level of networks with explicit domain information.

5   Discussion

In the BraTS challenge, we hypothesize that the scanner harmonization problem is less important than we initially assumed and can be learned implicitly. The state-of-the-art usually addresses scanner differences and inter-patient variance together by normalization and bias-field correction in the preprocessing. In contrast to the brain MRIs, the data of the cell nuclei datasets visually appears quite different. However, there is a chance that the mapping to an internal uniform feature representation is quite simple. Basically, a projection on the different common stain components: white, violet, pink, blue and brown, and accumulating the respective channels would enable the network to learn domain-independent features quite easily. Some indication to support this (keeping in mind that the individual means do not vary significantly) may be observed in the PPnet, which provides such a basic mapping for preprocessing the data. With the exception of the centroid prediction task in IHC and FLM, the PPnet predictions are consistently closer to the single-domain U-net performance than the U-net and DSnet. Grayscale and thermal infrared images are again quite different in appearance. Due to the lack of texture information in the infrared domain, it is reasonable to assume a more complex dependency between the domains, that could explain DSnet outperforming U-net and, in case of the small dataset, even the single-domain networks. On the larger dataset, there is still a consistent improvement compared to the multi-domain U-net (grayscale), while the single-domain network is either better (grayscale) or equally well (thermal infrared).

6   Conclusion

The proposed domain switch has the capability to improve detection results, when learning from multiple domains with little available label information. On large or very similar dataset the effect is less visible and a conventional U-net achieves similar results. However, employing domain switches in the networks has not lead to a significant drop in performance either. In our experiments the observed worst case was a non-significant performance change while the best case was a significant performance improvement.

Acknowledgements. This work was partially supported by the Federal Ministry of Education and Research – BMBF, Germany (grant no. 031 B0006B) and by the German Research Foundation – DFG (grant no. ME3737/3-1).

References

1. Bakas, S., et al.: Advancing the cancer genome atlas glioma MRI collections with expert segmentation labels and radiomic features. Sci. Data **4**, 170117 (2017)
2. Bug, D., Grote, A., Schüler, J., Feuerhake, F., Merhof, D.: Analyzing immunohistochemically stained whole-slide images of ovarian carcinoma. Bildverarbeitung für die Medizin 2017. I, pp. 173–178. Springer, Heidelberg (2017). https://doi.org/10.1007/978-3-662-54345-0_41
3. Gadermayr, M., Appel, V., Klinkhammer, B.M., Boor, P., Merhof, D.: Which way round? A study on the performance of stain-translation for segmenting arbitrarily dyed histological images. In: Frangi, A.F., Schnabel, J.A., Davatzikos, C., Alberola-López, C., Fichtinger, G. (eds.) MICCAI 2018. LNCS, vol. 11071, pp. 165–173. Springer, Cham (2018). https://doi.org/10.1007/978-3-030-00934-2_19
4. Kopaczka, M., Kolk, R., Merhof, D.: A fully annotated thermal face database and its application for thermal facial expression recognition. In: 2018 IEEE International Instrumentation and Measurement Technology Conference (I2MTC), pp. 1–6. IEEE (2018)
5. Kopaczka, M., Schock, J., Merhof, D.: Super-realtime facial landmark detection and shape fitting by deep regression of shape model parameters. arXiv preprint arXiv:1902.03459 (2019)
6. Kumar, N., Verma, R., Sharma, S., Bhargava, S., Vahadane, A., Sethi, A.: A dataset and a technique for generalized nuclear segmentation for computational pathology. IEEE Trans. Med. Imaging **36**(7), 1550–1560 (2017)
7. Maška, M., et al.: A benchmark for comparison of cell tracking algorithms. Bioinformatics **30**(11), 1609–1617 (2014)
8. Menze, B.H., et al.: The multimodal brain tumor image segmentation benchmark (BRATS). IEEE Trans. Med. Imaging **34**(10), 1993–2024 (2015)
9. Myronenko, A.: 3D MRI brain tumor segmentation using autoencoder regularization. In: Crimi, A., Bakas, S., Kuijf, H., Keyvan, F., Reyes, M., van Walsum, T. (eds.) BrainLes 2018. LNCS, vol. 11384, pp. 311–320. Springer, Cham (2019). https://doi.org/10.1007/978-3-030-11726-9_28
10. Ronneberger, O., Fischer, P., Brox, T.: U-Net: convolutional networks for biomedical image segmentation. In: Navab, N., Hornegger, J., Wells, W.M., Frangi, A.F. (eds.) MICCAI 2015. LNCS, vol. 9351, pp. 234–241. Springer, Cham (2015). https://doi.org/10.1007/978-3-319-24574-4_28
11. Sagonas, C., Antonakos, E., Tzimiropoulos, G., Zafeiriou, S., Pantic, M.: 300 faces in-the-wild challenge: database and results. Image Vis. Comput. **47**, 3–18 (2016)
12. Sagonas, C., Tzimiropoulos, G., Zafeiriou, S., Pantic, M.: 300 faces in-the-wild challenge: the first facial landmark localization challenge. In: Proceedings of the IEEE International Conference on Computer Vision Workshops, pp. 397–403 (2013)
13. Sagonas, C., Tzimiropoulos, G., Zafeiriou, S., Pantic, M.: A semi-automatic methodology for facial landmark annotation. In: Proceedings of the IEEE Conference on Computer Vision and Pattern Recognition Workshops, pp. 896–903 (2013)
14. Ulman, V., et al.: An objective comparison of cell-tracking algorithms. Nat. Methods **14**(12), 1141 (2017)

Real-Time 3D Reconstruction of Colonoscopic Surfaces for Determining Missing Regions

Ruibin Ma, Rui Wang$^{(\boxtimes)}$, Stephen Pizer, Julian Rosenman, Sarah K. McGill, and Jan-Michael Frahm

University of North Carolina at Chapel Hill, Chapel Hill, USA
wrlife@cs.unc.edu

Abstract. Colonoscopy is the most widely used medical technique to screen the human large intestine (colon) for cancer precursors. However, frequently parts of the surface are not visualized, and it is hard for the endoscopist to realize that from the video. Non-visualization derives from lack of orientations of the endoscope to the full circumference of parts of the colon, occlusion from colon structures, and intervening materials inside the colon. Our solution is real-time dense 3D reconstruction of colon chunks with display of the missing regions. We accomplish this by a novel deep-learning-driven dense SLAM (simultaneous localization and mapping) system that can produce a camera trajectory and a dense reconstructed surface for colon chunks (small lengths of colon). Traditional SLAM systems work poorly for the low-textured colonoscopy frames and are subject to severe scale/camera drift. In our method a recurrent neural network (RNN) is used to predict scale-consistent depth maps and camera poses of successive frames. These outputs are incorporated into a standard SLAM pipeline with local windowed optimization. The depth maps are finally fused into a global surface using the optimized camera poses. To the best of our knowledge, we are the first to reconstruct dense colon surface from video in real time and to display missing surface.

Keywords: Colonoscopy · SLAM · Reconstruction · RNN

1 Introduction

Colorectal cancer is the third most common cancer in men and the second in women worldwide [6]. Colonoscopy is an effective method of detecting and removing pre-malignant polyps.

Electronic supplementary material The online version of this chapter (https://doi.org/10.1007/978-3-030-32254-0_64) contains supplementary material, which is available to authorized users.

© Springer Nature Switzerland AG 2019
D. Shen et al. (Eds.): MICCAI 2019, LNCS 11768, pp. 573–582, 2019.
https://doi.org/10.1007/978-3-030-32254-0_64

There is strong evidence to support the assertion that polyps and adenomas of all kinds are missed at colonoscopy (pooled miss-rate 22% [8] among multiple studies). An important cause is that the colonic mucosal surface was not entirely surveyed [5]. However, it is very difficult to detect missing colonic surface from video alone, let alone quantify its extent, because one sees only a tiny fraction of the colon at any given time rather than a more global view. The solution is to build a system to visualize missing colon surface area by reconstructing the streaming video into a fully interactive dense 3D textured surface that reveals holes in the surface if regions were not visualized (Fig. 1). This should be done in real time so that the endoscopist can be alerted to the unseen surface in a timely manner so that the situation can be remedied.

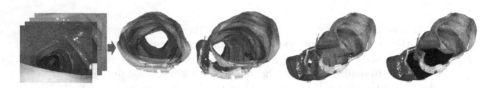

Fig. 1. 3D reconstruction for visualization of missing colonic surface (highlighted in black in the last image, 25% surface), small colon pouches that are occluded by ridges.

Hong et al. [4] used haustral geometry to interpolate the virtual colon surface so as to find missing regions. However, their work only provided single-frame reconstruction and haustral occlusion (without fusion), which is inadequate to determine what has been missed during the procedure. Also, there is no inter-frame odometry being used, which could boost reconstruction accuracy. Armin et al. [1] produced a 2D visibility map which was less intuitive than a 3D dense reconstruction. Zhao et al. [15] used Shape From Motion and Shading for dense endoscopy reconstruction but is not real time.

The SLAM (simultaneous localization and mapping) [2,3,7] and the Structure-from-Motion (SfM) methods [9] take a video as input and generate both 3D point positions and a camera trajectory. However, besides the fact that most of them do not generate dense reconstructions, they work poorly on colonoscopy images for the following reasons: (1) colon images are very low-textured, which is a disadvantage for the feature-point-based methods, e.g., ORBSLAM [7]; (2) photometric variations (caused by moving light source, moist surface and occlusions) and geometric distortions make tracking (predicting camera pose and 3D point positions for each frame) too difficult; (3) lack of translational motion and poor tracking leads to severe camera/scale drift (Fig. 2) and noisy 3D triangulation.

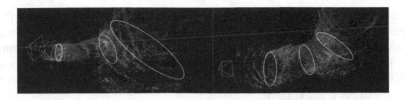

Fig. 2. Left: Sparse point cloud of a chunk of colonoscopy video produced by a standard SLAM pipeline (DSO) [2]; Right: Sparse point cloud produced by ours (intermediate result). The cross sections are approximated by yellow ellipses. The diameters of the DSO result are dramatically decreasing (scale drift), which is non-realistic. Our result has a much more consistent scale thanks to the depth maps predicted by the RNN. (Color figure online)

Convolutional neural networks (CNN) have been used for SLAM tasks and predicting dense depth maps [12, 14, 16]. However, these end-to-end networks are subject to accumulated camera drift because there is no optimization used during prediction as in standard SLAM systems. In contrast, there are works that use CNN to improve a standard SLAM system [11, 13]. CNN-SLAM [11] incorporated CNN depth prediction to the LSD-SLAM [3] pipeline to provide robust depth initialization. The dense depth maps are finally fused into a global mesh. Yang et al. [13] used CNN-predicted depth (trained on stereo image pairs) to solve the scale drift problem in Direct Sparse Odometry (DSO) [2]. However, there are neither stereo images nor groundtruth depth for colonoscopy images. Also, training a CNN on colonoscopy images will be difficult due to the aforementioned challenges.

In this paper, we present a deep-learning-driven colonoscopic SLAM system. We develop a recurrent neural network (RNN) to predict both depth and camera poses and combine it in a novel fashion with a SLAM pipeline to improve the stability and drift of successive frames' reconstructions. The RNN training addresses the difficulties of reconstructing from colonoscopy images. The SLAM pipeline optimizes the depth and camera poses provided by the RNN. Based on these optimized camera poses, the depth maps of the keyframes are fused into a textured global mesh using a nonvolumetric method. Our method produces a high-quality camera trajectory and colon reconstruction which can be used for missed region visualization in colonoscopy. The whole system runs in real time.

2   Methodology

2.1   Full Pipeline

The full pipeline includes the following steps: (1) Deep-learning-driven tracking: predicting frame-wise depth map and tentative camera pose which are used to initialize the photoconsistency-based tracking; (2) Keyframe selection: upon enough camera motion, creating a new keyframe as the new tracking reference and updating the neural network; (3) Local windowed optimization: the camera poses and sparsely sampled points' depth values of the latest N (e.g., 7) keyframes are jointly optimized; (4) Marginalization: the oldest keyframe in window is finalized, i.e., marginalized from the optimization system; (5) Fusion: using optimized camera pose, the image and the depth map of the marginalized keyframe is fused with existing surface. We will detail item 1 in Sect. 2.2, items 2–4 in Sect. 2.3 and item 5 in Sect. 2.4 (Fig. 3).

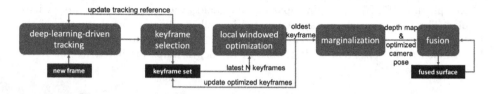

Fig. 3. Flow chart of presented deep-learning-driven colonoscopic SLAM system

2.2 Deep-Learning-Driven Tracking

Our deep-learning-driven tracking is developed upon RNN-DP (a recurrent neural network for depth and pose estimation [12]) that predicts a depth map and a camera pose for each image in the video. However, it cannot be directly trained on colonoscopy videos because there is no groundtruth depth available. In addition, the pose estimation network in RNN-DP is trained based on image reprojection error, which is severely affected by the specular points and occlusions in colonoscopy videos. Therefore, in this section we present several new strategies that allow RNN-DP to be successfully trained on colonoscopy videos.

To solve the problem of the lack of groundtruth depth, we used SfM [9] to produce a sparse depth map for each individual colonoscopy video frame. These sparse depth maps are then used as groundtruth for RNN-DP training. We collected 60 colonoscopy videos, each containing about 20K frames. Then we grouped every 200 consecutive frames into a subsequence with an overlap of 100 frames with the previous subsequence. Thereby we generated about 12K subsequences from 60 colonoscopy videos. Then we ran SfM [9] on all the subsequences to generate sparse depth maps for each frame. Following the training pipeline in RNN-DP [12], these sparse depth maps are used as ground-truth for training.

To avoid the error from specularity (saturation), we computed a specularity mask M^t_{spec} for each frame based on an intensity threshold. Image reprojection error at saturated regions are explicitly masked out by M^t_{spec} during training.

Colonoscopy images also contain severe occlusions by haustral ridges, so a point in one image may not have any matching point in other images. The original RNN-DP did not handle occlusion explicitly. In order to properly train it on colonoscopy video, we compute an occlusion mask M^t_{occ} to explicitly mask out image reprojection error at occluded regions. The occlusion mask is determined by a forward-backward geometric consistency check, which was introduced in [14].

Our improved RNN-DP outputs frame-wise depth maps and tentative camera poses (relative to the previous keyframe). They are used to initialize the photoconsistency-based tracking [2] that refines the camera pose.

2.3 Keyframe Management and Optimization

In this subsection, we will briefly review how a vanilla SLAM pipeline (DSO) works and then introduce how RNN-DP interacts with the system.

Besides (deep-learning-driven) tracking, the other three main modules of the SLAM system are keyframe selection, local windowed optimization and marginalization. The SLAM system keeps a history of all keyframes. The latest keyframe is used as the tracking reference for the incoming frames. In the keyframe selection module, if the relative camera motion or the change of visual content (measured by photoconsistency) is large enough, the new frame will be inserted into the keyframe set. It will then be used as a new tracking reference.

When a keyframe is inserted, the local windowed optimization module is triggered. The local window contains the latest 7 keyframes. From each of these keyframes, 2000 2D active points are sampled in total, preferring high-gradient regions. Each active point is based on exactly one keyframe but is projected to other keyframes to compute a photometric error. By minimizing the total photometric loss, the camera poses (7×6 parameters) and the depth values of the sampled points (2000 parameters) are jointly optimized. In addition, to tolerate global brightness change of each keyframe, two lighting parameters per frame are added to model the affine transform of brightness. The purpose of the sampling is to enable efficient joint optimization by maintaining sparsity.

After optimization, the oldest keyframe is excluded from the optimization system by marginalization based on the Schur complement [2]. The finalized reconstructed keyframe is to be fused into the global mesh.

The SLAM system is improved using our RNN-DP network. In the keyframe selection module, when a new keyframe is established, the original DSO used the dilated projections of existing active points to set the depth map for this keyframe, which is used in the new tracking tasks. The resulting depth map is sparse, noisy and is subject to scale drift. In our method we set the depth map for this keyframe using the depth prediction from the network. Our depth maps are dense, more accurate and scale consistent. As a result, it makes the SLAM system easier to bootstrap, which is known to be a common problem for SLAM. On the other hand, the SLAM system also improves the result of raw RNN-DP predictions by optimization, which is very important to eliminate accumulated camera drift of RNN-DP. In summary, this is a win-win strategy.

Our RNN-DP network is integrated into the SLAM system. Its execution is directed by the keyframe decisions made by the system. After tracking, the hidden states of the RNN-DP remain at the stage of the latest keyframe. They are updated only when a new keyframe is inserted.

2.4   Fusion into a Chunk

The independent depth maps predicted by the RNN-DP need to be fused into a global mesh. We use a point-based (nonvolumetric) method called SurfelMeshing [10]. It takes a RGB+depth+camera sequence as input and generates a 3D surface. Since SurfelMeshing requires well-overlapped depth maps, we add a preprocessing step to further align the depths.

Windowed depth averaging: the fusion module keeps a temporal window that keeps the latest 7 marginalized keyframes. In parallel, the depth map of the 6 old keyframes are first projected to the latest keyframe. Second, the new keyframe replaces its depth with the weighted average of the projected depth maps and its current depth. The weights are inversely proportional to time intervals. The average depth is used for fusion. This step effectively eliminates the non-overlapping between depth maps at a cost of slight smoothing.

The fusion result (a textured mesh) is used for missing region visualization and potentially for region measurement.

3   Experiments

Our algorithm is currently able to reconstruct a colon in chunks when the colon structure is clearly visible. The end of a chunk is determined by recognizing a sequence of non-informative frames, e.g., frames of intervening material or bad lighting, whose tracking photoconsistencies are all lower than a threshold. The chunks we reconstructed are able to visualize the missing regions. We provide quantitative results estimating the trajectory accuracy and qualitative results on the reconstruction and missing region visualization.

3.1   Trajectory Accuracy

To evaluate the trajectory accuracy, we compare our method to DSO [2] and RNN-DP [12]. Since there is no groundtruth trajectory for colonoscopic video, to generate high quality camera trajectories in an offline manner, we use colmap [9], which is a state-of-the-art SfM software that incorporates pairwise exhausted matching and global bundle adjustment. These trajectories are then used as "groundtruth" for our evaluation.

Evaluation Metrics. We use the absolute pose error (APE) to evaluate global consistency between the real-time system estimated and the colmap-generated "groundtruth" trajectory. We define the relative pose error E_i between two poses $P_{gt,i}, P_{est,i} \in \mathrm{SE}(3)$ at timestamp i as

$$E_i = (P_{gt,i})^{-1} P_{est,i} \in \mathrm{SE}(3) \tag{1}$$

The APE is defined as

$$APE_i = ||trans(E_i)|| \tag{2}$$

where $trans(E_i)$ refers to the translational components of the relative pose error. Then different statistics can be calculated on the APEs of all timestamps, e.g., the RMSE:

$$\text{RMSE} = \sqrt{\frac{1}{N} \sum_{i=1}^{N} APE_i^2} \tag{3}$$

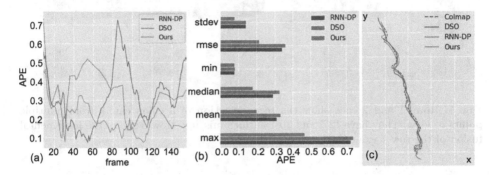

Fig. 4. Evaluation result on one colonscopy sequence. (a) APE of the three approaches across the whole sequence. (b) Statistics based on APE. (c) A bird's-eye view of the full trajectories. (Color figure online)

Table 1. Average statistics based on the APE across 12 colonoscopic sequences

Method	rmse	std	min	median	mean	max
RNN-DP	0.617	0.253	0.197	0.518	0.560	1.229
DSO	0.544	0.278	0.096	0.413	0.465	1.413
Ours	**0.335**	**0.157**	**0.074**	**0.272**	**0.294**	**0.724**

Figure 4 shows evaluation results on one colonoscopic sequence. Figure 4a compares the absolute pose error (APE) of the three approaches on the example sequence: our result (red) has the lowest APE at most times. Figure 4b shows APE statistics of the three approaches: our result is better than the other two approaches. Figure 4c shows the trajectories of the three approaches together with the groundtruth. Table 1 shows the statistics of Fig. 4b but averaged across 12 colonoscopic sequences: we achieve the best result on all the metrics.

3.2 Reconstructions and Missing Regions

Figure 5 shows two high-quality examples of fused surfaces. The two chunks are dense and textured. It also shows the incremental fusion process of the first example. The snapshots are captured in real time.

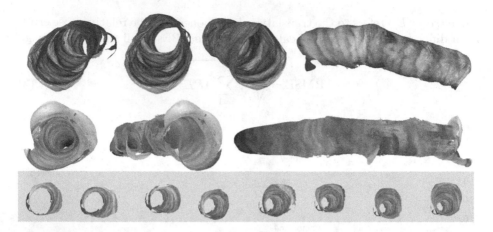

Fig. 5. Rows 1 and 2 each show the reconstruction of a colon chunk from multiple points of view. They have 12% and 10% surface missing. Row 3 shows the incremental fusion of the row 1 example.

There are multiple reasons for missing regions. Two important ones are lack of camera orientations to the full circumference of parts of a colon and haustral occlusion. These two reasons are respectively illustrated in Figs. 6 and 1. For the four chunks shown in this paper the missing area fraction was notable: 25%, 12%, 10%, and 33% respectively, as verified on the video by our colonoscopiist co-author, Dr. McGill.

Limitations and Future Work. We currently reconstruct in chunks because the tracking will fail upon very large camera motion or deformation. Loop closure is not included in our current system; it could be useful for backward motion. Making the tracking more robust to large deformation and adding loop closure are two future directions.

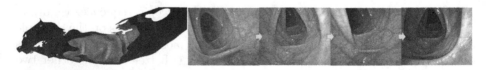

Fig. 6. A part of the colon chunk is missing (33% surface) due to the lack of camera orientations. This can be verified by checking the respective video frames (the upper part of the colon was not seen). However, this might not be realized during a colonoscopy.

4   Conclusion

We developed a deep-learning-driven dense SLAM system for colonoscopy. It is the first to reconstruct chunks of a colon as fused surface from a video sequence (vs. existing single-frame methods) in real time. The reconstructions can be used for the visualization of missed colonic surfaces that lead to potential missed adenomas. Our technical contributions include (1) a recurrent neural network that predicts depth and camera poses for colonoscopic images; (2) integrating the recurrent neural network into a standard SLAM system to improve tracking and eliminate drift, and (3) fusion of colonoscopic frames into a global high-quality mesh. Clinically, it should help endoscopists to realize missed colonic surface and resect more pre-cancerous polyps.

References

1. Armin, A., Chetty, G., De Visser, H., Dumas, C., Grimpen, F., Salvado, O.: Automated visibility map of the internal colon surface from colonoscopy video. Int. J. Comput. Assist. Radiol. Surg. **11** (2016). https://doi.org/10.1007/s11548-016-1462-8
2. Engel, J., Koltun, V., Cremers, D.: Direct sparse odometry. IEEE Trans. Pattern Anal. Mach. Intell. **40**, 611–625 (2018)
3. Engel, J., Schöps, T., Cremers, D.: LSD-SLAM: large-scale direct monocular SLAM. In: Fleet, D., Pajdla, T., Schiele, B., Tuytelaars, T. (eds.) ECCV 2014. LNCS, vol. 8690, pp. 834–849. Springer, Cham (2014). https://doi.org/10.1007/978-3-319-10605-2_54
4. Hong, D., Tavanapong, W., Wong, J., Oh, J., De Groen, P.C.: 3d reconstruction of virtual colon structures from colonoscopy images. Comput. Med. Imaging Graph. **38**(1), 22–33 (2014)
5. Hong, W., Wang, J., Qiu, F., Kaufman, A., Anderson, J.: Colonoscopy simulation. In: Proceedings of SPIE (2007)
6. Jemal, A., Center, M.M., DeSantis, C., Ward, E.M.: Global patterns of cancer incidence and mortality rates and trends. Cancer Epidemiol. Prev. Biomark. **19**(8), 1893–1907 (2010)
7. Mur-Artal, R., Montiel, J.M.M., Tardós, J.D.: ORB-SLAM: a versatile and accurate monocular SLAM system. IEEE Trans. Robot. **31**(5), 1147–1163 (2015)
8. van Rijn, J.C., Reitsma, J.B., Stoker, J., Bossuyt, P., van Deventer, S., Dekker, E.: Polyp miss rate determined by tandem colonoscopy: a systematic review. Am. J. Gastroenterol. **101**, 343 (2006)
9. Schönberger, J.L., Frahm, J.M.: Structure-from-motion revisited. In: Conference on Computer Vision and Pattern Recognition (CVPR) (2016)
10. Schöps, T., Sattler, T., Pollefeys, M.: Surfelmeshing: online surfel-based mesh reconstruction. CoRR abs/1810.00729 (2018). http://arxiv.org/abs/1810.00729
11. Tateno, K., Tombari, F., Laina, I., Navab, N.: CNN-SLAM: real-time dense monocular SLAM with learned depth prediction. In: 2017 IEEE Conference on Computer Vision and Pattern Recognition (CVPR), pp. 6565–6574, July 2017
12. Wang, R., Pizer, S.M., Frahm, J.M.: Recurrent neural network for (un-)supervised learning of monocular video visual odometry and depth. In: Proceedings of the IEEE Conference on Computer Vision and Pattern Recognition (CVPR) (2019)

13. Yang, N., Wang, R., Stückler, J., Cremers, D.: Deep virtual stereo odometry: leveraging deep depth prediction for monocular direct sparse odometry. In: Ferrari, V., Hebert, M., Sminchisescu, C., Weiss, Y. (eds.) ECCV 2018. LNCS, vol. 11212, pp. 835–852. Springer, Cham (2018). https://doi.org/10.1007/978-3-030-01237-3_50

14. Yin, Z., Shi, J.: GeoNet: unsupervised learning of dense depth, optical flow and camera pose. In: CVPR, pp. 1983–1992 (2018)

15. Zhao, Q., Price, T., Pizer, S., Niethammer, M., Alterovitz, R., Rosenman, J.: The endoscopogram: a 3D model reconstructed from endoscopic video frames. In: Ourselin, S., Joskowicz, L., Sabuncu, M.R., Unal, G., Wells, W. (eds.) MICCAI 2016. LNCS, vol. 9900, pp. 439–447. Springer, Cham (2016). https://doi.org/10.1007/978-3-319-46720-7_51

16. Zhou, T., Brown, M., Snavely, N., Lowe, D.G.: Unsupervised learning of depth and ego-motion from video. In: CVPR (2017)

Human Pose Estimation
on Privacy-Preserving Low-Resolution
Depth Images

Vinkle Srivastav[1]([✉]) [ID], Afshin Gangi[1,2] [ID], and Nicolas Padoy[1] [ID]

[1] ICube, University of Strasbourg, CNRS, IHU Strasbourg, Strasbourg, France
{srivastav,padoy}@unistra.fr
[2] Radiology Department, University Hospital of Strasbourg, Strasbourg, France

Abstract. Human pose estimation (HPE) is a key building block for developing AI-based context-aware systems inside the operating room (OR). The 24/7 use of images coming from cameras mounted on the OR ceiling can however raise concerns for privacy, even in the case of depth images captured by RGB-D sensors. Being able to solely use low-resolution privacy-preserving images would address these concerns and help scale up the computer-assisted approaches that rely on such data to a larger number of ORs. In this paper, we introduce the problem of HPE on low-resolution depth images and propose an end-to-end solution that integrates a multi-scale super-resolution network with a 2D human pose estimation network. By exploiting intermediate feature-maps generated at different super-resolution, our approach achieves body pose results on low-resolution images (of size 64×48) that are on par with those of an approach trained and tested on full resolution images (of size 640×480).

Keywords: Human pose estimation · Privacy preservation · Depth images · Low-resolution data · Operating room

1 Introduction

Modern hospitals could highly benefit from the use of smart assistance systems that are able to support the workflow by exploiting digital data from equipment and sensors through artificial intelligence and surgical data science [11,12]. This is illustrated by the recent development of new applications, such as patient activity monitoring inside intensive care units (ICU) [10], staff hand-hygiene recognition [5], radiation exposure monitoring during hybrid surgery [13] and workflow steps recognition in the operating room (OR) [18].

These systems, which have a huge potential to improve safety and care, all rely on machine intelligence using computer vision models to extract semantic

---

Electronic supplementary material The online version of this chapter (https://doi.org/10.1007/978-3-030-32254-0_65) contains supplementary material, which is available to authorized users.

D. Shen et al. (Eds.): MICCAI 2019, LNCS 11768, pp. 583–591, 2019.
https://doi.org/10.1007/978-3-030-32254-0_65

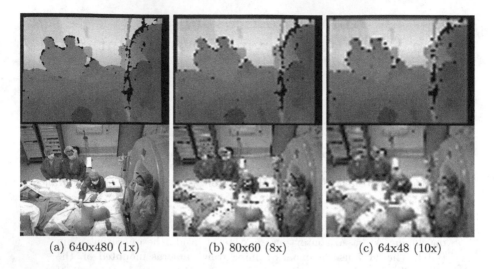

(a) 640x480 (1x)   (b) 80x60 (8x)   (c) 64x48 (10x)

Fig. 1. Depth and color images from MVOR dataset [17] down-sampled at different resolutions using bicubic interpolation (resized for better visualization). Low-resolution depth images contain little information for the identification of patient and health professionals. Corresponding color images in the second row are shown for better appreciation of the downsampling process. (Color figure online)

information from visual data. In particular, human detection and pose estimation in the operating room [1,6,8] is one of the key components to develop such applications. Constant monitoring by the use of cameras raises however potential concerns for the privacy of patients and health professionals. Cameras usually capture the color, depth or both types of images for visual processing. Color images appear to be the most privacy-intrusive, but even textureless depth images can also intrude the privacy when used at sufficiently high-resolution [3,4]. This is particularly relevant in environments where the number of persons is limited and where the persons could potentially be more easily identified. Figure 1 shows depth images at different resolutions. It suggests that low-resolution images could be used for more privacy-compliant computer-vision applications and that their recording could be better accepted by clinical institutions. In [4], it has been shown that activity recognition can be performed on low-resolution depth images captured for the tasks of hand-hygiene classification and ICU activity logging. In this work, we investigate whether low-resolution depth images contain sufficient information for accurate human pose estimation (HPE).

HPE consists of localizing human keypoints in images. Methods for human pose estimation are different for color and depth images both in terms of model architectures and complexity of training datasets. In the case of color images, deep learning models have recently shown remarkable progress with the help of large scale *in the wild* annotated datasets, such as COCO [9]. Deep learning models for HPE can generally be grouped into bottom-up and top-down approaches.

Bottom-up approaches first detect the keypoints and then group them to form skeletons [2], whereas top-down approaches first detect the person using person detectors and then use single person pose estimator to estimate body joints in each detected box [19]. Top-down approaches are often more accurate due to their two-stage design but slower in comparison to bottom-up approaches. For depth images, Shotton et al. [16] use high-resolution synthetic depth dataset to train the models, while Haque et al. [6] focus on single person pose estimation using datasets recording actors performing simulated actions. Recently, Srivastav et al. [17] have introduced the MVOR dataset, which contains color and depth images captured in the OR along with ground truth human poses. They have also evaluated recent HPE methods. This is therefore an interesting testbed for multi-person pose estimation on depth data captured during real surgical activities, which we will use in this work.

Current methods for HPE inside the OR have been developed using standard resolution images [1,8]. We have found that state-of-the-art models, which are trained on the high-resolution images, perform poorly on the corresponding low-resolution images. In this paper, we therefore propose an approach for the human pose estimation problem on low-resolution depth images. To the best of our knowledge, this is the first work that attempts to solve this task.

To train our system, we use a non-annotated dataset of synchronized RGB-D images captured in the OR environment. Unlike conventional approaches, which use either manual or synthetically rendered annotations challenging to generate, we propose to use the detections from a state-of-the-art method applied to the color images as pseudo ground truth for the corresponding depth images. This simple idea turns out to be very effective. Indeed, as our approach only requires a set of RGB-D images at train time, it can be easily retrained in any facility since no annotation process is needed. Then, it can run round the clock on low-resolution depth images from the same facility. Our HPE approach is a network which integrates super-resolution modules with a 2D multi-person body keypoint estimator based on RTPose [2]. It utilizes intermediate super-resolution feature maps to better learn the high-frequency features. With the proposed architecture, we achieve the same results as a network trained on the standard resolution images and improve by 6.5% the results of a baseline method which up-samples the low-resolution images with bicubic interpolation before feeding them to the pose estimation network.

2 Methodology

2.1 Architecture

Our approach is inspired by the recent developments in the area of super-resolution and multi-person human pose estimation. We propose to integrate a super-resolution image estimator and a 2D multi-person pose estimator in a joint architecture, illustrated in Fig. 2. This architecture is based on modification from the RTPose network [2]. Besides yielding competitive results on COCO and MVOR, RTPose has the advantage to perform multi-person pose estimation

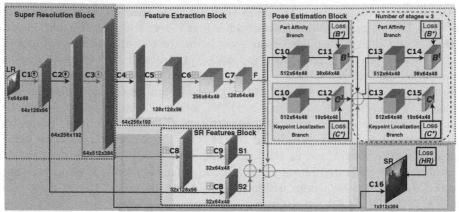

⊕: 2x2 upsampling using pixel-shuffle ⊞: 2x2 maxpooling ⊕: feature concatination

C1: c3(1,64)->c3(64,128)->c3(128, 256) **C2:** c3(64,64)->c3(64,128)->c3(128, 256) **C3:** c3(64,64)->c3(64,128)->c3(128, 256)->c3(256, 256)

C4: c3(64,64)->c3(64,64) **C5:** c3(64,64)->c3(64,128) **C6:** c3(128,256)->c3(256,256)->c3(256,256)->c3(256,256)

C7: c3(256,512)->c3(512,512)->c3(512,256)->c3(256,128) **C8:** c3(64,32) **C9:** c3(32,32)

C10: c3(128,128)->c3(128,128)->c3(128,128)->c1(128,512) **C11:** c1(512,38) **C12:** c1(512,19)

C13: c7(249,128)->c7(128,128)->c7(128,128)->c7(128,128)->c7(128,128)->c1(128,128) **C14:** c1(128,38) **C15:** c1(128,19) **C16:** c3(64,1)

Fig. 2. Proposed architecture. The super-resolution block increases the spatial resolution by a factor of 8x and generates intermediate SR feature maps (S1, S2) used by the pose estimation block to learn high-frequency features. All losses are mean square error losses. C1 to C16 are convolution layers grouped together for better visualization and described below the figure, where c1(n1, n2), c3(n1, n2), c7(n1, n2) each represent a convolution layer with kernel size 1×1, 3×3, 7×7 and padding 0, 1, 3, respectively. Parameters n1 and n2 are the numbers of input and output channels and all convolution layers are followed by RELU non-linearity.

in a single step, thereby simplifying the integration and training of the super-resolution modules. It is composed of a `feature extraction block` and a `pose estimation block` shown in Fig. 2. We introduce a `super-resolution block`, which does not only increase the spatial resolution but also generates super-resolution (SR) feature maps (S1, S2). These intermediate feature-maps contain high-frequency details, which are lost during the low-resolution (LR) image generation process and used in the `pose estimation block` for better localization. The `super-resolution block` uses a multi-stage design, where each stage increases the spatial resolution of the features maps by a factor of two using the pixel-shuffle algorithm [15] (while reducing the number of channels by four). During training, a complete SR image is generated to compute the auxiliary loss **L_HR**, which compares the SR image to the ground truth high-resolution (HR) depth image using the L2 norm. This helps to train the `super-resolution block` and refines the input to the `SR features block`. Note that during training, errors from the pose estimation are also back-propagated to these blocks. Furthermore, at test time only LR images are used and no SR images need to be generated by the network since only the SR feature maps are used.

RTPose was originally developed for color images. Since depth images contain fewer texture details, we have made the architecture more computationally efficient by reducing the number of iterative refinement stages from five to three. The network uses two separate branches, one for keypoint localization and another to compute part affinity maps [2]. In our architecture, these two branches consume the 3 types of features (F, S1, S2), where F are the features extracted from the high-resolution feature maps provided by the super-resolution block. The final skeleton is generated from the part affinity and keypoint localization heatmaps using the bipartite graph matching algorithm presented in [2]. Losses in the pose estimation network are used as in [2], but now take the input from the SR feature maps (S1, S2). At each stage t, two L2 losses L_B^t and L_C^t are computed from the predicted part affinity/keypoint localization heatmaps (B^t/C^t) and the ground truth heatmaps (B^*/C^*). All the L_B^t and L_C^t losses are summed together to form the pose estimation loss **L_P**. Finally, the total loss is the sum of **L_HR** and **L_P**. We have chosen to weigh both terms equally as we observe that their magnitudes are similar. The complete network is trained end-to-end jointly for both super-resolution and pose estimation.

2.2 Ground-Truth Generation

In the literature, authors have either used manually annotated or synthetically generated datasets to train for HPE on depth images. Manual annotations can be expensive and time-consuming, and synthetic annotations are difficult to generate due to the constraint of realistic rendering and do not always generalize well to real scenarios. Therefore, we use an alternate approach to generate annotations. This approach is based on the observation that the RGBD cameras capture synchronized color and depth streams, and recent HPE methods trained on the COCO dataset [9] work remarkably well on the color images. Therefore, we use detections from the color images to train the model for the depth images. To facilitate this approach, we collected an unlabeled RGBD dataset containing synchronized 80k color and depth images captured in the OR during real surgical procedures. Then, we used the state-of-art person detector Mask-RCNN [7] and a single person pose estimator MSRA [19] on color images to generate detections. We filter out the false positives and retain high-quality detections in both the stages using thresholds selected from the qualitative results on a small set of images. This approach generates pseudo ground truth automatically without using any human annotation efforts. It is therefore scalable and can be deployed to any facility. For human pose estimation, we choose here a two steps method based on Mask-RCNN and MSRA for their state-of-the-art performance on the public COCO dataset. Note that such a two-step method would be less convenient to use in our approach, due to the large architectures involved and the fact that super-resolution would need to be integrated into both.

3 Experiments and Results

Training Setup: We use the dataset of 80k images and the pseudo ground truth described in Sect. 2.2 for training. It contains 20k images from four categories, where each category includes images with one, two, three and four or more persons. We split the dataset into 77k training and 3k validation images. When downsampling the images to sizes 80×60 and 64×48, we use bicubic interpolation. To generate pseudo ground truth, we use a threshold of 0.7 in the person-detector stage and then select the skeleton if at least 4 keypoints are detected with a score greater than 0.35. We use PyTorch deep learning framework in our experiments. The depth images are normalized in the range [0, 255] and we train our networks using the stochastic gradient descent optimizer with a momentum of 0.9. The initial learning rate is set to 0.001 with a step decay of 0.1 after 12k iterations and each model is trained for 32k iterations with a batch size of 12. We use the pre-trained weights from the authors of RTPose to initialize the pose-estimator networks. Note that these weights were originally obtained using the color images from the COCO dataset. For the layers that have been modified in the pose-estimation network and contain a larger number of channels (e.g. to accommodate S1 and S2), we repeated the same weights and perturbed them by a small random number. The weights of the super-resolution network are initialized using orthogonal initialization [14].

Testing Setup: We evaluate our method on the publicly available depth images of the MVOR dataset [17], which contains images of size 640×480 captured in an OR from 3 different viewpoints during actual clinical interventions. The training dataset comes from the same environment and camera setup but contains data captured on different days. During testing, we use the flip-test, namely average the original heatmaps with the heatmaps obtained after flipping the images horizontally to refine the predictions. We use the percentage of correct keypoints (PCK) [20] as an evaluation metric, which is widely used to measure the localization accuracy of the detected skeletons in multi-person scenarios.

3.1 Results

We show our results in Table 1. RTPose_640x480, RTPose_80x60, and RTPose_64x48 are baseline RTPose models that do not use any super-resolution and are trained on 640×480 (full-size), 80×60, and 64×48 size depth images, respectively. These RTPose variants are the original models modified to take a 1-channel input. The degraded 80×60 and 64×48 images are resampled to the original size using bicubic interpolation to match the input size of the network. DepthPose_80x60 and DepthPose_64x48 are our proposed networks directly trained on 80×60 and 64×48 low-resolution images. Results show that the DepthPose_64x48 network, which uses 10x downsampled images, performs on par with the baseline trained on full-size image. Accuracy is improved by over 6.5% compared to the baseline RTPose_64x48. DepthPose_80x60 performs even better than RTPose_640x480 (an interesting fact also observed in [4] in the context of activity classification) and is 3.6% better than RTPose_80x60.

Table 1. Results of our proposed method (DepthPose) compared to the baselines (RTPose and SR+RTPose) for different image resolutions.

	Head	Shoulder	Hip	Elbow	Wrist	Average
RTPose_640x480	82.9	82.2	57.0	68.5	42.8	66.7
RTPose_80x60	81.1	80.0	54.7	65.3	37.3	63.7
RTPose_64x48	77.8	76.4	52.9	60.7	32.0	60.0
DepthPose_80x60	84.3	83.8	55.3	69.9	43.3	67.3
DepthPose_64x48	84.1	83.4	54.3	69.0	41.4	66.5
SR+RTPose_80x60	83.5	82.7	54.1	68.1	40.5	65.8
SR+RTPose_64x48	82.5	81.3	51.0	66.3	37.8	63.8

We have also evaluated the quality of the pseudo ground truth by running the Mask-RCNN and MSRA models on the color images from MVOR. The resulting PCK value is 76.2, showing that there still exists a gap of around 9% to be filled between the depth and color images. This may also explain the improved results of DepthPose_80x60 model, which takes advantage of an improved architecture compared to the full-size RTPose_640x480 model. Figure 3 shows some qualitative results of the DepthPose_64x48 model. Additional qualitative comparisons are available in the supplementary material.

Comparative Study Without SR Feature Maps: We also experiment to better understand the effect of using super-resolution. Instead of giving to the baselines RTPose_80x60 and RTPose_64x48 images that are up-sampled with bicubic interpolation, we feed and train these networks with images up-sampled separately using a super-resolution network. The super-resolution network corresponds to the super-resolution block trained independently using loss L_HR.

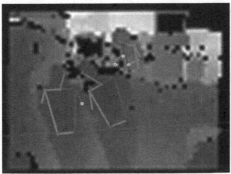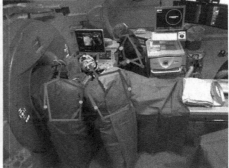

Fig. 3. Qualitative results of the DepthPose_64x48 model on a 64 × 48 LR depth image with 3 persons. Ground truth is overlaid on the color images for better visualization. (Color figure online)

We observe in Table 1 that this procedure (SR+RTPose) improves the overall accuracy, but yields result inferior to DepthPose by 1.5% and 2.7% for 80×60 and 64×48 images, respectively. This shows that the use of intermediate SR feature maps in the pose estimation network helps to better localize keypoints. Also, SR+RTPose has the disadvantage to explicitly generate super-resolution images, the privacy compliance of which would need to be considered.

4   Conclusion

In this paper, we present an approach for high-resolution multi-person 2D pose estimation from low-resolution depth images. Our evaluation on the public MVOR dataset shows that even with a 10x subsampling of the depth images, our method achieves results equivalent to a pose estimator trained and tested on the original-size images. Furthermore, we show that by exploiting high-quality pose detections on the color images of a non-annotated RGB-D dataset, we can generate pseudo ground truth for the depth images and train a decent OR pose estimator. These results suggest the high potential of low-resolution images for scaling up and deploying privacy-preserving AI assistance in hospital environments.

Acknowledgements. This work was supported by French state funds managed by the ANR within the Investissements d'Avenir program under references ANR-16-CE33-0009 (DeepSurg), ANR-11-LABX-0004 (Labex CAMI) and ANR-10-IDEX-0002-02 (IdEx Unistra). The authors would also like to thank the members of the Interventional Radiology Department at University Hospital of Strasbourg for their help in generating the dataset.

References

1. Belagiannis, V., et al.: Parsing human skeletons in an operating room. Mach. Vis. Appl. **27**(7), 1035–1046 (2016)
2. Cao, Z., Simon, T., Wei, S.E., Sheikh, Y.: Realtime multi-person 2D pose estimation using part affinity fields. In: CVPR, pp. 7291–7299 (2017)
3. Cheng, Z., Shi, T., Cui, W., Dong, Y., Fang, X.: 3D face recognition based on kinect depth data. In: 4th International Conference on Systems and Informatics (ICSAI), pp. 555–559 (2017)
4. Chou, E., et al.: Privacy-preserving action recognition for smart hospitals using low-resolution depth images. In: NeurIPS-MLH (2018)
5. Haque, A., et al.: Towards vision-based smart hospitals: a system for tracking and monitoring hand hygiene compliance. In: Proceedings of Machine Learning for Healthcare, vol. 68 (2017)
6. Haque, A., Peng, B., Luo, Z., Alahi, A., Yeung, S., Fei-Fei, L.: Towards viewpoint invariant 3D human pose estimation. In: Leibe, B., Matas, J., Sebe, N., Welling, M. (eds.) ECCV 2016. LNCS, vol. 9905, pp. 160–177. Springer, Cham (2016). https://doi.org/10.1007/978-3-319-46448-0_10
7. He, K., Gkioxari, G., Dollár, P., Girshick, R.: Mask R-CNN. In: ICCV, pp. 2961–2969 (2017)

8. Kadkhodamohammadi, A., Gangi, A., de Mathelin, M., Padoy, N.: Articulated clinician detection using 3D pictorial structures on RGB-D data. Med. Image Anal. **35**, 215–224 (2017)

9. Lin, T.Y., et al.: Microsoft COCO: common objects in context. In: Fleet, D., Pajdla, T., Schiele, B., Tuytelaars, T. (eds.) ECCV 2014. LNCS, vol. 8693, pp. 740–755. Springer, Cham (2014). https://doi.org/10.1007/978-3-319-10602-1_48

10. Ma, A.J., et al.: Measuring patient mobility in the ICU using a novel noninvasive sensor. Crit. Care Med. **45**(4), 630 (2017)

11. Maier-Hein, L., et al.: Surgical data science: enabling next-generation surgery. Nat. Biomed. Eng. **1**, 691–696 (2017)

12. Padoy, N.: Machine and deep learning for workflow recognition during surgery. Minim. Invasive Ther. Allied Technol. **28**(2), 82–90 (2019)

13. Rodas, N.L., Barrera, F., Padoy, N.: See it with your own eyes: markerless mobile augmented reality for radiation awareness in the hybrid room. IEEE Trans. Biomed. Eng. **64**(2), 429–440 (2017)

14. Saxe, A.M., McClelland, J.L., Ganguli, S.: Exact solutions to the nonlinear dynamics of learning in deep linear neural networks. arXiv:1312.6120 (2013)

15. Shi, W., et al.: Real-time single image and video super-resolution using an efficient sub-pixel convolutional neural network. In: CVPR, pp. 1874–1883 (2016)

16. Shotton, J., et al.: Real-time human pose recognition in parts from single depth images. Commun. ACM **56**(1), 116–124 (2013)

17. Srivastav, V., Issenhuth, T., Abdolrahim, K., de Mathelin, M., Gangi, A., Padoy, N.: MVOR: a multi-view RGB-D operating room dataset for 2D and 3D human pose estimation. In: MICCAI-LABELS Workshop (2018)

18. Twinanda, A.P., Shehata, S., Mutter, D., Marescaux, J., de Mathelin, M., Padoy, N.: Multi-stream deep architecture for surgical phase recognition on multi-view RGBD videos. In: M2CAI-MICCAI Workshop (2016)

19. Xiao, B., Wu, H., Wei, Y.: Simple baselines for human pose estimation and tracking. In: Ferrari, V., Hebert, M., Sminchisescu, C., Weiss, Y. (eds.) ECCV 2018. LNCS, vol. 11210, pp. 472–487. Springer, Cham (2018). https://doi.org/10.1007/978-3-030-01231-1_29

20. Yang, Y., Ramanan, D.: Articulated human detection with flexible mixtures of parts. IEEE Trans. Pattern Anal. Mach. Intell. **35**(12), 2878–2890 (2012)

A Mesh-Aware Ball-Pivoting Algorithm for Generating the Virtual Arachnoid Mater

Hirofumi Seo[1][✉], Taichi Kin[2], and Takeo Igarashi[1]

[1] Department of Creative Informatics, The University of Tokyo,
7-3-1 Hongo, Bunkyo-ku, Tokyo, Japan
hseo-tky@umin.ac.jp,takeo@acm.org
[2] Department of Neurosurgery, The University of Tokyo,
7-3-1 Hongo, Bunkyo-ku, Tokyo, Japan
tkin-tky@umin.ac.jp
https://www-ui.is.s.u-tokyo.ac.jp/en/

Abstract. We introduce the Mesh-Aware Ball-Pivoting Algorithm (MABPA), which generates a concave hull triangle mesh, taking one or more oriented, manifold triangle surfaces as input. All vertices of the concave hull mesh output consist of some of the vertices of the input meshes, and the output includes outmost triangle polygons from the input meshes. The MABPA was developed for synthesizing the virtual arachnoid mater around the brain, but is also useful for computationally generating a virtual membrane mesh around any internal organ in general. The arachnoid mater by the MABPA is useful for deformable brain simulation such as a virtual cerebral aneurysm clipping surgery, because collision detection between the membrane and the brain is basically unnecessary. They seldom intersect with each other, because each vertex of the membrane is associated with a vertex from the input.

Keywords: Surface reconstruction · Concave hull · Triangle mesh · Polygon · Cerebral aneurysm · Clipping surgery · Arachnoid mater · Wrapping membrane · Deformable simulation

1 Introduction

Several attempts at simulating a cerebral aneurysm clipping surgery exist, but most of them focus on the clipping after cutting the arachnoid mater [1,2]. One of the reasons is that the arachnoid mater is too thin to be detected by medical images, so it would have to be virtually created whenever a representation is needed. It is present in Shono et al. [5], but is rudimentarily represented by several tiny square planes manually placed on the Sylvian fissure. Cutting is represented by the deletion of individual polygons as the user selects them.

We introduce a new approach, the Mesh-Aware Ball-Pivoting Algorithm (MABPA), based on the Ball-Pivoting Algorithm (BPA) [3] to produce a more

© Springer Nature Switzerland AG 2019
D. Shen et al. (Eds.): MICCAI 2019, LNCS 11768, pp. 592–600, 2019.
https://doi.org/10.1007/978-3-030-32254-0_66

highly convincing arachnoid mater around the brain. MABPA constructs a concave hull triangle mesh (Fig. 1b) around one or more oriented, manifold triangle surface meshes (Fig. 1a). User-specified radius values are taken as parameters. The original BPA uses a set of vertices (a point cloud) as input, and does not consider vertex connectivity or surface, even if the input is represented as a polygonal mesh (or meshes). So, the output mesh created by the original BPA often intersects the input meshes (Fig. 1c), while the one created by the MABPA does not (Fig. 1b). In addition, each vertex of the output mesh created by the MABPA is placed at exactly the same position of a vertex from the input, and the outmost triangle polygons of the input are used as a part of the output mesh. This feature makes it possible to avoid costly collision detection when we want to deform both the input meshes (the brain) and the concave hull mesh (the virtual arachnoid mater) at the same time during simulation. A total of 10 different brain input meshes were tried, and all resulted in reasonable virtual arachnoid maters; each generated within five seconds.

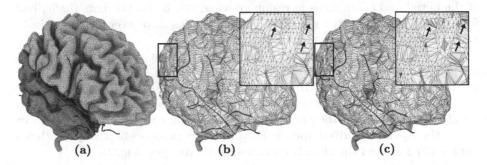

Fig. 1. Mesh-Aware Ball-Pivoting Algorithm overview. (a) The input meshes: the partial frontal lobe (beige), the partial temporal lobe (orange), arteries (pink), and veins (blue). (b) The output mesh created by the MABPA. (c) The output mesh created by the original BPA. Some parts of the input meshes intersect the output mesh. In addition, (b) is smoother than (c) (black arrows). (Color figure online)

2   Methods

2.1   Pre-processing

The original BPA was developed by Bernardini et al. in [3], and how to implement it has been well documented in [4]. The MABPA takes one or more oriented, manifold triangle surface meshes as input. Oriented means the front and back side of each triangle is consistently defined by the order of the three vertices of the triangle. This is necessary for placing the circumscribed sphere of radius ρ (ρ-ball) of the triangle outside of the mesh. Manifold in this context means each edge of a mesh is adjacent to only one or two triangle polygons of the mesh. Each mesh can be either open or closed. The MABPA requires manifold input because it uses information from adjacent polygons on each edge. A single or multiple scalar values $\rho_0, \rho_1, \ldots, \rho_n$ ($\rho_0 > \rho_1 > \ldots > \rho_n > 0$) are also necessary as radii of each ρ-ball. Typically, the values have to be defined manually by the user. In addition, all polygons in the input mesh that are intersecting or penetrating each other should be removed beforehand. This allows the seed triangles to be collected properly, and to prevent such inappropriate polygons from being used as a part of the resulting concave hull.

The first step is to extract seed triangles from the input meshes. An initial ρ_0-ball is placed on the front side of every triangle of the input meshes as its circumscribed sphere. The ρ_0-ball cannot be placed if ρ_0 is smaller than the radius of the circumscribed circle of the triangle. A triangle ABC is added as a seed triangle only when the circumscribed sphere exists and no vertices are on or inside the sphere except for the vertex A, B and C. The radius ρ_0 should be large enough to prevent the ρ_0-ball from going deep inside any concave part of the input meshes, but too large of a ρ_0 tends to make the seed triangles too sparse. So after extracting the initial seed triangles, it is better to try with smaller ρ_n-balls ($n = 1, 2, \ldots, N$). We limit the candidates to adjacent polygons of the initial seed triangles as in region growing, which also prevents the ρ_n-ball from going deep inside the structure. We repeat this step several times (Fig. 2) and the result is used as the initial output mesh.

In order to reuse as many triangles from the input meshes as possible, a triangle filling process is then performed. This process adds an input triangle to the output mesh if all three vertices of the triangle are also the vertices of seed triangles (Fig. 2b). Triangles added by this process are not guaranteed to satisfy the condition of the original BPA; some other vertices might be on or inside the ρ_n-circumscribed sphere. However, this process effectively fills holes between and around the already extracted seed triangles (Fig. 2).

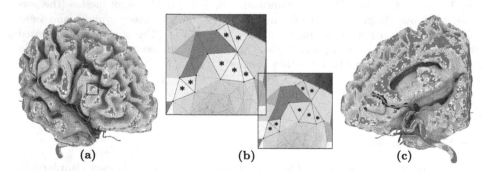

(a)   (b)   (c)

Fig. 2. Seed triangles by $\rho_0 = 12.0$ (red), $\rho_1 = \frac{3}{4}\rho_0 = 9.0$ (orange), $\rho_2 = \frac{3}{4}\rho_1 = 6.75$ (yellow), $\rho_3 = \frac{3}{4}\rho_2 = 5.0625$ (green) and $\rho_4 = \frac{3}{4}\rho_3 = 3.796875$ (light blue), and triangles by filling (white). 17,475 seed triangles, and 3,047 triangles by filling out of 122,510 input triangles. (b) The enlarged view of (a). All vertices of triangle marked by * are also the vertices of seed triangles, so they become a part of the output mesh. (Color figure online)

2.2 Mesh-Aware Ball-Pivoting Algorithm (MABPA)

For each boundary edge of the current output mesh, the MABPA tries to find a vertex to generate a triangle from the vertex and the boundary edge just as in BPA [3,4]. All vertices the ρ_n-ball hits when it pivots around the edge are collected and kept in hit order as candidate vertices. If the ball does not hit a vertex or is too small to be placed at the initial position, no candidate vertex is selected for this edge.

The 2D case is easier to understand (Fig. 3). Let AB one of the seed edges, let BX be one of the input contour edges but not a seed edge, and let Y and Z be the remaining input vertices. Now the ρ-ball (blue) is initially placed on AB as the circumscribed circle with its center at O_A, and pivots around B (clockwise in this case). The ball first hits Y followed by Z and then X, so those are the candidate vertices in that order. The sorting order can be determined by calculating the rotation angle from the initial position of the center of the ρ-ball (B–O_A) to the center of each hitting ρ-ball position (B–O_Y, B–O_Z, and B–O_X respectively). Let us call these angles θ_*, pivoting angles.

However, whenever there are input contour edges like BX, some candidate vertices might be placed under the input contour like Y. So, the MABPA also calculates the angle from the base edge B–A to each candidate edge B–Y, B–Z, and B–X if the pivoting center connects to an input edge (B to BX). Let us call these angles ϕ_*, face angles (edge angles in 2D). In Fig. 3, ϕ_X is the base face angle, because BX is one of the input contour edges. The MABPA removes the vertices whose face angles are larger than the base face angle from the candidate vertices. Y is removed because $\phi_Y > \phi_X$. So the candidate vertices are now Z and X in that order. Z is then selected and BZ is added to the output edge.

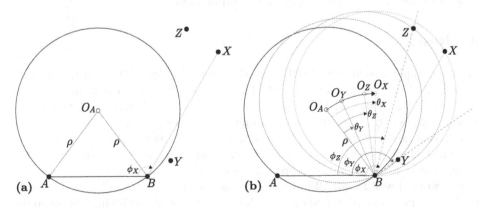

Fig. 3. The MABPA in 2D. (Color figure online)

The 3D case is similar to the 2D case (Fig. 4). Suppose the ρ-ball (not shown in Fig. 4) is initially placed on the triangle ABC as the circumscribed sphere with its center at O_{ABC}, and pivots around the edge BC in contact with B and

C. The center of the ρ-ball moves on the circle of its radius $\sqrt{\rho^2 - (a/2)^2}$ with its center at the midpoint M of BC and perpendicular to BC. Suppose the ρ-ball hits X, we can calculate the pivoting angle θ_X as the angle from M–O_{ABC} to M–O_{XCB}. The face angle ϕ_X is equal to the dihedral angle from the triangle ABC to the candidate triangle XCB.

Vertices which are already in the current output mesh but not on the boundary (let us call them internal mesh vertices) are also removed from the candidate vertices, because the candidate triangle would then make the surface non-manifold. While the original BPA also discards candidate vertices if the ρ-ball placed on each candidate triangle has any other vertices inside it, the MABPA does not if the vertices inside the ρ-ball are internal mesh vertices. This tends to result in a smoother output mesh. The MABPA also discards candidate vertices if the candidate triangle would cause a non-manifold surface, or overlaps with the current output mesh (Fig. 5). Then, the triangle formed with the remaining first candidate vertex is added to the output mesh. This process is executed for all the boundary edges of the current output mesh. The order of selecting an edge from the boundary might result in a different output mesh, but the output meshes look very similar in the cases we examined.

2.3   Post-processing

There often remain some holes after the MABPA as in the original BPA. We fill each hole using a heuristic method as shown in Fig. 6a–c. We also apply an edge flip. If two adjacent triangles of the input meshes (ABC and DCB, the beige lower image in Fig. 6d) have been replaced by two other triangles in the output mesh (ABD and DCA, the purple upper image in Fig. 6d), we flip the edges in order to reuse the two triangles from the input meshes.

3   Results

We have implemented the MABPA on Microsoft Windows 10 PC with an Intel Core i7-7700K CPU running at 4.2 GHz, with 64 GB of RAM and an NVIDIA GeForce GTX 1080Ti GPU running Epic Games Unreal Engine 4.16 (UE4.16). The calculation time for the virtual arachnoid mater shown in Fig. 7 from the input meshes shown in Fig. 1a (containing 77,798 vertices, 231,524 edges, and 153,816 triangles) was approximately 1.7 s. There were no remaining holes and no intersections between the output mesh and the input meshes. The same ρ_n values worked well for all 10 input brain cases we tried because the size of each patient brain was similar, and each mesh had been generated by images taken by the same medical equipment and using the same algorithm. This is an advantage of the MABPA in clinical use.

Figure 8 provides a visual comparison of the effect of varying the ρ-ball values. As we add smaller ρ_n balls, the number of triangles generated increases, but the calculation time decreases. This is because when the pivoting ρ_n-ball is larger, more vertices have to be checked as to whether they lie inside the ρ_n-ball or not.

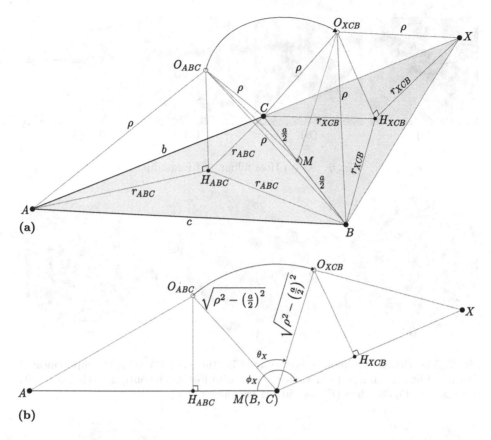

Fig. 4. The MABPA in 3D. Compare this figure with Fig. 3.

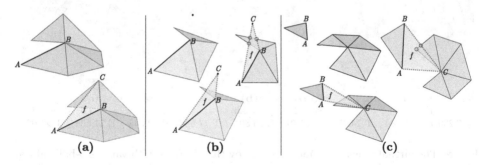

Fig. 5. AB: the current base edge for MABPA (thick black line) and ABC (f, transparent cyan): the candidate triangle. (a) A non-manifold case. (b) and (c) Overlapping cases. (Color figure online)

We integrated the virtual arachnoid mater generated by the MABPA with a virtual cerebral aneurysm clipping surgery. Figure 9 shows images from a real-time rendering of the simulation on UE4.16. The region where the membrane

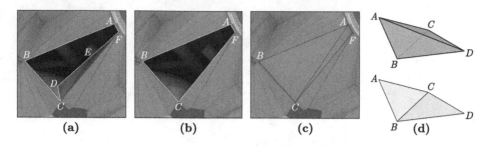

Fig. 6. (a)–(c) Hole filling. (d) Edge flip.

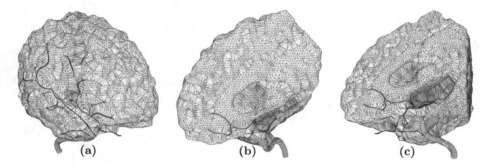

Fig. 7. The virtual arachnoid mater created by the MABPA from the input meshes shown in Fig. 1a, using ρ_0 to ρ_4 values as shown in Fig. 2. The output mesh has 15,104 vertices (V), 45,306 edges (E) and 30,204 triangles (T).

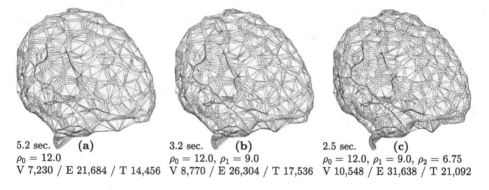

5.2 sec.   (a)   3.2 sec.   (b)   2.5 sec.   (c)
$\rho_0 = 12.0$ $\rho_0 = 12.0, \rho_1 = 9.0$ $\rho_0 = 12.0, \rho_1 = 9.0, \rho_2 = 6.75$
V 7,230 / E 21,684 / T 14,456   V 8,770 / E 26,304 / T 17,536   V 10,548 / E 31,638 / T 21,092

Fig. 8. The virtual arachnoid mater created by the MABPA with various ρ-ball values.

wraps the brain has been displayed with some blurring effect, which creates a more realistic look when the incised area is rendered clearly (Fig. 9c). The virtual arachnoid mater seldom intersect with the brain and the blood vessels during the deformable simulation because each vertex of the virtual arachnoid mater is associated with a vertex from the brain and the blood vessels. However,intersection occurs if the virtual arachnoid mater *above* the brain (instead of *on* the brain) is pushed strongly inwards.

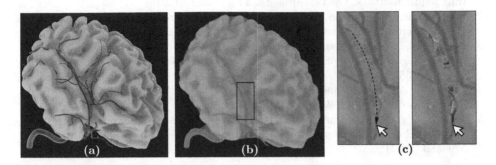

Fig. 9. Real-time rendering of a virtual cerebral aneurysm clipping surgery. (a) and (b) Before and after adding the virtual arachnoid mater. (c) Cutting the virtual arachnoid mater by moving the cursor.

4   Limitations and Future Work

The MABPA cannot be fully automatic because $\rho_0 \ldots \rho_n$ need to be set manually to obtain a desirable result. However, it is possible to precompute for every triangle of the input meshes the maximum circumscribed sphere on the front side of it inside which there is no vertex (sometimes there will be no such sphere, and sometimes the radius of the sphere will be $+\infty$). Using this precomputed information, the system can quickly show which triangles become seed triangles for a given ρ (specified by the user interactively using a slider). Such a feature allows the user to find desirable ρ efficiently.

The main limitation is that there is no guarantee that the MABPA always produces a water-tight mesh (i.e. a mesh with no hole). The original BPA also shares the same problem.

The concave hull mesh created by the MABPA will be useful not only for other virtual surgical simulations in providing membrane wrapping around other internal organs, but also for video games as a roughly wrapped collision mesh, because the shape is much closer to the input mesh in comparison with the convex hull tequniques that are now widely used in games.

Acknowledgements. This research was supported by AMED under Grant Number JP18he1602001. The authors would like to thank Dr. Naoyuki Shono of The Department of Neurosurgery at The University of Tokyo for providing brain meshes, and Miyu Hashimoto for assisting implementations.

References

1. Alaraj, A., et al.: Virtual reality cerebral aneurysm clipping simulation with real-time haptic feedback. Oper. Neurosurg. **11**(1), 52–58 (2015)
2. Bambakidis, N.C., Selman, W.R., Sloan, A.E.: Surgical rehearsal platform: potential uses in microsurgery. Neurosurgery **73**(suppl-1), S122–S126 (2013)
3. Bernardini, F., Mittleman, J., Rushmeier, H., Silva, C., Taubin, G.: The ball-pivoting algorithm for surface reconstruction. IEEE Trans. Vis. Comput. Graph. **5**(4), 349–359 (1999)
4. Digne, J.: An analysis and implementation of a parallel ball pivoting algorithm. Image Process. Line **4**, 149–168 (2014)
5. Shono, N., et al.: Microsurgery simulator of cerebral aneurysm clipping with interactive cerebral deformation featuring a virtual arachnoid. Oper. Neurosurg. **14**(5), 579–589 (2017)

Attenuation Imaging with Pulse-Echo Ultrasound Based on an Acoustic Reflector

Richard Rau[✉], Ozan Unal, Dieter Schweizer, Valery Vishnevskiy, and Orcun Goksel

Computer-assisted Applications in Medicine, ETH Zurich, Zurich, Switzerland
rrau@ee.ethz.ch

Abstract. Ultrasound attenuation is caused by absorption and scattering in tissue and is thus a function of tissue composition, hence its imaging offers great potential for screening and differential diagnosis. In this paper we propose a novel method that allows to reconstruct spatial attenuation distribution in tissue based on computed tomography, using reflections from a passive acoustic reflector. This requires a standard ultrasound transducer operating in pulse-echo mode, thus it can be implemented on conventional ultrasound systems with minor modifications. We use calibration with water measurements in order to normalize measurements for quantitative imaging of attenuation. In contrast to earlier techniques, we herein show that attenuation reconstructions are possible without any geometric prior on the inclusion location or shape. We present a quantitative evaluation of reconstructions based on simulations, gelatin phantoms, and *ex-vivo* bovine skeletal muscle tissue, achieving contrast-to-noise ratio of up to 2.3 for an inclusion in *ex-vivo* tissue.

Keywords: Ultrasound · Attenuation · Computed tomography · Speed of sound · Limited angle tomography

1 Introduction

Changes in tissue characteristics may be a prominent indication of pathology, which can be probed by sonography. For instance, shear-wave elastography aims to estimate tissue shear-modulus [5,16], while speed-of-sound imaging relates to tissue bulk modulus [4,15].

Typical B-mode ultrasound images the amplitude of echos from tissue. The ultrasound (US) intensity *attenuates* during acoustic propagation via several mechanisms: US waves may *reflect* and *scatter*, respectively, from large and small tissue structures of differing acoustic impedance. Frictious losses in tissue cause *viscous absorption*. Additionally, a main mode of energy loss in tissue is via *relaxation absorption*, which is due to consecutive wave-fronts "hitting" the tissue

© Springer Nature Switzerland AG 2019
D. Shen et al. (Eds.): MICCAI 2019, LNCS 11768, pp. 601–609, 2019.
https://doi.org/10.1007/978-3-030-32254-0_67

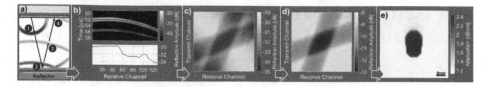

Fig. 1. Processing chain for the attenuation reconstruction with the reflector setup. (a) Schematic of the passive reflector setup with exemplary wavefronts. (b) k-Wave simulated received echos from the passive reflector. (c/d) Reflected amplitudes for all $M = 128^2$ transmit/receive channel combinations before (c) and after calibration (d). (e) Reconstruction of the UA distribution.

that is locally recovering (bouncing back) from the push of an earlier wavefront [17]. Overall, the effects above lead to *ultrasound attenuation* (UA), i.e. the amplitude decay of US signals, dependent on tissue composition; e.g. UA is known to differ between malignant and benign tissues such as in breast tumors [1, 2,7,8]. Therefore, imaging of UA can serve as a diagnostic bio-marker.

Successful imaging of UA has so far only been achieved using complex, dedicated imaging setups using transmission mode, e.g. a ring transducer scanning the breast suspended in a water bath [4,10]. Such transmission mode setups cannot be implemented with conventional clinical US systems with hand-held transducers, making UA imaging inaccessible for most clinical practice. In this paper we propose a novel method for imaging spatial UA distribution based on *limited-angle computed tomography* (LA-CT) with a conventional linear array transducer. The only additional hardware required is a passive reflector, similarly to those proposed for speed-of-sound imaging in [11]. A reflector setup was also proposed earlier for quantifying UA [3,9], which was however not suitable for imaging (reconstructing) arbitrary spatial distributions, but shown only for quantifying values for known geometries. Furthermore, due to reconstruction instabilities, only synthetic and phantom examples could be quantified, but no actual tissue samples. In this work we present for the first time the image reconstruction of acoustic attenuation in tissue using a single, conventional ultrasound transducer.

2   Methods

In Fig. 1 an overview of the acquisition and processing chain for the UA reconstruction is illustrated. A plexiglas plate (density: $\rho = 1180\,\text{kg/m}^3$, speed-of-sound: $c = 2700\,\text{m/s}$) is placed at a distance d away from the transducer. We employ a full-matrix (multistatic) acquisition sequence, where following each single element transmit (Tx), echo on all elements is received (Rx) in parallel. Such process is then repeated for the transmission of all channels. A sample wavefront path is shown in Fig. 1a at different time-points: after transmission (1), while being reflected from the plate (2), during echo travel (3), and during reception at the transducer (4). The echo from the passive reflector's top surface is then delineated across Rx channels for each transmit event and the amplitude of the signal envelope along this delineated reflection is recorded as seen in Fig. 1b. Reflection amplitude for all Tx-Rx combinations are shown in Fig. 1c. With the approximation that the ultrasound pulses propagate as rays, the amplitude of the reflector when transmitting with channel t and receiving with channel r is described by

$$A_{t,r} = A_{t,\theta} \cdot R(\theta) \cdot S_r \cdot \exp\left(-\int_{\mathrm{ray}_{t,r}} \alpha(x,y)\,\mathrm{d}l\right), \tag{1}$$

where S_r is the sensitivity of Rx element r, $R(\theta)$ is the incident-angle dependent reflection coefficient at the reflector interface, $A_{t,\theta}$ is the initial amplitude of channel t in ray-direction θ, and the exponent describes the amplitude decay based on the line integral of attenuation α along $\mathrm{ray}_{t,r}$ from element t to r.

2.1 Calibration

In order to isolate the attenuation effects from $A_{t,r}$, one needs to estimate or compensate for any other influences in (1) such as from the impulse response of the transducer (affecting $A_{0,t}$ and S_r) and reflection characteristics (i.e., $R(\theta)$). To that end, we normalize the measurements with a calibration experiment in water, for which the speed-of-sound $c_{\mathrm{water}} = 1482.5\,\mathrm{m/s}$ and the attenuation coefficient $\alpha_{\mathrm{water}} \approx 0.05\,\mathrm{Np/cm}$ are known from the literature, given water temperature $T = 20\,^\circ\mathrm{C}$ and imaging frequency of $5\,\mathrm{MHz}$. For the calibration experiment and an actual acquisition, $A_{t,\theta}$ and S_r can be assumed to be similar; however, $R(\theta)$ may differ due to a speed-of-sound mismatch between water and tissue. Nevertheless, such reflection coefficient at the acoustic reflector interface can be analytically estimated using Snell's law, because the wavelength is smaller compared to the reflector dimensions. For the reflector interface:

$$R_k(\theta) = \frac{m_k \cos(\theta) - n_k \sqrt{1 - \frac{\sin^2(\theta)}{n_k^2}}}{m_k \cos(\theta) + n_k \sqrt{1 - \frac{\sin^2(\theta)}{n_k^2}}}, \tag{2}$$

where speed-of-sound ratio $n_k = c_{\mathrm{reflector}}/c_k$ and density ratio $m_k = \rho_{\mathrm{reflector}}/\rho_k$. We herein assume $\rho_{\mathrm{tissue}} \approx \rho_{\mathrm{water}} \approx 1000\,\mathrm{kg/m^3}$. The normalized reflection amplitude matrix (cf. Fig. 1d) can therefore be computed as:

$$b_{t,r} = \ln \frac{A_{t,r,\mathrm{tissue}}(\theta) R_{\mathrm{water}}(\theta)}{A_{t,r,\mathrm{water}}(\theta) R_{\mathrm{tissue}}(\theta)} = -\int_{\mathrm{ray}_{t,r}} \alpha\,\mathrm{d}l \approx -\sum_{i \in \mathrm{ray}_{t,r}} l_i \alpha_i, \tag{3}$$

where the ray integral is discretized as summation over a reconstruction grid, with each attenuation value α_i weighted by path length l_i within grid element i.

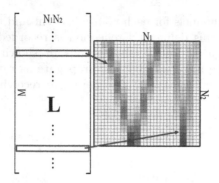

Fig. 2. Reconstruction matrix $\mathbf{L}$ with two representative paths depicted.

2.2 Attenuation Reconstruction

Given M logarithms of normalized reflection amplitudes $\mathbf{b} \in \mathbb{R}^M$, we perform a tomographic reconstruction of the spatial UA distribution on a $N_1 \times N_2$ spatial grid by formulating the following convex optimization problem:

$$\hat{\boldsymbol{\alpha}} = \arg\min_{\boldsymbol{\alpha}} \|\mathbf{L}\boldsymbol{\alpha} + \mathbf{b}\|_1 + \lambda\|\mathbf{D}\boldsymbol{\alpha}\|_1, \tag{4}$$

where $\mathbf{L} \in \mathbb{R}^{M \times N_1 N_2}$ is the sparse ray path matrix (cf. Fig. 2) that implements (3) and $\boldsymbol{\alpha} \in \mathbb{R}^{N_1 N_2}$ is the reconstructed image. A regularization weight λ controls the amount of spatial smoothness and is essential due to the ill-conditioning of $\mathbf{L}$. The regularization matrix $\mathbf{D}$ implements LA-CT specific image filtering aimed to suppress streaking artifacts along wave propagation directions via anisotropic weighting of horizontal, vertical and diagonal gradients as described in [13]. In this paper we empirically set λ=0.6 for all experiments, and use an unconstrained optimization package `minFunc`[1] to numerically solve (4).

3 Experiments

Metrics. We used the following metrics for quantitative analysis:

- Contrast-ratio fraction: CRF $= \hat{C}/C^*$, where $C = 2|\mu_{\mathrm{inc}} - \mu_{\mathrm{bkg}}|/(|\mu_{\mathrm{inc}}| + |\mu_{\mathrm{bkg}}|)$ with the mean inclusion value μ_{inc} and mean background value μ_{bkg}. The ^ and * indicate the reconstruction and ground truth, respectively.
- Contrast-to-noise ratio: CNR $= |\mu_{\mathrm{inc}} - \mu_{\mathrm{bkg}}|/\sqrt{\sigma_{\mathrm{inc}}^2 + \sigma_{\mathrm{bkg}}^2}$, variance σ^2.
- Root-mean-squared-error: RMSE $= \sqrt{\|\hat{\boldsymbol{\alpha}} - \boldsymbol{\alpha}^*\|_2^2/N}$.
- Peak signal-to-noise ratio: PSNR $= 20\log_{10}(\hat{\alpha}_{\mathrm{max}}/\mathrm{RMSE})$.

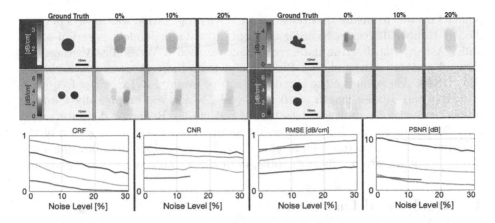

Fig. 3. Evaluation results for k-Wave simulated datasets at different noise settings. Box colors on the top correspond to the colors in the evaluation plots at the bottom. The purple case is only plotted up to 13% noise, due to reconstruction failure at a higher noise level. The scale-bars represent 10 mm. (Color figure online)

Note that only CNR above can be computed without a given ground truth UA.

Simulation Study. To evaluate and quantify the accuracy of the UA reconstructions, four different simulations with increasing complexity in the UA patterns were performed, which are shown in Fig. 3. Simulations were performed using the k-Wave ultrasound simulation toolbox [18] using a spatial grid resolution of 37.5 μm. Full-matrix acquisition was simulated at a center frequency of 5 MHz with pulses of 10 half cycles, where longer pulse lengths allow for narrower bandwidth and more accurate estimation of the reflection amplitude based on the envelope at reflector delineation. The transducer was simulated containing 128 channels (yielding $M = 128^2$) with a pitch of 300 μm. To investigate the effect of noise on reconstructions, we added zero-mean Gaussian noise on simulated measurements, with a standard deviation as a percentage of the normalized reflection amplitude matrix, an example of which is illustrated in Fig. 1d.

***Ex-vivo* and Phantom Study.** Gelatin phantoms were prepared with 10% gelatin in water per weight. We created pure and scattering phantoms; the latter with 1% Sigmacell Cellulose Type 50 (Sigma Aldrich, St. Louis, MO, USA). Fresh bovine skeletal muscle was used as an *ex-vivo* tissue sample. Using combinations of the above, we created four different phantoms: *ex-vivo* muscle inclusions in gelatin phantom (a) with and (b) without cellulose for scattering; and *ex-vivo* muscle tissue with embedded gelatin inclusions (c) with and (d) without cellulose, as shown in Fig. 4(left).

Measurements were carried out with the samples submerged in distilled water at room temperature, with muscle fibers oriented orthogonal to the imaging

---

plane. This was to ensure that the acoustic wave propagation was always perpendicular to fiber direction, in order to avoid direction-dependent speed-of-sound and UA variation. For the data acquisition we used a Verasonics Vantage 128 channel system connected to a Philips L7-4 transducer (Verasonics, Kirkland, WA, USA). Analogous to the simulation setup, we used a Tx center frequency of 5 MHz and a pulse length of 10 half cycles, which was empirically found to be best suited for amplitude detection of reflections. Reflector distance varied from 30 mm to 46 mm depending on the sample size. For normalization of the acquired *ex-vivo*/phantom amplitude matrices, we conducted calibration measurements at the given reflector depths, in distilled water at room temperature.

4   Results and Discussion

The four representative cases of the simulation study in Fig. 3 demonstrate that our method accurately reconstructs the background UA values, the inclusion locations, and their approximate shape. Due to the regularization, the inclusion UA values are slightly underestimated w.r.t. the background, which is also reflected in CRF values being <1. At higher noise levels as well as with increasing complexity of the ground truth UA distribution, the accuracy of the reconstruction decreases, yielding higher RMSE and lower PSNR and CNR as one might expect. A generally observed feature is that the reconstructed inclusion shapes are axially elongated, which is a known problem for LA-CT reconstructions [13], especially at relatively higher noise levels. It can also be observed that the laterally separated inclusions are reconstructed more accurately than axially separated ones (Fig. 3). This demonstrates a general limitation of the LA-CT imaging: decreased resolution in axial direction due to insufficient spatial encoding in the transverse plane. Still, it can be seen that even for this very challenging case, an approximate reconstruction of inclusion locations and attenuation characteristics is possible, at least at relatively lower noise levels.

For the *ex-vivo*/phantom experiments the results are shown in Fig. 4 with the normalized amplitude matrices, UA reconstructions and B-Mode images. For the pure gelatin phantom (b), UA values are expected to be very low, which is corroborated with our finding of $\mu_{bkg} = (0.15 \pm .47)$ dB/cm as the mean background attenuation value. UA is expected to increase with added cellulose and hence scattering, which again is confirmed by our finding of $\mu_{bkg} = (0.84 \pm 0.42)$ dB/cm for the phantom (a). Furthermore, the tissue inclusions in (a&b) are reconstructed successfully, with high CNR values of 3.05 (a) and 6.92 (b), when the inclusion is delineated using the B-Mode images.

For the cases where the gelatin inclusions are placed in the muscle tissue, the reconstructions also perform well, even though the amplitude matrices show no clear and distinct profile, as was observed above for the cases (a&b). The inclusions in UA reconstructions are observed to be axially elongated, similarly to the simulated cases. This smearing results in an underestimation of UA inclusion values in the delineated regions compared to the background values, thus leading to a decrease in CNR. To verify the robustness of our method for the *ex-vivo*

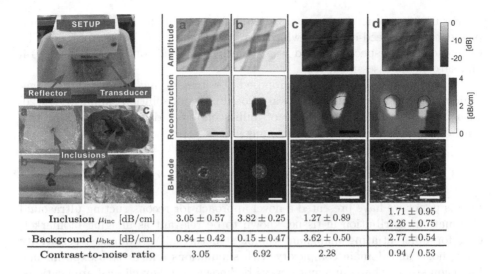

	a	b	c	d
Inclusion μ_{inc} [dB/cm]	3.05 ± 0.57	3.82 ± 0.25	1.27 ± 0.89	1.71 ± 0.95 2.26 ± 0.75
Background μ_{bkg} [dB/cm]	0.84 ± 0.42	0.15 ± 0.47	3.62 ± 0.50	2.77 ± 0.54
Contrast-to-noise ratio	3.05	6.92	2.28	0.94 / 0.53

Fig. 4. *Ex-vivo* bovine skeletal muscle results. On the left, the experimental setup is shown with the different study cases: muscle inclusion in gelatin (a) with and (b) without cellulose; and muscle samples with gelatin inclusions (c) with and (d) without cellulose. The scale-bars represent 10 mm.

experiments, muscle UA values across all four experiments (a–d) are compared in the table in Fig. 4. All muscle values (which are inclusion in a and b, and background in c and d) are seen to lie within (3.21 ± 0.67) dB/cm, which is in agreement with the values reported in the literature for bovine skeletal muscle when measured perpendicular to fibers [7].

Note that local speed-of-sound variations cause US wavefront aberrations; for instance for inclusions, an acoustic lens effect is observed where the amplitude readings from straight ray approximation are inaccurate. This is visible in Fig. 4a in the amplitude matrix, where higher amplitudes are observed right on the margin of the relatively higher attenuating (darker) cross pattern. To improve the reconstructions further, a possibility would be to correct ray refractions based on speed-of-sound estimations, which can be derived from timing deviations [11].

In this study we only compensate for the speed-of-sound effects on the reflection coefficient differences at the reflector interface, based on (3). However, tissue speed-of-sound variations may additionally be affecting the angular beam profile of Tx/Rx transducer elements, thus introducing deviations in the amplitude matrix hindering its effective normalization. Nevertheless, given the successful reconstruction results, we believe such effect on the beam profile to be minimal.

UA is dependent on the frequency of the US pulse, i.e. $\propto f^y$, where y is tissue dependent. Thus, using narrowband pulses, reconstructions could be carried out at different frequencies to estimate the frequency dependence parameter y as yet another imaging biomarker and tissue characteristic.

For multi-parametric characterization, UA can be an imaging biomarker complementary to speed-of-sound, which may be superior to elastography [6]. The quantification of speed-of-sound was recently proposed for breast density [14] and sarcopenia assessment [12].

A practical limitation of our proposed UA imaging method is that an algebraic reconstruction is utilized. A variational network solution similar to [19,20] with inference times on the order of milliseconds could help to overcome this limitation towards real-time UA imaging.

5   Conclusion and Outlook

In this paper we have presented a novel approach for reconstructing ultrasound attenuation distribution in tissue, known to be relevant as imaging biomarker, e.g., for differentiating malignant tumor structures. We evaluated sensitivity w.r.t. noise and domain complexity with simulations and *ex-vivo* experiments. Inclusion size or shape may not always be known in many clinical applications. We show herein, to best of our knowledge for the first time, accurate reconstruction of attenuation without prior knowledge using conventional ultrasound linear arrays. Since our proposed method can be implemented in standard ultrasound systems and requires only minimal hardware addition of a passive acoustic reflector, it is readily translatable to clinical setting. Prospective applications could be the anatomical locations that allow two-sided access, such as the imaging of the breast and the extremities.

Funding. It was provided by the Swiss National Science Foundation and Innosuisse.

References

1. Bamber, J.C., Hill, C.R.: Ultrasonic attenuation and propagation speed in mammalian tissues as a function of temperature. Ultras. Med. Biol. **5**(2), 149–157 (1979)
2. Bamber, J.C., Hill, C.R., King, J.A.: Acoustic properties of normal and cancerous human liver: dependence on tissue structure. Ultras. Med. Biol. **7**(2), 135–144 (1981)
3. Chang, C.H., Huang, S.W., Yang, H.C., Chou, Y.H., Li, P.C.: Reconstruction of ultrasonic sound velocity and attenuation coefficient using linear arrays: clinical assessment. Ultras. Med. Biol. **33**(11), 1681–1687 (2007)
4. Duric, N., et al.: Detection of breast cancer with ultrasound tomography: first results with the Computed Ultrasound Risk Evaluation (CURE) prototype. Med. Phys. **34**(2), 773–785 (2007)
5. Eby, S.F., Song, P., Chen, S., Chen, Q., Greenleaf, J.F., An, K.N.: Validation of shear wave elastography in skeletal muscle. J. Biomech. **46**(14), 2381–2387 (2013)
6. Glozman, T., Azhari, H.: A method for characterization of tissue elastic properties combining ultrasonic computed tomography with elastography. J. Ultras. Med. **29**(3), 387–398 (2010)
7. Goss, S.A., Johnston, R.L., Dunn, F.: Comprehensive compilation of empirical ultrasonic properties of mammalian tissues. J. Acoust. Soc. Am. **64**, 423–457 (1978)

8. Goss, S.A., Johnston, R.L., Dunn, F.: Compilation of empirical ultrasonic properties of mammalian tissues. II. J. Acoust. Soc. Am. **68**(1), 93–108 (1980)

9. Huang, S.W., Li, P.C.: Ultrasonic computed tomography reconstruction of the attenuation coefficient using a linear array. IEEE Trans. Ultras. Ferr. Freq. Control **52**(11), 2011–2022 (2005)

10. Li, C., Sandhu, G.Y., Boone, M., Duric, N.: Breast imaging using waveform attenuation tomography. In: Procs SPIE Med Imaging, vol. 10139, p. 101390A (2017)

11. Sanabria, S.J., Rominger, M.B., Goksel, O.: Speed-of-sound imaging based on reflector delineation. IEEE Trans. Biomed. Eng. **66**(7), 1949–1962 (2019)

12. Sanabria, S., et al.: Speed of sound ultrasound: a novel technique to identify muscle loss in seniors. Eur. Radiol. **29**(1), 3–12 (2019)

13. Sanabria, S.J., Goksel, O.: Hand-held sound-speed imaging based on ultrasound reflector delineation. In: Ourselin, S., Joskowicz, L., Sabuncu, M.R., Unal, G., Wells, W. (eds.) MICCAI 2016. LNCS, vol. 9900, pp. 568–576. Springer, Cham (2016). https://doi.org/10.1007/978-3-319-46720-7_66

14. Sanabria, S.J., et al.: Breast-density assessment with handheld ultrasound: a novel biomarker to assess breast cancer risk and to tailor screening? Eur. Radiol. **28**(8), 3165–3175 (2018)

15. Sanabria, S.J., Ozkan, E., Rominger, M., Goksel, O.: Spatial domain reconstruction for imaging speed-of-sound with pulse-echo ultrasound: simulation and in vivo study. Phys. Med. Biol. **63**(21), 215015 (2018)

16. Sandrin, L., Tanter, M., Catheline, S., Fink, M.: Shear modulus imaging with 2-D transient elastography. IEEE Trans. Ultras. Ferr. Freq. Control **49**(4), 426–435 (2002)

17. Smith, N.B., Webb, A.G.: Introduction to Medical Imaging: Physics, Engineering, and Clinical Applications. Cambridge University Press, Cambridge (2011)

18. Treeby, B.E., Cox, B.T.: k-Wave: MATLAB toolbox for the simulation and reconstruction of photoacoustic wave fields. J. Biomed. Opt. **15**(2), 021314 (2010)

19. Vishnevskiy, V., Rau, R., Goksel, O.: Deep variational networks with exponential weighting for learning computed tomography. In: MICCAI (2019, accepted). arXiv:1906.05528

20. Vishnevskiy, V., Sanabria, S.J., Goksel, O.: Image reconstruction via variational network for real-time hand-held sound-speed imaging. In: Knoll, F., Maier, A., Rueckert, D. (eds.) MLMIR 2018. LNCS, vol. 11074, pp. 120–128. Springer, Cham (2018). https://doi.org/10.1007/978-3-030-00129-2_14

SWTV-ACE: Spatially Weighted Regularization Based Attenuation Coefficient Estimation Method for Hepatic Steatosis Detection

Farah Deeba[1]([⊠]) [iD], Caitlin Schneider[1], Shahed Mohammed[1] [iD],
Mohammad Honarvar[1], Edward Tam[2], Septimiu Salcudean[1],
and Robert Rohling[1,3]

[1] Department of Electrical and Computer Engineering,
The University of British Columbia, Vancouver, BC, Canada
farahdeeba@ece.ubc.ca
[2] The Lair Centre, Vancouver, BC, Canada
[3] Department of Mechanical Engineering, The University of British Columbia,
Vancouver, BC, Canada

Abstract. We present a spatially weighted total variation regularization based method for measuring the ultrasonic attenuation coefficient estimate (ACE). We propose a new approach to adapt the local regularization by employing envelope signal-to-noise-ratio deviation, an indicator of tissue inhomogeneity. We evaluate our approach with simulations and demonstrate its utility for hepatic steatosis detection. The proposed method significantly outperforms the reference phantom method in terms of accuracy (9% reduction in ACE error) and precision (52% reduction in ACE standard deviation) for the homogeneous phantom. The method also exceeds the performance of uniform TV regularization in inhomogeneous tissue with high backscatter variation. The ACE computed using the proposed method showed a strong correlation of 0.953 (p = 0.003) with the MRI proton density fat fraction, whereas the reference phantom method and uniform TV regularization yield correlations of 0.71 (p = 0.11) and 0.44 (p = 0.38), respectively. The equivalence of SWTV-ACE with MRI proton density fat fraction, which is the current gold standard for hepatic steatosis detection, shows the potential of the proposed method to be a point-of-care tool for hepatic steatosis detection.

Keywords: Attenuation coefficient estimate · Nonalcoholic fatty liver disease · Steatosis · Proton density fat fraction · Envelope signal-to-noise ratio deviation

1 Introduction

Accompanying the pandemic spread of obesity, nonalcoholic fatty liver disease (NAFLD) is emerging as the most common cause of chronic liver disease with an

© Springer Nature Switzerland AG 2019
D. Shen et al. (Eds.): MICCAI 2019, LNCS 11768, pp. 610–618, 2019.
https://doi.org/10.1007/978-3-030-32254-0_68

estimated global prevalence of 25% [5]. From the early stage defined as simple hepatic steatosis (excessive fat accumulation in liver cells), NAFLD can potentially progress into advanced fibrosis, cirrhosis and malignancy. Liver biopsy is not feasible for routine screening due to its potential risk and prohibitive cost. Thus, there is a significant interest in developing reliable, inexpensive and non-invasive biomarkers to detect and monitor the progression of NAFLD.

Fat droplets in the fatty liver cause cellular ballooning, which affects the ultrasonic scattering process, resulting in an increase in attenuation coefficient estimate (ACE). Based on this principle, ACE can be utilized as a promising tool to detect and quantify hepatic steatosis [9]. Unfortunately, ACE methods based on a sliding window approach suffer from the trade-off between image resolution and estimation precision and accuracy. Larger windows improve accuracy and precision by reducing the spatial variation noise inherent in ultrasonic scattering, whereas smaller windows better resolve the underlying structure [7]. More recently, researchers have shown that regularization incorporating a spatial prior can improve ACE results in terms of precision and resolution in homogeneous regions [1,11]. However, variation in scatterer size and concentration inevitably creates inhomogeneity in tissue, which results in a large error in ACE estimation [8]. This issue, while unaddressed in [1], was tackled using different regularization weights for inhomogeneous phantoms (variable backscatter with uniform ACE) than that used for homogeneous phantoms (variable ACE with uniform backscatter) in [11]. Clearly, different regularization weights for different phantoms would not be applicable for biological tissue, where variation in ACE and backscatter may occur simultaneously. Moreover, using uniform regularization across the image as in [1,11], would lead to over-smoothing in homogeneous regions in an attempt to compensate for the local inhomogeneities.

In this work, we propose, for the first time, a spatially weighted total variation regularization based reference phantom method for ACE estimation. The contributions of the paper are: (1) modulating the amount of regularization depending on the inhomogeneity information, (2) derivation of the spatially weighted regularization parameters from the tissue inhomogeneity indicator: envelope signal-to-noise ratio deviation [2], and (3) introducing the novel use of spatially weighted regularization within the ACE computation framework. We validate the proposed method on simulation and phantom data. Finally, we demonstrate the successful application of the proposed method in computing ACE for liver *in vivo* and in assessing the extent of hepatic steatosis with Magnetic Resonance Imaging Proton Density Fat Fraction (MRI-PDFF) imaging as a reference.

2   Method

2.1   Spatially Weighted Regularization Based ACE (SWTV-ACE)

The ultrasound ACE is a measure of ultrasound amplitude dissipation due to the combined effect of scattering and absorption, whereas the dissipation associated with the scattering is small compared to absorption (less than 10% for typical biological tissue) [3]. The standard way is to compute ACE using the reference phantom method [12]. According to this method, the radiofrequency (RF) data are acquired from both the tissue sample and a reference phantom using the same transducer and system settings.

ACE is computed in a $m \times n$ grid using a frequency band discretized at r points. For a RF signal window centered at $(i, j)[i \in (1, m), j \in (1, n)]$ location, the ratio of the power spectrum S from the sample to the reference phantom at frequency $f_k, k \in (1, r)$ can be written as [2,11]:

$$RS_{i,j,k} = \frac{S^s_{i,j,k}}{S^r_{i,j,k}} = \frac{A^s_{i,j,k}B^s_{i,j,k}}{A^r_{i,j,k}B^r_{i,j,k}} = \frac{e^{-4\alpha^s_{i,j}f_k z_{i,j}}}{e^{-4\alpha^r_{i,j}f_k z_{i,j}}} \cdot \frac{B^s_{i,j}}{B^r_{i,j}}. \tag{1}$$

Here, the s and r superscript denote sample and reference, respectively. A is the total attenuation effect from the transducer surface to the center of the respective RF signal window, B is the backscatter coefficient (BSC), z is the axial distance from the transducer surface to the center of the corresponding time-gated RF signal window, and α is the effective ACE for the total ultrasound propagation path z. After taking the natural logarithm, Eq. 1 reduces to:

$$\ln[RS_{i,j,k}] = -4(\alpha^s_{i,j} - \alpha^r_{i,j})f_k z_{i,j} + \ln \frac{B^s_{i,j}}{B^r_{i,j}}. \tag{2}$$

Substituting the following variables in Eq. 2 as: $\ln[RS_{i,j,k}] = Y_{i,j,k}, \alpha^r_{i,j} - \alpha^s_{i,j} = \alpha_{i,j}, \ln \frac{B^s_{i,j}}{B^r_{i,j}} = \beta_{i,j}$, we get,

$$Y_{i,j,k} = -4\alpha_{i,j}f_k z_{i,j} + \beta_{i,j}. \tag{3}$$

The above equation can be written in a matrix form: $y = Ax + \eta$, where η denotes Gaussian noise with zero mean and standard deviation σ, where

$$A = \begin{bmatrix} 4z_{1,1}f_1 \cdots & 0 & 1 \cdots 0 \\ \vdots & \ddots & \vdots & \vdots \ddots \vdots \\ 0 & \cdots 4z_{m,n}f_1 & 0 \cdots 1 \\ \vdots & \vdots & \vdots & \vdots \vdots \vdots \\ 4z_{1,1}f_r \cdots & 0 & 1 \cdots 0 \\ \vdots & \ddots & \vdots & \vdots \ddots \vdots \\ 0 & \cdots 4z_{m,n}f_r & 0 \cdots 1 \end{bmatrix}, y = \begin{bmatrix} Y_{1,1,1} \\ \vdots \\ Y_{m,n,1} \\ \vdots \\ Y_{1,1,r} \\ \vdots \\ Y_{m,n,r} \end{bmatrix}, x = \begin{bmatrix} \alpha_{1,1} \\ \vdots \\ \alpha_{m,n} \\ \beta_{1,1} \\ \vdots \\ \beta_{m,n} \end{bmatrix}.$$

We propose to solve the following spatially weighted optimization problem for the reconstruction of $x = [\alpha, \beta]$ from the noisy estimation Y:

$$\hat{x} = \arg \min_{x}\{\|y - Ax\|^2_2 + \lambda_1 TV(\alpha) + \lambda_2 SWTV(\beta)\}, \tag{4}$$

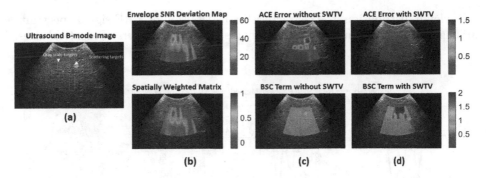

Fig. 1. Feasibility test of the proposed SWTV-ACE method on a tissue-mimicking phantom. (a) Ultrasound image of the phantom with backscatter variation; (b) Spatially weighted matrix formation as a function of the envelope SNR deviation map; (c) & (d) ACE and BSC results with and without SWTV.

where the first term is the data fidelity term, the second and third terms are the anisotropic TV based regularization term, and λ_1 and λ_2 are the regularization weights. The TV operator is defined as: $TV(\alpha) = \sum_{i,j} |\alpha_{i+1,j} - \alpha_{i,j}| + |\alpha_{i,j+1} - \alpha_{i,j}|$, and

$$SWTV(\beta) = \sum_{i,j} W_\beta^{i,j} (|\beta_{i+1,j} - \beta_{i,j}| + |\beta_{i,j+1} - \beta_{i,j}|).$$

Here we have employed a spatially weighted total variation regularization on the BSC term, β. The reason is that a change in scattering affects the power spectrum of the ultrasound RF data, which should be accounted into the BSC term, β. However, the assumption of constant backscatter in the reference phantom method and uniform piece-wise homogeneity in uniform TV regularization fail to account for the change in scattering into the BSC term and consequently result in inaccurate computation of ACE. For the regions associated with changes in backscatter, β should be lightly regularized to decrease the penalty on their variation. Therefore, we propose incorporating a spatially weighted matrix W_β into the regularization of β to account for the backscatter variation.

2.2 Derivation of Spatially Weighted Matrix

According to a previous study, envelope SNR deviation is a useful criterion to indicate inhomogeneity, i.e., variation in backscatter. Envelope SNR Deviation, ΔSNR_e is defined as:

$$\Delta SNR_e = \frac{|SNR_e - SNR_{opt}|}{SNR_{opt}} \times 100\%, \tag{5}$$

where SNR_e is defined as the ratio of the mean to the standard deviation of the RF signal envelope. $SNR_{opt} = 1.91$, which is the average envelope SNR of a Rayleigh distribution, the characteristic distribution of a RF signal spectrum, arising from a large number of randomly distributed scatterers of identical sizes.

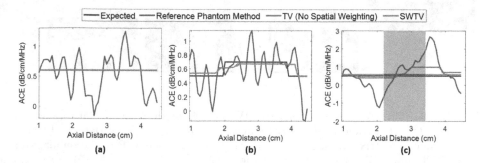

Fig. 2. ACE results for simulated phantoms: (a) phantom 1 (uniform ACE and BSC); (b) phantom 2 (variable ACE and uniform BSC); and (c) phantom 3 (uniform ACE and variable BSC).

To validate the applicability of ΔSNR_e as an indicator of inhomogeneity, we performed a feasibility analysis of RF data acquired from an ultrasound phantom (Model 040GSE) manufactured by CIRS (Norfolk, VA, USA). The phantom contains two different types of targets: scattering targets and gray scale targets (Fig. 1a). The scattering targets are made of nylon monofilaments and contain scatterers of different size, whereas the gray scale targets contain scatterers with a different density. As we plot the ΔSNR_e map, the targets can be distinguished with high ΔSNR_e values (Fig. 1b). Ideally, the phantom has a uniform ACE value of 0.7 dB/cm/MHZ, and variable BSC values at the locations of the targets (BSC values were not reported by the manufacturer). Interestingly, computing the ACE and BSC using both the reference phantom and the uniform TV regularization yield high ACE errors at the target locations while both the methods fail to identify the variation in the BSC term (Fig. 1c). As a solution to this problem, we propose to form a spatially weighted matrix, W_β as a function of ΔSNR_e, to adaptively regularize the BSC parameter:

$$W_\beta(\Delta SNR_e) = \frac{a}{1 + \exp[b.(\Delta SNR_e - \Delta SNR_e^{\min})]}, \tag{6}$$

where a and b are constants. $\Delta SNR_e^{\min}$ is a nominal ΔSNR_e value for which the associated regions can be considered to be homogeneous. As ΔSNR_e remains much smaller than $\Delta SNR_e^{\min}$, the weighting has little effect on the regularization. On the other hand, the weight will decrease as ΔSNR_e increases resulting in relaxation of the regularization effect on the BSC term. By applying the proposed spatially weighted TV regularization, the ACE error was significantly reduced, where the BSC term captures the backscatter variation at the target locations (Fig. 1d).

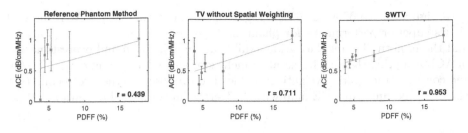

Fig. 3. *In vivo* human liver ACE from six patients and their correlation with proton density fat fraction. The error bars show the standard deviation whereas the square represents the mean calculated over a region-of-interest.

3 Experiments and Results

The proposed method was implemented in MATLAB 2018a (The MathWorks Inc., Natick, MA, USA). The optimization problem was solved using the convex optimization toolbox CVX in MATLAB [4]. We evaluated the proposed SWTV-ACE method on several datasets including simulations and liver *in vivo*. We compared the performance of the proposed method against the reference phantom method [12] and uniform TV regularization. The dimensions of the sliding windows were selected to be 15 scanlines (10 wavelengths) laterally and 8.5 mm (10 wavelengths) axially with an 80% overlap in both directions for all the methods. We set $\lambda_1 = 2^1$, $\lambda_2 = 2^{-1}$ for the regularization weights and $a = 5, b = 0.09$, and $\Delta SNR_e^{\min} = 15$ as the parameters of the spatially weighted matrix, W_β (Fig. 3; Eqs. 4 and 6).

3.1 Simulations

We used the k-Wave toolbox to simulate three numerical phantoms [10]. Phantom 1 consisted of homogeneous medium with uniform ACE (0.6 dB/cm/MHz) and uniform BSC. Phantom 2 had uniform BSC and variable ACE, where the background ACE was 0.5 dB/cm/MHz, and the inclusion ACE was 0.7 dB/cm/MHz. Phantom 3 had variable BSC and uniform ACE (0.5 dB/cm/MHz), where the inside inclusion had a higher BSC compared to the background. Also, we simulate a phantom with uniform ACE (0.6 dB/cm/MHz) and uniform BSC, which would be used as the reference phantom to compensate for the system dependence.

For phantom 1 and phantom 2, the SWTV-ACE method gives similar performance as that obtained from the uniform TV regularization as these phantoms have uniform BSC. In both methods, ACE error is reduced significantly (<1%) compared to the reference phantom method (10%), whereas the ACE variance is reduced to ∼1% from 53% obtained using the reference phantom method (Fig. 2(a)). For phantom 2, both uniform TV and SWTV-ACE method can identify the ACE transition in the center inclusion (standard deviation ∼11%) opposed to the reference phantom method where the transition remains occluded with high variance of ACE (63%) (Fig. 2(b)). Finally, the SWTV-ACE method shows superior performance for phantom 3 where both the reference phantom and the uniform TV regularization exhibit underestimation and overestimation of ACE centering the high backscatter inclusion (shaded area in Fig. 2(c)) [8]. On the contrary, the spatial weighting enables the proposed method to reconstruct the expected uniform ACE map with 16% error and standard deviation <1%.

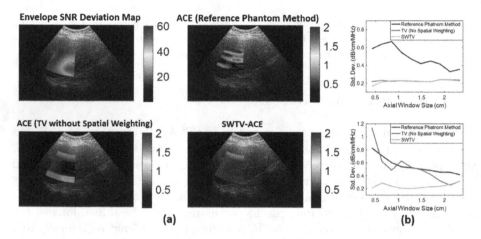

Fig. 4. (a) An example of ACE computation for *in vivo* human liver using three different methods. (b) Effect of window size on estimation variance of ACE for a homogeneous region-of-interest (top) and inhomogeneous region-of-interest (bottom).

3.2   *In Vivo* Liver: Steatosis Detection

We validated the efficacy of the proposed method to detect hepatic steatosis based on six patients, who underwent MRI in a 3.0 T system (Philips Achieva, Philips Medical Systems). MRI proton density fat fraction (MRI-PDFF) computed from the MRI data was used as a gold standard for hepatic steatosis quantification, which strongly correlates with histological steatosis grading [6]. The patients also underwent ultrasound examination with an Ultrasonix SonixTouch machine (Analogic, Canada), the RF data from which were used to compute ACE. The correlation between MRI-PDFF and ACE values was calculated to evaluate the performance of the SWTV-ACE method to detect hepatic steatosis.

The correlation between ACE computed using the reference phantom method to MRI-PDFF was 0.44 (p = 0.3838). The TV method yields a better correlation performance (r = 0.71, p = 0.1132). The SWTV-ACE method outperforms both of these methods with a correlation of 0.953 (p =.003). Therefore, SWTV-ACE method demonstrated an improved correlation with MRI-PDFF even with small window size, therefore extending the trade-off between window size and precision inherent in conventional ACE computation.

We also showed an example of ACE computation for *in vivo* liver, where an inhomogeneity indicated by high envelope SNR deviation causes significant variation of ACE (including negative ACE values) computed using the reference phantom method and the uniform TV regularization method (Fig. 4(a)). However, SWTV-ACE method yields positive ACE values with low estimation variance. Additionally, we investigated the effect of axial window size on the the estimation variation of ACE for a homogeneous region-of-interest $(\max(\Delta SNR_e) < 20\%)$ and an inhomogeneous region-of-interest in liver $(mean(\Delta SNR_e) > 20\%)$. For the homogeneous case, both uniform TV regularization and SWTV-ACE methods maintain similar standard deviation for different window sizes, whereas the reference phantom method exhibits the trade-off where estimation precision improves with increasing window size. For the inhomogeneous case, however, SWTV-ACE method outperforms both the reference phantom method and the uniform TV regularization by maintaining similar standard deviation for different window sizes (Fig. 4(b)). Therefore, SWTV-ACE effectively improves the quality of ACE computation by reducing the variability in the estimates irrespective of window size. The improved resolution will be beneficial to provide information about the local variation within the liver, whereas the improved precision would be required to qualify as a reliable diagnostic tool.

4   Conclusion

We propose a new spatially weighted regularization based ACE estimation method. The goal was to modulate the regularization in the inhomogeneous regions using a weight function formulated as a function of envelope signal-to-noise ratio, an indicator of tissue heterogeneity. The proposed method was able to attain improved precision without compromising the resolution of ACE for both homogeneous and inhomogeneous regions with high backscatter variation. The strong correlation of the ACE measurements with the current gold-standard MRI-PDFF demonstrated the potential application of the proposed method for the detection of liver steatosis.

Acknowledgements. This work was supported by the Natural Sciences and Engineering Research Council of Canada (NSERC) and the Canadian Institutes of Health Research (CIHR) (Grant CPG-146490).

References

1. Coila, A.L., Lavarello, R.: Regularized spectral log difference technique for ultrasonic attenuation imaging. IEEE Trans. Ultrason. Ferroelectr. Freq. Control **65**(3), 378–389 (2017). https://doi.org/10.1109/TUFFC.2017.2719962
2. Deeba, F., et al.: Attenuation coefficient estimation of normal placentas. Ultras. Med. Biol. **45**(5), 1081–1093 (2019). https://doi.org/10.1016/j.ultrasmedbio.2018.10.015

3. Flax, S.W., Pelc, N.J., Glover, G.H., Gutmann, F.D., McLachlan, M.: Spectral characterization and attenuation measurements in ultrasound. Ultrason. Imaging **5**(2), 95–116 (1983). https://doi.org/10.1016/0161-7346(83)90013-5
4. Grant, M., Boyd, S., Ye, Y.: CVX: Matlab software for disciplined convex programming (2008)
5. Loomba, R., Sanyal, A.J.: The global NAFLD epidemic. Nat. Rev. Gastroenterol. Hepatol. **10**(11), 686 (2013). https://doi.org/10.1038/nrgastro.2013.171
6. Noureddin, M., et al.: Utility of magnetic resonance imaging versus histology for quantifying changes in liver fat in nonalcoholic fatty liver disease trials. Hepatology **58**(6), 1930–1940 (2013). https://doi.org/10.1002/hep.26455
7. Oelze, M.L., O'Brien Jr., W.D.: Defining optimal axial and lateral resolution for estimating scatterer properties from volumes using ultrasound backscatter. J. Acoust. Soc. Am. **115**(6), 3226–3234 (2004). https://doi.org/10.1121/1.1739484
8. Pawlicki, A.D., O'Brien Jr., W.D.: Method for estimating total attenuation from a spatial map of attenuation slope for quantitative ultrasound imaging. Ultrason. Imaging **35**(2), 162–172 (2013). https://doi.org/10.1177/0161734613478695
9. Pohlhammer, J.D., O'Brien Jr, W.D.: The relationship between ultrasonic attenuation and speed in tissues and the constituents: water, collagen, protein and fat. In: Medical physics of CT and Ultrasound: Tissue Imaging and Characterization. American Institute of Physics (1980)
10. Treeby, B.E., Jaros, J., Rendell, A.P., Cox, B.: Modeling nonlinear ultrasound propagation in heterogeneous media with power law absorption using a k-space pseudospectral method. J. Acoust. Soc. Am. **131**(6), 4324–4336 (2012). https://doi.org/10.1121/1.4712021
11. Vajihi, Z., Rosado-Mendez, I.M., Hall, T.J., Rivaz, H.: Low variance estimation of backscatter quantitative ultrasound parameters using dynamic programming. IEEE Trans. Ultrason. Ferroelectr. Freq. Control **65**(11), 2042–2053 (2018). https://doi.org/10.1109/TUFFC.2018.2869810
12. Yao, L.X., Zagzebski, J.A., Madsen, E.L.: Backscatter coefficient measurements using a reference phantom to extract depth-dependent instrumentation factors. Ultrason. Imaging **12**(1), 58–70 (1990). https://doi.org/10.1177/016173469001200105

Deep Learning-Based Universal Beamformer for Ultrasound Imaging

Shujaat Khan[ID], Jaeyoung Huh[ID], and Jong Chul Ye[✉][ID]

Department of Bio and Brain Engineering,
Korea Advanced Institute of Science and Technology (KAIST),
335 Gwahangno, Yuseong-gu, Daejeon 305-701, Korea
{shujaat,woori93,jong.ye}@kaist.ac.kr

Abstract. In ultrasound (US) imaging, individual channel RF measurements are back-propagated and accumulated to form an image after applying specific delays. While this time reversal is usually implemented using a hardware- or software-based delay-and-sum (DAS) beamformer, the performance of DAS decreases rapidly in situations where data acquisition is not ideal. Herein, for the first time, we demonstrate that a single data-driven adaptive beamformer designed as a deep neural network can generate high quality images robustly for various detector channel configurations and subsampling rates. The proposed deep beamformer is evaluated for two distinct acquisition schemes: focused ultrasound imaging and planewave imaging. Experimental results showed that the proposed deep beamformer exhibit significant performance gain for both focused and planar imaging schemes, in terms of contrast-to-noise ratio and structural similarity.

Keywords: Ultrasound · Adaptive beamforming · Deep neural network

1 Introduction

Due to minimal invasiveness from non-ionizing radiations and excellent temporal resolution, ultrasound (US) imaging is an indispensable tool for various clinical applications such as cardiac, fetal imaging, etc. The basic imaging principle of US imaging is based on the time-reversal [2,11], which is based on a mathematical observation that the wave operator is self-adjoint. For example, in focused B-mode US imaging, the return echoes from individual scan-line are recorded by the receiver channels, after which delay-and-sum (DAS) beamformer applies the

This work is supported by National Research Foundation of Korea, Grant Number: NRF-2016R1A2B3008104.

Electronic supplementary material The online version of this chapter (https://doi.org/10.1007/978-3-030-32254-0_69) contains supplementary material, which is available to authorized users.

© Springer Nature Switzerland AG 2019
D. Shen et al. (Eds.): MICCAI 2019, LNCS 11768, pp. 619–627, 2019.
https://doi.org/10.1007/978-3-030-32254-0_69

time-reversal delay to the channel measurement and additively combines them for each time point to form images at each scan-line. Although sonic inhomogeneities can cause wavefront aberrations in ultrafast imaging [1], the estimation of the time delay in the DAS beamformer is based primarily on the assumption of a constant sound speed. Due to the simplicity, high-speed analog-to-digital converters (ADCs) and large number of receiver elements are often necessary in to reduce side lobes which otherwise degrade image resolution and contrast. To address this problem, various adaptive beamforming techniques have been developed over the several decades [5, 7, 10].

Recently, inspired by the tremendous success of deep learning, the authors in [3, 13] use deep neural networks for the reconstruction of high-quality US images from limited number of received radio frequency (RF) data. For example, the work in [3] uses deep neural network for coherent compound imaging from small number of plane wave illumination. In focused B-mode ultrasound imaging, [13] employs the deep neural network to interpolate the missing RF-channel data with multiline aquisition for accelerated scanning. While these recent deep neural network approaches provide impressive reconstruction performance, the current design is not universal in the sense that they are designed and trained for specific acquisition scenario.

Therefore, one of the most important contributions of this paper is to demonstrate that a single end-to-end beamformer implemented by a deep neural network (DeepBF) can generate high quality images robustly for various detector channel configurations and subsampling rates. The main innovation of our universal deep beamformer comes from one of the most exciting properties of deep neural network - exponentially increasing expressiveness with respect to the channel and depth [12]. Thanks to the expressiveness of neural networks, our DeepBF can learn large number of mappings between various cases of RF measurements and images, and exhibits superior image quality for all sub-sampling rates. Moreover, unlike [13] that interpolates the missing RF data and uses standard DAS beamformer, the novelty of this work is the end-to-end deep learning to replace the standard BF, which was never considered in [13]. Consequently, our approach is much simpler and can be easily incorporated to replace the standard beamforming pipeline. Inspite of the simplicity, we will show that this approach outperforms the interpolation approach in [13]. Another important byproduct of the proposed method is that the trained neural network can further improve the image contrast even for the full rate cases. The origin of this performance enhancement is also analyzed.

2   Method

2.1   Dataset

Multiple RF data were acquired using a linear array transducer (L3-12H) with a center frequency of 8.48 MHz on E-CUBE 12R US system (Alpinion Co., Korea). The configuration of the probe is given in Table 1.

Table 1. Probe configuration

Parameter	Linear probe
Probe model no.	L3-12H
Carrier wave frequency	8.48 MHz
Sampling frequency	40 MHz
No. of probe elements	192
No. of Tx elements	128
No. of TE events (focused mode)	96
No. of Rx elements (focused/unfocused mode)	64/192
No. of PWs (unfocused mode)	31
Elements pitch	0.2 mm
Elements width	0.14 mm
Elevating length	4.5 mm

Using a linear probe, we acquired RF data from the carotid area of 10 volunteers. In focused mode imaging experiment the *in-vivo* data consists of 40 temporal frames per subject, providing 400 sets of Depth-Receiver channels-transmit events (Depth-Rx-TE) data cube. The dimension of each Rx-TE plane was 64×96. A set of 30,000 Rx-TE planes was randomly selected from the 4 subjects datasets, and data cubes (Depth-Rx-TE) are then divided into 25,000 datasets for training and 5000 datasets for validation. The remaining dataset of 360 frames was used as a test dataset.

In plane wave imaging experiments, we acquire 109 frames, among which only 8 frames (images) from in-vivo data were used for training and 1 for validation purpose while remaining 100 were used as test dataset. Each US image raw data consist of 31 PWs and 192-channels, and each frame have different depth ranges varying from 25–60 mm consist of 2000–9000 depth planes.

For quantitative evaluation, we also acquired RF data from the ATS-539 multipurpose tissue mimicking phantom. These datasets were only used for test purpose and no additional training of CNN was performed on it. The phantom datasets were used to verify the generalization power of the proposed method.

2.2   RF Sub-sampling Scheme

For focused mode imaging, we generated six sets of sub-sampled RF data at different down-sampling rates. In addition to the full RF data (i.e. 64-channels), we use several sub-sampling cases using 32, 24, 16, 8 and 4 Rx-channels. Since the active receivers at the center of the scan-line get RF data from direct reflection, two channels that are in the center of active transmitting channels were always included to improve the performance, and remaining channels were randomly selected from the receiving channels. For each depth plane, a different sampling pattern (mask) is used. The non-active Rx channels are zero-padded.

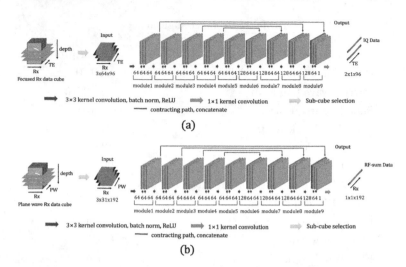

Fig. 1. Proposed CNN architecture for sub-sampled (a) focused US B-mode imaging. (b) planewave US B-mode imaging.

For unfocused planar wave imaging, in addition to the full RF data, we generated six sets of sub-sampled RF data at different down-sampling rates. In particular, we used two subsampling schemes: variable down-sampling of RF-channel data pattern across the depth to reduce high data-rate and power requirements, and uniform sub-sampling of PWs angles to accelerate acquisition speed. Here we use the following subsampling cases: (1) 64, 32, 16, and 8 Rx-channels with 31 PWs. (2) 31, 11, 7, and 3 PWs with 64 Rx-channels.

2.3   Network Architecture

In focused mode imaging, $3 \times 64 \times 96$ data-cube in the Depth-Rx-TE subspace was used for CNN training to generate a $2 \times 3 \times 96$ I and Q data in the Depth-TE plane. Here IQ data is the Hilbert transformed data before envelope detection. The input cube consist of three adjacent depth planes and the target IQ data of middle plane is obtained from two output channels each representing real and imaginary parts. The proposed CNN consists of 27 convolution layers composed of a contracting path with concatenation, batch normalization, ReLU except for the last convolution layer. The first 26 convolution layers use 3×3 convolutional filters (i.e., the 2-D filter has a dimension of 3×3), and the last convolution layer uses a 1×1 filter and contract the $3 \times 64 \times 96$ data-cube from Depth-Rx-TE sub-space to $2 \times 1 \times 96$ IQ-Depth-TE plane as shown in Fig. 1(a).

In plane wave imaging a multi-channel CNN was trained using $3 \times 31 \times 192$ data-cube in the Depth-PW-Rx sub-space to generate a 1×192 RF sum data in the Depth-TE plane. Three input channels were used to process three adjacent depth planes to generate target RF sum data of the central depth plane. The proposed CNN consists of 27 convolution layers composed of a contracting path with concatenation, batch normalization, and ReLU except for the last convolution layer. The first 26 convolution layers use 3×3 convolutional filters (i.e., the 2-D filter has a dimension of 3×3), and the last convolution layer uses a 1×1 filter and contract the $3 \times 31 \times 192$ data-cube from Depth-PW-Rx sub-space to $1 \times 1 \times 192$ Depth-Rx plane as shown in Fig. 1(b).

Both networks were implemented with MatConvNet [9] in the MATLAB 2015b environment. Specifically, for network training, the parameters were estimated by minimizing the l_2 norm loss function using a stochastic gradient descent with a regularization parameter of 10^{-4}. The learning rate started from 10^{-3} and gradually decreased to 10^{-5} in 200 epochs. The weights were initialized using Gaussian random distribution with the Xavier method [4].

3 Experimental Results

To quantitatively show the advantages of the proposed deep learning method, we used the contrast-to-noise ratio (CNR), generalized CNR (GCNR) [8], and structure similarity (SSIM).

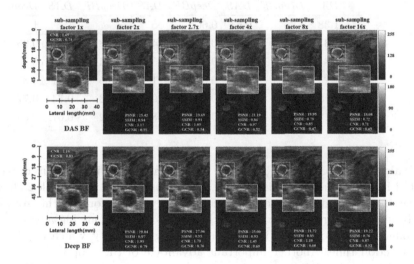

Fig. 2. Focused B-mode imaging reconstruction results of standard DAS beam-former and the proposed method for in-vivo carotid region.

Focused Mode Imaging. Figure 2 show the results of an *in vivo* example for the full data (i.e. 64 channel) as well as 32, 24, 16, 8 and 4 Rx-channels down-sampling schemes. Since 64 channels are used as a full sampled data, this corresponds to $1\times, 2\times, 2.7\times, 4\times, 8\times$ and $16\times$ sub-sampling factors. The images are generated using the proposed DeepBF and the standard DAS beam-former method. Our method significantly improves the visual quality of the US images by estimating the correct dynamic range and eliminating artifacts for both sampling schemes. From difference images, it is evident that the quality degradation of images in DAS is higher than the DeepBF. Note that the proposed method successfully reconstruct both the near and the far field regions with equal efficacy, and only minor structural details are imperceivable. Furthermore, it is remarkable that the CNR and GCNR values are significantly improved by the DeepBF even for the fully sampled case (eg. from 1.69 to 2.16 in CNR and from 0.74 to 0.83 in GCNR), which clearly shows the advantages of the proposed method. It is believed that this is due to performance boosting behavior similar to super-resolution deep neural networks in which the authors have found that multiple-magnification training outperforms fixed-magnification cases [6]. Additional results on phantom dataset are available in supplemental document.

Table 2. Focus B-mode imaging performance comparison for *in vivo* data using variable sampling pattern

Sub-sampling factor	CNR		GCNR		PSNR (dB)		SSIM	
	DAS	*DeepBF*	*DAS*	*DeepBF*	*DAS*	*DeepBF*	*DAS*	*DeepBF*
1	1.38	1.45	0.64	0.66	∞	∞	1	1
2	1.33	1.47	0.63	0.66	24.59	27.38	0.89	0.95
2.7	1.3	1.44	0.62	0.66	23.15	25.54	0.86	0.92
4	1.25	1.38	0.6	0.64	21.68	23.55	0.81	0.87
8	1.18	1.26	0.58	0.6	19.99	21.03	0.74	0.77
16	1.12	1.17	0.56	0.58	18.64	19.22	0.67	0.69

We also compared the CNR, GCNR, PSNR, and SSIM distributions of reconstructed B-mode images obtained from 360 *in-vivo* test frames. Table 2 showed that the proposed deep beamformer consistently outperformed the standard DAS beamformer for all subsampling schemes and ratios. One big advantage of ultrasound image modality is it run-time imaging capability, which require fast reconstruction time. Another important advantage of the proposed method is the run-time complexity. The average reconstruction time for each depth planes is around 4.8 (ms), which could be easily reduce by optimized implementation and reconstruction of multiple depth planes in parallel.

In contrast to [13] where deep learning approach was designed for interpolating missing RF data to be used as input for standard beamformer (BF), the proposed method is an end-to-end CNN-based beamforming pipeline, without requiring additional BF. To verify that the new approach does not sacrifice any performance, we performed quantitative study using test dataset. As shown in Supplementary Material, the proposed network outperform the method in [13] in both CNR and GCNR.

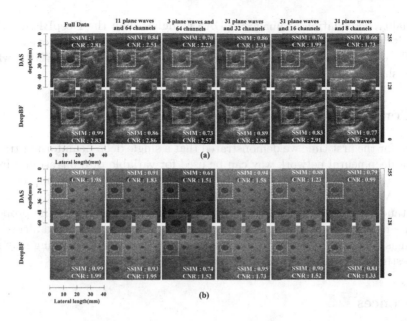

Fig. 3. Planewave B-mode imaging reconstruction results of standard DAS beamformer and the proposed method for: (a) in-vivo carotid region (b) tissue mimicking phantom.

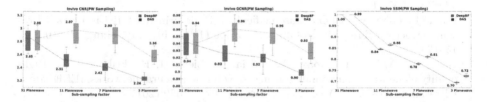

Fig. 4. Quantitative comparison using invivo data on different subsampling schemes in plane wave imaging: (first column) CNR value distribution, (second column) GCNR value distribution, (third column) SSIM value distribution.

Planewave US Imaging. Figure 3(a) and (b) show the results *in vivo* and phantom image examples for different down-sampling schemes. The images are generated using the proposed DeepBF and the standard DAS beam-former method. Our method significantly improves the visual quality of the US images by estimating the correct dynamic range and eliminating artifacts for both sampling schemes. From zoomed region images, it can be seen that the quality of the DeepBF images is relatively unchanged for variable sampling scenarios. Note that the proposed method successfully reconstruction both the near and the far field regions with equal efficacy, and only minor structural details are imperceivable. In addition, we compared the CNR, GCNR, and SSIM distributions of reconstructed B-mode images obtained from 100 invivo test frames. Our method shows significant performance gain in all measures. From Fig. 4, it is evident that the quality degradation of images in DAS is higher than the DeepBF. Furthermore, it is remarkable that the CNR value are significantly improved by the DeepBF even for the fully sampled case (eg. from 2.85 to 2.86 in CNR), which clearly shows the advantages of the proposed method.

4   Conclusion

Herein, for the first time we demonstrated that a single deep beamformer trained using a deep neural network way can be used for variable rate ultrasound imaging. Even for fully sampled data, the proposed method further improves the images. Moreover, CNR, GCNR, PSNR, and SSIM were significantly improved over standard DAS method across various subsampling schemes. The proposed schemes may substantially help in designing low-powered accelerated ultrasound imaging systems. Runtime implementation for cardiac or fetus imaging may help in investigating clinical significance of the proposed method.

References

1. Dahl, J.J., Mcaleavey, S.A., Pinton, G.F., Soo, M.S., Trahey, G.E.: Adaptive imaging on a diagnostic ultrasound scanner at quasi real-time rates. IEEE Trans. Ultrason. Ferroelectr. Freq. Control 53(10), 1832–1843 (2006). https://doi.org/10.1109/TUFFC.2006.115
2. Fink, M.: Time reversal of ultrasonic fields. I. Basic principles. IEEE Trans. Ultrason. Ferroelectr. Freq. Control 39(5), 555–566 (1992). https://doi.org/10.1109/58.156174
3. Gasse, M., Millioz, F., Roux, E., Garcia, D., Liebgott, H., Friboulet, D.: High-quality plane wave compounding using convolutional neural networks. IEEE Trans. Ultrason. Ferroelectr. Freq. Control 64(10), 1637–1639 (2017)
4. Glorot, X., Bengio, Y.: Understanding the difficulty of training deep feedforward neural networks. In: Proceedings of the Thirteenth International Conference on Artificial Intelligence and Statistics, pp. 249–256 (2010)
5. Jensen, A.C., Austeng, A.: The iterative adaptive approach in medical ultrasound imaging. IEEE Trans. Ultrason. Ferroelectr. Freq. Control 61(10), 1688–1697 (2014). https://doi.org/10.1109/TUFFC.2014.006478
6. Kim, J., Lee, J.K., Lee, K.M.: Accurate image super-resolution using very deep convolutional networks. In: Proceedings of the IEEE Conference on Computer Vision and Pattern Recognition, pp. 1646–1654 (2016)
7. Kim, K., Park, S., Kim, J., Park, S., Bae, M.: A fast minimum variance beamforming method using principal component analysis. IEEE Trans. Ultrason. Ferroelectr. Freq. Control 61(6), 930–945 (2014). https://doi.org/10.1109/TUFFC.2014.2989
8. Rodriguez-Molares, A., Hoel Rindal, O.M., D'hooge, J., Måsøy, S., Austeng, A., Torp, H.: The generalized contrast-to-noise ratio. In: 2018 IEEE International Ultrasonics Symposium (IUS), pp. 1–4, October 2018. https://doi.org/10.1109/ULTSYM.2018.8580101
9. Vedaldi, A., Lenc, K.: MatConvNet: convolutional neural networks for MATLAB. In: Proceedings of the 23rd ACM International Conference on Multimedia, pp. 689–692. ACM (2015)

10. Viola, F., Walker, W.F.: Adaptive signal processing in medical ultrasound beam-forming. In: IEEE Ultrasonics Symposium, 2005, vol. 4, pp. 1980–1983, September 2005. https://doi.org/10.1109/ULTSYM.2005.1603264
11. Wu, F., Thomas, J., Fink, M.: Time reversal of ultrasonic fields. II. Experimental results. IEEE Trans. Ultrason. Ferroelectr. Freq. Control **39**(5), 567–578 (1992). https://doi.org/10.1109/58.156175
12. Ye, J.C., Sung, W.K.: Understanding geometry of encoder-decoder CNNs. In: Chaudhuri, K., Salakhutdinov, R. (eds.) Proceedings of the 36th International Conference on Machine Learning. Proceedings of Machine Learning Research, vol. 97, pp. 7064–7073. PMLR, Long Beach, 09–15 June 2019
13. Yoon, Y.H., Khan, S., Huh, J., Ye, J.C.: Efficient B-mode ultrasound image recon-struction from sub-sampled RF data using deep learning. IEEE Trans. Med. Imag-ing **38**(2), 325–336 (2018)

Towards Whole Placenta Segmentation at Late Gestation Using Multi-view Ultrasound Images

Veronika A. Zimmer[1]([✉]), Alberto Gomez[1], Emily Skelton[1], Nicolas Toussaint[1], Tong Zhang[1], Bishesh Khanal[1,2], Robert Wright[1], Yohan Noh[1,3], Alison Ho[4], Jacqueline Matthew[1], Joseph V. Hajnal[1], and Julia A. Schnabel[1]

[1] School of Biomedical Engineering and Imaging Sciences, King's College London, London, UK
veronika.zimmer@kcl.ac.uk
[2] Nepal Applied Mathematics and Informatics Institute for Research (NAAMII), Kathmandu, Nepal
[3] Department of Mechanical and Aerospace Engineering, Brunel University London, Uxbridge, UK
[4] Department of Women and Children's Health, School of Life Course Sciences, King's College London, London, UK

Abstract. We propose a method to extract the human placenta at late gestation using multi-view 3D US images. This is the first step towards automatic quantification of placental volume and morphology from US images along the whole pregnancy beyond early stages (where the entire placenta can be captured with a single 3D US image). Our method uses 3D US images from different views acquired with a multi-probe system. A whole placenta segmentation is obtained from these images by using a novel technique based on 3D convolutional neural networks. We demonstrate the performance of our method on 3D US images of the placenta in the last trimester. We achieve a high Dice overlap of up to 0.8 with respect to manual annotations, and the derived placental volumes are comparable to corresponding volumes extracted from MR.

1 Introduction

Fetal ultrasound (US) is the primary imaging modality to monitor fetal development. While the fetal body, especially the fetal brain, are subjects of intensive research, only few methods exist to study the placenta in utero [1]. Placental development and function influence fetal health yet only placental site and cord insertion are routinely assessed using US. Limiting factors are the large size of the placenta at late gestation, high variation in shape and position, the limited field-of-view (FoV) and the lack of contrast in US. Placenta magnetic resonance image (MRI) acquisition overcomes some of those challenges as it provides a large FoV and an excellent soft-tissue contrast. Recently, the first method to assess the placenta in utero in a standardized way was presented using fetal MRI [2].

© Springer Nature Switzerland AG 2019
D. Shen et al. (Eds.): MICCAI 2019, LNCS 11768, pp. 628–636, 2019.
https://doi.org/10.1007/978-3-030-32254-0_70

However, fetal MRI is corrupted by motion artifacts due to fetal motion and maternal breathing and fetal MRI reconstruction is an active field of research [3]. US is still the standard screening tool because, in contrast to MRI, it is performed in real-time, is relatively inexpensive, and widely available. MRI is generally only used upon referral from the US clinic to gain insight into specific conditions. US based placenta segmentation could therefore lead to automatic volume quantification, morphology and function, in clinical routine scans. In [4], a semi-automatic method based on the random walker algorithm was proposed to segment the placenta. State-of-the-art segmentation methods using convolutional neural networks (CNNs) have been used in [5,6] and in [7] additionally for the fetus and the gestational sac. These methods focused on early pregnancies between 10–14 weeks of gestational age (GA), when the placenta is small enough to fit in the limited FoV of US. Routine anomaly screening is performed at 20 weeks GA but placental volume at later gestations may be of benefit in predicting/monitoring fetal development. Therefore a larger field of view is required to capture the whole placenta by US.

Multi-view imaging can be used to extend the FoV of a single image. For example, the entire placenta can be captured by acquiring, aligning and fusing multiple 3D US images (Fig. 1). In previous works [8–10], registration algorithm and/or tracker information were employed to align the images and provide multi-view US. The resulting image has an extended FoV, and view-dependent artifacts such as shadows can be minimized through the additional signal information from multiple views [11]. Aligning US placenta remains however challenging, due to the lack of salient features to drive the registration process. External tracking, on the other hand, can provide position information of the US probe but is oblivious to maternal and fetal motion.

In this work, we introduce, for the first time, a pipeline to extract the whole placenta at late gestation. The approach consist of three stages: first, multi-view image acquisition, second, multi-view image fusion, and third, multi-view placenta segmentation. The multi-view US images are acquired using a time-interleaved multi-probe US system without the need of image registration. We present a voxel-wise image fusion method to combine the images and to reduce view-dependent artifacts, and compare four approaches based on CNNs to extract the whole placenta from the multi-view images.

We test our pipeline on a dataset of 3D US images to estimate placental volume in the last trimester of pregnancy. We successfully fuse multi-view images to get an extended FoV and are able to extract the placenta. The derived placental volumes are comparable to corresponding volumes extracted from MR. To the best of our knowledge, this is the first time the placenta is segmented at late gestation from US imaging.

2   Methods and Materials

The three stages of the proposed pipeline for whole placenta extraction (multi-view acquisition, fusion and segmentation) are described below.

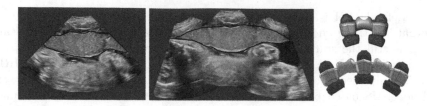

Fig. 1. Ultrasound placenta imaging using a multi-probe system. Left: slice of 3D US image (30.6 weeks GA) covering only part of the placenta; Middle: slice of 3D multi-view image of the whole placenta; Right: physical multi-probe holder for two and three US probes.

2.1 Multi-probe Ultrasound Imaging

We acquire multiple US images using an in-house US signal multiplexer which allows to connect multiple Philips X6-1 probes to a Philips EPIQ V7 US system. The multiplexer switches rapidly between up to three probes so that images from each probe are acquired in a time-interleaved fashion. The manual operation of the transducers is very slow compared to the acquisition frame rate. Therefore, for the purpose of data processing, consecutive images are assumed to have been acquired simultaneously over a small time window. We designed a physical device that fixes the probes in an angle of 30° to each other, which ensures a large overlap between the images, and allows easy and comfortable operation (see Fig. 1).

2.2 Multi-view Image Fusion

In our application, the goal is to combine multiple images of the placenta to extend the FoV while minimizing view-dependent artifacts. The multi-view fusion method proposed in [11] produces high quality fusion but is computationally expensive. We propose a simplification of that method by replacing the B-spline based fusion for a voxel-wise fusion as follows.

Let $I_1, \ldots, I_V$, with $I_v : \Omega \subset \mathbb{R}^d \to \mathbb{R}, i = 1, \ldots, V$ be images of the same object taken from V views. Their spatial correspondences are known through spatial transformations $\phi_v : \Omega_v \subset \mathbb{R}^d \to \Omega \subset \mathbb{R}^d$. The fused image $I_F : \Omega_F \to \mathbb{R}$ with $\Omega_1, \ldots, \Omega_V \subset \Omega_F$ at point $\mathbf{x} \in \Omega_F$ is obtained by

$$I_F(\mathbf{x}) = \frac{\sum_{v=1}^{V} w_v(\mathbf{x}) \cdot \mathbb{1}_{\mathbf{x} \in \Omega_v} \cdot (I_v \circ \phi_v)(\mathbf{x})}{\sum_{v=1}^{V} w_v(\mathbf{x})}$$

with weight function $w : \mathbb{R}^d \to \mathbb{R}$. In other words, the intensity of a point $\mathbf{x}$ of the fused image is calculated by the weighted mean of corresponding points in the single images. The weight of a (transformed) data point $\mathbf{x}$ are formulated as a function of the depth in the US image with respect to the probe position $\mathbf{b} \in \mathbb{R}^d$ and the beam angle $\alpha \in [-\frac{\pi}{2}, \frac{\pi}{2}]$ in the same way as in [11]. In effect, image points with a strong signal (to correct for shadow artifacts) and at a position close to the center of the US frustum (where the quality of the image is typically the best) will receive higher weights.

2.3 Whole Placental Segmentation

Semantic Segmentation Using Neural Networks. In recent years, convolutional neural networks (CNNs) have shown excellent segmentation results, outperforming conventional methods in quality of the segmentation and in speed [12,13]. In a supervised CNN approach, the segmentation of an object is learned only driven by the data from a training dataset $T = \{(I_n, S_n), n = 1, \ldots, N\}$, with images $I_n : \mathbb{R}^d \to \mathbb{R}$ and ground truth segmentations $S_n : \mathbb{R}^d \to \{0, 1\}$ (in our case US images with $d = 3$ and manual annotations of the placenta). The model f estimates for an input image I the segmentation map S: $S = f(I, \Theta)$. During the training process of model $f(I, \Theta)$ with the training set T, the parameters of the network $\Theta \in \mathbb{R}^P$ are optimized to minimize a loss function $\mathcal{L}$, which measures the agreement between the ground truth S_n and the estimated segmentation of the model. The parameters Θ include the connection weights, biases and convolutional kernel weights.

Our segmentation network is based on the widely used U-net architecture [12] which is a fully convolutional neural network with an encoder-decoder architecture, a bottleneck layer in between and skip connections from encoder layers to decoder. We use ReLUs, strided convolution using max pooling for downsampling, and zero padding. We set [32, 64, 128, 256] feature maps per layer where all the convolutional kernels and feature maps are in 3D.

For training, we resample all images to size $128 \times 128 \times 128$. During training, we minimize the Dice loss using the Adam optimizer and a learning rate of 0.001. We augment our dataset by image flipping in x- and z-axis (avoid flipping the image upside down to keep the correct positioning of the US frustum), intensity rescaling by $\pm 10\%$ and small random translation (up to five pixels in all directions). Rotations are avoided because that would produce non-realistic view direction-dependent image features.

Multi-view Image Segmentation. At later gestation, the FoV of US is too small to capture the whole placenta with a single US probe. Multiple probes, as described above, or placenta sweeps using an appropriate registration or tracking method to align the images, can be used to visualize the whole placenta in one US volume. Those images differ not only in the view of the placenta, but also in view-dependent artifacts, such as shadows or attenuation. To provide a consistent segmentation of the whole placenta across multiple images, we propose four CNN-based variants, which make use of the multi-view information in different ways (see Fig. 2).

(S1) The model f_1 is trained on N single US images I_n^s with manual annotations $S_n^s, n = 1, \ldots, N$ of the placenta, without using any information of correspondences between different views of the same placenta. The resulting segmentations for the individual images are aligned and fused using maximum intensity voting to obtain the segmentation of the whole placenta.

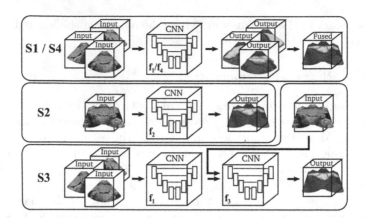

Fig. 2. Illustration of strategies to obtain multi-view placenta segmentation using 3D convolutional networks.

(S2) The model f_2 is trained on $M < N$ fused multi-view images I_m^{mv} with manual annotations $S_m^{mv}, m = 1, \ldots, M$. The training set is smaller compared to approach (S1) since one image I_m^{mv} is the fusion of two or three images I_n^s. The fused images are resampled to size $192 \times 128 \times 128$. The larger size in the first dimension is to account for the larger FoV in the fused images.

(S3) The model f_1, trained on individual images, is re-trained as model f_3 using fused multi-view images (re-sampled to the size of individual images) which have been separately annotated. Using pre-trained weights from f_1 as initialization allows to train on the smaller dataset of fused images.

(S4) The last model f_4 is trained in a similar manner as f_1, except that the individual annotations are obtained from the manual segmentations of the fused multi-view images by mapping them from the fused image space back to the single image space. This reduces the amount of manual segmentations to carry out for the same amount of training data. The manual segmentation task is easier since fused images have better image quality and larger FoV.

3   Experimental Results

3.1   Dataset

We used a dataset of 127 3D US images to test our pipeline, which were selected from 4D (3D+time) image streams from 30 patients covering different parts of the placenta. Each acquisition was performed as part of a defined scan protocol by one of two operators. A subset of 94 images were acquired with a two-transducer (64) or a three-transducer (30) holder device, and the rest were acquired using a single transducer. Two patients were in the second trimester (24 and 25 weeks GA) and the others in the third trimester (29–34 weeks GA). We split the dataset into training (85 images), validation (16 images) and test

Table 1. Segmentation accuracy measured using the Dice coefficient and relative volume difference (mean±std.).

		Train	Validate	Test (single)	Test (multi-view)
S1	# images	85	16	26	12
	Dice	0.80 ± 0.09	0.75 ± 0.15	0.74 ± 0.15	**0.81 ± 0.05**
	Δ vol (%)	16.1 ± 17.9	27.9 ± 22.5	26.2 ± 22.1	**16.5 ± 12.2**
S2	# images	27	3	–	12
	Dice	0.75 ± 0.12	0.84 ± 0.10	–	0.76 ± 0.17
	Δ vol (%)	23.8 ± 18.7	13.2 ± 19.5	–	20.7 ± 27.1
S3	# images	85/27	16/3	–	12
	Dice	0.86 ± 0.04	0.83 ± 0.11	–	**0.80 ± 0.11**
	Δ vol (%)	11.9 ± 7.7	16.8 ± 21.3	–	**15.9 ± 19.9**
S4	# images	85	16	26	12
	Dice	0.70 ± 0.15	0.61 ± 0.24	0.65 ± 0.18	0.72 ± 0.12
	Δ vol (%)	28.6 ± 25.7	44.7 ± 29.5	37.1 ± 25.2	20.8 ± 15.8

set (26 images). When trained only on multi-view images (approaches (S2) and (S3)), the sets reduce to 27, 3 and 12 images for training, validation and testing, respectively.

3.2 Results

The results for placenta segmentation are shown in Table 1 and a representative example of whole placenta segmentations is shown in Fig. 3. The accuracy of the segmentation during training, validation and inference are calculated using the Dice overlap and the absolut volume difference relative to the ground truth segmentation. Methods (S1) and (S3) both achieve the best results with a mean Dice of 0.8 and a volume difference of around 16% for the multi-view images of the whole placenta with the smallest volume difference obtained by (S3) at 15.9%. The additional CNN in (S3) did not improve the results from (S1) further. For (S2), the training was performed only on the multi-view images, and therefore fewer images were used for training. Unsurprisingly, this yields worse results than (S3), which was pre-trained. The worst results were obtained using (S4). This can be explained by the fact that although the ground truth segmentation incorporates information from all views, the network is trained on individual images and therefore not capable of learning the relation between different views of the same object. To test for significance, we performed a paired Wilcoxon signed-rank test on the Dice overlaps. The results for single images (only S1 and S4) are significantly different with $p < 0.001$. On multi-view images, we found a significant difference between S1 and S4 ($p = 0.018$) and S2 and S3 ($p = 0.02$).

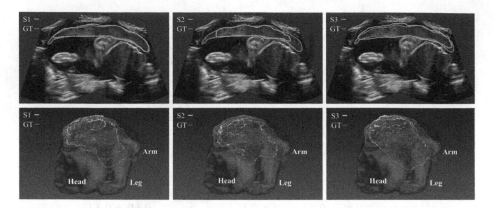

Fig. 3. Top row: 2D slice showing a cut of the 3D whole-placenta segmentation (24.4 weeks GA); Bottom row: 3D visualization of fetus and placenta. Automatic segmentations (in green) using (S1) (left), (S2) (centre) and (S3) (right). Ground truth is shown in red. (Color figure online)

Table 2. Comparison of placental volume (PV, in mm^3) extracted from US (manual and automatic) and MR (manual) segmentations (seg.). (S1) US: automatic seg. from US using method (S1); GT US: manual ground truth seg.; MR: manual MR seg.

	GA	(S1) US PV	GT US PV	MR PV	(S1)/MR	GT/MR
1	32+2	549.6	583.9	588.8	−6.66	**−0.83**
2	30+1	505.5	539.9	534.1	−5.35	**1.09**
3	33+1	616.6	605.5	664.1	**−7.15**	−8.82
4	31+2	584.8	614.5	578	**−1.18**	6.31

Additionally, we compared the placental volume measured in MRI and US for a subset of the data. Table 2 shows the results using manual expert segmentations of the MRI data, the multi-view US data and automatic segmentation with method (S1). All US volumes differ less than 10% from the corresponding MR volume, suggesting that nearly the whole placenta is covered by the multi-view US images.

4   Conclusions

We proposed a fully automatic method for the extraction of whole placenta volumes at late gestation. The method consists of three stages, namely multi-view image acquisition, image fusion and placenta segmentation. We used CNNs with a standard architecture (U-net) for the segmentation procedure. We showed with four approaches how this can be adapted to multi-view placenta segmentation with a dice overlap of 0.8 and placental volumes comparable to MR.

The automatic segmentation underestimates the placental volume, both for the manual annotation in US (see Fig. 3) and the MR volume (see Table 2).

This consistent negative bias could be explained by the poor contrast in US and requires further investigation. The manual annotation is challenging and thin parts of the placenta, especially at the boundaries, as shown in Fig. 3, are hard to delineate. Future work will include the refinement of the segmentation method. However, the negative bias with respect to the MR volume is also present in the manual annotations from US [14]. Apart from the poor contrast in US, some part of the placenta might still be missing in the multi-view images. In this work, the placental MR volume is extracted from the raw MR volume prior to motion correction and reconstruction, which explains also some of the differences between US and MR annotations. Our method enables future work for the comparison of US and MR placenta in more detail.

Our approach is suitable for real-time application, with an inference time of 40 ms. Enabling automatic placenta extraction from US in clinical routine can pave the way for placenta-based abnormality detection.

Acknowledgements. This work was supported by the Wellcome Trust IEH Award [102431], by the Wellcome/EPSRC Centre for Medical Engineering [WT203148/Z/16/Z] and by the National Institute for Health Research (NIHR) Biomedical Research Centre at Guy's and St Thomas' NHS Foundation Trust and King's College London. The views expressed are those of the author(s) and not necessarily those of the NHS, the NIHR or the Department of Health.

References

1. Torrents-Barrena, J., et al.: Segmentation and classification in MRI and US fetal imaging: recent trends and future prospects. Med. Imag. Anal. **51**, 61–88 (2019)
2. Miao, H., et al.: Placenta maps: in utero placental health assessment of the human fetus. IEEE Trans. Vis. Comp. Graph. **23**(6), 1612–1623 (2017)
3. Torrents-Barrena, J., et al.: Fully automatic 3D reconstruction of the placenta and its peripheral vasculature in intrauterine fetal MRI. Med. Imag. Anal. **54**, 263–279 (2019)
4. Stevenson, G.N., Collins, S.L., Ding, J., Impey, L., Noble, J.A.: 3-D ultrasound segmentation of the placenta using the random walker algorithm: reliability and agreement. Ultras. Med. Biol. **41**(12), 3182–3193 (2015)
5. Oguz, B.U., et al.: Combining deep learning and multi-atlas label fusion for automated placenta segmentation from 3DUS. In: Melbourne, A., et al. (eds.) PIPPI/DATRA -2018. LNCS, vol. 11076, pp. 138–148. Springer, Cham (2018). https://doi.org/10.1007/978-3-030-00807-9_14
6. Looney, P., et al.: Fully automated, real-time 3D ultrasound segmentation to estimate first trimester placental volume using deep learning. JCI Insight **3**(11), e120178 (2018). https://doi.org/10.1172/jci.insight.120178
7. Yang, X., et al.: Towards automated semantic segmentation in prenatal volumetric ultrasound. IEEE Trans. Med. Imag. **38**(1), 180–193 (2018)
8. Wachinger, C., Wein, W., Navab, N.: Three-dimensional ultrasound mosaicing. In: Ayache, N., Ourselin, S., Maeder, A. (eds.) MICCAI 2007. LNCS, vol. 4792, pp. 327–335. Springer, Heidelberg (2007). https://doi.org/10.1007/978-3-540-75759-7_40

9. Ni, D., et al.: Volumetric ultrasound panorama based on 3D SIFT. In: Metaxas, D., Axel, L., Fichtinger, G., Székely, G. (eds.) MICCAI 2008. LNCS, vol. 5242, pp. 52–60. Springer, Heidelberg (2008). https://doi.org/10.1007/978-3-540-85990-1_7

10. Gomez, A., Bhatia, K., Tharin, S., Housden, J., Toussaint, N., Schnabel, J.A.: Fast registration of 3D fetal ultrasound images using learned corresponding salient points. In: Cardoso, M.J., et al. (eds.) FIFI/OMIA -2017. LNCS, vol. 10554, pp. 33–41. Springer, Cham (2017). https://doi.org/10.1007/978-3-319-67561-9_4

11. Zimmer, V.A., et al.: Multi-view image reconstruction: application to fetal ultrasound compounding. In: Melbourne, A., et al. (eds.) PIPPI/DATRA -2018. LNCS, vol. 11076, pp. 107–116. Springer, Cham (2018). https://doi.org/10.1007/978-3-030-00807-9_11

12. Ronneberger, O., Fischer, P., Brox, T.: U-net: convolutional networks for biomedical image segmentation. In: Navab, N., Hornegger, J., Wells, W.M., Frangi, A.F. (eds.) MICCAI 2015. LNCS, vol. 9351, pp. 234–241. Springer, Cham (2015). https://doi.org/10.1007/978-3-319-24574-4_28

13. Litjens, G., et al.: A survey on deep learning in medical image analysis. Med. Imag. Anal. **42**, 60–88 (2017)

14. Gomez, A., et al.: Regional differences in end-diastolic volumes between 3D echo and CMR in HLHS patients. Front. Pediatr. **4**, 133 (2016)

Single Shot Needle Tip Localization in 2D Ultrasound

Cosmas Mwikirize[1]([✉])[iD], John L. Nosher[2], and Ilker Hacihaliloglu[1,2]

[1] Department of Biomedical Engineering, Rutgers University,
Piscataway, NJ 08854, USA
cosmas.mwikirize@rutgers.edu
[2] Department of Radiology, Rutgers Robert Wood Johnson Medical School,
New Brunswick, NJ 08901, USA

Abstract. We present a novel real-time technique for dynamic localization of the needle tip in 2D ultrasound during challenging interventions in which the tip is imperceptible or shaft information is unavailable. We first enhance the needle tip from time-series ultrasound data through digital subtraction of consecutive frames. The enhanced tip image is then fed to a cascade of similar convolutional neural networks: a tip classifier and a tip location regressor. The classifier ascertains tip motion and the regressor directly outputs the coordinates of the tip. Since we do not require needle shaft information, the method achieves efficient localization of both in-plane and out-of-plane needles. Our approach is trained and evaluated on an *ex vivo* dataset collected using two different ultrasound machines, with in-plane and out-of-plane insertion of 17G and 22G needles in bovine, porcine and chicken tissue. We use $12,000$ frames extracted from 40 video sequences for training and validation, and 500 frames from 20 sequences as test data. The framework achieves a tip localization error of 0.55 ± 0.07 mm, and overall processing time of 0.015 s (67 fps). Validation studies against state-of-the-art achieved 29% and 509% improvement in accuracy and processing rate respectively. Because of the real-time execution time and accurate tip localization, we believe that our approach is potentially a breakthrough for real-time needle tip localization in challenging ultrasound-guided interventions.

Keywords: Needle enhancement · Needle localization · Ultrasound · Deep learning

1 Introduction

Although two-dimensional (2D) ultrasound (US) has become the standard-of-care for guidance of minimally invasive procedures such as regional anesthesia and percutaneous interventional oncology, the success of these procedures is still

Electronic supplementary material The online version of this chapter (https://doi.org/10.1007/978-3-030-32254-0_71) contains supplementary material, which is available to authorized users.

D. Shen et al. (Eds.): MICCAI 2019, LNCS 11768, pp. 637–645, 2019.
https://doi.org/10.1007/978-3-030-32254-0_71

hindered by technical limitations of US. For instance, in-plane needles are difficult to align with the US beam especially at steep insertion angles. Further, thin needles do not give adequate reflection of the US beam. These challenges often lead to a low intensity shaft and tip, thus making needle localization difficult. For needles inserted out-of-plane, the tip is even more difficult to discern from the image in absence of shaft information.

To address this challenge, learning based methods for localizing needles in US have recently become prominent. For instance, Pourtaherian et al. demonstrated semantic needle segmentation in 3D US using orthogonal-plane convolutional networks [5], but their approach required computationally expensive processing routines for volumetric data (4–5 min for patch classification and 2–3 s for semantic segmentation). Still targeting 3D US, Arif et al. have achieved an automatic needle detection and tracking method that runs at 3 fps [4]. For 2D US, Beigi et al. proposed imperceptible needle tracking using spatiotemporal and spectral features [3]. Although their method achieves a good tip localization error of 0.82 mm, it has a processing rate of <1 fps and localizes only in-plane needles. Mwikirize et al. proposed a detection and tracking method for partially visible needles, achieving a localization error of 0.23 mm, and processing rate of ≈2 fps for in-plane needles [2]. Recently, Mwikirize et al. also demonstrated localization of both in-plane and out-of-plane needles, with a localization error of 0.72 mm and processing time of 10 fps [1]. In [1], the needle tip is enhanced from two consecutive frames, augmented by solving a total variation regularization problem to minimize irrelevant motion effects, and localized using a deep learning framework that inserts a bounding box around the tip. Tip location is then estimated as the center of this bounding box. Despite these recent advances, a method that accurately localizes needles in US at a real-time processing rate is yet to be demonstrated.

In this paper, we are motivated by the two-frame foreground detection model reported in [1] to develop a framework for needle tip localization with superior localization accuracy and computational efficiency. From a sequence of 2D US frames, we enhance the needle tip using a technique similar to [1]. In the enhanced tip images, we are interested in the frames in which substantial needle motion has occurred. Therefore, we formulate a deep learning model that sequentially performs classification (we want to know if an enhanced tip exists) and direct needle tip localization (if it exists, show us where it is). We treat the enhanced needle tip as a landmark which we define using two keypoints. Our main contribution here is a novel framework consisting of a cascade of a classification and a vanilla regression Convolutional Neural Network (CNN) for learning needle tip descriptors in 2D US.

Using a combination of the classification and regression networks achieves better performance than prior art. This is the first needle localization approach to achieve true real-time performance (67 fps) with clinically acceptable accuracy (0.55 ± 0.07) mm. The proposed method could be useful for localizing needles in interventional procedures where there are limited external motion events, for

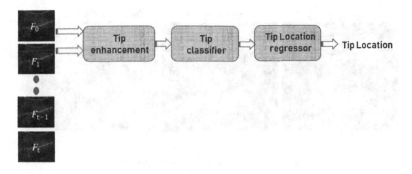

Fig. 1. Hierarchy of the proposed method. F_0 to F_t are US frames in a sequence.

example during peripheral nerve blocks. Next, we describe our framework in detail.

2 Methods

Our objective is a framework that automatically localizes the needle tip in temporal US data. The framework should be robust to intensity variations between images captured under different imaging scenarios and needle insertion profiles. The proposed methods targets both out-of-plane and in-plane inserted needles in which the tip exhibits low contrast to the rest of the US image. The proposed approach consists of three stages illustrated in Fig. 1: (a) enhancement of the needle tip from 2 consecutive US frames, (b) determining whether the enhanced image contains substantial needle tip information, using a classifier network, and (c) estimating the needle tip location using a keypoint regression CNN. The classification step is necessary because the hand-inserted needle tip does not move smoothly through space and hence there will be frames in the sequence where the needle tip has not changed spatial location. Next, we describe these processes.

2.1 Dataset Overview

The 2D B-mode US images we used in our learning experiments were collected using two imaging systems: SonixGPS (Analogic Corporation, Peabody, MA, USA) with a hand-held C5-2/60 curvilinear probe, and 2D hand-held wireless US (Clarius C3, Clarius Mobile Health Corporation, Burnaby, BC, Canada). We inserted needles of types: a 17G SonixGPS vascular access needle (Analogic Corporation, Peabody, MA, USA) and a 22G spinal Quincke-type needle (Becton, Dickinson and Company, Franklin Lakes, NJ, USA) in freshly excised bovine and porcine tissue, as well as chicken breast overlaid on a lumbosacral spine phantom. The needles were inserted both in-plane (30° to 70° insertion angle) and out-of-plane up to a depth of 70 mm. For the SonixGPS needle, we collected tip localization data from the electromagnetic (EM) tracking system (Ascension Technology Corporation, Shelburne, VT, USA). During the experiments,

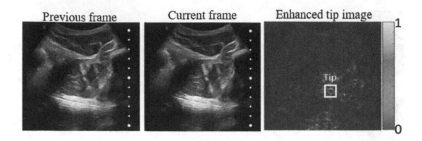

Fig. 2. The tip enhancement process.

minor motion events were simulated by exerting pressure on the tissue with the probe, and probe rotation. In total, we collected 60 volumes (30 in-plane, 30 out-of-plane: 40 with SonixGPS system and 20 with Clarius C3 system), with each video sequence having more than 600 frames. For the training and validating the tip classifier, we used a total of 7000 positive examples (enhanced images with the tip) and 5000 negative examples (enhanced images without tip information). For tip location regression, we used 7000 images (only positive examples) for training and validation, and for testing, we used 500 images from 20 sequencies not used for training and validation.

2.2 Needle Tip Enhancement

The needle enhancement process follows [1]. From a US frame sequence $F_0, F_1...F_{t-1}, F_t$ where the subscript denotes the respective temporal position and F_0 is the first frame, we compute $z(x, y)$, the logical difference of consecutive frames: For a current frame $n(x, y)$ and a previous frame $m(x, y)$,

$$z(x, y) = m^c(x, y) \wedge n(x, y). \tag{1}$$

Here, $m^c(x, y)$ is the bitwise complement of $m(x, y)$, while $\wedge$ is the bitwise AND logical operation. This logical differencing routine will produce intensities $T : [0, 255]$ representative of the difference between the two frames. Therefore, subtle motion between the two frames will be captured. It is expected that the needle tip will give us the most prominent feature in $z(x, y)$. Different than [1], to compensate for irrelevant motion events, we apply a 12×12 median filter to $z(x, y)$ and do not perform any further tip augmentation. Figure 2 shows the result of the tip enhancement process.

2.3 Tip Classification Network

The architecture of the tip classification network is shown in Fig. 3. The network consists of 6 blocks of convolution, ReLU, batch normalization and max pooling layers, 2 blocks of convolution, ReLU and batch normalization layers, and 3 fully connected layers. The input consists of a 256×256 image. All convolution layers

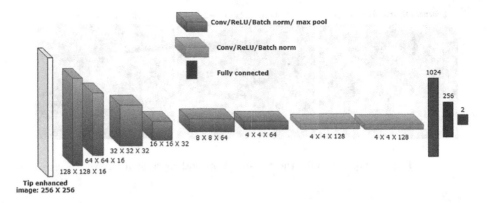

Fig. 3. The tip classification network. The tensor dimensions of the activation feature maps after each block are indicated.

utilize a 3 × 3 kernel, and a stride/padding of 1 pixel. The max pooling layers utilize a 2 × 2 kernel.

Positive and negative examples for the enhanced needle tip (Fig. 4) are labeled by an expert radiologist with over 30 years of experience in interventional radiology, while referring to the corresponding original US sequences and EM tracking information for tracked needles. In positive examples, the tip exists as a distinct high intensity feature, a few pixels thick, against a low intensity background. Such a feature is lacking from the negative training examples. If other high intensity noisy artifacts exist, the classifier can differentiate them from the needle. Note that last feature map for the classification task, from the last fully connected (FC) layer, is a vector of dimension $1 \times 1 \times 2$, i.e., it is meant to differentiate images of two classes: those with an enhanced tip and those without it. We apply Softmax activation to this feature map and use the Log Loss to calculate deviations between the network output and the ground-truth. During training, we use stochastic gradient descent with momentum (SGDM) optimizer, and initial learning rate of 10^{-2}.

2.4   Tip Regression Network

The architecture of the tip regression network mirrors the classification network (Fig. 3), with the exception of terminating in a 4-output FC layer (the needle tip location is defined by 2 keypoints as we will describe shortly). In essence, we have a cascade of two twin CNNs which share all the learned layers but differ only in the output. During training and testing, the classification task and the tip location regression task are run in series.

The input to the regression network is the tip enhanced image and the corresponding location labels. Keypoints for the needle tip are labeled as shown in Fig. 4. We use 2 keypoints on the needle tip, i.e., $t_p : (x_1, y_1), (x_2, y_2)$. The use of 2 keypoints constrains the spatial likelihood of the tip since the enhanced tip feature is not geometrically definable for labeling purposes. The keypoint labels

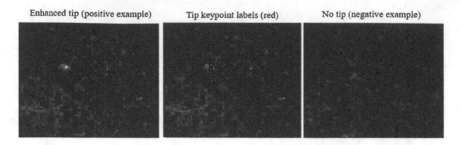

Enhanced tip (positive example)   Tip keypoint labels (red)   No tip (negative example)

Fig. 4. Tip labels for the classification and regression CNNs.

are placed geometrically opposite along a line through the center of the enhanced tip feature and the pixel at the distal end.

The enhanced images are augmented by rotating them through 90°, 180° and 270°. The labels are computationally manipulated to match the rotated images. From the original 7000 enhanced images, this yields 28,000 training examples. Further, the labels are normalized to be in the range $Q : [-1, 1]$. Since the initial labels are in the range $[1, 256]$, scaling reduces the magnitude of the Mean Squared Error (MSE), which we use as the loss function metric, and the magnitude of the gradients. This quickens the training process and ensures stable convergence. At test time, the outputs are rescaled to match the original data.

The last feature map for the regression task, from the last FC layer is a vector of dimension $1 \times 1 \times 4$, containing the four ordinates of the two labels: $(x_1, y_1), (x_2, y_2)$. During training, we use RMSprop optimizer, an initial learning rate of 10^{-3}, and a mini batch size of 32.

At test time, the tip location $T(x_t, y_t)$ is directly obtained from the network outputs as the average of the x and y outputs, i.e., $x_t = (x_1 + x_2)/2, y_t = (y_1 + y_2)/2$. Since we do not need a region-proposal step or anchor boxes to tell the network where to look, our framework provides a single-shot approach for tip localization.

3   Results and Analysis

Qualitative Results: Figure 5 shows examples of tip enhancement and localization. Note that tip has low contrast and shaft information is not visible, but our framework accurately localizes the tip. This is because our method detects subtle intensity changes arising from tip motion, that are otherwise not easily discernible with the naked eye. Further, localization accuracy is generally resilient to high intensity artifacts in the rest image.

Classification Accuracy: The classification network achieved an overall sensitivity and specificity of 88% and 82% respectively on test sequences. By comparison, the method in [1] achieved sensitivity and specificity of 95% and 90% respectively. Specifically, the method in [1] outperforms the proposed method

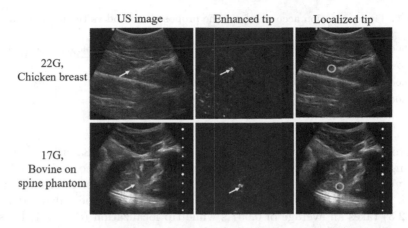

Fig. 5. Needle tip localization results. The red arrow points to the tip location while the green circle shows the localized tip. (Color figure online)

in presence of increased motion artifacts in the imaging medium ([1] includes a computationally expensive step for noise removal). However, in relatively stable sequences, the classification accuracy was similar (98% vs 97%). Therefore, the proposed method is suitable for procedures where there is minimal motion from physiological events, for example lumbar facet injections and peripheral nerve blocks. Nevertheless, we believe a larger training dataset would improve classification accuracy, even in the presence of motion artifacts.

Tip Localization Error: The groundtruth tip location is determined from the original US sequences by our expert radiologist, with augmentation from the EM tracking system. Localization error is determined from the Euclidean Distance (ED) between the automatically determined tip location from our approach and the ground truth. We evaluated the proposed method for both in-plane (IP) and out-of-plane (OP) needle insertions, and achieved an overall tip localization error of 0.55 ± 0.07 mm. A comparative analysis with other localization approaches is shown in Table 1. The proposed method outperforms the methods in [1,2] with a statistically significant improvement ($p < 0.005$). Since [2] requires shaft information, we used 250 test images from the sequences with in-plane needle insertion for its evaluation. For all the methods, we imposed an error cap of 2 mm as a measure of localization success. By dropping the worst 3% cases of the data analyzed with the method in [1] in order to obtain a 94% success rate similar to proposed method, the localization error dropped to 0.73 ± 0.07 mm which shows that our method still achieves improved results ($p < 0.005$). Most of the failed cases (6%) resulted from the tip localization network regressing onto a false artifact in the enhanced image. We anticipate that performance in this regard can be improved with a bigger training dataset.

Computation Time: All our experiments were ran on an NVIDIA GeForce GTX 1060 6 GB GPU, 3.6 GHz Intel(R) CoreTM i7 16 GB CPU Windows PC.

Table 1. Tip localization accuracy from the proposed method vs the methods in [1,2]

Method	Test data	Error (mm)	Processing time (s)	Success rate
Proposed method	500(250 IP, 250 OP)	0.55 ± 0.07	0.015 (67 fps)	94%
Method in [1]	500(250 IP, 250 OP)	0.78 ± 0.08	0.091 (11 fps)	97%
Method in [2]	250 (IP)	1.23 ± 0.45	0.42 (2 fps)	52%

The proposed method was implemented in MATLAB 2018a using the Deep Learning Toolbox. The learning framework is trained offline and tested with offline video sequences of US data. Average processing time for the enhancement process (Sect. 2.2) is 0.002 s per image. Classification of the enhanced image (Sect. 2.3) takes an average of 0.007 s while tip localization (Sect. 2.4) lasts for 0.006 s. The overall processing time is thus 0.015 s (67 fps), a real time speed. This is a 509% improvement, in fps, on the method in [1].

Network Ablation Studies: For the regression component of our learning framework, we investigated different network structures, consisting of different numbers of convolution and pooling layers and evaluated the relative performance using the normalized Root Mean Square Error (RMSE) on the validation dataset. The proposed method achieved a normalized RMSE of 0.006. This was better than that achieved by the maximum network depth for the 256×256 image input consisting of 8 convolution layers with pooling after each layer (0.014) and a network with only 6 convolution layers (0.05). We compared performance of different optimizers in the regression network. The following optimizers achieved the correspondingly indicated normalized RMSE: RMSprop (0.006), Adam (0.05), and SGDM (0.14). We also investigated the effect of using dropout layers in our network but there was no significant improvement in performance. Lastly, we compared the proposed regression network with other state-of-the-art regression methods: PoseCNN [6] and NaimishNet [7]. These achieved normalized RMSE of 0.029 and 0.303 respectively on the validation dataset compared to 0.006 from the proposed method. These comparative studies informed the design and fine-tuning of our regression network for optimal tip localization performance.

4   Conclusion

We have introduced a novel real-time approach for needle tip localization from 2D US sequences. The approach combines three subprocesses: tip enhancement from digital subtraction of consecutive frames, tip classification to determine whether an enhanced image contains tip information, and regression to automatically output the tip spatial coordinates. We demonstrate experimentally that our novel learning framework outperforms state-of-the-art methods [1,2] in computational efficiency and tip localization accuracy. To the best of our knowledge, this is the fastest needle enhancement and localization approach ever reported.

Given more data and computing resources, performance of the proposed method can further be improved.

Note that since our method relies on subtraction of consecutive frames, it is prone to interference from motion artifacts arising from physiological activity such as breathing or pulsation in the clinical setting. We hypothesize that with a larger training dataset, sensitivity to motion would be further reduced. This will form part of our future work. We will also extend our algorithm for localization of surgical tools for US-based spinal fusion surgery.

Acknowledgments. This work was accomplished with funding support from the North American Spine Society 2017 young investigator award.

References

1. Mwikirize, C., Nosher, J.L., Hacihaliloglu, I.: Learning needle tip localization from digital subtraction in 2D ultrasound. Int. J. CARS **14**(6), 1017–1026 (2019)
2. Mwikirize, C., Nosher, J.L., Hacihaliloglu, I.: Convolution neural networks for real-time needle detection and localization in 2D ultrasound. Int. J. CARS **13**(5), 647–657 (2018)
3. Beigi, P., Rohling, R., Salcudean, S., Ng, G.: CASPER: computer-aided segmentation of imperceptible motion-a learning-based tracking of an invisible needle in ultrasound. Int. J. CARS **12**(11), 1857–66 (2017)
4. Pourtaherian, A., et al.: Robust and semantic needle detection in 3D ultrasound using orthogonal-plane convolutional neural networks. Int. J. CARS **13**(9), 1321–1333 (2018)
5. Arif, M., Moelker, A., Walsum, T.V.: Automatic needle detection and real-time bi-planar needle visualization during 3D ultrasound scanning of the liver. Med. Image Anal. **53**, 104–110 (2019)
6. Xiang, Y., Schmidt, T., Narayanan, V., Fox, D.: PoseCNN: a convolutional neural network for 6D object pose estimation in cluttered scenes arXiv:1711.00199v3 (2017)
7. Agarwal, N., Krohn-Grimberghe, A., Vyas, R.: Facial key points detection using deep convolutional neural network - NaimishNet arXiv:1710.00977v1 (2017)

Discriminative Correlation Filter Network for Robust Landmark Tracking in Ultrasound Guided Intervention

Chunxu Shen[1,2], Jishuai He[1,2], Yibin Huang[3], and Jian Wu[2(✉)]

[1] Tsinghua University, Beijing 100084, China
{scxl6,hjsl8}@mails.tsinghua.edu.cn
[2] Graduate School at Shenzhen, Tsinghua University, Shenzhen 518055, China
wuj@sz.tsinghua.edu.cn
[3] Shenzhen Traditional Chinese Medicine Hospital, Shenzhen 518034, China
huangyb2004@126.com

Abstract. Due to uncertainties from breathing and drift in image-guided abdominal intervention, surgeon would add margins around target so that it can be adequately covered and treated. To mitigate the uncertainties and make motion management more effective, we develop a real-time and high accuracy algorithm for anatomical landmark tracking in liver ultrasound sequences. In this paper, we firstly generate a feature extractor based on an end-to-end network by embedding fully convolutional network (FCN) into discriminative correlation filter (DCF). Meanwhile, we reformulate traditional DCF as a differentiable neural layer (DCF layer) to guarantee generated convolutional features are tightly coupled to DCF. Then we train the end-to-end network by encoding millions of ultrasound images and optimizing an elaborate designed loss function. Finally, we utilize the tailored feature extractor and DCF tracker to perform online tracking. Proposed algorithm is evaluated on 85 landmarks across 39 ultrasound sequences by the organizers of the Challenge on Liver Ultrasound Tracking (CLUST), and yielding 1.11 ± 0.91 mm mean and 2.68 mm 95%ile tracking error. The processing speed for per landmark is about 44–47 frames per second with GPU implementation. Extensive evaluation is performed among proposed and published state-of-the-art algorithms, and results show our algorithm significantly reduces maximum error and achieves a leading performance. Ablation study further supports the benefit from the tailored feature extractor. Clinical application analysis proves our tracker can lessen the heavy burden on surgeon and reduce dependence on medical experience.

Keywords: Fully convolutional network · Discriminative correlation filter · Abdominal interventional therapy

1 Introduction

In the past years, minimally invasive therapy, such as image guided radiotherapy [1], has large potential for reducing complication rates, minimizing surgical trauma and reducing hospital stay. During abdominal intervention, ultrasound is attractive to guide

© Springer Nature Switzerland AG 2019
D. Shen et al. (Eds.): MICCAI 2019, LNCS 11768, pp. 646–654, 2019.
https://doi.org/10.1007/978-3-030-32254-0_72

puncture needle or other medical devices due to its less radiation exposure and rich temporal resolution. Further, image-guided abdominal intervention can benefit from accurate motion tracking, in order to minimize treatment margins and deal with moving anatomical targets, due to breathing and drift. However, ultrasound imaging suffers from low signal-to-noise ratio and low spatial resolution, which makes surgeon spend more time to localize anatomical target. Therefore, accuracy and real-time anatomical landmark tracking can be helpful during the operations.

Several ultrasound based tracking approaches have been proposed in the literature during the past years, like learned metric [2, 3], block matching [4, 5], optical-flow [6, 7], kernel correlation filter [8] and supporter [9]. Nevertheless, these approaches often require substantial parameter tuning or severely depend on fine initial anatomical contours. Therefore, they are incompetent to complex anatomical surroundings, and even potentially increase extra burden on surgeon when employing them into clinical application. Recently, convolutional neural network (CNN) has achieved success in ultrasound-based tracking [2, 3]. Nouri utilizes CNN-based feature to perform anatomical landmark tracking [2], and they train a tracker by minimizing the distance between patches including the same landmark at the center in adjacent frames. Because they employ fully connected network, the processing speed of their tracker severely depends on initial patch size. Additionally, Nouri does not carefully consider deformation and temporal constrains, so that the tracker fails in some complex anatomical cases. Alternatively, Gomariz uses siamese network to design a landmark detection framework [3], and then they skillfully design a temporal consistency model to improve detection performance. While they achieve a promising results, how to decrease maximum tracking error and improve stability needs further discussion. Therefore, real-time, accuracy and robust tracking of the landmark is important for ultrasound-guided intervention, requiring a further improvement.

In order to achieve a high tracking precision while keeping a real-time processing speed, FCN and DCF based landmark tracker is introduced to this paper. Our contributions mainly focus on four aspects: first, we train a tailored feature extractor for DCF tracker using an end-to-end network by combining FCN and DCF. Second, proposed tracker achieves a leading results on CLUST dataset by evaluating on 85 landmarks across 39 ultrasound sequences. Third, ablation study on network architecture proves our tracker significantly benefits from the tailored feature extractor. And fourth, clinical application analysis illustrates proposed approach is robust when initial patch size changes in a relative large scale, which means our tracker is potential to lessen burden on surgeon and decrease dependency on medical experience.

2 Method

2.1 Foundation of DCF

Let $\varphi(\mathrm{x})$, $\varphi(\mathrm{z})$ represent features transformation of target image patch $\mathbf{x}$ and search image patch $\mathbf{z}$ respectively. Then a discriminative correlation classifier [10] can be trained based on $\varphi(\mathrm{x})$ and its ideal probability map y (namely labels). Therefore, the DCF can be determined by minimizing the output of ridge loss [10]:

$$\min_{\mathbf{w}_i}\left\{\sum_{i=0}^{D}(\mathbf{w}_i \star \varphi_i(\mathbf{x}) - y_i)^2 + \lambda\|\mathbf{w}_i\|^2\right\} \tag{1}$$

Where $\star$ is circular correlation and $\mathbf{w}_i$ denotes the i-th channel coefficient of DCF. Besides, $\lambda > 0$ is regularization coefficient which prevents tracker from overfitting. According to [10], Eq. (1) has a close-form solution in Fourier space:

$$\widehat{\mathbf{w}}_i = \frac{(\varphi_i(\mathbf{x}))^* \odot \widehat{\mathbf{y}}}{\sum_{i=0}^{D}\widehat{\varphi}_i(\mathbf{x}) \odot (\widehat{\varphi}_i(\mathbf{x}))^* + \lambda} \tag{2}$$

Here, $\widehat{\mathbf{y}} = \mathbf{F}(\mathbf{y})$ means Discrete Fourier Transform (DFT); $\widehat{\mathbf{y}}^*$ is the complex conjugate of $\widehat{\mathbf{y}}$. Additionally, $\odot$ is Hadamard product operator; and $\widehat{\mathbf{w}}_i$ is the DFT of $\mathbf{w}_i$.

With $\widehat{\mathbf{w}}_i$, the displacement of landmarks $\mathrm{d}(x, y)$ between adjacent frames can be determined by calculating maximum in the probability map [10]. In Eq. (2), $\mathbf{R}_s$ represents the location probability maps of targets in search patches.

$$\mathbf{R}_s = \mathbf{F}^{-1}\left(\sum_{i=0}^{D}(\widehat{\mathbf{w}}_i)^* \odot \varphi_i(\mathbf{z}_s)\right) \tag{3}$$

Where, $\mathbf{z}_s = s(\mathbf{z})$ denotes scale transformation on search patch, which is employed to alleviate anatomical structure deformation.

In this work, we employ FCN to extract convolutional features for target patch $\mathbf{x}$ and search patch $\mathbf{z}$ respectively.

2.2   Tailored Feature Extractor

DCF can be accelerated by transforming it into Fourier domain and is differentiable. Therefore, in order to achieve a high tracking precision while keeping a real-time processing speed, we firstly present an end-to-end network to generate tailored feature extractor for DCF tracker. Then we introduce the loss function and back-propagation process in detail.

End-to-End Network. We develop an end-to-end network to generate tailored feature for DCF tracker, as depicted in Fig. 1. Firstly, we utilize FCN to extract the convolutional features by coding millions of clinical ultrasound patch pairs, i.e. target patch in current frame and search patch in next frame. Then DCF layer is used to calculate location probability maps. With the loss function optimized, the location probability maps would be close to the labels.

The FCN structure we use has following blocks: ConvBlock ($3 \times 3 \times 48/1$) - ConvBlock ($3 \times 3 \times 48/1$) - ConvBlock ($3 \times 3 \times 48/1$) - Local Response Normalization (LRN) layer. The shorthand notation: ConvBlock (k $\times$ k $\times$ N/s) consists of a convolution layer with N filters of size k $\times$ k with stride s, a batch normalization and a Rectified Linear Units (ReLU). Here we employ LRN layer to improve the

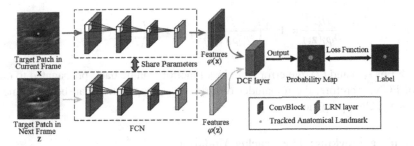

Fig. 1. The end-to-end training network for tailored convolutional feature extractor generation. The red dots in target patch and search patch are manual annotation landmarks (Color figure online)

representation ability of convolutional features. Additionally, the DCF layer originates from traditional DCF, i.e. the Eqs. (2) and (3), which is reformulated as a differentiable neural layer.

Loss Function and Back-Propagation. As a crucial step in proposed network, reformulating traditional DCF as a differentiable layer and achieving end-to-end training can make convolution features tightly coupled to DCF tracker. Let d denotes real landmark displacements in adjacent frames; d_s denotes the displacement prediction by Eq. (3); then the objective function is:

$$L(\boldsymbol{\theta}) = \sum_{s=1}^{S} \|d - d_s\|^2 + \chi \|\boldsymbol{\theta}\|^2 \tag{4}$$

Where $\boldsymbol{\theta}$ is the hyper-parameter in network, and $\chi > 0$ is weight decay, in order to ensure Eq. (4) get convergence. For avoiding sparsity, furthermore, we use ideal probability map $\mathbf{R}$ and the output of proposed network $\mathbf{R}_s$ to rewrite the Eq. (4) as:

$$E(\boldsymbol{\theta}) = \sum_{s=1}^{S} \|\mathbf{R} - \mathbf{R}_s\|^2 + \chi \|\boldsymbol{\theta}\|^2 \tag{5}$$

Because of $\partial E/\partial \mathbf{R}_s = \mathbf{F}^{-1}\left(\partial E/\partial \widehat{\mathbf{R}}_s^*\right)$ [12], Therefore, if we regard $\widehat{\varphi}_i(\mathbf{x})$ and $\left(\widehat{\varphi}_i(\mathbf{x})\right)^*$ as independent variables, the back-propagation of target branch (i.e., the upper branch in Fig. 1) can be written as:

$$\frac{\partial E}{\partial \varphi_i(\mathbf{x})} = \mathbf{F}^{-1}\left(\frac{\partial E}{\partial(\widehat{\varphi}_i(\mathbf{x}))^*} + \left(\frac{\partial E}{\partial \widehat{\varphi}_i(\mathbf{x})}\right)^*\right) \tag{6}$$

Similarly, the back-propagation of search branch (i.e. the lower branch in Fig. 1) is calculated as:

$$\frac{\partial E}{\partial \varphi_i(\mathbf{z}_s)} = \mathbf{F}^{-1} \left(\frac{\partial E}{\partial (\widehat{\varphi}_i(\mathbf{z}_s))^*} \right) = \mathbf{F}^{-1} \left(\frac{\partial E}{\partial \widehat{\mathbf{R}}_s^*} (\widehat{\mathbf{w}}_i) \right) \tag{7}$$

With Eqs. (6) and (7), the error from loss function can be back-propagated to output port of FCN, therefore, the remainder of error back-propagation can be performed by traditional FCN optimization.

2.3   Online Tracking: The Tracker Updating

When the end-to-end network has been trained, we use FCN part to generate convolutional features for target and search patches respectively, and then employ DCF to perform online tracking, as Fig. 2 shows. Meanwhile, in order to ensure DCF competent for ultrasonic revenue variation, we update the tracker online by combining the new correlation filter $\widehat{\mathbf{w}}_{i,t+1}$ with old one $\widehat{\mathbf{w}}_{i,t}$ linearly. In free breathing, the motion pattern of abdominal anatomical landmarks is approximate periodic. When the tracker updates, it is reasonable that we pay attention on the first correlation filter $\widehat{\mathbf{w}}_{i,t=1}$. Therefore, we utilize the update rule, i.e. Equation (8), to prevent tracking performance from degrading in long-term tracking.

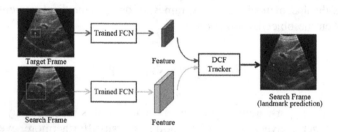

Fig. 2. Online tracking based on DCF tracker and the tailored convolutional feature. The yellow boxes in target and search frame mean target and search patch extraction respectively. The red dots in target and search frame are manual annotation and algorithm output respectively (Color figure online)

$$\widehat{\mathbf{w}}_{i,t+1} = (1 - \beta) \cdot \left(\mu \cdot \widehat{\mathbf{w}}_{i,t} + (1 - \mu) \cdot \widehat{\mathbf{w}}_{i,t+1} \right) + \beta \cdot \widehat{\mathbf{w}}_{i,t=1} \tag{8}$$

Where $\mu \geq 0$ denotes linear interpolation factor; and recurrence factor $\beta \geq 0$ means the attention we pay on $\widehat{\mathbf{w}}_{i,t=1}$.

3 Experiments

3.1 Implementation Details

We train the end-to-end network and evaluate online tracking performance on CLUST dataset [11]. We utilize the training set to train proposed end-to-end network. Firstly, the adjacent frames in same sequence are cropped into target and search patches, whose size both are 71×71. Then ideal probability maps (namely labels) are generated using Gaussian distribution with the bandwidth of 0.50. Additionally, to combat overfitting we augment all training patches by flipping horizontally and vertically, along with rotating them to 90, 180, 270°. We set learning rate to exponential decay $e^{-1.5*n}$, where n indicates epoch. The network is trained 30 epochs with stochastic gradient decent (momentum is 0.9) and a mini-batch size of 32. All hyper-parameters in network are initialized randomly and trained from scratch.

Moreover, we fix scale transformation $S = \{m^k | m = 1.05, k = -2, -1, 0, 1, 2\}$ both in offline training and online tracking process. Empirically, we assign the linear Interpolation factor μ and recurrence factor β to 0.01 and 0.25 respectively. The regularization coefficient λ and weight decay χ both are 1e−4.

Our algorithm is developed in MATLAB (2017a). All experiments are conducted with Intel Core i7-6700 at 3.4 GHz and a single NVIDAI Quadro M4000 GPU.

3.2 Results and Analysis on CLUST Test Datasets

CLUST organizers perform performance evaluation when we submit all tracking results. Euclidean distance is employed to evaluate tracking performance between each manual annotation and our algorithm output. Then mean, standard deviation (SD), 95% ile and maximum error are counted. Additionally, we consider processing speed seriously, measured by frames per second (FPS), to ensure real-time landmarks tracking in clinical intervention. We show all the tracking results in Table 1.

Table 1. Performance summary for proposed tracker on CLUST test dataset in millimeter

Dataset	Min	Mean	SD	95%ile	Maximum	FPS
CIL	0.01	1.25	1.15	4.03	6.55	46.18
ETH	0.00	0.98	0.60	2.16	4.45	47.13
ICR	0.01	1.02	0.73	2.61	7.13	45.06
MED1	0.01	1.54	1.49	4.76	10.48	44.77
MED2	0.02	1.04	0.67	2.18	4.88	45.02
Total	**0.01**	**1.11**	**0.91**	**2.68**	**10.48**	**44.74**

Further, we compare the tracking performance, shown in Table 2, among existing published works and our. Our tracking results achieve an improvement in SD of 0.12 mm (approximately 11.65%) and maximum error 9.52 mm (approximately

47.07%) over the previous best results [5] and [7] respectively. In particular, we focus on the revenue from a substantial reduction in maximum error, which means proposed tracker can provide a more reliable target prediction.

Table 2. Performance comparison of published the-state-of-art with ours in millimeter. #means that no access to 20% of all data before computation of the tracking results. More details please see https://clust.ethz.ch/results.html (the first anonymous)

Method	Tracked objects	Mean	SD	95%ile	Maximum
#Nouri [2]	80%	3.35	5.21	14.19	39.39
#Kondo [8]	80%	2.91	10.52	5.18	17.29
#Makhinya [6]	80%	1.44	2.80	3.62	25.55
#Hallack [4]	80%	1.21	3.17	2.82	35.20
Ozkan [9]	100%	1.04	1.48	2.26	21.41
Shepard [5]	100%	**0.72**	1.25	**1.71**	24.30
Williamson [7]	100%	0.74	1.03	1.85	19.80
This work	100%	1.11	**0.91**	2.68	**10.48**

3.3 Ablation Study for Network Architecture

In this part, we employ CLUST training set ($\sim 80\%$ for training, 20% for testing) to perform ablation study for network architecture, in order to understand the benefit from the tailored convolutional extractor. First, we replace proposed end-to-end network by Siamese network [3] (with three ConvBlock) to analysis the benefit from DCF layer. Then we employ proposed end-to-end network with different number of ConvBlock to explore the revenue from deep convolutional feature. Table 3 shows all online tracking results. Results show our algorithm significantly benefits from the tailored feature extractor for DCF tracker. Besides, as shown in Table 3, four ConvBlocks are most suitable for ultrasound feature extraction, which may provide a reference for other studies.

Table 3. Performance evaluation with different feature extractor networks in millimeter. / means there are cases of tracking failure.

Feature extractor network	Mean	SD	95%ile	Maximum	FPS
Siamese network	/	/	/	/	/
Proposed (1 × ConvBlock)	2.11	1.75	2.32	14.13	**50.84**
Proposed (2 × ConvBlock)	1.68	1.42	1.74	14.18	48.65
Proposed (3 × ConvBlock)	1.46	1.23	1.67	**13.71**	46.88
Proposed (4 × ConvBlock)	**1.33**	**1.12**	**1.59**	14.75	45.08
Proposed (5 × ConvBlock)	1.56	1.31	1.84	13.17	43.21

3.4   Clinical Application Analysis for the Initial Patch Size

Given ultrasound images are acquired in real time and the size of tracked anatomical tissue varies, nevertheless, surgeons have no extra time to initialize the outline of anatomical structure. Therefore, we perform clinical application analysis for initial patch size when employ proposed algorithm to perform online tracking. Figure 3 shows proposed tracker can achieve robust location performance when tracked anatomical patch size changes in a large scale, which is potential to lessen burden on surgeon and reduce dependence on medical experience.

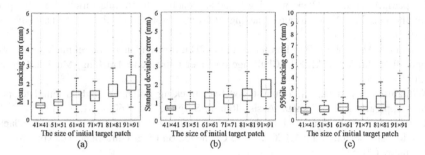

Fig. 3. Tracking error distribution on 53 landmarks with different initial patch size. (a), (b) and (c) are mean, standard deviation and 95%ile tracking error respectively

4   Conclusion and Discussion

In this paper, we develop a real time and high accuracy tracker for robust anatomical landmark tracking in ultrasound-guided abdominal intervention. By training an end-to-end network, tailored convolutional feature extractor is generated after coding millions of ultrasound images. When compared to other state-of-the-art works, proposed algorithm achieves a leading mean tracking error, along with the best standard deviation and maximum tracking error. In particular, our maximum tracking error deceases nearly 47.07% over the previous best result. Abundant ablation study on end-to-end network architecture proves the tailored feature extractor can significantly improve online tracking performance. Extra clinical application analysis shows our tracker is robust for initial patch size, though it changes in a large scale. This result is in favor of lessening surgical burden on doctors and reducing dependency on medical experience. Further study with longer ultrasound sequence, including more complex anatomical landmark and using different feature fusion approaches, is needed.

Acknowledgement. This work is supported in part by Knowledge Innovation Program of Basic Research Projects of Shenzhen under Grant JCYJ20160428182053361, in part by Guangdong Science and Technology Plan under Grant 2017B020210003 and in part by National Natural Science Foundation of China under Grant 81771940, 81427803.

References

1. Riley, C., et al.: Dosimetric evaluation of the interplay effect in respiratory-gated RapidArc radiation therapy. Med. Phys. **41**(1), 011715 (2014)
2. Nouri, D., Rothberg, A.: Liver ultrasound tracking using a learned distance metric. In: MICCAI 2015 Challenge on Liver Ultrasound Tracking, Munich, Germany (2015)
3. Gomariz, A., et al.: Siamese networks with location prior for landmark tracking in liver ultrasound sequences. arXiv preprint arXiv:1901.08109 (2019)
4. Hallack, A., et al.: Robust liver ultrasound tracking using dense distinctive image features. In: MICCAI 2015 Challenge on Liver Ultrasound Tracking, Munich, Germany (2015)
5. Shepard, A., et al.: A block matching based approach with multiple simultaneous templates for the real-time 2D ultrasound tracking of liver vessels. Med. Phys. **44**(11), 5889–5900 (2017)
6. Makhinya, M., Goksel, O.: Motion tracking in 2D ultrasound using vessel models and robust optic-flow. In: MICCAI 2015 Challenge on Liver Ultrasound Tracking, Munich, Germany (2015)
7. Williamson, T., et al.: Ultrasound-based liver tracking utilizing a hybrid template/optical flow approach. Int. J. Comput. Assist. Radiol. Surg. **13**(10), 1605–1615 (2018)
8. Kondo, S.: Liver ultrasound tracking using kernelized correlation filter with adaptive window size selection. In: MICCAI 2015 Challenge on Liver Ultrasound Tracking, Munich, Germany (2015)
9. Ozkan, E., et al.: Robust motion tracking in liver from 2D ultrasound images using supporters. Int. J. Comput. Assist. Radiol. Surg. **12**(6), 941–950 (2017)
10. Henriques, J., et al.: High-speed tracking with kernelized correlation filters. IEEE Trans. Pattern Anal. Mach. Intell. **37**(3), 583–596 (2015)
11. Luca, V., et al.: The 2014 liver ultrasound tracking benchmark. Phys. Med. Biol. **60**(14), 5571–5599 (2015)
12. Christoph, B., et al.: On the computation of complex valued gradientxs with application to statistically optimum beamforming. arXiv preprint arXiv:1701.00392 (2019)

Echocardiography Segmentation by Quality Translation Using Anatomically Constrained CycleGAN

Mohammad H. Jafari[1]([✉]), Zhibin Liao[1], Hany Girgis[1,2], Mehran Pesteie[1], Robert Rohling[1], Ken Gin[1,2], Terasa Tsang[1,2], and Purang Abolmaesumi[1]

[1] University of British Columbia, Vancouver, BC, Canada
mohammadj@ece.ubc.ca
[2] Vancouver General Hospital, Vancouver, BC, Canada

Abstract. Segmentation of an echocardiogram (echo) is favorable for assessment of cardiac functionality and disease. The quality of the captured echo is a key factor that affects the segmentation accuracy. In this paper, we propose a novel generative adversarial network architecture, which aims to improve echo quality for the segmentation of the left ventricle (LV). The proposed model is anatomically constrained to the structure of the LV in apical four chamber (AP4) echo view. A set of discriminative features are learned through unpaired translation of low to high quality echo using adversarial training. The anatomical constraint regularizes the model during end-to-end training to preserve the corresponding shape of the LV in the translated echo. Experiments show that leveraging information in the translated high quality echocardiograms by the proposed method improves the robustness of the segmentation, where the worst-case Dice similarity score is improved by a margin of 15% over the baseline.

Keywords: Adversarial networks · Image translation · Quality improvement · Segmentation · Echocardiography

1 Introduction

Transthoracic echocardiography (echo) is one of the most widely used mediums to study heart since it is non-invasive, cost-effective, and readily accessible. Accurate segmentation of left ventricle (LV) in the echo is an important step leading to obtaining clinically important biomarkers such as left ventricle end-diastolic (ED) and end-systolic (ES) volumes and left ventricular ejection fraction (LVEF).

Conventional non-deep learning methods for ultrasound image segmentation can be categorized into active contour models, deformable templates, and level

---

M. H. Jafari, Z. Liao, and H. Girgis—Joint first authorship.
T. Tsang and P. Abolmaesumi—Joint senior authorship.

© Springer Nature Switzerland AG 2019
D. Shen et al. (Eds.): MICCAI 2019, LNCS 11768, pp. 655–663, 2019.
https://doi.org/10.1007/978-3-030-32254-0_73

sets [5]. In addition, several deep models have been recently proposed for this task. Oktay *et al.* and Degel *et al.* incorporated anatomical shape priors for echo segmentation learned via joint embedding [2,6]. Also, variations of the U-Net model [7] have been proposed for the LV segmentation [9]. In a comprehensive study, Leclerc *et al.* evaluated the segmentation performance of deep convolutional models in 2D echo [4]. Their study showed that deep encoder-decoder architectures, outperform state-of-the-art non-deep learning methods. In particular, U-Net indicated the most effective segmentation performance with respect to its parameter size. However, despite advances in model development, low quality echocardiography data remains a burden on the robustness of segmentation models. Quality is determined by the visibility of the anatomical structures in the captured echo, which is affected by factors such as expertise of the sonographer obtaining the view, patient's acoustic properties, and device settings. Poor quality can lead to faulty segmentation, leakage to adjacent chambers, or shrinkage of the LV mask.

Conventional imaging methods for echo enhancement are usually hard to generalize across patients and ultrasound machines. Improving the quality of the echo can be defined as translation of images from low- to high-quality domain. Various deep learning methods have been investigated to highlight attributes of a target domain in samples of a source domain. In the absence of paired data, Zhu *et al.* proposed CycleGAN, a cycle consistent generative adversarial network (GAN) for image translation across two domains [11]. Variations of CycleGAN have been investigated for medical data translation, where there is a high cost associated with data acquisition and annotation. In [3], given two domains (CT and MRI), and ground-truth segmentation in MRI, CycleGAN is used to transfer MRI to CT, and the synthesized CTs with MRI labels are used to train a segmentation network. In [10], the objective is to train separate segmentation networks in CT and MRI, where CycleGAN is used to transfer one domain to another and augment the data in each domain.

In this paper, we propose a method to improve echo quality for the purpose of LV segmentation in apical four chamber (AP4) view. We introduce an anatomically constrained CycleGAN (ACCGAN) in which a structure-wise regularization is considered to constrain the model to retain LV structure during unpaired echo quality translation. A dataset of 427 patients is used for the experiments, showing that ACCGAN can improve the robustness of LV segmentation, with the worst-case Dice score increasing by 15% over the baseline.

2   Material and Method

The AP4 is one of the primary views to study the left ventricle. The echocardiography data is collected from Picture Archiving and Communication System at Vancouver General Hospital, with ethics approval of the Clinical Medical Research Ethics Board, in consultation with the Information Privacy Office. Data is captured using Philips iE33 and GE Vivid ultrasound machines. The dataset comprises 854 annotated AP4 frames by expert cardiologist from echo

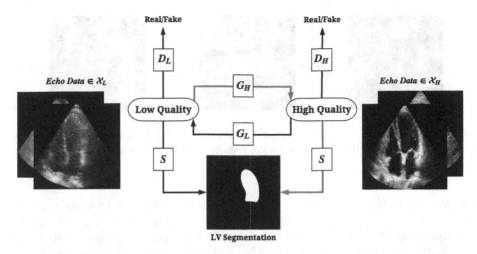

Fig. 1. Design of the proposed method. G_H and G_L denote low to high and high to low quality translation networks, respectively. D_H and D_L are the high and low quality discriminator networks, respectively. The LV segmentation network is denoted by S. After end to end training, the path shown by blue arrays is used for LV segmentation, in which the input is first translated to high quality echo, and then, is passed to S for segmentation. (Color figure online)

studies of 427 patients. For each study, the LV is annotated at the end-diastolic (ED) and end-systolic (ES) phases. In addition, an auxiliary set of echo studies is gathered, for which an expert cardiologist has examined each cine loop and scored its quality as *Poor*, *Fair*, *Good*, or *Excellent*. The quality scores are based on criterion such as visibility of anatomical structures and echo gain. A number of 4,112 frames from 87 cine series scored as *Excellent* are grouped as high quality echo, and a number of 6,059 frames from 131 cine series with score of *Poor* or *Fair* are grouped as low quality echo.

2.1 Quality Translation for LV Segmentation by ACCGAN

We hypothesize that segmentation of high quality data is more accurate, since anatomical structures are better visible in high quality echo. To this end, we first translate an input frame to high quality domain and then perform the segmentation. We tackle the echo quality improvement as an unpaired image to image translation by a cycle-consistent generative adversarial network (Cycle-GAN) [11], using unpaired images in groups of low quality and high quality echo. However, using cycle-consistency bound alone, the LV may arbitrary be altered through translation, which negatively affects the segmentation accuracy. To tackle this problem, we introduce an anatomy-wise regularization to the end-to-end training to explicitly ensure preserving LV anatomy during quality translation. The extended model is named anatomically constrained CycleGAN (Fig. 1).

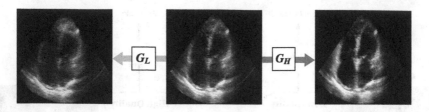

Fig. 2. Sample echo quality translation by ACCGAN. Middle column is a raw input frame, left column is the translation to low quality, and right column is the translation to high quality.

Problem Formulation: Suppose we have a set of segmentation training samples as $\mathcal{X}_S = \{(f_i, m_i)\}_{i=1}^{N_S}$, where each pair in $\mathcal{X}_S$ is an AP4 echo frame (f_i) and its corresponding LV segmentation mask (m_i). The auxiliary training set includes low quality echo samples $\mathcal{X}_L = \{f_{L_i}\}_{i=1}^{N_L}$ and high quality echo samples $\mathcal{X}_H = \{f_{H_i}\}_{i=1}^{N_H}$. $\mathcal{X}_H$ and $\mathcal{X}_L$ are unpaired frames with no LV segmentation available. Also, there is no assumption about the quality score of the echo in $\mathcal{X}_S$. We define $G_H : L \to H$ and $G_L : H \to L$ as networks translating echo from low (L) to high (H), and high to low quality domains, respectively. D_H and D_L are discriminator models for real and translated data, in high and low echo quality domains, respectively, and S is the LV segmentation model.

Adversarial Loss: The translator networks G_H and G_L and the discriminator networks D_H and D_L are trained by an adversarial loss of $\mathcal{L}_{adv}$. D_H and D_L are trained by feature matching GAN objective function [8]. G_H and G_L translate frame's quality such that D_H and D_L cannot distinguish between features of real versus the quality translated echo.

$$\mathcal{L}_{adv}(G_H, G_L, D_H, D_L) = \|\mathbb{E}_{f_H \in \mathcal{X}_H} D_H(f_H) - \mathbb{E}_{f_L \in \mathcal{X}_L} D_H(G_H(f_L))\|_2^2$$
$$+ \|\mathbb{E}_{f_L \in \mathcal{X}_L} D_L(f_L) - \mathbb{E}_{f_H \in \mathcal{X}_H} D_L(G_L(f_H))\|_2^2. \quad (1)$$

Cycle-Consistency Loss: Following the argument in [11], in theory, using adversarial loss alone maps a frame in the source domain to an arbitrary data point within the target domain. To limit the space of translation, forward and backward cycle-consistency losses are added to the training:

$$\mathcal{L}_{cyc}(G_H, G_L) = \mathbb{E}_{f_L \in \mathcal{X}_L} \|G_L(G_H(f_L)) - f_L\|_1 + \mathbb{E}_{f_H \in \mathcal{X}_H} \|G_H(G_L(f_H)) - f_H\|_1. \quad (2)$$

Identity Loss: We define an identity loss for G_H and G_L, *i.e.*, $G_H(f_H) \approx f_H$ and $G_L(f_L) \approx f_L$. For segmentation data, the quality label of the frame is not known, hence, the translator should learn that if the input is already in the target quality domain, the alterations by translation should be minimized:

$$\mathcal{L}_{id}(G_H, G_L) = \mathbb{E}_{f_L \in \mathcal{X}_L} \|G_L(f_L) - f_L\|_1 + \mathbb{E}_{f_H \in \mathcal{X}_H} \|G_H(f_H) - f_H\|_1. \quad (3)$$

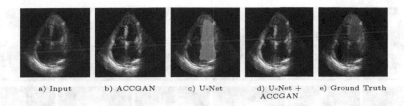

a) Input   b) ACCGAN   c) U-Net   d) U-Net +   e) Ground Truth
ACCGAN

Fig. 3. Effect of echo quality on LV segmentation. (a) Sample low quality echo, (b) translation to high quality by ACCGAN, (c) segmentation of the original input, (d) segmentation of the quality improved frame, and (e) cardiologist segmentation of LV as the ground truth.

Segmentation Loss: The segmentation model S is pretrained to minimize a binary segmentation Dice loss ($\mathfrak{D}$) between predicted LV segmentation mask and the segmentation ground truth:

$$\mathcal{L}_{s_{pretrain}}(S) = \mathbb{E}_{(f,m)\in\mathcal{X}_S}\mathfrak{D}(S(f),m). \tag{4}$$

Anatomy-Wise Regularization Loss: The L_{cyc} provides a bound on the translation output space. However, we observe that using L_{cyc} alone may result in arbitrary alterations to the LV structures during quality transformation. To further regularize the translators toward preserving the LV boundaries during quality transformation, we introduce an anatomy-wise regularization $\mathcal{L}_{awr}$ to the training. We ensure that the LV segmentation is matched to the ground truth segmentation after an echo is translated to a target quality domain, *i.e.*, $S(G_H(f)) \approx m$ and $S(G_L(f)) \approx m$:

$$\mathcal{L}_{awr}(G_H, G_L) = \mathbb{E}_{(f,m)\in\mathcal{X}_S}[\mathfrak{D}(S(S(G_H(f))),m) + \mathfrak{D}(S(G_L(f)),m)]. \tag{5}$$

The anatomically targeted loss term in Eq. (5) regularizes both low to high and high to low quality translation mappings using $\mathcal{X}_S$. During training iterations, the segmentation model S is also kept updated by $\mathcal{L}_s$ trained on original and quality translated frames:

$$\mathcal{L}_s(S) = \mathbb{E}_{(f,m)\in\mathcal{X}_S}[\mathfrak{D}(S(f),m) + \mathfrak{D}(S(G_H(f)),m) + \mathfrak{D}(S(G_L(f)),m)]. \tag{6}$$

Full Objective Function: Now we can put the parts together to define our full objective function as:

$$\mathcal{L} = \mathcal{L}_{adv} + \mathcal{L}_{cyc} + \mathcal{L}_{id} + \mathcal{L}_{awr} + \mathcal{L}_s. \tag{7}$$

The model is trained by solving the minmax optimization problem given by:

$$\min_{G_H,G_L,S} \max_{D_H,D_L} \mathcal{L}(G_H, G_L, D_H, D_L, S). \tag{8}$$

After end-to end training, the mapping $S(G_H(f))$, *i.e.*, segmentation of the translated frame to high quality, is used to obtain segmentation for the input frame f.

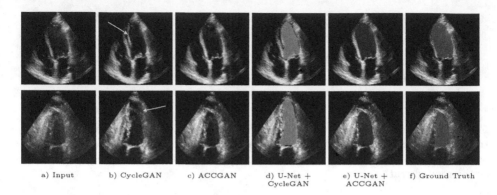

a) Input   b) CycleGAN   c) ACCGAN   d) U-Net +   e) U-Net +   f) Ground Truth
                                                      CycleGAN   ACCGAN

Fig. 4. Sample visual comparisons between CycleGAN and ACCGAN. (a) Input frame, (b) translation to high quality by CycleGAN, (c) translation to high quality by ACC-GAN, (d) segmentation of translated echo by CycleGAN, e) segmentation of translated echo by ACCGAN, and (f) cardiologist segmentation of LV as the ground truth. The cyan arrows on (b) show the locations where the LV wall is distorted by CycleGAN. (Color figure online)

3   Implementation and Experimental Results

3.1   Networks Architecture and Training Details

G_H, G_L, and S networks have the same architecture following U-Net [7]. The input is an image of size 128×128. The model has four down sampling and four inverse up sampling steps, with bypass connections concatenating feature maps from contracting layers to the expansion path. The number of kernels in the first layer is 16, doubled after each down sampling step. All convolutional layers have filter size 3×3. Down sampling and up sampling is done by strided convolution and strided transposed convolution with size 2×2, respectively. All convolutional layers are followed by instance normalization and *ReLu* activation function. The non-linearity in the last layer is selected to be *sigmoid*. D_H and D_L networks include four convolutional layers with kernel size 4×4, each followed by an instance normalization layer, LeakyReLu with $\alpha = 0.2$, and average pooling of size 2×2 with stride of two. The first convolutional layer has 32 filters, doubled after each pooling layer. The model is ended with a convolutional layer with one kernel and no non-linearity, which outputs an 8×8 feature map used in feature matching adversarial loss. Dropout with the ratio of 0.2 is applied to the output of activation functions in D_H, D_L, G_H, and G_L. Instance normalization is not used in the first layer of D_H and D_L, and the last layer of G_H, G_L, and S.

The segmentation dataset described at the beginning of Sect. 2, is randomly split into two non-overlapping groups for train and test. Also, 10% training data is set aside as validation to search for optimal hyperparameters. Train, validation, and test data is split based on mutually exclusive patients. The method is implemented in python and Keras with TensorFlow backend. Through hyperparameter optimization, we applied a weighting of 10 and 0.1 for L_{cyc} and L_{id} in

Table 1. Evaluation of the methods for LV segmentation. Best results are in bold.

Method	Hausdorff (mm)				Dice Score (%)			
	ED		ES		ED		ES	
	Mean	Max	Mean	Max	Mean	Min	Mean	Min
U-Net [9]	7.4 ± 4.7	42.8	8.8 ± 6.7	62.8	93.4 ± 3.5	66.5	90.0 ± 5.3	60.8
U-Net + CycleGAN [11]	7.9 ± 4.5	36.9	9.2 ± 4.9	52.0	92.9 ± 3.6	72.7	89.2 ± 5.5	50.1
U-Net + ACCGAN (Proposed)	**7.1 ± 3.2**	**16.6**	**7.8 ± 3.0**	**19.9**	**93.6 ± 2.9**	**82.8**	**90.2 ± 4.3**	**75.0**

Eq. 7, respectively, where the other loss terms are equally weighted by one. An *Adam* optimizer with initial learning rate of $1e − 3$, $\beta_1 = 0.5$, and $\beta_2 = 0.999$ is used to optimize the model weights.

3.2   Quantitative Evaluation

Dice score and Hausdorff distance for LV segmentation are presented in Table 1. The first row is U-Net applied on the original images. The second and third rows are the U-Net applied on quality translated echo to high quality by Cycle-GAN and ACCGAN, respectively, where U-Net is fine tuned on original images and their translation to high quality. The ACCGAN and CycleGAN had the same network architecture and experiment setup. The quality translation by the proposed method significantly improves the mean Hausdorff distance and Dice score compared to the U-Net and U-Net + CycleGAN (t-test, p-value < 0.05). Specifically, we would like to highlight the improvement in the robustness of the segmentation, where the standard deviation of the results is reduced in both metrics. We also estimated the quality of test data using the method of [1]. Comparing ACCGAN with U-Net baseline, ACCGAN improves the baseline by mean and max Hausdorff by 1.1 mm and 44.9 mm in low quality group, while the improvement is 0.4 mm and 22.9 mm in high quality group, respectively. It shows the effectiveness of quality improvement through ACCGAN, where the improvement in segmentation for low quality group is much more pronounced.

4   Conclusion and Discussion

Quality of the echo could directly affect the accuracy of LV segmentation. In this paper, we proposed a novel method to improve the quality of the echo in order to enhance the robustness of LV segmentation. We introduced a structured regularization to CycleGAN to transform echo from low to high quality, while specifically preserving LV anatomy. Experiments showed that leveraging ACCGAN could noticeably reduce the standard deviation of the obtained results shown in Dice score and Hausdorff distance, and could improve the LV segmentation performance in the worst-case samples.

A sample visual result of quality translation by ACCGAN is shown in Fig. 2. As can be seen, the quality translation networks have learned discriminative features regarding echo quality. Translation to high quality has improved the visibility of LV, and some missing parts of the anatomy are completed by the network. The translation to low quality has resulted in fuzzy borders, synthetic lower echo gain, and less visibility of anatomy, which are expected discriminative features for low quality echo. Figure 3 shows the effect of quality translation on LV segmentation. As can be seen for the low quality input, U-Net has produced a faulty segmentation mask with a large leakage to the right atrium. After quality improvement, the LV border is intensified and the LV anatomy is better visualized, which in turn has improved the validity of the segmentation. Figure 4 shows the quality translation by the proposed method (ACCGAN), compared to CycleGAN. As is shown, quality translation by CycleGAN might result in arbitrary changes to the anatomy of LV. On the other hand, the proposed ACCGAN has increased echo quality and LV visibility while preserving the LV structure.

The ACCGAN network runs in real time in an implemented ejection fraction estimation platform. In the future, we follow the extension of the proposed method to other echo views and multiple anatomy segmentation. Also, we will investigate the impact of echo quality on the acquisition of cardiac biomarkers such as stroke volume and detection of wall motion abnormalities.

Acknowledgements. This work is supported in part by the Canadian Institutes of Health Research (CIHR) and in part by the Natural Sciences and Engineering Research Council of Canada (NSERC). The authors would like to acknowledge the support provided by Dale Hawley and the Vancouver Coastal Health in providing us with the anonymized, deidentified data.

References

1. Abdi, A.H., et al.: Automatic quality assessment of echocardiograms using convolutional neural networks: feasibility on the apical four-chamber view. IEEE TMI **36**(6), 1221–1230 (2017)
2. Degel, M.A., Navab, N., Albarqouni, S.: Domain and geometry agnostic CNNs for left atrium segmentation in 3D ultrasound. In: Frangi, A.F., Schnabel, J.A., Davatzikos, C., Alberola-López, C., Fichtinger, G. (eds.) MICCAI 2018. LNCS, vol. 11073, pp. 630–637. Springer, Cham (2018). https://doi.org/10.1007/978-3-030-00937-3_72
3. Huo, Y., et al.: Adversarial synthesis learning enables segmentation without target modality ground truth. In: IEEE ISBI, pp. 1217–1220 (2018)
4. Leclerc, S., et al.: Deep learning for segmentation using an open large-scale dataset in 2D echocardiography. IEEE TMI **38**, 2198–2210 (2019)
5. Noble, J.A., Boukerroui, D.: Ultrasound image segmentation: a survey. IEEE TMI **25**(8), 987–1010 (2006)
6. Oktay, O., et al.: Anatomically constrained neural networks (ACNNs): application to cardiac image enhancement and segmentation. IEEE TMI **37**(2), 384–395 (2018)
7. Ronneberger, O., Fischer, P., Brox, T.: U-Net: convolutional networks for biomedical image segmentation. In: Navab, N., Hornegger, J., Wells, W.M., Frangi, A.F. (eds.) MICCAI 2015. LNCS, vol. 9351, pp. 234–241. Springer, Cham (2015). https://doi.org/10.1007/978-3-319-24574-4_28
8. Salimans, T., et al.: Improved techniques for training GANs. In: NIPS, pp. 2234–2242 (2016)

9. Zhang, J., et al.: Fully automated echocardiogram interpretation in clinical practice: feasibility and diagnostic accuracy. Circulation **138**(16), 1623–1635 (2018)
10. Zhang, Z., et al.: Translating and segmenting multimodal medical volumes with cycle- and shape-consistency generative adversarial network. In: IEEE CVPR (2018)
11. Zhu, J.Y., et al.: Unpaired image-to-image translation using cycle-consistent adversarial networks. In: IEEE CVPR, pp. 2223–2232 (2017)

Matwo-CapsNet: A Multi-label Semantic Segmentation Capsules Network

Savinien Bonheur[1(✉)], Darko Štern[2,3], Christian Payer[2,3], Michael Pienn[1], Horst Olschewski[1,4], and Martin Urschler[1,5]

[1] Ludwig Boltzmann Institute for Lung Vascular Research, Graz, Austria
savinien.bonheur@lvr.lbg.ac.at
[2] Ludwig Boltzmann Institute for Clinical Forensic Imaging, Graz, Austria
[3] Institute of Computer Graphics and Vision, Graz University of Technology, Graz, Austria
[4] Department of Internal Medicine, Medical University of Graz, Graz, Austria
[5] School of Computer Science, University of Auckland, Auckland, New Zealand

Abstract. Despite some design limitations, CNNs have been largely adopted by the computer vision community due to their efficacy and versatility. Introduced by Sabour et al. to circumvent some limitations of CNNs, capsules replace scalars with vectors to encode appearance feature representation, allowing better preservation of spatial relationships between whole objects and its parts. They also introduced the dynamic routing mechanism, which allows to weight the contributions of parts to a whole object differently at each inference step. Recently, Hinton et al. have proposed to solely encode pose information to model such part-whole relationships. Additionally, they used a matrix instead of a vector encoding in the capsules framework. In this work, we introduce several improvements to the capsules framework, allowing it to be applied for multi-label semantic segmentation. More specifically, we combine pose and appearance information encoded as matrices into a new type of capsule, i.e. Matwo-Caps. Additionally, we propose a novel routing mechanism, i.e. Dual Routing, which effectively combines these two kinds of information. We evaluate our resulting Matwo-CapsNet on the JSRT chest X-ray dataset by comparing it to SegCaps, a capsule based network for binary segmentation, as well as to other CNN based state-of-the-art segmentation methods, where we show that our Matwo-CapsNet achieves competitive results, while requiring only a fraction of the parameters of other previously proposed methods.

Keywords: Capsules network · Convolutional neural network · Chest X-ray · Multi-label · Semantic segmentation

1 Introduction

Widely adopted by the computer vision and medical image analysis communities, convolutional neural networks (CNNs) have enabled huge progress in many

© Springer Nature Switzerland AG 2019
D. Shen et al. (Eds.): MICCAI 2019, LNCS 11768, pp. 664–672, 2019.
https://doi.org/10.1007/978-3-030-32254-0_74

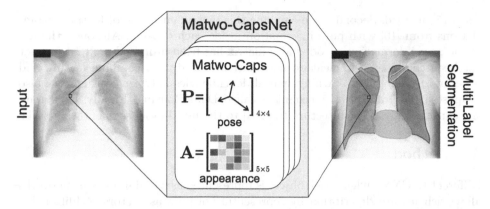

Fig. 1. Overview of our proposed multi-label semantic segmentation method, which incorporates Matwo-Caps consisting of a matrix **P** encoding pose information and a matrix **A** encoding appearance information.

applications related to these areas, e.g. image classification, computer aided diagnostics or semantic segmentation [5,6]. However, CNNs also suffer from some limitations by design. Firstly, its formulation with consecutive convolution combined with pooling layers does not readily support the preservation of spatial dependencies of object parts in relation to the whole object. Especially in semantic segmentation applications, such dependencies may be crucial to encode constraints regarding anatomical information with the minimal amount of parameters, e.g. composing an X-ray image of the thorax by left and right lung structures as well as the heart, which are all anatomically constrained by each other in their relative locations. Secondly, CNNs max-pooling operation additionally leads not only to a loss of fine spatial information, but also potentially discards relevant information. Thirdly, the scalar representation of feature activations extracted with a CNN obscures its interpretability, which participates to the CNNs "black box" nature. Tackling these problems, Sabour et al. [10] proposed to replace scalar representations of feature activations with vectors encoding the feature instantiations, i.e. capsules [2]. Differently from CNNs, these capsules are coupled through dynamically calculated weights in each forward pass. This optimization mechanism, i.e. dynamic routing [10], allows to weight the contributions of parts to a whole object differently not just during training but also during inference. This interesting concept of capsule based networks has been mainly adapted for image classification applications, however, it has never been shown to be in line or go beyond state-of-the-art results. Moreover, up to now the capability of capsules being used for semantic segmentation has only been shown on binary segmentation tasks [4].

In this work we introduce Matwo-CapsNet, a multi-label semantic segmentation network that is based on the concept of capsules. Our proposed capsule network extends upon the related work as follows: Firstly, differently from the vector encoding of feature instantiations from [10], in our work we use a matrix encoding instead. Secondly, we combine this matrix encoding of feature instantiations from [10] with pose information inside each capsule. Although the use of the pose information encoded as a matrix has been proposed in [3], it has not yet been combined with feature information. Thirdly, to combine feature and pose information when learning spatial dependencies between capsules, we also propose a novel attention mechanism called Dual Routing. Finally, we extend the capsule network architecture from [4] to the multi-label segmentation task.

2   Method

Different to CNNs, where each object is represented as a scalar, capsule networks allow rich feature description by representing objects as vectors. Additionally, capsule networks are based on the hypothesis that a complex object (i.e. parent capsule) can be described through a weighted contribution of simpler objects (i.e. child capsules) after they are transformed into the feature space of the complex object. In the dynamic routing procedure, weights are dynamically calculated such that they correspond to the agreement of each transformed child capsule being a part of the complex parent capsule.

Thus, for each child-parent combination, a matrix $\mathbf{T}_{i\rightarrow n}$ of size $N \times N$ that transforms the child vector $\boldsymbol{v}_i$ of size N to the parent vector $\boldsymbol{v}_n$ of size N needs to be learned. Although in most of the previous works, capsules are represented as vectors, in [3] appearance encoding is replaced with a matrix $\mathbf{P}_i$ describing the object's pose.

Matwo-Capsule. In this work, we combine these two concepts of representing an object by both appearance and pose, each having its own transformation matrix from child i to parent n. We encode as a matrix not just the pose $\mathbf{P}$, but also the appearance features $\mathbf{A}$, see Fig. 1. Thus, for the same number of transformation parameters $(N \times N)$, we extend the representation of the appearance features $\mathbf{A}$ from a vector of size N to a matrix of size $N \times N$. The transformations of the child i pose $\mathbf{P}_i$ as well as appearance $\mathbf{A}_i$ matrices to the parent n matrices $\mathbf{P}_{i\rightarrow n}$ and $\mathbf{A}_{i\rightarrow n}$ are defined as

$$\mathbf{P}_{i\rightarrow n} = \mathbf{P}_i \mathbf{T}^{\mathbf{P}}_{i\rightarrow n} \quad \text{and} \quad \mathbf{A}_{i\rightarrow n} = (\mathbf{A}_i + b_{i\rightarrow n}) \, \mathbf{T}^{\mathbf{A}}_{i\rightarrow n}, \tag{1}$$

where $b_{i\rightarrow n}$ is a learned bias for the appearance matrix $\mathbf{A}_i$. $\mathbf{T}^{\mathbf{A}}_{i\rightarrow n}$ and $\mathbf{T}^{\mathbf{P}}_{i\rightarrow n}$ are the transformation matrices for appearance and pose, respectively. Same as the coordinate addition step in [3], we combine image coordinates x, y with each $\mathbf{T}^{\mathbf{P}}$.

In order to create the pose $\mathbf{P}_n$ and appearance matrix $\mathbf{A}_n$ of the parent capsule, the transformed matrices of all of its children need to be combined, i.e.,

$$\mathbf{P}_n = Psquash\left(\sum_i \alpha_{i\rightarrow n}\mathbf{P}_{i\rightarrow n}\right) \quad \text{and} \quad \mathbf{A}_n = squash\left(\sum_i \alpha_{i\rightarrow n}\mathbf{A}_{i\rightarrow n}\right), \tag{2}$$

where $Psquash$ and $squash$ are non-linear functions used to bound the values between -1 and 1. While we use the $squash$ function as proposed in [10] for

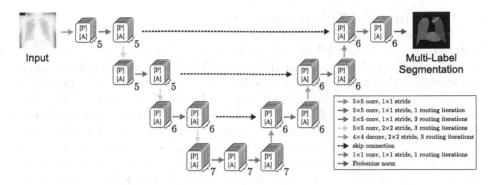

Fig. 2. Our proposed Matwo-CapsNet architecture for multi-label segmentation. The number of capsules in each layer is indicated below the respective layer.

appearance matrices, we propose to use $Psquash(\mathbf{P}) = \frac{\mathbf{P}}{\max(abs(\mathbf{P}))}$, a special squashing function dedicated to pose matrices. The weighting factor $\alpha_{i \to n}$ of (2) defines how much each child contributes to the parent and is defined during the routing procedure.

Dual-Routing. The dynamic routing mechanism of [10] follows an iterative optimization strategy based on the cross correlation between vectors of child and parent capsules to define their agreement $c_{i \to n}$. We extend this concept in our Dual Routing mechanism by treating the pose and appearance features separately before combining them via multiplication, i.e.,

$$c_{i \to n} = \langle \mathbf{P}_{i \to n}, \mathbf{P}_n \rangle_F \cdot \langle \mathbf{A}_{i \to n}, \mathbf{A}_n \rangle_F, \tag{3}$$

where $\langle \cdot, \cdot \rangle_F$ denotes the Frobenius inner product. Finally, the weighting factors $\alpha_{i \to n}$ for each child of Eq. (2) are calculated by applying the sigmoid function to $c_{i \to n}$.

Matwo-CapsNet Architecture. We extend the SegCaps network architecture [4] for multi-label segmentation and integrate our Matwo-Caps into our proposed Matwo-CapsNet, see Fig. 2. Similarly as in SegCaps, for each pixel (x, y) of either the input image or the intermediate layers, a set of Matwo-Caps is defined, i.e. $\mathbf{P}_i(x, y)$ and $\mathbf{A}_i(x, y)$. To incorporate local neighborhood information inside of our Matwo-CapsNet, a convolution kernel of size $k \times k$ (see Fig. 2) is learned for the pose and appearance matrices $\mathbf{P}_i$ and $\mathbf{A}_i$. The predicted multi-label segmentation L at each location (x, y) corresponds to the index of the capsule of the last layer with the highest activation, i.e.,

$$L(x, y) = \arg \max_i (\|\mathbf{P}_i(x, y)\|_F \cdot \|\mathbf{A}_i(x, y)\|_F). \tag{4}$$

3 Experimental Setup and Results

Dataset. We evaluate our Matwo-CapsNet on the Japanese Society of Radiological Technology (JSRT) dataset [11]. The JSRT dataset consists of 247 chest radiographs with a resolution of 2048×2048 and a pixel size of 0.175 mm. The groundtruth segmentation labels were provided by van Ginneken et al. [1], who manually annotated left and right lungs, left and right clavicles and the heart, leading to six labels including the background. We split the JSRT dataset into two equally sized training and testing sets. Due to memory limitations, all images are scaled to a resolution of 128×128 pixels. As intensity preprocessing, the input images are rescaled such that the pixels of each image are within -1 and 1. To prevent overfitting, we apply random data augmentation in the form of spatial (translation, scaling, rotation, elastic deformations) and intensity (shift, scaling) transformations on the input images, as described in [8].

Evaluated Networks. To ensure a fair comparison between capsule networks and CNNs, we also evaluate our implementation of the state-of-the-art *U-Net* [9] segmentation architecture. Differently to the original U-Net, we exchanged the deconvolution operations with linear upsampling, reduced the number of intermediate convolution outputs to 16, and reduced the number of levels to 4, leading to the approximate same number of parameters as our proposed Matwo-CapsNet. As a loss function, we use a pixel-wise softmax cross entropy.

We compare our proposed Matwo-CapsNet[1] with the *SegCaps* network [4], which was originally proposed for binary segmentation. We used the author's implementation from their source code repository[2] and reimplemented it in our network training framework to be consistent with our data augmentation. We also extend SegCaps to multi-label segmentation by increasing the number of output capsules from one to six. Furthermore, we increase the capacity of the multi-label SegCaps by having at least six capsules at any given layer, as well as increasing the length of the feature vector of each capsule to be at least $N = 32$. Different to [4], we do not incorporate a reconstruction loss and adapt SegCaps to the multi-label segmentation task by replacing the weighted binary cross-entropy loss with either a weighted softmax cross-entropy loss or a weighted spread loss.

To evaluate different contributions of our Matwo-CapsNet, we introduce two additional variants of the network, in which we replace the appearance matrix with a vector and use either dynamic routing as proposed by [10] (*MatVec-CapsNet O_r*) or our proposed Dual Routing (*MatVec-CapsNet D_r*). All our networks use the spread loss function.

Training our Matwo-CapsNet on the JSRT dataset with an NVidia Titan XP equipped with 12 GB RAM takes approximately 45 h, while testing one image requires approximately one second.

---

[1] Our code is available at https://github.com/savinienb/Matwo-CapsNet.
[2] https://github.com/lalonderodney/SegCaps.

Table 1. The multi-label Dice scores of the evaluated networks in % on the JSRT dataset. The used loss function for each of our networks is shown within brackets. Number of network parameters are shown as multiples of thousands.

Network	#Params	Lungs		Clavicles		Heart
		L	R	L	R	
U-Net (Softmax)	42K	97.36	97.87	90.87	90.64	94.49
SegCaps (weighted Softmax)	2,129K	21.18	35.79	4.49	2.93	32.83
SegCaps (weighted Spread)	2,129K	30.74	0	0.06	0	23.23
MatVec-CapsNet O_r (Spread)	43K	95.57	96.43	82.89	82.56	92.37
MatVec-CapsNet D_r (Spread)	43K	96.60	97.15	86.41	86.38	93.42
Matwo-CapsNet (Spread)	43K	97.01	97.45	88.32	87.82	94.37
U-Net [7]	31,000K	96.4		83.4		93.4
InvertedNet [7]	3,141K	96.6		88.9		94.0

Results. To verify that the original SegCaps-Net implementation is working within our augmentation and training framework, we evaluated SegCaps-Net on a binary task using the JSRT dataset, where the foreground object is defined as both left and right lungs and background as everything else. The results of this experiment show a Dice score of 95.38% for the foreground object. As outcome of our multi-label segmentation experiments, in Table 1 we show results in terms of multi-label Dice scores for the U-Net, our multi-label adaptations of the SegCaps-Net, and different variants of our proposed network, together with the state-of-the-art segmentation method for this dataset [7]. Note that different evaluation setups are used in [7]. Qualitative results are shown in Fig. 3, where the first row shows results where both U-Net and Matwo-CapsNet perform very well. The other rows show more challenging examples, where errors from the two methods are visualized.

4   Discussion and Conclusion

To the best of our knowledge, we are the first to show that multi-label semantic segmentation can be performed with a capsule based network architecture. The only other capsule based segmentation network proposed in the literature, i.e. SegCaps-Net [4], showed promising results but solely for binary lung segmentation when applied on a dataset of thoracic 2D CT slices. We tested their code within our framework on the JSRT dataset adapted for a binary segmentation task by setting left and right lung as foreground. This resulted in a Dice score of 95.38%, which is a competitive result when compared to state-of-the-art methods like the U-Net (see left and right lungs in Table 1). However, a direct extension of the SegCaps-Net to the multi-label segmentation task did not achieve satisfactory results, although we tested two different loss functions and compensated

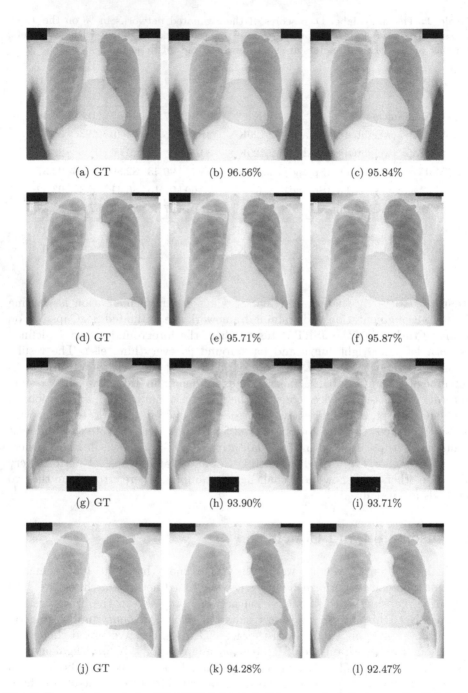

Fig. 3. Example images for the JSRT dataset. Left images show the groundtruth labels (GT), center images show results and mean Dice scores of our U-Net implementation and right images show results and mean Dice scores of our proposed Matwo-SegCaps.

class label imbalances present in the JSRT dataset through the use of weighted loss functions.

Using the same appearance vector encoding and dynamic routing mechanism as in [10], but by introducing a pose matrix and by extending the SegCaps architecture, we show how to successfully apply the capsule concept to multi-label segmentation (see *MatVec-CapsNet O_r* in Table 1). Simultaneously, the experiment shows that this performance is possible with a heavily reduced amount of network parameters as compared to SegCaps. Further, by replacing the routing mechanism used in [4,10] with our proposed Dual Routing (*MatVec-CapsNet D_r*), we show that performance can be improved, especially for small anatomical structures, i.e. the clavicles. Finally, we receive our best results with the Matwo-CapsNet architecture, which additionally encodes the appearance information as a matrix instead of a vector. These results are very close to our heavily optimized U-Net implementation and both U-Net and Matwo-CapsNet outperform the currently best reported results on the JSRT dataset for images with the same resolution [7], while solely requiring a fraction of the network parameters. Our qualitative results presented in Fig. 3, show that both U-Net and Matwo-CapsNet have limitations with small structures like the right clavicle in (f) or the top of the right lung in (h) as well as with challenging pathological cases like the bottom of the left lung in (k) and (l).

In conclusion, our work has shown that representing appearance and pose information as matrix encodings, as well as combining both kinds of information using our novel Dual Routing mechanism, enables capsule based architectures to be used for multi-label segmentation. Moreover, we introduce a novel state-of-the-art U-Net architecture for multi-label segmentation of the JSRT dataset, which is highly optimized regarding its number of parameters. We compare our proposed capsule network with this architecture and demonstrate results that are in line for the multi-label segmentation task with a similar number of parameters. In future work, we will explore different, more complex routing schemes, e.g. EM-routing [3], and extend our Matwo-CapsNet to volumetric data.

References

1. van Ginneken, B., Stegmann, M.B., Loog, M.: Segmentation of anatomical structures in chest radiographs using supervised methods: a comparative study on a public database. Med. Image Anal. **10**(1), 19–40 (2006)
2. Hinton, G.E., Krizhevsky, A., Wang, S.D.: Transforming auto-encoders. In: Honkela, T., Duch, W., Girolami, M., Kaski, S. (eds.) ICANN 2011. LNCS, vol. 6791, pp. 44–51. Springer, Heidelberg (2011). https://doi.org/10.1007/978-3-642-21735-7_6
3. Hinton, G.E., Sabour, S., Frosst, N.: Matrix capsules with EM routing. In: International Conference on Learning Representations (ICLR) (2018)
4. LaLonde, R., Bagci, U.: Capsules for Object Segmentation. In: International Conference on Medical Imaging with Deep Learning (MIDL) (2018)
5. LeCun, Y., Bottou, L., Bengio, Y., Haffner, P.: Gradient-based learning applied to document recognition. Proc. IEEE **86**(11), 2278–2324 (1998)

6. LeCun, Y., Bengio, Y., Hinton, G.: Deep learning. Nature **521**, 436–444 (2015)
7. Novikov, A.A., Lenis, D., Major, D., Hladuvka, J., Wimmer, M., Bühler, K.: Fully convolutional architectures for multiclass segmentation in chest radiographs. IEEE Trans. Med. Imaging **37**(8), 1865–1876 (2018)
8. Payer, C., Štern, D., Bischof, H., Urschler, M.: Multi-label whole heart segmentation using cnns and anatomical label configurations. In: Pop, M., et al. (eds.) STACOM 2017. LNCS, vol. 10663, pp. 190–198. Springer, Cham (2018). https://doi.org/10.1007/978-3-319-75541-0_20
9. Ronneberger, O., Fischer, P., Brox, T.: U-Net: convolutional networks for biomedical image segmentation. In: Navab, N., Hornegger, J., Wells, W.M., Frangi, A.F. (eds.) MICCAI 2015. LNCS, vol. 9351, pp. 234–241. Springer, Cham (2015). https://doi.org/10.1007/978-3-319-24574-4_28
10. Sabour, S., Frosst, N., Hinton, G.E.: Dynamic routing between capsules. In: Neural Information Processing Systems (NIPS) (2017)
11. Shiraishi, J., et al.: Development of a digital image database for chest radiographs with and without a lung nodule. Am. J. Roentgenol. **174**(1), 71–74 (2000)

LumiPath – Towards Real-Time Physically-Based Rendering on Embedded Devices

Laura Fink[1,2], Sing Chun Lee[1], Jie Ying Wu[1], Xingtong Liu[1], Tianyu Song[1], Yordanka Velikova[1], Marc Stamminger[2], Nassir Navab[1], and Mathias Unberath[1(✉)]

[1] Johns Hopkins University, Baltimore, USA
unberath@jhu.edu
[2] Friedrich-Alexander University Erlangen-Nuremberg, Erlangen, Germany

Abstract. With the increasing computational power of today's workstations, real-time physically-based rendering is within reach, rapidly gaining attention across a variety of domains. These have expeditiously applied to medicine, where it is a powerful tool for intuitive 3D data visualization. Embedded devices such as optical see-through head-mounted displays (OST HMDs) have been a trend for medical augmented reality. However, leveraging the obvious benefits of physically-based rendering remains challenging on these devices because of limited computational power, memory usage, and power consumption. We navigate the compromise between device limitations and image quality to achieve reasonable rendering results by introducing a novel light field that can be sampled in real-time on embedded devices. We demonstrate its applications in medicine and discuss limitations of the proposed method. An open-source version of this project is available at https://github.com/lorafib/LumiPath which provides full insight on implementation and exemplary demonstrational material.

Keywords: Light field · Fibonacci · Augmented reality

1 Introduction

Real-Time Physically-Based Rendering. Conventional rasterization methods generate images by artificially shading objects but mostly limit considerations to direct illumination. In contrast, physically-based rendering aims to synthesize images by simulating light propagation. To this end, these methods consider how light quanta are emitted from light sources and interact with the environment before impinging on a camera's image plane. As a direct

Electronic supplementary material The online version of this chapter (https://doi.org/10.1007/978-3-030-32254-0_75) contains supplementary material, which is available to authorized users.

D. Shen et al. (Eds.): MICCAI 2019, LNCS 11768, pp. 673–681, 2019.
https://doi.org/10.1007/978-3-030-32254-0_75

consequence, physically-based rendering additionally provides indirect illumination effects which have a high impact on perceived realism. One such method, *ray tracing* [12], simulates light rays in a reverse order. Incoming radiance is integrated for each pixel by following rays that are emitted from the camera. These rays hit objects in the scene which they interact with, based on the physical simulation of illumination phenomena such as reflection, refraction, and shadowing. From these hit-points, again all incoming radiance is integrated and rays are repeatedly traced until they eventually reach a light source (or exit the scene).

Accurately accounting for imaging physics can result in rendered images that are indiscernible from real ones. However, integrating incoming radiance for each pixel is computationally expensive and barely real-time. Hardware, like the *Nvidia GeForce RTX*, made a big step towards real-time ray tracing by incorporating deep learning technology, drastically reducing the required computations. This is achieved by aggressively limiting light-scene interactions; resulting artifacts are masked with machine learning-based post-processing.

The increase in compute capabilities of graphics processing units (GPUs) and advances of rendering algorithms have fueled the recent interest in adopting real-time physically-based rendering in daily applications. Unfortunately, these advances do not translate well to applications on embedded devices. This is because (1) GPU hardware cannot easily be miniaturized and integrated, and (2) remote-computation and streaming is not necessarily desirable (particularly in the medical context). In the remainder of this manuscript, we describe methods that aim at bringing real-time physically-based rendering to embedded devices.

Related Work. We limit our non-exhaustive review of related work to plenoptic functions (light fields), and physically-based rendering on embedded devices.

The Plenoptic Function. Light transport in a 3D static scene can be expressed as tracing the set of all possible rays; rays are defined by their origin $(x, y, z) \in \mathbb{R}^3$ and direction $(\theta, \phi) \in [0, \pi] \times [0, 2\pi]$, yielding five degrees of freedom (DoFs). This description is referred to as *light field* or *plenoptic function*. Hardware limitations led to precomputing a subset of the plenoptic function in a domain of interest rather than simulating light-scene interaction on the fly. Image synthetization is then performed by sampling and interpolating the precomputed results. Such approaches are referred to as *image based rendering* [10] and are capable of highly reducing the computations needed at runtime.

Among the most well-known representatives of such approaches is the Lumi-Graph [3], which reduces the five DoFs of the plenoptic function to four. The LumiGraph is based on the assumption that the medium surrounding an object of interest is transparent (radiance is constant along the ray), and therefore, the plenoptic function can be parameterized in terms of a bounding surface, namely a cube. By heavily constraining possible camera-object arrangements, this surface can be further reduced by only considering two opposite sides of the cube, i.e. two planes. Two point sets P_o and P_d discretize the first and second plane, respectively. The set of precomputed rays can then be determined by connecting every point $p_o \in P_o$ with each point $p_d \in P_d$. This arrangement may lead to artifacts [1] due to a non-uniform sampling of the light field.

Camahort et al. [1] examined sampling on a sphere to provide more uniform light fields. They perform a binning approach based on a Bresenham-style discretization of the spherical surface which, in addition to not being perfectly uniform, has the major drawback of the runtime complexity or radiance information query being dependent on the number of bins.

Physically-Based Rendering on Embedded Devices. A patent [14] out of Siemens Healthineers is one of the closest works we are aware of that aims to achieve physically-based rendering on embedded devices. Their method is similar to ours in that it partly front-loads computations to accelerate image generation. However, the application still seems to depend on ray casting at runtime which is found to be a quite demanding task for today's embedded devices, including head-mounted displays, in its own right [4].

Contributions. In summary, our contributions are:

- An algorithm for real-time physically-based rendering-like results on embedded devices based on uniformly sampled light fields, which, to the best of our knowledge, is the first algorithm to do so.
- A new 2D plenoptic function representation using two *Spherical Fibonacci point sets* [9], which are sampled uniformly and with arbitrary sampling size providing flexibility in tweaking memory to any embedded device.
- Fast neighborhood query of our domain using an extended version of the *Keinert Inverse Fibonacci Mapping* [7]. It has constant time complexity per pixel, does not require additional query structures and is decoupled from the light field's discretization granularity. The runtime only depends on the fixed number of queried neighbors needed during color interpolation.
- An effective machine learning-based post processing filter which is well designed for the execution on embedded devices that trend to incorporate inferencing acceleration and its evaluation.

2   Method

In order to allow for physically-based rendering on embedded devices, our prototype consists of a two-step algorithm. First, we compute all values of a reformulated plenoptic function and save the outcome as texture, which trades off hardware resources for rendering quality (see Fig. 1). Second, we transform the computationally expensive rendering task into a fast data query and interpolation task using this new representation (see Fig. 2). Additionally, we present a neural network that performs post-rendering correction in order to resolve artifacts and vastly enhance image quality.

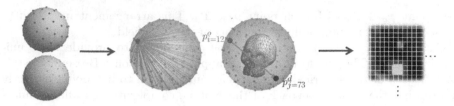

Fig. 1. $\hat{L}(i,j)$ and filling the texture. The surface of the bounding sphere **S** is discretized by the two point sets P_o^M and P_d^N. Rays are traced from each p_i^o to each p_j^d resulting in re-parameterization and discretization of the plenoptic function, referred to as $\hat{L}(i,j)$. The value of $\hat{L}(i,j)$ is written to a 2D texture at position (i,j).

LumiPath-Based Rendering. The parameterization of the plenoptic function $L(x, y, z, \theta, \phi)$ implies that we consider our scene as static. Further, we assume that the medium outside of a bounding sphere **S** which encapsulates our domain of interest (DOI) is totally transparent. Thus, radiance along a ray remains constant and consequently, the radiance emitted from the DOI is equal to the radiance at the intersection point of a ray with **S**. We reparameterize and discretize the plenoptic function L according to the surface of **S** (with radius R and origin O) and hence reduce the domain of L to our DOI.

For uniform discretization of the surface of **S**, we use *Spherical Fibonacci (SF) point sets* P_{SF}^n [9]. A point p_i of a SF point set P_{SF}^n is given by

$$p_i = C(\phi_i, \cos^{-1}(z_i)), \text{with } \phi_i = 2\pi \left[\frac{i}{\Phi}\right], z_i = 1 - \frac{2i+1}{n},$$

where $[x]$ is the fractional part of x : $[x] = x - \lfloor x \rfloor$, C is the conversion of unit vectors from polar to Cartesian coordinates $C(\theta, \phi) = (x, y, z)^T = (\cos(\phi)\sin(\theta), \sin(\phi)\sin(\theta), \cos(\theta))^T$ and $i \in \{0, \ldots, n-1\}$. We have two SF point sets P_o^M and P_d^N, where M is the number of ray origins o and N is the number of directions d. The set of all rays R^K is determined by the two spherical Fibonacci point sets P_o^M and P_d^N. The each-to-each connection of P_o^M and P_d^N yields $M \times N$ as the cardinality of R^K. A ray $r_k \in R^K$ acts as camera ray for the path tracing and is given by

$$r_k = (O + Rp_i^o) + t\hat{d}_{i,j}, \text{with } d_{i,j} = p_j^d - p_i^o, i \in \{0, \ldots, M-1\}, j \in \{0, \ldots, N-1\}.$$

We use a conventional path tracer comparable to [11]. During the tracing, ray origins are uniformly jittered on a disk with area $A = {}^A\mathbf{S}/M$ to substantially reduce rendering noise at the cost of additional blurring of the result. The captured radiance for each r_k is stored in a two dimensional texture. Each dimension of the texture corresponds to one of the point sets P_o^M and P_d^N and thus, the indices i and j not only identify a point given by the Fibonacci sequence but also the texel coordinates for memory accesses. Therefore, our reparameterized, discrete form of the plenoptic function is in fact 2D (parameterized by 2 indices of the point sets), denoted by $\hat{L}(i,j)$.

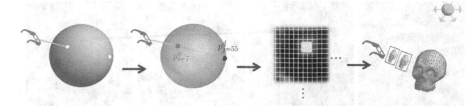

Fig. 2. Process of image synthetization by sampling $\hat{L}(i,j)$. A rasterization ray yields two hitpoints h_o and h_d (white dots). In case of nearest sampling, h_o and h_d are mapped to their nearest neighbors p_i^o and p_j^d. (i,j) in the point sets P_o^M and h_d from P_d^N are used as coordinates to fetch a texel from the texture, and thus sampling $\hat{L}(i,j)$. The mapping is performed for each pixel of the displayed image.

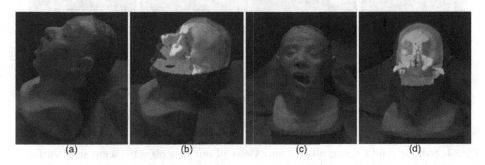

Fig. 3. A human head phantom without overlay (a, c) augmented with representative LumiPath-based renderings without post processing (c, d).

To synthesize images on the embedded device, we retrieve the precomputed physically-based rendering result from $\hat{L}(i,j)$ during the rasterization process of very simple sphere geometry, which is a simple texturing process (see Fig. 2). For each rasterization ray that hits the sphere $\mathbf{S}$, we find two hit points, h_o and h_d for the front and back face, respectively (discarding tangential rays). Given a point h on the sphere $\mathbf{S}$, we use Keinert's inverse mapping [7] to find the nearest neighbor in an SF point set P in constant time. Hence, sampling of $\hat{L}$ queries the nearest neighbor of h_o from P_o^M and h_d from P_d^N, denoted by i and j, and retrieves the sampled value $\hat{L}(i,i)$ from our plenoptic function.

Unfortunately, nearest neighbor sampling yields images that are piece-wise constant and thus, unpleasant in appearance. We modify the query to return up to nine neighbors of a point h instead. We observe that considering five neighbors for each point h_o and h_d leads to sufficient results, for 25 samples of $\hat{L}$ per pixel of the displayed image. Neighbors are weighted by their distance to the original hitpoints via a filter kernel of size $R\sqrt[4]{5}\sqrt{\frac{4\pi}{\sqrt{5}N}}$, where N is the size of the SF point set. As the inverse mapping has constant time complexity and the number of samples is fixed, our image generation algorithm has constant time complexity for each pixel. Figure 3 shows representative images obtained with this method.

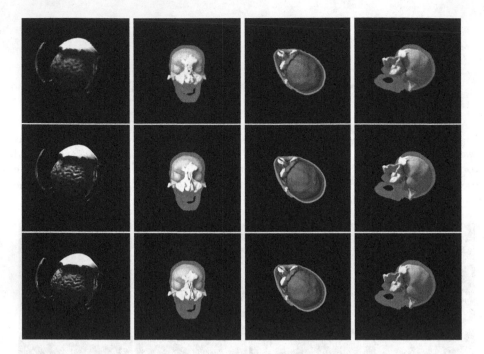

Fig. 4. Sample rendering results for four views of our test objects (segmented surfaces from CT data and skull model [2]). Top: Lumipath-based without post processing (pp). Middle: Lumipath-based with pp. Bottom: Conventionally path traced.

Generative Adversarial Network-Based Post Processing. Analyzing the higher frequency components of a LumiPath-based image clearly reveals a deterministic pattern of artifacts as shown in Fig. 4. A known method to improve image-based renderings is a view point or parallax correction which takes into account the distance of a hitpoint to the rendered surface [3]; however, this is non-trivial in use cases such as volume rendering, where the depth of hitpoints is ill-defined.

We use non-linear filtering in the form of a generative adversarial network (GAN) to improve image quality. Our network structure is adapted from [5]. We use a 3-layer U-Net as generator. The generative loss is the weighted sum of the *Structural Similarity Index* (SSIM) and L2 loss to encourage smooth structural and color reconstruction. The discriminator is made of 7 blocks of 2D convolution followed by ReLU and dropout. We modify the discriminator's last layer to be average pooling, which emphasizes local patterns, as observed in our artifacts. We use the relativistic GAN, which assigns confidence value to whether a sample is fake or real, with mean-squared loss to speed up convergence [6]. The renderings of our dataset were generated from alternating viewpoints with uniformly sampled distances and view angles withing reasonable ranges and facing the object of interest. The renderings were randomly distributed into train (2220 image pairs), validation (204 image pairs) and test set (195 image pairs). Areas that the LumiPath did not cover were masked out in the reference image during training to prevent the network from hallucinating missing image parts and rather concentrate on local artifact patterns.

3   Results

Figure 4 shows representative images that were synthesized using a conventional path tracer and our *LumiPath* plenoptic function with and without learning-based post-processing. We evaluated our rendering results with respect to the conventionally path traced image (1024 samples per pixel) using quantitative image quality metrics, namely the SSIM and the *Complex Wavelet SSIM* [13], which are commonly used for image quality assessment. In contrast to the SSIM, the CWSSIM performs a complex wavelet transform of the image to a steerable pyramid (with 8 levels in total) prior to the analysis of contrast, structure and luminance [13]. Therefore, the CWSSIM is especially interesting as image-quality trade-offs for our LumiPath-based renderings are most prominent in higher frequency domains, e.g. along edges and specular highlights (see Fig. 4). Considering ten representative views, we obtain average SSIM values of 0.972/0.975 and a CWSSIM of 0.997/0.998 with/without post-processing post-processing.

The cardinality of the point sets P_o^M and P_d^N were set to $M = 12288$ and $N = 23576$, with points of P_o^M limited to the upper hemisphere. Consequently, the precomputed texture had a size of 576 MB ($0.5 \times 12288 \times 23576 \times 4$ Byte). We evaluated the performance of our (naïve) prototype on the Microsoft Hololens v1. We measured framerates between $\approx$5.2 to 9.1 fps ($\approx$14 to 15 fps in the emulator) for both eyes in total and views similar to the ones shown in Fig. 3. In comparison, rendering one frame of our ground truth as shown in Fig. 4 took about 3 min on a *Nvidia GTX 980M*. Our path tracing framework is based on the *Nvidia Optix Engine*.

4   Discussion and Conclusion

We present first steps towards a physically-based rendering pipeline on embedded devices that show promising results. The proposed method achieves $\approx$7.5 fps for both views on a Hololens v1. More work to optimize the code and enable GPU use will further improve performance.

As our prototype is currently designed in two disjoint parts, rendering is limited to static objects. In case of changing conditions, the light field has to be recalculated. Further, our current prototype visualizes surfaces rather than volumes. We will investigate how our approach translates to volume rendering applications that, ultimately, we consider our method most useful for.

While both the rendering and network run on the HoloLens, limited memory restricts them to run sequentially, with network execution not currently real-time capable. This can be mitigated by further code optimization, but as embedded devices become more powerful, their increased memory bandwidth and dedicated tensor processing units will enable more concurrency. We show that using a generative network to perform non-linear filtering, we can remove artifacts from our interpolation method. Our renderings were based on a lightfield that was below 600 MB, which seems appropriate for today's embedded devices. Additionally, during the quantitative comparison to the pathtraced ground truth, we observe that our network implicitly denoises our rendering, which further enhances the perceived quality.

Future work in post-processing may explore network architectures that directly sample from our plenoptic function to synthesize the desired image and can be trained end-to-end. Such approach would be appealing since the origin and direction can be taken into account during the inference process. Doing so is not possible with the post-rendering correction described here that operates on already interpolated color values. In addition, a network that is aware of our light field structure might be helpful to further reduce the number of texture accesses, which we observed as one of the biggest bottlenecks in our current prototype (texture reads made up $\approx 33.3\%$ of the frametime).

While we currently use machine learning-based post-rendering corrections, other approaches can also be incorporated into our pipeline to improve image quality. A promising approach would be the investigation of non-uniform sampling patterns of the Fibonacci Spheres, e.g. based on specific object properties. However, adaptive sampling of Fibonacci Spheres is complex and requires sophisticated handling of boundaries.

In summary, we understand our results as promising, yet preliminary evidence that our LumiPath algorithm can achieve reasonable real-time physically-based rendering results on untethered compute-limited devices such as OST HMDs. Finally, these developments may prove useful for light field displays which bring dynamic focal lengths to OST HMDs and solve the vergence-accommodation conflict [8].

Acknowledgements. The Titan V used for this research was donated by the Nvidia Corporation. The authors would like to thank Benjamin Keinert for helping to understand the inverse Fibonacci mapping and Arian Mehrfard for his help in acquiring screenshots.

References

1. Camahort, E., Lerios, A., Fussell, D.: Uniformly sampled light fields. In: Drettakis, G., Max, N. (eds.) Rendering Techniques 1998, pp. 117–130. Springer, Vienna (1998). https://doi.org/10.1007/978-3-7091-6453-2_11
2. Coretti, M.: Study and implementation of a decomposable virtual skull in 54 anatomically correct elements. Thesis
3. Gortler, S.J., Grzeszczuk, R., Szeliski, R., Cohen, M.F.: The lumigraph. In: Proceedings of the 23rd Annual Conference on Computer Graphics and Interactive Techniques, SIGGRAPH 1996, pp. 43–54. ACM, New York (1996)
4. Hajek, J., et al.: Closing the calibration loop: an inside-out-tracking paradigm for augmented reality in orthopedic surgery. In: Frangi, A.F., Schnabel, J.A.,

Davatzikos, C., Alberola-López, C., Fichtinger, G. (eds.) MICCAI 2018. LNCS, vol. 11073, pp. 299–306. Springer, Cham (2018). https://doi.org/10.1007/978-3-030-00937-3_35

5. Isola, P., Zhu, J.Y., Zhou, T., Efros, A.A.: Image-to-image translation with conditional adversarial networks. In: CVPR, pp. 5967–5976. IEEE (2017)

6. Jolicoeur-Martineau, A.: The relativistic discriminator: a key element missing from standard GAN. arXiv preprint arXiv:1807.00734 (2018)

7. Keinert, B., Innmann, M., Sänger, M., Stamminger, M.: Spherical fibonacci mapping. ACM Trans. Graph. **34**(6), 193:1–193:7 (2015)

8. Kramida, G.: Resolving the vergence-accommodation conflict in head-mounted displays. IEEE Trans. Vis. Comput. Graphics **22**(7), 1912–1931 (2015)

9. Marques, R., Bouville, C., Ribardière, M., Santos, L.P., Bouatouch, K.: Spherical Fibonacci point sets for illumination integrals. Comput, Graph. Forum **32**, 134–143 (2013)

10. McMillan, L., Bishop, G.: Plenoptic modeling: an image-based rendering system. In: SIGGRAPH, pp. 39–46. Citeseer (1995)

11. Pharr, M., Jakob, W., Humphreys, G.: Physically Based Rendering: From Theory to Implementation. Morgan Kaufmann, Burlington (2016)

12. Rademacher, P.: Ray tracing: graphics for the masses. XRDS **3**(4), 3–7 (1997)

13. Sampat, M.P., Wang, Z., Gupta, S., Bovik, A.C., Markey, M.K.: Complex wavelet structural similarity: a new image similarity index. IEEE Trans. Image Process. **18**(11), 2385–2401 (2009)

14. Zhou, S.K., Engel, K.: Method and system for volume rendering based on 3D image filtering and real-time cinematic rendering. US Patent 9,984,493 (2018)

An Integrated Multi-physics Finite Element Modeling Framework for Deep Brain Stimulation: Preliminary Study on Impact of Brain Shift on Neuronal Pathways

Ma Luo[1]($\boxtimes$), Paul S. Larson[2], Alastair J. Martin[2], Peter E. Konrad[1], and Michael I. Miga[1]

[1] Vanderbilt University, Nashville, TN 37235, USA
{m.luo,michael.i.miga}@vanderbilt.edu
[2] University of California, San Francisco, CA 94143, USA

Abstract. Deep brain stimulation (DBS) is an effective therapy for movement disorders. The efficacy of DBS depends on electrode placement accuracy and programming parameter optimization to modulate desired neuron groups and pathways. Compounding the challenge of surgical targeting and therapy delivery is brain shift during DBS burr hole surgery. Brain shift introduces potentially significant misalignment between intraoperative anatomy and preoperative imaging data used for surgical planning and targeting. Brain shift may also impact the volume of tissue activation (VTA) and consequently neuronal pathway recruitment for modulation. This work introduces an integrated framework of patient specific biomechanical and bioelectric models to account for brain shift and examines its impact on DBS delivery. Specifically, the biomechanical model was employed to predict brain shift via an inverse problem approach, which was driven by sparse data derived from interventional magnetic resonance (iMR) imaging data. A bioelectric model consisting of standard conductive physics was employed to predict electric potential maps in the presence of the deformed patient anatomy. The electrode leads for creating the potential maps were reconstructed from iMR visualized trajectory and a known lead model geometry. From the electric potential distribution, the VTA was estimated. In an effort to understand changes to neuronal pathway recruitment, the model displacement field was used to estimate shift impact on the VTA intraoperatively. Finally, VTAs in patient space with and without shift consideration were transformed to an atlas available via the Human Connectome Project where tractography was performed. This enabled the observation and comparison of neuronal pathway recruitment due to VTA distributions with and without shift considerations. Preliminary results using this framework in 2 patients indicate that brain shift impacts the extent, number, and volume of neuronal pathways affected by DBS. Hence consideration of brain shift in DBS burr hole surgery is desired to optimize outcome.

Keywords: Deep brain stimulation · Brain shift · Finite element modeling

© Springer Nature Switzerland AG 2019
D. Shen et al. (Eds.): MICCAI 2019, LNCS 11768, pp. 682–690, 2019.
https://doi.org/10.1007/978-3-030-32254-0_76

1 Introduction

Deep brain stimulation (DBS) is an effective surgical treatment for movement disorders such as Parkinson's disease (PD). The efficacy of DBS therapy is dependent on the accuracy of surgical targeting and the optimization of stimulation parameters. For the former, complicating the challenge of accurate surgical targeting is brain shift, which occurs from an alteration to intracranial mechanical equilibrium due to the introduction of a burr hole and opening of the dura. Brain shift compromises the alignment between intraoperative patient anatomy and the preoperative magnetic resonance (MR) image volume of the patient, which is used for surgical planning and targeting. Using interventional magnetic resonance (iMR) imaging, Ivan et al. found shift ranging from 0.0 to 10.1 mm throughout the brain with the greatest shift observed in the frontal lobe; 9% of the patients had shift over 2 mm in deep brain structures and 20% over 1 mm [1]. This misalignment between the preoperative presentation and intraoperative anatomy of the patient is particularly problematic for DBS therapy as its targets are often relatively small. Ivan et al. suggested misplacement of the target by as little as 2 mm can introduce inadequate treatment [1]. Current clinical approaches to address brain shift are microelectrode recording (MER) in awake procedures and iMR in asleep procedures. A biomechanical model-based approach that leverages sparse intraoperative measurements, if accurate, could potentially offer another avenue of brain shift correction that could either complement or eliminate the need for MER, or reduce the workflow and economic burdens posed by iMR. Comprehensive efforts of brain shift compensation in DBS surgery via model-based approach are quite limited, especially with respect to validation studies using clinical patient data and possible intraoperative deployment. Early works (e.g. Hamzé et al.) have largely focused on the feasibility of forward solution or preliminary validation with simulated data [2]. In recent work by Luo et al. and followed independently by Li et al., both examined model-based approaches with clinical data: with the former, iMR data was available for comparison, and in the latter only two subsurface targets using preop- and postop- CTs were analyzed; both however, were limited to one patient [3, 4]. The motivation of this work is to refine a model-based approach for brain shift correction that presents minimal disruption to existing workflow for possible intraoperative deployment, and examine model prediction using high fidelity clinical iMR imaging data.

Our emphasis on the feasibility of intraoperative deployment also stems from the desire to further explore the second aspect of a successful DBS therapy, i.e. optimization of programming parameters. To facilitate the optimization of modulation parameters in DBS treatment, previously groups, most notably McIntyre et al., have constructed bioelectric finite element (FE) models to estimate voltage or electric field distribution, which can be used to predict volume of tissue activation (VTA) and its overlap with anatomical structures for surgical planning and target selection [5]. Similarly, we have pursued a bioelectric FE modeling approach based on bioelectric conductive physics; however, unlike previous studies that focus on reconstructing and optimizing stimulation parameters postoperatively, this work aims to establish a framework that bridges the aforementioned biomechanical model with patient-specific bioelectric model with the objective that better surgical navigation and targeting will be facilitated by adjusting for brain shift, and long-term post-implant electrode positions will be enhanced by estimating shifts during intraoperative electrode evaluation. By accounting for both biomechanical and bioelectric effects, the therapeutic and functional impact of DBS therapy can be better planned and predicted. In particular, the impact of shift on neuronal pathway recruitment can be predicted and adjusted without the need of MER assistance or iMR guidance. In the work presented here, we are examining the feasibility of this integrated multi-physics framework of patient-specific biomechanical and bioelectric models and investigating the differences in VTA and neuronal pathway recruitment with and without considering brain shift.

2   Methodology

2.1   Data

Two patients undergoing iMR-guided DBS procedures were studied where preoperative MR and iMR after bilateral DBS implantations were acquired with patient consent and Institutional Review Board approval; details of surgical and imaging procedures can be found in [1]. Examples of acquired data are shown in Fig. 1, noting significant asymmetric shift in frontal lobe, and crosshair indicating the deformed lateral ventricle.

2.2   Biomechanical Model-Based Approach for Brain Shift Estimation

The developed model-based shift compensation approach relies on the construction of a deformation atlas, which is a pre-computed collection of intraoperative shift possibilities. Subsequently an inverse problem approach driven by sparse intraoperative measurements is employed to provide volumetric shift estimation.

Patient preoperative MR was used to construct a FE mesh incorporating internal structures such as falx, tentorium and brain stem [6]. Displacement and pressure boundary conditions were prescribed as: (1) brain surface above a preset level is given stress free (freely deforming); (2) brain stem is fixed in displacement; (3) the rest of brain surface and dural septa are given slip (tangential movement allowed yet no normal motion) conditions; (4) nodes above a fluid drainage level have a defined pressure reference value and below have a Neumann condition, i.e. no drainage allowed [6, 7]. Moreover, with the observation of ventricular shape change and hemispheric asymmetric deformation, additional boundary conditions were given to the ventricle. Specifically, the lateral ventricle was modeled as a void and further divided into four segments spatially. For the ipsilateral ventricle associated with the largest asymmetric shift, the ventricle was separated into two segments. Each segmental portion was allowed to assume a type 1 pressure condition with 3 different possible nonzero pressure levels considered, where the introduced pressure gradients reflected ranges within ~ 7.5 mmHg. Given the combinations available, this provided a total of 9 pressure configurations for consideration in our solution distribution. With respect to the contralateral ventricle, while also having two segments, both were given type 1 pressure level of zero. This pressure treatment described the apparent presence of a pressure gradient due to pneumocephalus. Combining this mode of deformation and the modeled effect of asymmetric CSF drainage, two important factors considered to contribute to asymmetric shift in DBS are compensated for. To account for variability in surgery, different CSF drainage levels and modestly varied head configurations relative to gravity were created assuming the patient was in supine position [3]. Finally, with model-driving conditions reflecting the aforementioned configurations defined, a biphasic biomechanical model was used to resolve the volumetric displacement field for each configuration to form an atlas of deformation [6]. To drive the inverse problem, homologous surface and subsurface points were designated on preoperative and iMR images and served as the source for a least squared error fitting process (n = 27 points for case 1 and n = 31 for case 2). It should be noted here that the rationale for the use of such sparse data (rather than the whole iMR data set) is in anticipation of an approach that would not require iMR, i.e. transcranial or burr hole ultrasound. The optimization involves a linear combination of the deformation atlas solutions evaluated at the sparse data points for fit [3, 6]. Once optimized, the same weighting is used with the entire atlas to provide a volumetric brain shift estimation. As the purpose of this study is to examine the model's ability to recover subsurface shift, the deformed position of the subsurface points was used to quantitatively evaluate performance. This model predicted volumetric displacement field was also used to update the preoperative MR. This model updated MR was then compared to preoperative MR and iMR for qualitative assessment of model performance as well.

2.3 Bioelectric Model for Volume of Tissue Activation Estimation

Once the updated patient MR is obtained from the biomechanical component of the integrated framework, a bioelectric FE model is constructed via Poisson's equation:

$$\nabla \cdot (-\sigma \nabla V_e) = I \tag{1}$$

where Ve is the electrical potential (Volts), σ is the conductivity tensor (Siemens/meter), and I is the injected current from an electrical source.

With the insertion path of the electrode leads visible on the iMR image, shown in Fig. 1(b), the trajectory of the electrode leads was determined by identifying two points along the aforementioned path in order to establish a vector. Furthermore, with the most distal end of the insertion visible on iMR assumed to be tip of the electrode lead and a known DBS model (Medtronic 3389) geometry, electrode leads can be reconstructed and incorporated into the patient-specific bioelectric model with mesh refinement around the electrode contacts. An illustration of the bioelectric model with bilateral electrode leads is shown in Fig. 2. In this preliminary study, a monopolar voltage stimulation was tested where one contact (contact 0) was set to −3 V while the outer brain surface was set to the ground. While patient diffusion tensor imaging (DTI) data was not available in this study, an DTI atlas (HCP1065 at 1 mm available via FSL) in MNI space was mapped to patient space via preservation of principal directions through registration of T1 weighted images in patient and MNI spaces via Advanced Normalization Tools (ANTs) [8, 9]. With simulated patient DTI data, the diffusion tensor of each model FE mesh element was computed via interpolation of the diffusion data from the 8 neighboring voxels with respect to the element centroid and then conductivity was determined from diffusion data via a linear relationship and assumed over the element domain [10], thus providing a heterogenous and anisotropic medium. In addition, the effect of tissue encapsulation surrounding the electrode contacts was considered by designating elements within 0.5 mm of the contacts with a conductivity of 0.1 S/m [11]. The electric potential solution was solved via Eq. (1) and the VTA was determined by a threshold of -0.5 V.

2.4   Integrated Framework—Impact of Shift on Neuronal Recruitment

With model estimated VTA in the intraoperative configuration determined and a model predicted brain shift displacement field obtained, active nodes forming the VTA could be mapped to preoperative space using the inverse of the model displacement field. This process provided estimates of surgical target shift; it also allowed for a comparison of VTAs with and without the consideration of brain shift. With active nodes forming the VTAs determined with and without shift consideration, these active nodes could be transformed to a standard MNI space. The transformation was achieved by registration of T1 weighted images in patient and MNI spaces (ICBM152) via ANTs [8]. Once VTAs were mapped to the standard space, a Human Connectome Project (HCP) dMRI population-averaged template (HCP1021 at 1 mm) available via DSI Studio (http://dsi-studio.labsolver.org) was used to perform tractography [12]. As an experiment to understand the shift impact on neuronal pathway recruitment, this transformation enabled the examination of the differences in pathway recruitment due to VTA differences introduced by shift. Tractography was performed in DSI Studio using the default quantitative anisotropy (qa) threshold, angular threshold of 60°, step size 0. 5 mm, smoothing parameter 0.2, length 20.0–200.0 mm with a 500,000 seed count [12]. The resulting fiber tracts were compared between the VTAs with and without shift considerations, qualitatively via visual examination, and quantitatively via number, length and volume coverage of recruited tracts.

3   Results

3.1   Brain Shift Compensation Performance

Qualitative assessment of model shift correction was performed by comparing preoperative MR, iMR and model updated MR on corresponding slices. An example is shown in Fig. 1. Model updated MR exhibits better feature agreements with only sparse data (particularly in the frontal lobe) with the iMR data as compared to preoperative MR. The crosshair in Fig. 1(a)–(c) indicate better shift recovery at the lateral ventricle by the model updated MR image. Also of note, the inverse problem that produced the model prediction and subsequent patient MR update were computed in <1 min.

With respect to a quantitative assessment, designated corresponding subsurface features near the trajectory of electrode leads were examined by comparing this intraoperative measurement to its model predicted counterpart. For each patient, 16 features were examined for a total of 32 measurements in gauging model performance.

The model reduced shift induced misalignment from 6.71 ± 1.89 to 1.87 ± 0.64 mm (∼72.1% correction) in case 1, and from 8.64 ± 1.42 to 2.89 ± 0.92 mm (∼66.47%) in case 2. Overall the model reduced misalignment from 7.67 ± 1.92 to 2.38 ± 0.94 mm (∼68.94%).

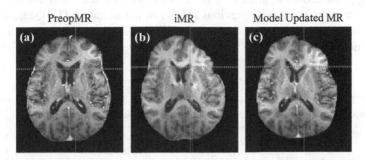

PreopMR   iMR   Model Updated MR

Fig. 1. (a) preopMR, (b) iMR and (c) model updated MR. Better feature agreement exhibited by iMR and model updated MR vs. preopMR, particularly in the frontal lobe. Crosshair indicates agreement at lateral ventricle between model updated MR and iMR vs. preopMR

3.2 VTA Estimation

The bioelectric model with reconstructed electrode leads are shown in Fig. 2(a) and (b), here noting model predicted asymmetric shift. With contact 0 (red in Fig. 2(b)) set to −3 V for both implants, the VTAs are obtained by thresholding at −0.5 V. The estimated VTAs are shown in yellow and superimposed onto the model updated MR in Fig. 2(c)–(d) for case 1 and case 2, respectively.

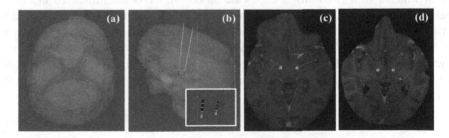

Fig. 2. (a) and (b) Bioelectric model built via model updated MR accounting for shift with reconstructed electrode leads. (c) and (d) VTAs (yellow) superimposed onto model updated MR (Color figure online)

3.3 Neuronal Pathway Recruitment with and without Shift Consideration

The mean computed shift experienced by VTAs (surgical targets) across 2 cases was 1.13 mm. VTA shift was 0.20 and 1.19 mm for case 1 for left and right implants respectively, and 2.60 and 0.52 mm for case 2 for left and right implants. These magnitudes are consistent with previous reports in the literature [1]. Quantitative difference of neuronal pathways resulted from VTAs with and without shift considerations is summarized in Table 1.

Table 1. Comparison of number of recruited tracts, tract length and tract volume for VTA distributions with and without shift considerations (left implant/right implant)

		Number of tracts (left/right)	Tract length (mean ± std) (mm) (left/right)	Tract volume (mm^3) (left/right)
Case 1	VTA with shift consideration	1119/908	100.82 ± 15.60/ 56.54 ± 14.50	5511/2998
	VTA without shift consideration	1158/826	99.60 ± 15.73/ 58.81 ± 18.36	5720/3376
Case 2	VTA with shift consideration	866/895	96.66 ± 22.87/ 64.46 ± 16.59	5320/3348
	VTA without shift consideration	1477/820	109.49 ± 7.37/ 65.07 ± 15.98	5530/3034

Figure 3(e) provides a 3D view of the recruited pathways for both cases without shift consideration. For qualitative visual comparison, recruited pathways of the target with significant shift (>1 mm) in each case based on VTAs are illustrated in Fig. 3, where results with shift consideration are shown in the top panels and without shift consideration in the bottom panels (axial, sagittal, and coronal views are shown in Fig. 3(a), (b), and (c), respectively). Figure 3(d) further provides a zoomed coronal view highlighting the difference in the extent of recruited pathways with and without shift consideration at target with significant shift (1.19 mm for case 1 and 2.60 mm for case 2).

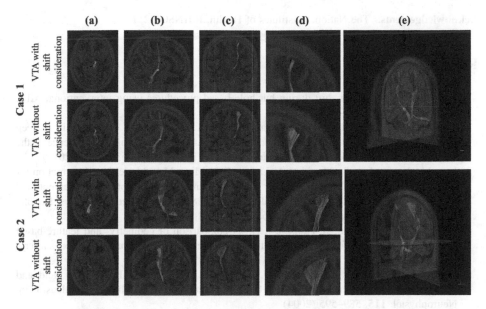

Fig. 3. Compare neuronal pathway recruitment for VTAs with shift consideration (top) vs. without (bottom) in axial (a), sagittal (b) and coronal view (c). Notable difference in extent in (d). (e) 3D view of neuronal pathways with bilateral implants without shift consideration

4 Discussion and Conclusions

In this work, we presented an integrated framework of patient specific biomechanical and bioelectric models for DBS burr hole procedures. A model-based brain shift correction approach was developed that can provide updated patient MR image volumes and demonstrated good agreement in comparison to iMR data. The correction methodology presents minimal disruption to existing workflow and enables the potential intraoperative deployment of this system in aiding surgical navigation, targeting and direct visualization. Furthermore, by coupling this biomechanical model to a patient specific bioelectric model, VTAs could be estimated and neuronal pathway recruitment could be predicted, which has implications regarding functional outcome and therapy quality. Interestingly, differences in neuronal pathway recruitment are readily observable with and without shift consideration, both qualitatively (different extents in Fig. 3) and quantitatively (e.g. tract number in Table 1). This potentially highlights the need for intraoperative shift correction with the complement of a tool capable of providing bioelectric information to assist surgical targeting and functional therapy. Regarding limitations of the work, the methods must be implemented on a larger population with likely efforts using MER for validation of neuronal recruitment impact. For the biomechanical model, better understanding of the interplay of pneumocephalus and ventricular effects are needed. For the bioelectric model, increased sophistication, e.g. accounting for the frequency-dependency of the stimulation, and enhanced VTA modeling, is desired. Nevertheless, the work herein is provocative in that even small deformations are shown to induce considerable functional change in neuronal pathway recruitment.

Acknowledgements. The National Institutes of Health, R01NS049251.

References

1. Ivan, M.E., et al.: Brain shift during bur hole-based procedures using interventional MRI. J. Neurosurg. **121**, 149–160 (2014)
2. Hamzé, N., Bilger, A., Duriez, C., Cotin, S., Essert, C.: Anticipation of brain shift in deep brain stimulation automatic planning. In: 2015 37th Annual International Conference of the IEEE Engineering in Medicine and Biology Society (EMBC), pp. 3635–3638 (2015)
3. Luo, M., Narasimhan, S., Martin, A.J., Larson, P.S., Miga, M.I.: Model-based correction for brain shift in deep brain stimulation burr hole procedures: a comparison using interventional magnetic resonance imaging. In: Medical Imaging 2018: Image-Guided Procedures, Robotic Interventions, and Modeling, vol. 10576, p. 10 (2018)
4. Li, C., Fan, X., Aronson, J., Paulsen, K.D.: A comparison of geometry- and feature-based sparse data extraction for model-based image updating in deep brain stimulation surgery. SPIE (2019)
5. McIntyre, C.C., Mori, S., Sherman, D.L., Thakor, N.V., Vitek, J.L.: Electric field and stimulating influence generated by deep brain stimulation of the subthalamic nucleus. Clin. Neurophysiol. **115**, 589–595 (2004)
6. Sun, K., Pheiffer, T.S., Simpson, A.L., Weis, J.A., Thompson, R.C., Miga, M.I.: Near real-time computer assisted surgery for brain shift correction using biomechanical models. IEEE J. Transl. Eng. Health Med. **2**, 1–13 (2014)
7. Miga, M.I., et al.: Model-updated image guidance: initial clinical experiences with gravity-induced brain deformation. IEEE Trans. Med. Imaging **18**, 866–874 (1999)
8. Avants, B.B., Tustison, N.J., Song, G., Cook, P.A., Klein, A., Gee, J.C.: A reproducible evaluation of ANTs similarity metric performance in brain image registration. Neuroimage **54**, 2033–2044 (2011)
9. Jenkinson, M., Beckmann, C.F., Behrens, T.E., Woolrich, M.W., Smith, S.M.: FSL. Neuroimage **62**, 782–790 (2012)
10. Tuch, D.S., Wedeen, V.J., Dale, A.M., George, J.S., Belliveau, J.W.: Conductivity tensor mapping of the human brain using diffusion tensor MRI. Proc. Natl. Acad. Sci. U. S. A. **98**, 11697–11701 (2001)
11. Butson, C.R., Maks, C.B., McIntyre, C.C.: Sources and effects of electrode impedance during deep brain stimulation. Clin. Neurophysiol. **117**, 447–454 (2006)
12. Yeh, F.C., Verstynen, T.D., Wang, Y.B., Fernandez-Miranda, J.C., Tseng, W.Y.I.: Deterministic diffusion fiber tracking improved by quantitative anisotropy. PLoS ONE **8**, 16 (2013)

Author Index

Printed in the United States
By Bookmasters